Odell's Clinical Problem Solving in Dentistry

Odell's Clinical Problem Solving in Dentistry

4th Edition

Edited by

Avijit Banerjee, BDS MSc PhD (Lond) LDS FDS (Rest Dent) FDS RCS (Eng) FHEA

Chair of Cariology & Operative Dentistry / Honorary Consultant in Restorative Dentistry
Faculty of Dentistry, Oral & Craniofacial Sciences, King's College London
Guy's and St. Thomas' Hospitals NHS Foundation Trust,
London, UK

and

Selvam Thavaraj, BDS PhD FDS RCS FRCPath

Senior Lecturer/Honorary Consultant in Oral and Maxillofacial/Head and Neck Pathology,
Faculty of Dentistry, Oral & Craniofacial Sciences, King's College London
Guy's and St. Thomas' Hospitals NHS Foundation Trust,
London, UK

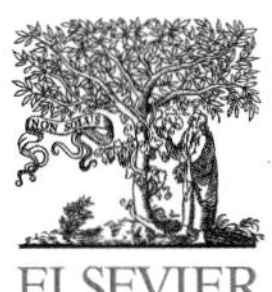

ELSEVIER Edinburgh London New York Oxford Philadelphia St Louis Sydney 2020

First edition 2000
Second edition 2004
Third edition 2010

ISBN: 978-0-7020-7700-5

Senior Content Strategist: Alison Taylor
Content Development Specialist: Carole McMurray
Content Coordinator: Susan Jansons
Senior Project Manager: Manchu Mohan
Design: Bridget Hoette
Illustration Manager: Paula Catalano
Marketing Manager: Deborah Watkins

Printed in China

Last digit is the print number: 9 8 7 6 5 4 3 2 1

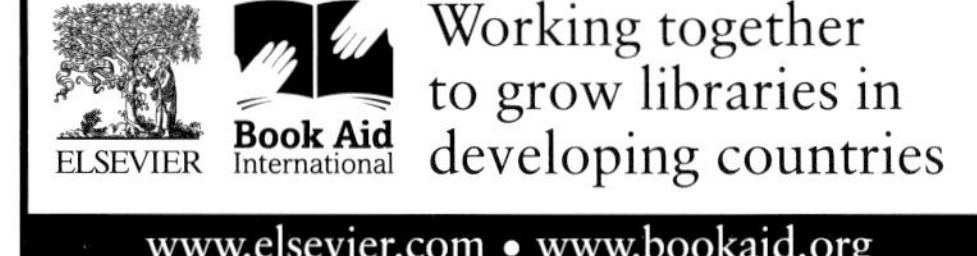

Contents

Preface, viii

Contributors, ix

1 **A High-Caries-Rate/High-Risk Patient, 1**
Avijit Banerjee

2 **A Multilocular Radiolucency, 9**
Eric Whaites and Edward Odell

3 **An Unpleasant Surprise, 15**
Martyn Ormond and Michael Escudier

4 **Gingival Recession, 21**
Mandeep Ghuman

5 **Multiple Missing Anterior Teeth and a Class III Incisor Relationship, 27**
Dirk Bister

6 **An Unsettled Patient, 35**
Yvonne M. Rooney

7 **A Dry Mouth, 39**
Pepe Shirlaw and Edward Odell

8 **Painful Trismus, 45**
Rodhri Davies and Luke Cascarini

9 **A Deep Carious Lesion, 51**
Avijit Banerjee

10 **A Lump On the Gingiva, 59**
Anwar R. Tappuni

11 **Pain On Biting, 63**
Francesco Mannocci

12 **CAD/CAM Fixed Prosthodontics, 67**
Rupert Austin and Deborah Bomfim

13 **Sudden Collapse, 75**
Emily Sherwin

14 **A Difficult Young Child, 79**
Wendy Bellis

15 **Pain After Extraction, 85**
Tara Renton

16 **A Numb Lip, 89**
Nicholas M. Goodger

17 **A Loose Anterior Tooth, 95**
Rupert Austin and Deborah Bomfim

18 **Oroantral Fistula, 101**
Tara Renton

19 **Troublesome Mouth Ulcers, 107**
Pepe Shirlaw and Shalini Nayee

20 **A Lump in the Neck, 111**
Nicholas M. Goodger and Selvam Thavaraj

21 **Trauma Causing Displacement of an Upper Central Incisor, 117**
Serpil Djemal and Ravi Chauhan

22 **Hypoglycaemia, 123**
Barbara Carey and Michael Escudier

23 **A Tooth Lost at Teatime, 127**
Vinod Patel and Alexander Crighton

24 **A Problem Overdenture, 135**
Jonathan Turner and David R. Radford

25 **Impacted Lower Third Molars, 139**
Tara Renton and Vinod Patel

26 **A Patient Presenting with an Avulsed Central Incisor, 147**
Serpil Djemal and Ravi Chauhan

27 **Discoloured Anterior Teeth, 151**
Michael Thomas

28 **A Very Painful Mouth, 157**
Pepe Shirlaw and Sandeep Joshi

29 **Caution! – X-Rays, 161**
Nicholas Drage and Eric Whaites

30 **Whose Fault Is It This Time?, 167**
Jonathan Turner and David R. Radford

31 **Ouch!, 173**
Chris Dickinson

32 **A Swollen Face and Pericoronitis, 179**
Tara Renton

33 **First Permanent Molars, 183**
Mike Harrison

34 **A Sore Mouth, 187**
Davinder Bains and Helen McParland

35 **A Failed Bridge, 193**
Sophie Watkins

36 **Skateboarding Accident?, 197**
Jennifer C. Harris

37 **An Adverse Reaction, 203**
Chris Dickinson

38 **Advanced Periodontitis, 207**
Mandeep Ghuman

39 **Fractured Incisors, 219**
Serpil Djemal and Ravi Chauhan

40 **An Anxious Patient, 223**
Emily Sherwin

41 **Blisters in the Mouth, 227**
Barbara Carey, Esther Hullah and Jane Setterfield

42 **Will *You* See My Son?, 231**
Wendy Bellis

43 **Bridge Design, 237**
Sophie Watkins

44 **Anticoagulation for a Prosthetic Heart Valve, 245**
Nicholas M. Goodger

45 **A White Patch on the Tongue, 251**
Helen McParland and Edward Odell

46 **Another White Patch On the Tongue, 257**
Edward Odell and Selvam Thavaraj

47 **Molar Endodontic Treatment, 261**
Francesco Mannocci

48 **An Endodontic Problem, 265**
Francesco Mannocci

49 **A Swollen Face, 271**
Tara Renton

50 **Missing Upper Lateral Incisors, 277**
Sophie Watkins

51 **Anterior Crossbite (Class III Malocclusion) with Displacement in the Mixed Dentition, 287**
Dirk Bister

52 **Localized Periodontitis?, 291**
Edward Odell and Mandeep Ghuman

53 **Unexpected Findings, 297**
Eric Whaites and Edward Odell

54 **A Gap Between the Front Teeth, 303**
Jonathan Turner, Mandeep Ghuman and David R. Radford

55 **A Lump in the Palate, 311**
Tara Renton

56 **Rapid Breakdown of First Permanent Molars (Molar–Incisor Hypomineralization), 315**
Mike Harrison

57 **Oral Cancer, 321**
Nicholas M. Goodger and Edward Odell

58 **A Complicated Extraction, 329**
Chris Dickinson

59 **Difficulty Opening the Mouth, 333**
Anand Lalli and Wanninayaka M. Tilakaratne

60 **Erosive Tooth Wear, 339**
Rupert Austin and Deborah Bomfim

61 **Worn Front Teeth, 343**
Rupert Austin and Deborah Bomfim

62 **A Case of Toothache, 349**
Eric Whaites

63 **A Child with a Swollen Face, 353**
Eric Whaites

64 **Recurrent Neck Swelling, 357**
Bethan Thomas, Niall O'Neill and Michael Escudier

65 **Failed Endodontic Treatment, 365**
Francesco Mannocci

66 **A Pain in the Head, 369**
Tara Renton

67 Aggressive Tooth Decay, 375
Mary Burke

68 Should I Repair or Replace These Restorations? – the '5 Rs', 381
Louis Mackenzie and Avijit Banerjee

69 Implant Planning, 391
Kalpesh A. Bavisha

70 Domiciliary Care, 397
Ellie Heidari

71 Managing Complaints, 405
Len D'Cruz

72 Loose Dentures/Resorbed Ridge Form, 409
Jonathan Turner and David R. Radford

73 'Invisible Custom-Made Braces', 415
Dirk Bister

74 Swollen Lips, 423
Martyn Ormond, Esther Hullah and Michael Escudier

75 Failing Implant Restoration, 427
Kalpesh A. Bavisha

Index, 431

Preface

It has been an honour and privilege to edit this latest edition of such an important and influential book in dentistry. The success of previous editions is testimony to Professor Odell's expertise, vast experience and hard work over many years, such that this book now sits as one of the most successful in its field, with a wide readership and professional acclaim. As its new editors, we believe it is absolutely appropriate that his name now becomes indelibly associated with this tome and we hope to do it justice in the future.

We have sought to maintain a format which encourages the reader to reorganize and apply knowledge and experience to 'real life' clinical scenarios. To this end, we have garnered the input from several new authors with expertise in their respective disciplines, to broaden the scope of clinical scenarios covered, updating cases with appropriate changes in national guidance, relevant legislation and advances in management practices. In so doing, this edition provides the reader with a wider mix of scenarios that falls within the scope of practice of a modern general oral healthcare practitioner and their team, including patient behaviour management issues, the use of digital dentistry, management and maintenance of dental implant cases and domiciliary care provision. We sincerely hope that the content appeals to undergraduates and newly qualified practitioners as well as our more experienced colleagues across the disciplines. As clinical cases do not vary globally, we also feel the content has an international appeal.

This book should not be seen as a substitute for subject texts and it is important for the reader to appreciate two things when reading this book. Firstly, it is impossible to cover all the varied scenarios that a busy oral health practitioner may face. Therefore, we as editors, have tried to select a broad range where helpful tips and hints may be applicable in other situations. The management of each scenario is not always set in stone and this book should not be taken as prescriptive. In all cases good clinical practice has centred on the patient's best interests. This path can and will vary from case to case and practitioner to practitioner, as no two patients or clinicians are the same or working in the same environment.

Secondly, this book draws heavily on the clinical knowledge and expertise of all contributing authors. We wish to acknowledge their massive effort in bringing their cases to life. Their sacrifice in personal time, energy and commitment must not be underestimated. Without this vital input from our friends and colleagues, this book simply could not exist and we are greatly indebted to them.

AB
ST

Contributors

The editors would like to acknowledge and offer grateful thanks for the input of all previous editions' contributors, without whom this new edition would not have been possible.

Rupert Austin, BDS MClinDent PhD MJDF RCS (Eng) MPros RCSEd FAcadMEd FHEA
Senior Clinical Lecturer and Honorary Consultant in Prosthodontics, Faculty of Dentistry, Oral & Craniofacial Sciences, King's College London, London, UK

Davinder Bains, BDS MFDS Edin
Specialty Doctor in Oral Medicine, Guy's and St Thomas' NHS Foundation Trust, London, UK

Avijit Banerjee, BDS MSc PhD (Lond) LDS FDS (Rest Dent) FDS RCS (Eng) FHEA
Chair of Cariology & Operative Dentistry / Honorary Consultant in Restorative Dentistry, Faculty of Dentistry, Oral & Craniofacial Sciences, King's College London, Guy's and St. Thomas' Hospitals NHS Foundation Trust, London, UK

Kalpesh A. Bavisha, BDS MSC FDS RCPS REST DENT
Consultant in Restorative Dentistry, Guy's and St. Thomas' NHS Foundation Trust, London, UK

Wendy Bellis, BDS MSc (Paeds) FHEA
Specialist Paediatric Dentist and Honorary Clinical Senior Teaching Fellow, Eastman Dental Institute, London, UK

Dirk Bister, MD DMD FDS RCS (Edin) FDSOrth MOrth MSc MA
Professor of Clinical Orthodontics, Consultant Orthodontist, Faculty of Dentistry, Oral & Craniofacial Sciences, Guy's and St. Thomas' NHS Trust, London, UK

Deborah Bomfim, BDS MSc (Cons Dent) MJDF RCS (Eng) FDS (Rest Dent) RCS (Eng)
Consultant Specialist and Honorary Clinical Lecturer in Restorative Dentistry, University College Hospitals NHS Foundation Trust, Eastman Dental Hospital, London, UK

Mary Burke, BDS FDS RCS (Eng)
Consultant in Special Care Dentistry, Guy's and St. Thomas' NHS Foundation Trust, London, UK

Barbara Carey, MB BCh BAO BDS NUI BA FDS (OM) RCS (Eng) FFDRCSI (Oral Medicine) FHEA
Consultant in Oral Medicine, Guy's and St Thomas' NHS Foundation Trust, London, UK

Luke Cascarini, BDS MBBCh FDS RCS FRCS (OMFS)
Consultant in Oral and Maxillofacial Surgery, Guy's and St Thomas' NHS Foundation Trust, London, UK

Ravi Chauhan, DDr Msc MJDF RCS FDS (Rest Dent) RCS
Consultant in Restorative Dentistry, John Radcliffe Hospital, Oxford, UK

Alexander Crighton, MB ChB (Edin) FDS (OM) RCSEd FDS RCPS
Consultant in Oral Medicine, NHS Greater Glasgow and Clyde, Glasgow, UK

Rodhri Davies, MBBS BDS MSc
Oral and Maxillofacial Surgery Specialty Registrar, Guy's and St Thomas' NHS Foundation Trust, London, UK

Len D'Cruz, BDS LDSRCS MFGDP LLM Dip FOd PGCert Med Ed
General Dental Practitioner and Senior Dento-Legal Advisor, British Dental Association, London, UK

Chris Dickinson, BDS MSc (Lond) DDPH MFDS LDS RCS (Eng) DipConSed (KCL)
Consultant and Honorary Senior Lecturer, Department of Sedation and Special Care Dentistry, Guy's and St Thomas' NHS Foundation Trust, London, UK

Serpil Djemal, BDS MSc DipED MRD FDS (Rest Dent) RCS
Consultant in Restorative Dentistry, King's College Hospital NHS Trust, London, UK

Nicholas Drage, BDS FDS RCS (Eng) FDS RCPS (Glas) DDRRCR
Consultant/Honorary Senior Lecturer in Dental and Maxillofacial Radiology, Department of Dental Radiology, University Dental Hospital, Cardiff and Vale University Health Board, Cardiff, UK

Michael Escudier, MD BDS MBBS FDS RCS FDS (OM) RCS FDS (OM) RCPSG FFDRCSI FFGDP (UK) FHEA
Professor of Oral Medicine and Education, Faculty of Dentistry, Oral & Craniofacial Sciences, King's College London, London, UK

Mandeep Ghuman, BSc (Hons) BDS MClinDent (Perio) PhD
Lecturer/Honorary Consultant in Periodontology, Faculty of Dentistry, Oral & Craniofacial Sciences, King's College London, London, UK

Nicholas M. Goodger, PhD BDS BSc (Hons) MBBS FRCSEd (OMFS) FDS RCS DLORCS
Consultant Oral and Maxillofacial Surgeon, East Kent Hospitals University NHS Foundation Trust, Ashford, Kent, UK

Jennifer C. Harris, BDS MSc FDS RCS FDS (Paed Dent)
Consultant/Honorary Senior Lecturer in Community Paediatric Dentistry, Sheffield Teaching Hospitals NHS Foundation Trust, University of Sheffield, Sheffield, UK

Mike Harrison, BDS MScD MPhil FDS (Paed Dent) RCS Edin
Consultant in Paediatric Dentistry, Guy's and St Thomas' NHS Foundation Trust, London, UK

Ellie Heidari, BDS MFDS RCS (Eng) MSc MA SFHEA
Department of Sedation and Special Care Dentistry, Faculty of Dentistry, Oral & Craniofacial Sciences, King's College London, London, UK

Esther Hullah, BDS MBBS FDS (OM) FHEA
Consultant in Oral Medicine, Honorary Clinical Senior Lecturer, Faculty of Dentistry, Oral & Craniofacial Sciences, King's College London, London, UK

Sandeep Joshi, BDS MFDS RCS
Specialist Dentist in Oral Medicine, Department of Oral Medicine, Guy's and St. Thomas' NHS Foundation Trust, London, UK

Anand Lalli, BDS MOralSurg PhD
Professor of Oral Surgery, School of Dentistry and Health Sciences, Charles Sturt University, Orange, NSW, Australia

Louis Mackenzie, BDS
General Dental Practitioner, Clinical Lecturer, School of Dentistry, University of Birmingham, UK
Lecturer (distance-learning), Faculty of Dentistry, Oral & Craniofacial Sciences, King's College London, UK

Francesco Mannocci, MD DDS PhD FHEA
Professor of Endodontology, Faculty of Dentistry, Oral & Craniofacial Sciences, King's College London, London, UK

Helen McParland, BDS FDS RCS Edin FHEA
Department of Oral Medicine, Consultant in Oral Medicine, Guy's and St Thomas' NHS Foundation Trust, London, UK

Shalini Nayee, BDS MBBS MSc
Academic Clinical Fellow, Specialty Trainee, Department of Oral Medicine, Guy's and St. Thomas' NHS Foundation Trust, London, UK

Niall O'Neill, BDS DDMFR
Locum Consultant in Dental and Maxillofacial Radiology, Guy's and St. Thomas' NHS Foundation Trust, London, UK

Edward Odell, PhD FDS RCS FRCPath
Professor of Oral Pathology and Medicine, Faculty of Dentistry, Oral & Craniofacial Sciences, King's College London, London, UK

Martyn Ormond, BDS MBBS FDS (OM) FHEA
Consultant in Oral Medicine, Guy's and St. Thomas' NHS Foundation Trust, London, UK

Vinod Patel, BSc (Hons) MFDS RCS (Ed) MOralSurg (Eng)
Consultant in Oral Surgery, Guy's and St. Thomas' NHS Foundation Trust, London, UK

David R. Radford, BDS PhD FDS RCS MRD
Retired Reader in Inter-professional Education and Multi-professional Care, Faculty of Dentistry, Oral & Craniofacial Sciences, King's College London, Director of Clinical Studies, University of Portsmouth Dental Academy, London, UK

Tara Renton, BDS MDSc PhD
Professor of Oral Surgery, Faculty of Dental, Oral & Craniofacial Sciences, King's College London, London, UK

Yvonne M. Rooney, BA BDentSc MJDFRCS DPDS MSc MSCDRCS
Specialist in Special Care Dentistry, King's College NHS Foundation Trust, London, UK

Jane Setterfield, BDS DCH DRCOG MD FRCP
Consultant in Dermatology in Relation to Oral Disease, Faculty of Dentistry, Oral & Craniofacial Sciences, St. John's Institute of Dermatology, King's College London, London, UK

Emily Sherwin, BDS MFDS MSc M Spec Care Dent PgCert MDTFEd
Consultant in Special Care Dentistry/Honorary Clinical Senior Lecturer, Department of Sedation and Special Care Dentistry, Guy's and St. Thomas' NHS Foundation Trust, London, UK

Pepe Shirlaw, BDS FDS RCPS
Consultant in Oral Medicine, Guy's and St. Thomas' NHS Foundation Trust and Faculty of Dentistry, Oral & Craniofacial Sciences, King's College London, London, UK

Anwar R. Tappuni, LDS RCS MRACDS (OM) PhD FHEA
Professor and Academic Lead for Oral Medicine, Institute of Dentistry, Queen Mary University of London, London, UK

Selvam Thavaraj, BDS PhD FDS RCS FRCPath
Senior Lecturer/Honorary Consultant in Oral and Maxillofacial/Head and Neck Pathology, Faculty of Dentistry, Oral & Craniofacial Sciences, King's College London, Guy's and St. Thomas' Hospitals NHS Foundation Trust, London, UK

Bethan Thomas, BDS BSc (Hons) PhD MFDS RCS DDMFR FHEA
Consultant in Dental and Maxillofacial Radiology, Guy's and St. Thomas' NHS Foundation Trust, London, UK

Michael Thomas, BDS MSc LDS RCS DGDP (UK) MRD RCS FICD
Senior Teaching Fellow / Senior Specialist Clinical Teacher, Faculty of Dentistry, Oral & Craniofacial Sciences, King's College London, London, UK

Wanninayaka M. Tilakaratne, BDS MS FDS RCS FRCPath PhD
Professor/Oral Pathology, Department of Oral and Maxillofacial Clinical Sciences, Faculty of Dentistry, University of Malaya, Kuala Lumpur, Malaysia

Jonathan Turner, BDS MSc MA (Ed) PhD
Senior Specialist Clinical Teacher, Faculty of Dentistry, Oral & Craniofacial Sciences, King's College London, London, UK

Sophie Watkins, BDS MSc FDS (Rest Dent) RCPS FDS RCS
Consultant in Restorative Dentistry, Guys' and St. Thomas' NHS Foundation Trust, London, UK

Eric Whaites, BDS MSc FDS RCS (Edin) FDS RCS (Eng) FRCR DDRRCR
Senior Lecturer/Honorary Consultant in Dental and Maxillofacial Radiology, Faculty of Dentistry, Oral & Craniofacial Sciences, King's College London, London, UK

Case 1
A High-Caries-Rate/High-Risk Patient

AVIJIT BANERJEE

Summary

A 17-year-old sixth-form college student presents at your general dental practice with several carious lesions, one of which is very large. How should you manage his condition?

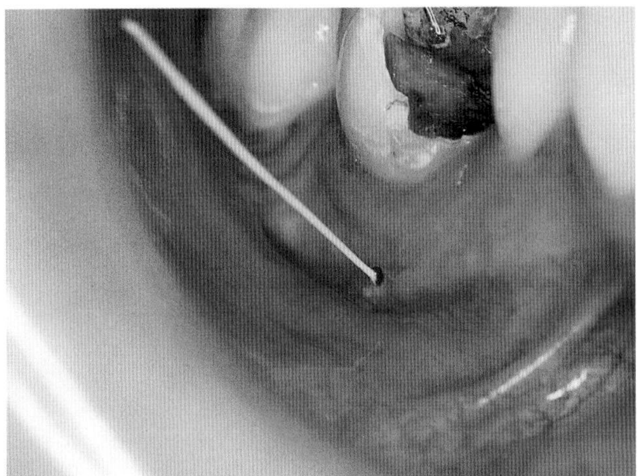

• **Fig. 1.1** The lower right first molar. The gutta percha point indicates a sinus opening.

History

Complaint

He complains that a filling has fallen out of a tooth on the lower right side and has left a sharp edge that irritates his tongue. He is otherwise asymptomatic.

History of Complaint

The filling was placed about a year ago at a casual visit to the dentist precipitated by acute toothache triggered by hot and cold foods and drink. He did not return to complete a course of treatment. He lost contact when he moved house and is not registered currently with a dental practitioner.

Medical History

The patient is otherwise fit and well.

Examination

Extraoral Examination

He is a fit and healthy-looking adolescent. No submental, submandibular or other cervical lymph nodes are palpable and the temporomandibular joints appear normal.

Intraoral Examination

The lower right quadrant is shown in Fig. 1.1. The oral mucosa is healthy, and the oral hygiene is satisfactory. There is gingivitis in areas, but no calculus is visible, and probing depths are 3 mm or less. The mandibular right first molar is grossly carious, and a sinus is discharging on its buccal aspect. There are no other restorations in any teeth. No teeth have been extracted, and the third molars are not visible. A small cavity is present on the occlusal surface of the mandibular right second molar.

Investigations

◆ What Further Examination Would You Carry Out?

Test of tooth sensibility (vitality) of the teeth in the region of the sinus. Even though the first molar is the most likely cause, the adjacent teeth should be tested because more than one tooth might be nonvital. The results should be compared with those of the teeth on the opposite side. Both hot/cold methods and electric pulp testing could be used because extensive reactionary (tertiary) dentine may moderate the response.

The first molar fails to respond to any test. All other teeth appear vital.

◆ What Radiographs Would You Take? Explain Why Each View is Required

See Table 1.1.

◆ What Problems are Inherent in the Diagnosis of Caries in This Patient?

Occlusal lesions are now the predominant form of caries in adolescents after the reduction in relative caries incidence over the past decades. Occlusal caries may go undetected on visual examination for two reasons. Firstly, it starts on the fissure walls and is obscured by sound superficial enamel, and secondly, lesions tend to cavitate late, if at all, probably because fluoride exposure reinforces the ionic structure of the overlying enamel. Superimposition of sound enamel also masks small- and medium-sized lesions on bitewing radiographs. The small occlusal cavity in the second molar arouses suspicion that other pits and fissures in the molars will be carious. Unless lesions are very large, extending into the middle third of dentine, they may not be detected on bitewing radiographs.

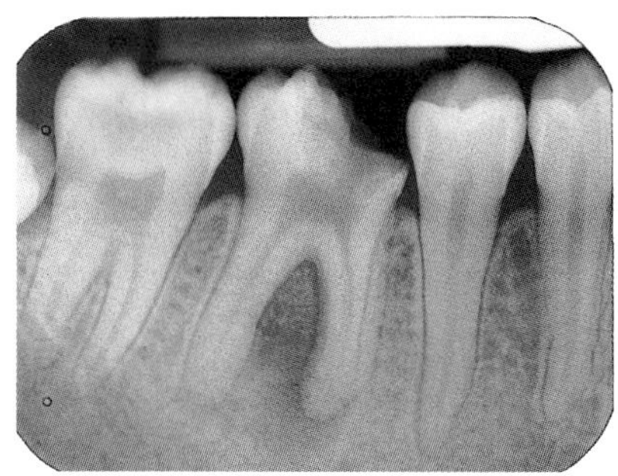
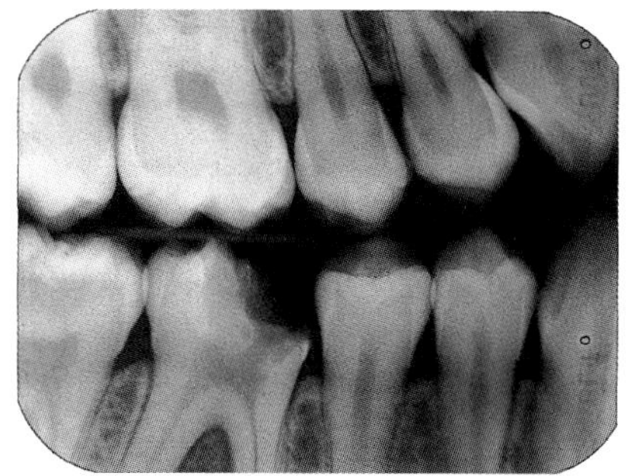
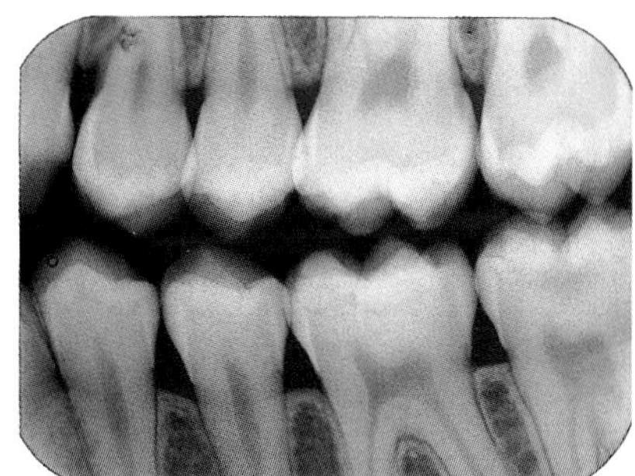

• **Fig. 1.2** Periapical and bitewing radiographs.

TABLE 1.1 Useful Radiographs and Their Clinical Benefit

Radiograph	Reason Taken
Bitewing radiographs	Primarily to detect proximal surface caries and, in this case, also required to help detect occlusal caries
Periapical radiograph of the lower right first molar tooth, taken with a paralleling technique	Preoperative assessment for endodontic treatment or for extraction, should it be necessary
Dental panoramic radiograph	Might be useful as a general survey view in a new patient and to determine the presence and position of third molars

◆ The Radiographs are Shown in Fig. 1.2. What Do You See?

The periapical radiograph shows the carious lesion in the crown of the lower right first molar to be extensive, involving the pulp. The mesial contact has been completely destroyed, and the molar has tilted mesially. There are periapical radiolucencies at the apices of both roots, that on the mesial root being larger. The radiolucencies are in continuity with the periodontal ligament, and there is loss of most of the lamina dura in the bifurcation and around the root apices.

The bitewing radiographs confirm the carious exposure and reveal occlusal carious lesions in all the maxillary and mandibular molars with the exception of the upper right first molar. No proximal caries is evident.

◆ If Two or More Teeth Were Possible Origins of the Sinus, How Might You Decide Between Them?

A gutta percha point could be inserted into the sinus prior to taking the radiograph, as shown in Fig. 1.1. A medium- or fine-sized point is flexible but resilient enough to pass along the sinus tract if twisted slightly on insertion. Points are radiopaque and can be seen on a radiograph extending to the source of the infection, as shown in a different case in Fig. 1.3.

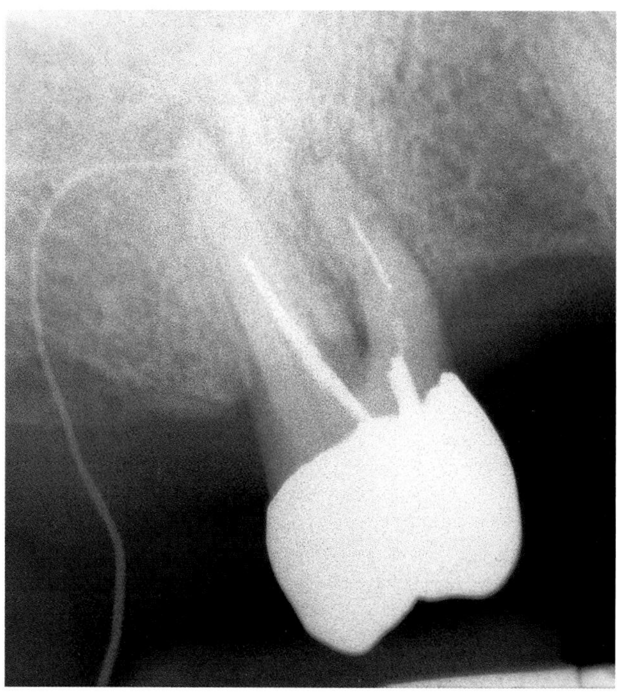

• **Fig. 1.3** A different case, showing a gutta percha point inserted through and tracing the path of a sinus.

Diagnosis

◆ What is Your Diagnosis?

The patient has a nonvital lower right first molar with a periapical abscess. In addition, he has a high caries rate in a previously almost caries-free dentition. He is, therefore, classified as 'high caries risk/susceptibility' (>2 new/active lesions in 2 years).

Management

The patient is horrified to discover that his dentition is in such a poor state, having experienced only one episode of toothache in the past. He is keen to do all that can be done to save all teeth, and a decision is made to try to restore the lower molar.

◆ How Will You Prioritize Treatment for This Patient? Why Should Treatment Be Provided in This Sequence?

See Table 1.2.

TABLE 1.2 Sequence of Care

Phase of Treatment	Items of Treatment	Reasons
Immediate phase	Caries removal from the lower right first molar, access cavity preparation for endodontics, drainage, irrigation with sodium hypochlorite and placement of a temporary restoration	Essential if the tooth is to be saved and to remove the source of the apical infection. There is also an urgent need to minimize further destruction of this tooth, which may soon be unrestorable. The temporary restoration is necessary to facilitate rubber dam isolation during future endodontic treatment, and it will also stabilize the occlusion and stop mesial drift.
Stabilization of caries	Removal of carious dentine in any cavitated lesions and placement of temporary restorations in all carious teeth in visits by quadrants or by two quadrants	To prevent further tooth destruction and progression to carious exposure while other phases of treatment are being carried out.
Preventive care (standard and active care nonoperative/noninvasive regimes) or operative/invasive prevention	Dietary analysis, oral hygiene instruction, fluoride advice, saliva analysis As occlusal lesions are noncavitated and asymptomatic (lesions within outer third of dentine radiographically), then consideration could be given to therapeutic sealants being placed into the carious fissures ± some caries excavation as needed ('preventive resin restoration')	Should start alongside the above and extend throughout the care plan, to reduce the high caries risk and ensure long-term oral health.
Definitive restoration	Will depend on what is found during or after placing any temporary or provisional restorations	Definitive restorations may be left until last; stabilization, prevention and risk reduction take priority.
Recall	Periodic review of treatments provided, patient adherence to behavioural changes; discuss individualized recall intervals with patient	Critical to review the patients' adherence to preventive advice and monitor the signs of caries risk/susceptibility fluctuation.

◆ What Temporary Restoration Materials are Available? What are Their Properties, and in What Situations are They Useful?

See Table 1.3.

◆ Why is One Molar So Much More Broken Down Compared with the Others?

It is difficult to be certain, but the extensive carious lesion is probably, in part, a result of a previous failed restoration. In view of the pattern of lesions in the other molars, it seems likely that this was a large occlusal restoration, and the history suggests that it was placed in a vital tooth. It probably undermined the mesial cusps or marginal ridge. Two factors could have contributed to the extensive carious lesion present only 1 year later: marginal leakage and/or undermining of the marginal ridge or mesial cusps leading to mechanical collapse of the tooth–restoration complex.

◆ Should You Ensure Removal of All Carious Tissue When Restoring the Vital Molars?

Removal of all softened carious tissue at the amelo-dentinal junction (cavity periphery) is essential, and only sound enamel/dentine or stained but firm dentine should be retained in the ideal situation.

Carious dentine removal over the pulp is treated differently. In a younger patient with relatively larger pulp chamber size, there is always a tendency for the operator to be more conservative. Very soft or flaky dentine (superficial, bacterially contaminated, caries-infected dentine) is ideally removed. Slightly soft dentine can be left in situ overlying the pulp, provided a good peripherally well-sealed adhesive restoration is placed over it. Deciding whether to leave the last layers of softened dentine can be difficult, and the decision rests, to a degree, on clinical experience. Physically interpreting softened dentine in rapidly advancing lesions is difficult. The deepest layers are soft through demineralization but are not necessarily grossly infected and can be retained over the pulp (demineralized, caries-affected dentine). Also, bacterial penetration of the dentine is not reliably indicated by staining in advancing lesions. Evidence shows that once a pulp is exposed during carious tissue removal procedures, the chances of medium-term pulp death in originally symptomatic teeth are increased significantly when compared with those cases where demineralized, caries-affected

TABLE 1.3 Temporary Restorative Materials*

Material	Examples	Properties	Situations
Zinc oxide and eugenol derivatives	Kalzinol	Bacteriocidal, easy to mix and place, cheap but not very strong; easily removed	Suitable for temporary restoration of most cavities, provided there is no significant occlusal load Endodontic access cavities
Self-setting zinc oxide cements	Cavit Coltosol	Harden in contact with saliva; reasonable strength and easily removed	Endodontic access cavities No occlusal load
Polycarboxylate cements	Poly-F	Adhesive to enamel and dentine; hard and durable	Used when mechanical retention is poor Strong enough to enable rubber dam placement when used in a badly broken down tooth
Glass ionomer cements (including silver-reinforced preparations)	Chem-fil Shofu Hi-Fi Ketac Silver	Adhesive to enamel and dentine; hard and durable; good appearance	As polycarboxylate cements and also useful in anterior teeth Could be used as a provisional restoration, lasting a few months

*Examples are not exhaustive.

dentine is retained as indirect pulp protection and the cavity sealed with an adhesive bio-interactive restorative material.

More detailed information on this minimally invasive (MI) operative selective carious tissue removal approach is discussed in Case 9.

◆ What Nonoperative Preventive Procedures Should Be Instigated for This Patient? Explain Why

Diet analysis and modification. The metabolically active caries process requires dietary sugars, in particular sucrose, glucose and fructose, an acidogenic plaque flora, a susceptible tooth surface and time, to encourage progression. Denying the plaque flora its substrate sugar is the most effective measure to halt the progression of existing lesions (secondary prevention) and prevent new ones forming (primary prevention). No preventive measure affecting the flora or tooth is as effective. A further advantage of emphasis on diet is that it forces patients to acknowledge that they must take responsibility for preventing disease and maintaining their own oral health. It is imperative that patients understand that dental caries is a lifestyle-related, behavioural, bacterially mediated, noncommunicable disease, which is wholly preventable by their actions alone.

◆ How Would You Evaluate a Patient's Diet?

Dietary analysis consists of two elements: enquiry into lifestyle and into the dietary components themselves. Information about the diet itself is of little value unless it is taken in context with the patient's lifestyle. Only dietary recommendations tailored to the patient's lifestyle are likely to be adopted. Using the COM-B ('capability', 'opportunity', 'motivation' and 'behaviour') model for behaviour management/change, patients need the capability to change their behaviour, as well as the opportunity within their current lifestyles (or a change that is practical for the patient to achieve is needed in this area) and motivation to do it. It is essential the oral healthcare team works with the patient in this regard. Also, using the GPS approach to modifying behaviour might be useful in this regard – patient-centred goal setting, planning and self-reflection of outcomes.

The diet record should include all the foods and drinks consumed, the amount (in readily estimated units) and the time of eating or drinking. It should encompass both weekdays and the weekend because behaviours can often be very different.

In this case, it should be noted that the patient is a 17-year-old student. Lifestyle often changes dramatically between ages 16 and 20 years. He may no longer be living at home and may be enjoying physical, financial and dietary independence from his parents. He may be eating a cheap carbohydrate-rich diet of snacks instead of regular meals. Long hours of studying may be accompanied by the frequent consumption of sweetened drinks and sugary snacks.

Analysis of the diet itself may be performed in a variety of ways. The patient can be asked to recall all foods consumed over the previous 24 hours. This is not very effective – relying, as it does, on a good memory and honesty – and is unlikely to give a representative account. Relying on memory recall events that occurred more than 24 hours ago is too inaccurate.

The most effective method is for patients to keep a written record of their diet for 4 consecutive days, including 2 working days and 2 leisure days (weekend). The need for patients to comply fully and assess their diet honestly must be stressed, and of course, the diet should not be changed because it is being recorded. Ideally, the analysis should be performed before any dietary advice is given. Even patients who do not keep an honest account have been made more aware of their diet. If they know what foods to omit from the sheet to make their dentist happy, at least the first step in an educative process has been taken.

◆ How Will You Analyse This Patient's 4-Day Diet Sheet Shown in Fig. 1.4? What is the Cause of His Caries Susceptibility?

Highlight sugar-rich foods and drinks as in Fig. 1.4. Note whether they are confined to meal times or whether they are eaten frequently and spaced throughout the day as snacks. The number of **sugar exposures should be counted** and discussed with the patient. Also, note the **consistency** of the food because dry and sticky foods take longer to be cleared from the mouth. Sugary drinks taken immediately before bed are highly significant because salivary flow is reduced during sleep, and, thus, clearance time is greater. Identify foods with a high **hidden sugar** content because patients often do not realize that such foods are significant; examples are baked beans, breakfast cereals, tomato ketchup and 'plain' biscuits.

The diet sheet shows that the main problem for this patient is too many sugar-containing drinks and frequent snacks of cake and biscuits. Most meals or snacks contain a high-sugar item and some more than one. The other typical cause of a high caries rate in this age group is sweets, especially mints.

A systematic review of the evidence linking sugar to caries incidence now highlights the importance of not only the frequency of sugar consumption per day but also the gross amount actually consumed. In both adults and children, the World Health Organization (WHO) recommends strongly that intake of free sugars should not exceed 10% of total energy consumption. This equates to approximately 50 g/person/day or 18 kg/person/year. Thus, it is important to read food labels to understand the relative sugar content as part of total energy consumed per day. Examples of dietary sugar content include one 200 ml carton of orange juice, 20 g; cup of tea with one teaspoon of sugar, 5 g; a small pot of low-fat fruit yogurt, 15 g.

◆ What Advice Will You Give the Patient?

The principles of a safer diet are shown in Table 1.4.

Dietary advice is provided by using the COM-B/GPS health-belief model of health education. However, it is well-known that education about the risks and consequences of lifestyle, habits and diet is often ineffective for the majority. It is important to judge the patient's likely adherence and provide dietary advice that can be used to make small but significant changes, rather than attempting to eradicate all sugar from the diet. As the diet improves, the advice should be adapted and extended during regular, and initially frequent, recall consultations, involving the patient in calculating the suitable intervals between appointments.

Advice must be acceptable, practical and affordable. In this case, the patient has already suffered the serious adverse consequences of his poor diet, and this may help change behaviour.

The patient must be made aware that damage to teeth continues for up to 1 hour after intake of a sugary food. The explanation given to some patients may be no more than this simple statement. Many other patients can comprehend the concept (if not the detail) of a Stephan curve without difficulty.

The patient should be advised to use a fluoride-containing toothpaste. During the period of dietary change, it would be beneficial to use a weekly fluoride rinse as well. This could be continued for as long as the diet is considered an unsafe one.

Oral hygiene instruction is also important and should be emphasized during all phases of care. It will not, by itself, stop caries progression, which is critical for this patient, and there is only mild gingivitis. However, continuously breaking up the plaque biofilm to prevent it from changing into an unhealthy, dysbiotic cariogenic biofilm will help maintain oral health in the long run. There is limited evidence to show that electric rotating/oscillating toothbrushes, when used effectively, can be more beneficial in comparison with their handheld counterparts.

◆ Assuming Good Adherence and Motivation, How Will You Restore the Teeth Definitively?

The mandibular right first molar requires orthograde endodontic root canal treatment and replacement of the temporary restoration with a core. Retention for the core can be provided by residual tooth tissue, provided the carious tissue destruction is not gross. The restorative material may be packed into the pulp chamber and the first 2–3 mm of the root canal (a form of Nayyar core). If insufficient natural crown remains, it may be supplemented with a preformed post in the usually more straight distal canals. The distal canal is not ideal in this case, being farther from the most extensively destroyed area, but it is larger.

The other molar teeth will need to have their temporary restorations replaced by definitive restorations. Caries has involved only the occlusal surface, but removal of these large lesions has probably left little more than an enamel shell. Restoration of such teeth with amalgam would require excessive removal of all the unsupported, undermined enamel, leaving little more than a root stump and a few spurs of tooth tissue. Restoration would be better achieved with a radiopaque glass ionomer cement and resin composite hybrid/layered restoration. The glass ionomer cement used to replace the missing dentine must be radiopaque so that it is not confused with residual or secondary caries on radiographs. A resin composite bonded to dentine with a dental adhesive would be an alternative to the glass ionomer cement. Alternatively, tricalcium silicate cements (e.g. Biodentine) may also be used to restore the bulk of the lost dentine, followed by a resin composite surface veneer, ideally placed a few weeks after placement of Biodentine, at a review appointment.

4 day diet analysis sheet for John Smith

	Thursday		Friday		Saturday		Sunday	
	Time	Item	Time	Item	Time	Item	Time	Item
Before breakfast			7.00	2 cups of tea with 2 sugars	7.30	4 chocolate biscuits tea with 2 sugars		
Breakfast	8.30	sausages pitta bread ketchup tea with 2 sugars	8.30	banana			8.00	chocolate puffed rice breakfast cereal 1 glass cola drink
Morning	9.20 11.15	1 glass cola drink hot chocolate chocolate bar	9.30	mug hot chocolate packet crisps can of diet cola drink	11.00	1 slice cherry cake	10.30	4 slices toast and peanut butter 1 piece cake
Mid-day meal	12.30	turkey salad sandwich 1 glass cola drink tea with 2 sugars	1.00 pm	2 pieces cheese on toast, garlic sausage 1 slice cake 1 glass cola drink	12.30	1 slice cake tea with 2 sugars	1.00 pm	fish pie 1 glass cola drink
Afternoon	4.00 pm	fizzy drink chocolate bar 1 slice cake	4.30 pm 5.00 pm	ham 1 piece cake tea with 2 sugars 1 glass cola drink	3.00 pm	sausages, beans, toast. an orange 1 can cola drink	2.00 pm 4.30 pm 6.00 pm	tea with 2 sugars 1 biscuit 1 piece cake tea with 2 sugars bar of chocolate
Evening meal	6.00 pm	salad, garlic sausage, ham, coleslaw	7.30 pm	burger and chips 1 can of cola drink	8.00 pm	spaghetti bolognaise ice cream	9.00 pm	fish and chips, peas 1 cola drink
Evening	10.30 pm	sausages crisps 1 glass fizzy drink			9.30 pm	tea with 2 sugars		

• **Fig. 1.4** The patient's diet sheet.

TABLE 1.4 Dietary Advice

Aims	Methods
Reduce the amount of sugar (<10% of total energy consumption; 50 g/person/day)	Check manufacturers' labels, and avoid foods with sugars such as sucrose, glucose and fructose, listed early in the ingredients. Natural sugars (e.g. honey, brown sugar) are as cariogenic as purified or added sugars. When sweet foods are required, choose those containing sweetening agents such as saccharin, acesulfame-K and aspartame. Diet formulations contain less sugar compared with their standard counterparts. Reduce the sweetness of drinks and foods. Become accustomed to a less sweet diet overall.
Restrict frequency of sugar intakes to meal times as far as possible	Try to reduce snacking. When snacks are required select 'safe snacks' such as cheese, crisps and fruit or sugar-free sweets such as mints or chewing gum (which not only has no sugar but also stimulates salivary flow and increases plaque pH). Use artificial sweeteners in drinks taken between meals.
Speed clearance of sugars from the mouth	Never finish meals with a sugary food or drink. Follow sugary foods with a sugar-free drink, chewing gum or a protective food such as cheese.

◆ Fig. 1.5 Shows the Restored Lower First Molar 2 Months After Endodontic Treatment. What Do You See, and What Long-Term Problem is Evident?

There is some bone healing around the apices and in the bifurcation. Complete healing would be expected after 6 months to 1 year, at which time the success of the overall root canal treatment can be judged.

As noted in the initial radiographs, the lower right first molar has lost its mesial contact, drifted and tilted. This makes it impossible to restore the normal contour of the mesial surface and contact point. The mesial surface is flat, and there is no defined contact point. In the long term, there is a risk of caries of the distal surface of the second premolar, and the caries is likely to affect a wider area of tooth and extend further gingivally compared with caries below a normal contact. The area will also be difficult to clean, and there is a risk of localized periodontitis. Tilting of the occlusal surface may also favour food packing into the contact unless the contour of the restoration includes an artificially enhanced marginal ridge.

Therefore, this tooth will probably require an indirect crown in the long term. Much of the enamel is undermined, and the tooth is weakened by endodontic treatment. A crown would allow the contact to have a better contour, but the problem is insoluble while the tooth remains in its present position. Orthodontic uprighting could be considered.

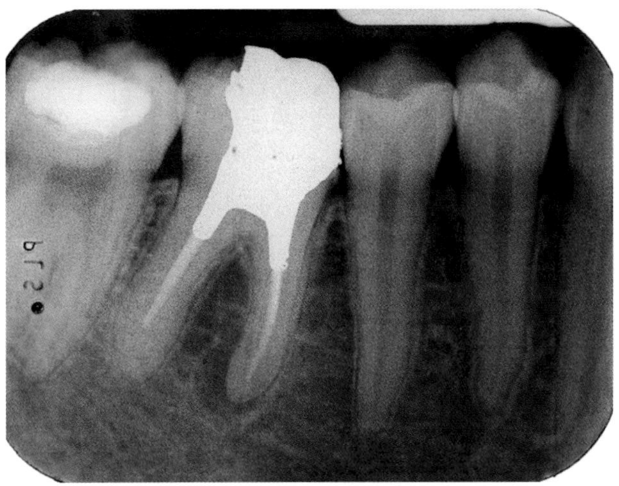

• **Fig. 1.5** Periapical radiograph of the restored lower first molar.

◆ Why Not Simply Extract the Lower Molar?

Extraction of the lower right first molar may well be the preferred treatment. The caries is extensive, restoration of the tooth will be complex and expensive and problems will probably ensue in the long term. The missing tooth might not be readily visible.

To a large degree, the decision will depend on the patient's wishes and the advice from the oral healthcare team. If the patient would be happy with an edentulous space, the extraction appears to be an attractive proposition. However, if a restoration is required, a bridge will require preparation of two further teeth. A denture-based replacement is probably not indicated, but an implant might be considered at a later date. Any hesitancy or uncertainty on the patient's part might well influence you to propose extraction.

Another factor affecting the decision is the condition and long-term prognosis of the other molars. If further molars are likely to be lost in the short or medium term, it makes sense to conserve whichever teeth can be successfully restored.

Medico-Legal Considerations of This Case

In terms of modifying the patient's caries susceptibility, it is imperative that contemporaneous records are kept of all consultations/appointments. The patient must be engaged with the preventive care philosophy for the greatest chance of success in the medium to long term. Details of all nonoperative and operative interventions must be recorded, along with their justification. All investigations must be fully reported, with relevant information including the dates when they were performed as well as their outcomes. Review consultation periodicity must be noted and explained, with evidence that the patient was fully informed, and consented to, the care episode.

Case 2

A Multilocular Radiolucency

ERIC WHAITES AND EDWARD ODELL

Summary

A 45-year-old African man presents in the dental accident and emergency department with an enlarged jaw (Fig. 2.1). You need to make a diagnosis and decide on treatment.

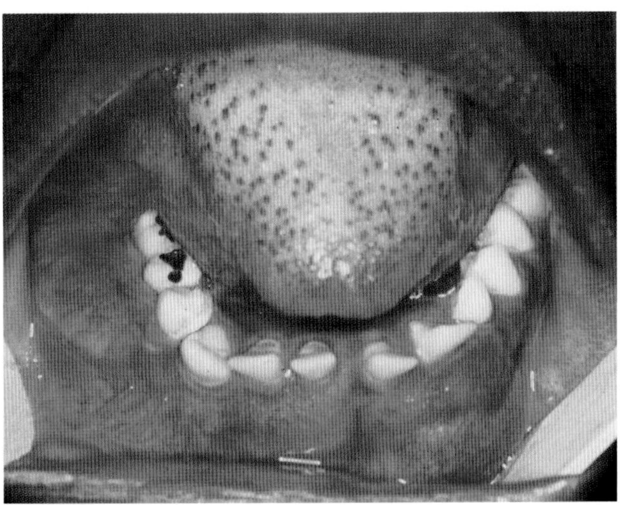

• **Fig. 2.1** The patient on presentation.

History

Complaint

The patient's main complaint is that his lower back teeth on the right side are loose and that his jaw on the right feels enlarged.

History of Complaint

The patient has been aware of his teeth slowly becoming looser over the previous 6 months. They seem to be 'moving' and are now at a different height from his front teeth, making eating difficult. He is also concerned that his jaw is enlarged and that there seems to be reduced space for his tongue. He has recently had the lower second molar on the right extracted. It was also loose, but extraction does not seem to have cured the swelling. Although not in pain, he has finally decided to seek treatment.

Medical History

He is otherwise fit and healthy.

Examination

Extraoral Examination

He is a fit-looking man with no obvious facial asymmetry but has a slight fullness of the mandible on the right. Palpation reveals a smooth, rounded, bony hard enlargement on the buccal and lingual aspects. Deep cervical lymph nodes are palpable on the right side. They are only slightly enlarged, soft, not tender and freely mobile.

Intraoral Examination

◆ What Do You See in Fig. 2.1?

There is a large swelling of the right posterior mandible visible in the buccal sulcus, its anterior margin is relatively well defined and level with the first premolar. The lingual aspect is not visible, but the tongue appears displaced upwards and medially, suggesting significant lingual expansion. The mucosa over the swelling is of normal colour, without evidence of inflammation or infection. There are two relatively small amalgams in the lower right molar and the second premolar.

If you could examine the patient, you would find that all his upper right posterior teeth have been extracted and that the lower molar and premolars are 2–3 mm above the height of the occlusal plane. These teeth are grade 3 mobile but still are vital.

◆ What are the Red Spots On the Patient's Tongue?

Fungiform papillae. They appear more prominent when the tongue is furred, as in this case, when the diet is not very abrasive.

◆ On the Basis of What You Know So Far, What Types of Condition Would You Consider is Present?

The history suggests a relatively slow-growing lesion, which is, therefore, likely to be benign. Although this is not a definitive relationship, there are no specific features suggesting malignancy, such as perforation of the cortex, soft tissue mass, ulceration of the mucosa, numbness of the lip or devitalization of teeth. The character of the lymph node enlargement does not suggest malignancy.

The commonest jaw lesions that cause expansion are odontogenic cysts. The commonest odontogenic cysts are the radicular (apical inflammatory) cyst, dentigerous cyst

TABLE 2.1 Radiographic Views

Radiographic View	Reason
Panoramic or oblique lateral radiograph	To show the lesion from the lateral aspect. The oblique lateral would provide the better resolution but might not cover the anterior extent of this large lesion. The panoramic radiograph would provide a useful survey of the rest of the jaws but only that part of this expansile lesion in the line of the arch will be in focus. An oblique lateral view was taken.
A postero-anterior (PA) view of the jaws	To show the extent of mediolateral expansion of the posterior body, angle or ramus.
A lower true (90°) occlusal view	To show lingual expansion, which will not be visible in the PA view of the jaws because of superimposition of the anterior body of the mandible.
A periapical view of the lower right second premolar and the first molar	To assess bone support and possible root resorption.

and odontogenic keratocyst. If this is a radicular cyst, it could have arisen from the first molar, although the occlusal amalgam is relatively small and there seems to be no reason to suspect that the tooth is not vital. A residual radicular cyst arising on the extracted second or third molar would be a possibility. A dentigerous cyst could be the cause if the third molar is unerupted. The possibility of an odontogenic keratocyst seems unlikely because these cysts do not normally cause much expansion. An odontogenic tumour is a possible cause, and an ameloblastoma would be the most likely one because it is the commonest and arises most frequently at this site and in this age group. There is a higher prevalence in Africans than in other racial groups. An ameloblastoma is much more likely than an odontogenic cyst to displace teeth and make them grossly mobile. A giant cell granuloma and numerous other lesions are possibilities but are all less likely.

Investigations

◆ Radiographs are Obviously Indicated. Which Conventional Views Would You Choose? Why?

Several different views are necessary to show the full extent of the lesion. These are listed in Table 2.1 and are shown in Figs 2.2–2.5.

Describe the radiographic features of the lesion.

The features are described in Table 2.2.

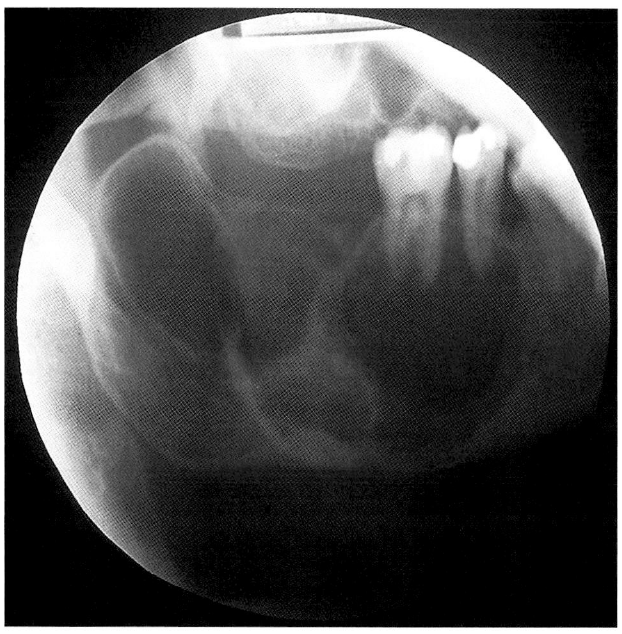

• **Fig. 2.2** Oblique lateral view.

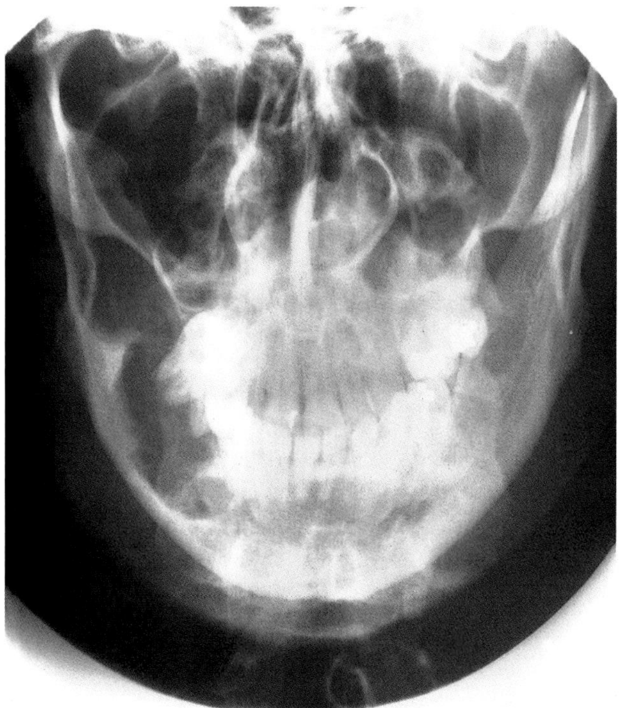

• **Fig. 2.3** Postero-anterior view of the jaws.

◆ Why Do the Roots of the First Molar and the Second Premolar Appear To Be So Resorbed in the Periapical View When the Oblique Lateral View Shows Minimal Root Resorption?

The teeth are foreshortened in the periapical view because they lie at an angle to the image receptor. This image has been taken by using the bisected angle technique and several factors contribute to the distortion:

- the teeth have been displaced by the lesion, so their crowns lie more lingually, and the roots more buccally;

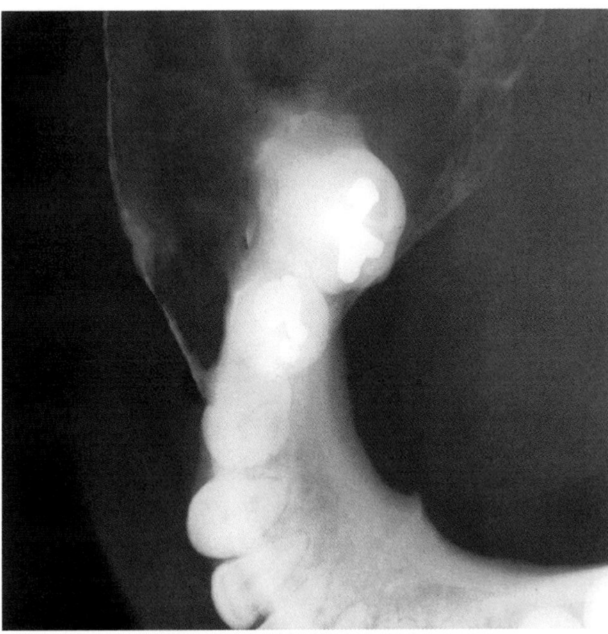

• **Fig. 2.4** Lower true occlusal view.

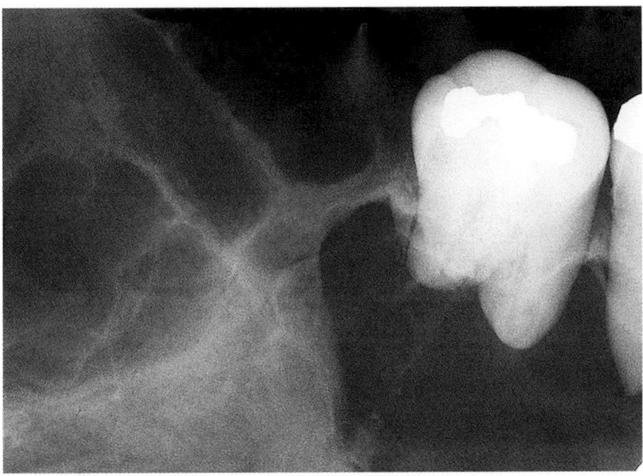

• **Fig. 2.5** Periapical view of the lower right first permanent molar.

- the lingual expansion of the jaw makes image receptor placement difficult, so it has had to be severely tilted away from the root apices;
- there was failure to take account of these two factors when positioning and angling the x-ray tubehead.

Radiological Differential Diagnosis

◆ What is Your Principal Differential Diagnosis?

1. Ameloblastoma
2. Giant cell lesion

◆ Justify This Differential Diagnosis

Ameloblastoma classically produces an expanding multilocular radiolucency at the angle of the mandible. As noted above, it most commonly presents at the age of this patient and is commoner in his racial group. The radiographs show the typical multilocular radiolucency, containing several large cystic spaces separated by bony septa, and the root resorption, tooth displacement and marked expansion are all consistent with an ameloblastoma of this size.

Giant cell lesion. A central giant cell granuloma is possible. These lesions can arise at almost any age, but the radiological features and site are slightly different, making ameloblastoma the preferred diagnosis. Central giant cell granuloma produces expansion and a honeycomb or multilocular radiolucency, but there would be no root resorption, and the lesion would be less radiolucent (because it consists of solid tissue rather than cystic neoplasm), often containing wispy osteoid or fine bone septa subdividing the lesion into a honeycomb-like pattern. However, these typical features are not always seen. The spectrum of radiological appearances range from lesions that mimic odontogenic and solitary bone cysts to those that appear identical to ameloblastoma or other odontogenic tumours. The aneurysmal bone cyst is another giant cell lesion that could produce this radiographic appearance with prominent expansion. Adjacent teeth are usually displaced but rarely resorbed. However, aneurysmal bone cyst is much rarer than central giant cell granuloma in the jaws.

TABLE 2.2 Features of Lesion

Feature of Lesion	Radiographic Finding
Site	Posterior body, angle and ramus of the right mandible
Size	Large, about 10 × 8 cm, extending from the second premolar, back to the angle and involving all of the ramus up to the sigmoid notch, and from the expanded upper border of the alveolar bone down to the inferior dental canal.
Shape	Multilocular, producing the soap bubble appearance.
Outline/edge	Smooth, well defined and mostly well corticated.
Relative radiodensity	Radiolucent with distinct radiopaque septa producing the multilocular appearance. There is no evidence of separate areas of calcification within the lesion.
Effects on adjacent structures	Gross lingual expansion of mandible, expansion buccally is only seen well in the occlusal films. Marked expansion of the superior margin of the alveolar bone and the anterior margin of the ascending ramus. The involved teeth have also been displaced superiorly. The roots of the involved teeth are slightly resorbed, but not as markedly as suggested by the periapical view. The cortex does not appear to be perforated.

◆ What Types of Lesion are Less Likely, and Why?

Several lesions remain possible but are less likely on the basis of either their features or their relative rarity.

Rarer odontogenic tumours, including particularly odontogenic fibroma and myxoma. These similar benign connective tissue odontogenic tumours are often indistinguishable from one another radiographically. Odontogenic myxoma is commoner than fibroma, but both are relegated to the position of unlikely diagnoses on the basis of their relative rarity and the younger age group affected. Both usually cause a unilocular or apparently multilocular expansive radiolucency at the angle of the mandible and displace adjacent teeth or sometimes loosen or resorb them. A characteristic, although inconsistent, feature in myxoma is that the internal dividing septa are usually fine and arranged at right angles to one another, in a pattern sometimes said to resemble the letters 'X' and 'Y' or the strings of a tennis racket. In myxoma, septa can also show the honeycomb pattern described in giant cell granuloma.

Odontogenic keratocyst. This is unlikely to be the cause of this lesion, but in view of its relative frequency, it might still be included at the end of the differential diagnosis. It should be included because it can cause a large multilocular radiolucency at the angle of the mandible in adults, usually slightly younger than this patient. However, the growth pattern of an odontogenic keratocyst is quite different from that of the present lesion. Odontogenic keratocysts usually extend a considerable distance into the body and/or ramus before causing significant expansion. Even when expansion is evident, it is usually a broad-based enlargement rather than a localized expansion. Adjacent teeth are rarely resorbed or displaced.

◆ What Lesions Have You Discounted, and Why?

Dentigerous cyst is a common cause of large radiolucent lesions at the angle of the mandible. However, the present lesion is not unilocular and does not contain an unerupted tooth. Similarly, the radicular cyst is unilocular but associated with a nonvital tooth.

Malignant neoplasms, either primary or metastatic. As noted above, the clinical features do not suggest malignancy, and the radiographs show an apparently benign, well-defined, slowly enlarging lesion.

Further Investigations

◆ Is a Biopsy Required?

Yes. If the lesion is an ameloblastoma, the treatment will be excision, whereas if it is a giant cell granuloma, curettage will be sufficient. A definitive diagnosis based on biopsy analysis is required to plan treatment.

◆ Would Aspiration Biopsy Be Helpful?

No. If an odontogenic keratocyst were suspected, this diagnosis might be confirmed by aspirating keratin. It would also be helpful in determining whether the lesion is solid or cystic. It would not be particularly helpful in the diagnosis of ameloblastoma.

◆ What Precautions Would You Take At Biopsy?

An attempt should be made to obtain a sample of the solid lesion. If this is an ameloblastoma and an expanded area of the jaw is selected for biopsy, it will almost certainly overlie a cyst in the neoplasm. A large part of many ameloblastomas is cyst space, and the stretched cyst lining is not always sufficiently characteristic histologically to make the diagnosis. If the lesion proves to be cystic on biopsy analysis, the surgeon should open up the cavity and explore it to identify solid tumour for sampling.

The surgical access must be carefully closed on bone to ensure that healing is uneventful and infection does not develop in the cyst spaces. The expanded areas may be covered by only a thin layer of eggshell-like periosteal bone. Once this is opened, it may be difficult to replace the margin of a mucoperiosteal flap back onto solid bone.

◆ The Histological Appearances of the Biopsy Specimen are Shown in Figs 2.6 and 2.7. What Do You See?

The specimen is stained with haematoxylin and eosin. At low power, the lesion is seen to consist of islands of epithelium separated by thin, pink, collagenous bands. Each

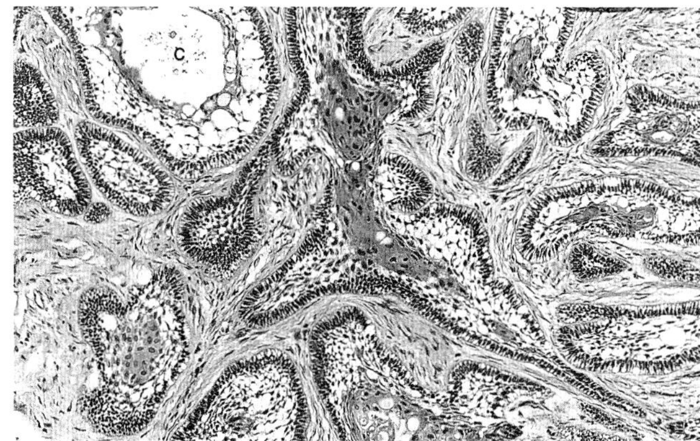

• **Fig. 2.6** Histological appearance of biopsy specimen at low power.

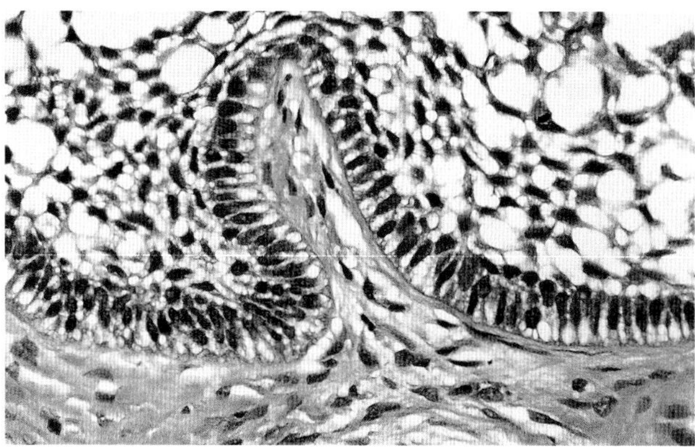

• **Fig. 2.7** Histological appearance of biopsy specimen at high power.

island has a prominent outer layer of basal cells, a paler staining zone within that, and sometimes a pink keratinized zone of cells centrally. One of the islands shows early cyst formation (as shown in Fig. 2.6, labelled 'c'). At higher power, the outer basal cell layer is seen to comprise elongate palisaded cells with reversed nuclear polarity (nuclei placed away from the basement membrane). Towards the basement membrane, many of the cells have a clear cytoplasmic zone, and the overall appearance resembles piano keys. Above the basal cell layer is a zone of very loosely packed stellate cells with large spaces between them. There is no inflammation.

◆ How Do You Interpret These Appearances?

The appearances are typical and diagnostic of ameloblastoma. The elongate basal cells bear a superficial resemblance to preameloblasts and the looser cells to stellate reticulum. The arrangement of the epithelium in islands with the stellate reticulum in their centres constitutes the follicular pattern of ameloblastoma.

Diagnosis

◆ The Final Diagnosis is Ameloblastoma, Conventional Type. Does the Type of Ameloblastoma Matter?

Yes, it is important for treatment planning. There are several different types of ameloblastoma, and not all exhibit extension into the surrounding medullary cavity. The characteristics of the main types are shown in Table 2.3.

Treatment

◆ What Treatment Will Be Required?

The ameloblastoma in this patient is classified as a benign neoplasm. However, it is locally infiltrative and, in some cases, permeates the medullary cavity around the main tumour margin. Ameloblastoma has to be excised with a 1 cm margin of normal bone and around any suspected perforations in the cortex to prevent recurrence. If ameloblastoma has escaped from bone, it may spread extensively in soft tissues and requires excision with an even larger margin. The lower border of the mandible may be intact and is sometimes left in place to avoid the need for full-thickness resection of the mandible and a bone graft. This carries a low risk of recurrence, but such recurrences are slow growing and may be dealt with conservatively after the main portion of the mandible has healed.

Excision with a bone margin, as described above, is considered the standard of care, but recently, some surgeons have been attempting more conservative treatment with curettage, as for unicystic ameloblastomas. This poses a risk of recurrence in those cases with bone permeation but avoids a major resection in other patients. In small mandibular ameloblastomas, such treatment can be successful. Close monitoring for follow-up is required, and small recurrences may be treated with further curettage. However, multifocal or second recurrence requires resection. Conservative treatment is not appropriate in the maxilla, where even conventional treatment carries a risk

TABLE 2.3 The Main Types of Ameloblastoma

Type	Features	Permeates Surrounding Bone?
Conventional ameloblastoma	The commonest type, previously called *solid/multicystic ameloblastoma*. Usually contains multiple cysts and has a multilocular radiographic appearance. Plexiform, follicular and mixed histological variants exist but have no bearing on behaviour or treatment. Desmoplastic ameloblastoma used to be considered a separate type but is now grouped with conventional ameloblastoma because intermediate conventional and desmoplastic types exist. However, it is worth being aware of this pattern because radiographically, it forms a fine honeycomb radiolucency that may resemble a fibro-osseous lesion with a margin that is difficult to define. No large cysts are present, and histologically, it comprises sparse islands of ameloblastoma dispersed in dense fibrous tissue. Unusually, this pattern is as frequent in the maxilla as in the mandible, and most cases exhibit spread into adjacent medullary spaces.	Yes, in a quarter or less of cases
Unicystic ameloblastoma	An ameloblastoma with only one cyst cavity and no separate islands of tumour, or just a few limited to the inner part of the fibrous wall. Presents radiographically as a cyst, sometimes in a dentigerous relationship. Can only be diagnosed definitively as a unicystic ameloblastoma by performing a complete histological examination after treatment.	No
Peripheral or extraosseous ameloblastoma	An ameloblastoma that develops as a soft tissue nodule outside bone, usually on the gingiva. Usually detected when small and readily excised. This variant is very rare.	No (the lesion is outside bone)

of recurrence, and occasionally, recurrent ameloblastoma can extend to the base of the skull and be inoperable. In this case, the lesion is clearly extensive and multilocular, filling almost the whole ramus and posterior body. In a case such as this, definitive resection in one operation is much better for the patient.

The fact that the ameloblastoma in this patient is of the follicular pattern is of no significance for treatment.

◆ What Other Imaging Investigations Would Be Appropriate for This Patient?

To plan the resection accurately, the extent of the tumour and any cortical perforations must be identified. Cone beam computed tomography (CBCT), computed tomography (CT) and/or magnetic resonance imaging (MRI) would show the full extent of the lesion in bone and surrounding soft tissue, respectively.

Case 3
An Unpleasant Surprise

MARTYN ORMOND AND MICHAEL ESCUDIER

Summary

A 17-year-old female patient becomes unwell, developing shortness of breath and a facial rash in your dental reception. What would you do?

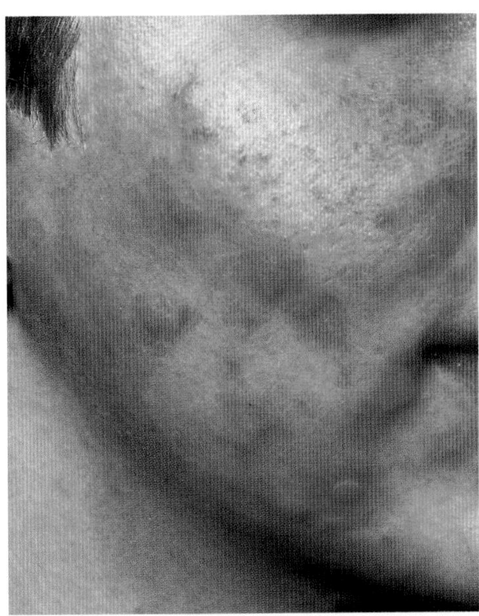

• **Fig. 3.1** The patient's face as she starts to feel unwell.

History

Complaint

The patient complains that she feels unwell, hot and breathless. Her face is itchy.

History of Complaint

The patient was attending for a planned restoration under local anaesthesia. Her symptoms developed whilst sitting in the waiting room eating a snack bought from a shop next door.

Medical History

You check your last medical history in the patient's notes and discover that the patient has asthma, which is well controlled, and is taking salbutamol on occasions. She also has eczema, as do her mother and brother, and she uses a topical corticosteroid cream, as prescribed. The patient has no known drug allergies.

Examination

◆ The Patient's Face is Shown in Fig. 3.1. What Do You See?

There is patchy erythema. In the most inflamed areas, there are well-defined raised oedematous weals, for instance, just above the lower border of the mandible below the commissure.

Diagnosis

◆ What is the Likely Diagnosis?

This is a typical urticarial rash, which indicates a type 1 hypersensitivity reaction. The rash, together with the systemic symptoms, indicates anaphylaxis arising from hypersensitivity to an unknown allergen. As the patient has not yet been exposed to any allergens in the dental surgery environment, the cause is most likely a food allergen, and the most likely cause of a severe reaction like this is peanuts.

◆ What Does Urticarial Mean?

The word *urticarial* comes from the Latin for nettle rash. An urticarial rash causes superficial oedema that may form separate, flat, raised blister-like patches (as in Fig. 3.1) or be diffuse. In the head and neck region, swelling is often diffuse because the tissues are lax. Markedly oedematous areas may become pale because of compression of their blood supply, but the background is erythematous. Patients often know an urticarial rash by the lay term *hives*.

◆ What are the Signs and Symptoms of Anaphylaxis?

The signs and symptoms vary with severity. The classic picture is of:

- a red urticarial rash
- oedema that may obstruct the airway
- hypotension caused by reduced peripheral resistance
- hypovolaemia caused by the movement of fluid out of the circulation into the tissues
- obstruction of small airways caused by oedema and bronchospasm.

Involvement of nasal and ocular tissues may cause rhinitis and conjunctivitis. There may also be nausea and vomiting.

◆ What is the Pathogenesis of Anaphylaxis?

Anaphylaxis is an acute type 1 hypersensitivity reaction triggered in a sensitized individual by an allergen. The allergen enters the tissues and binds to immunoglobulin E (IgE) acting as a receptor on the surface of mast cells, which are present in almost all tissues. Binding induces degranulation and the release of large amounts of inflammatory mediators, particularly histamine. These cause vasodilatation, increased capillary permeability and bronchospasm.

◆ Type 1 Hypersensitivity is Also Known As Immediate Hypersensitivity. Why?

Because acute anaphylactic reactions may occur within seconds. However, it is important to remember that reactions may be delayed for up to an hour, depending on the nature of the allergen and the route of exposure. In general, allergens administered intravenously cause immediate reactions, and those administered intramuscularly after approximately 30 minutes. It takes around 45 minutes for an orally administered allergen such as an antibiotic to be absorbed, pass through the circulation to the tissues and trigger a reaction. However, particular allergens can cause an anaphylactic reaction very quickly, whether applied topically or ingested, and important examples are peanuts and latex.

◆ What Would You Do Immediately?

The immediate cause of the reaction is not important, as all anaphylactic reactions are treated similarly.

- Reassure the patient.
- Assess vital signs, including blood pressure, pulse and respiratory rate.
- Have the patient lie flat (because there is no difficulty breathing).
- Call for help.
- Obtain oxygen and your practice's emergency drug box.

On examining for the signs noted above, you discover that the patient, previously breathing without difficulty, is now breathless, and a wheeze can be heard on expiration, indicating bronchospasm. She feels hot and has a pulse rate of 120 beats/min and blood pressure of 120/80 mmHg. She is conscious, but the effects are becoming more severe, and the rash now affects all the face and neck regions and has spread onto the upper aspect of the thorax and arms. The appearance of one arm is shown in Fig. 3.2. The erythematous areas seen are slightly raised.

Treatment

◆ What Would You Do Next?

Before the breathing problems were noted, you correctly laid the patient flat. However, her lungs must now be raised above the rest of her body to prevent oedema fluid collecting in the lungs.

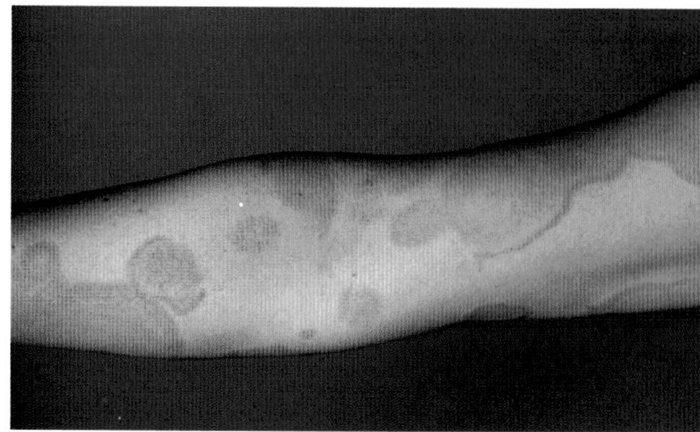

• **Fig. 3.2** The patient's arm 5 minutes after onset of the reaction.

Allow the patient to adopt the most comfortable position for breathing, and give:

- **oxygen** (5 l/min) via a facemask. Because there is bronchospasm, give the following drugs:
  - **Adrenaline/epinephrine.** 1:1000, 500 micrograms intramuscularly. The easiest form to administer is a pre-loaded 'EpiPen' or 'Anapen', both of which are available for adults (300 micrograms/dose) and children (150 micrograms/dose). Alternatively, a Min-I-Jet prepacked syringe and needle assembly or a standard vial of adrenaline/epinephrine solution, both containing 1 mg in 1 ml (1:1000), may be used. However, both these latter methods require a delay in administration to prepare the injection. You need to be familiar with whichever form is held in your practice because delay in calculating doses and volumes is clearly undesirable. Adrenaline/epinephrine may also be given subcutaneously, but the absorption is slower, and this route is no longer recommended. Note that autoinjectors are designed for self-administration and so provide a slightly lower dose than is recommended. The recommended site for the intramuscular injection is the anterolateral aspect of the middle of the thigh, where there is most muscle bulk. If clothing prevents access, the upper lateral arm, into the deltoid muscle, is an alternative site. In an emergency, it may be necessary to inject through clothing but this is not recommended. In the past, the tongue has been proposed as a potential site because it is familiar to dentists, but it is highly vascular, allowing rapid uptake of the drug and is unlikely to be acceptable to the conscious patient.
  - **Salbutamol.** This $\beta 2$ agonist may be helpful in patients experiencing respiratory distress. As the patient has asthma, she may have an inhaler with her and could be asked to take a dose. However, this is secondary to ensuring rapid delivery of adrenaline/epinephrine. Adrenaline/epinephrine is the life-saving drug and must be given without delay, before circulatory collapse. It is rapidly acting and will counteract pulmonary oedema or bronchospasm.

◆ After Giving a Single Dose of Adrenaline/Epinephrine with an Autoinjector, the Patient Recovers. What Would You Do Next?

- Continue to monitor the vital signs.
- Continue to administer oxygen.

- Arrange transfer of the patient to a hospital.
- Advise the patient of the need for formal investigation of her probable allergy.

◆ Can You Relax Now That the Immediate Crisis is Over?

No, definitely not. The response of the patient needs to be closely observed. Adrenaline/epinephrine is highly effective but has a very short half-life. Recurrence of bronchospasm, a drop in blood pressure or worsening oedema indicates a need for further adrenaline/epinephrine. In a severe reaction, this is likely to be needed about 5 minutes after the previous administration, and it can be repeated again as often as necessary.

Late relapse, hours later, is also possible. Mast cells release potent inflammatory mediators other than histamine, and some have long half-lives.

◆ Can an Anaphylactic Reaction Be Controlled Without Adrenaline/Epinephrine?

If the only features are a rash and mild swelling not involving the airway, it may be appropriate to give oral chlorphenamine (chlorpheniramine). However, if there is any suggestion of bronchospasm, hypotension or oedema around the airway, adrenaline/epinephrine will be needed. Adrenaline/epinephrine should be administered as early as possible to be effective, and it is better not to delay unless the signs and symptoms are very mild and of slow onset.

◆ What Additional Treatment Will Be Provided in the Hospital?

Once appropriate medical care arrives or the patient is admitted to the emergency department, the following treatment will be commenced:

- **Chlorphenamine** (chlorpheniramine) 10 mg intravenously will counteract the effects of histamine.
- **Hydrocortisone** 200 mg intravenously or intramuscularly.
- **Intravenous fluid** only required if hypotension develops. A suitable regime would be 500–1000 ml of normal saline infused over 5 minutes with continuous monitoring of vital signs.

The presentation of drugs useful for anaphylaxis is shown in Fig. 3.3.

Further Points

◆ Why is Adrenaline/Epinephrine Effective?

Adrenaline/epinephrine is the prototypical adrenergic agonist and has both α and β receptor activity. Alpha receptor–mediated action on arterioles causes vasoconstriction and, thus, reverses oedema. Beta receptor–mediated actions include increasing the cardiac output by increasing the force of contraction and heart rate ($\beta 1$) and bronchodilatation ($\beta 2$). Mast cell degranulation is also suppressed.

◆ Could You Have Predicted That This Patient Was At Risk of Anaphylaxis?

She has a history of asthma and a family history of eczema. This indicates atopy and carries an increased risk of developing hypersensitivity to a wide range of substances. However, not all patients with atopia develop severe reactions like this. It is important to take a thorough allergy history, particularly regarding drugs, rubber and other dental materials, as well as foods, in all patients. No patients with potential allergies should be exposed to their possible allergens until you have sought advice.

◆ Why Did This Patient Have No History of Severe Allergy?

This underlines the unpredictability of allergic reactions and why patients who have been administered any medication should be monitored for an appropriate time in case of adverse effects, the period depending on the route of administration (see above).

In this instance, the patient may have been sensitized by previous exposure to allergens such as peanut or other foods relatively recently. Although there is no evidence yet that peanut was the causative allergen, this is a definite possibility. Most dietary allergies start in childhood, but adults, even older adults, can develop allergy to nuts despite having consumed them without problems for many years. Adults who seem to have outgrown their childhood nut allergy can experience a relapse in later life.

Lack of an allergy history is also important with regard to penicillins because sensitization to very small quantities of penicillins in the environment may develop. Veterinary uses of penicillins leave residues in meat and milk, and these may be passed on to babies via their mother's milk. Penicillins are ubiquitous, and there is probably a genetic predisposition to explain why only a few individuals develop hypersensitivity.

◆ Can Patients Be Tested for the Causative Allergen?

Yes, but it carries a risk of anaphylaxis and must be performed with care in a specialized centre.

Unlike mild food allergies and intolerances, which are suspected in approximately twice as many individuals as those who actually suffer from them, severe food allergies are usually obviously authentic and often multiple. Testing is indicated because severe food allergy often strikes away from medical care and is not infrequently fatal.

For penicillin allergy, the most likely allergen to be administered by a dentist, only 10–20% of patients who report penicillin allergy are actually hypersensitive, and testing is reserved for those who give a convincing history of a type 1 reaction and who also have a definite requirement for penicillin. In most cases, a safe alternative antibiotic, for example, clindamycin, is available and so testing is not performed.

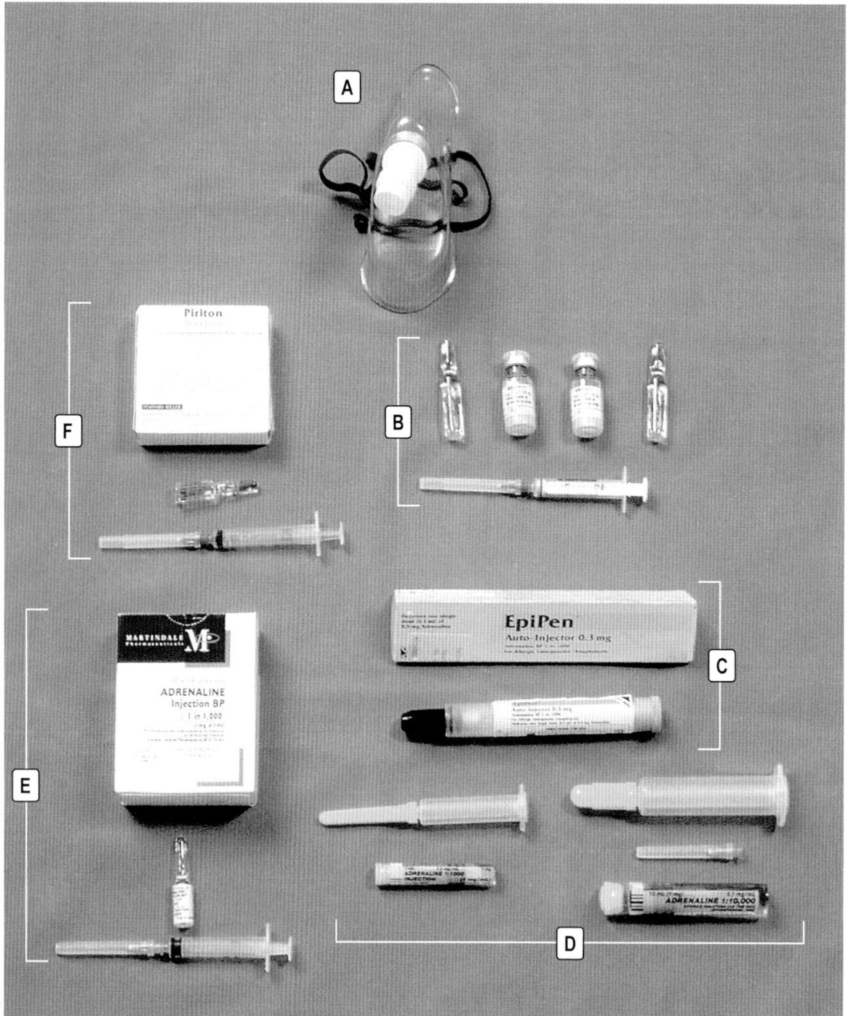

• **Fig. 3.3** Typical presentations of drugs used to treat anaphylaxis.

A. Oxygen mask.
B. Hydrocortisone. Vials of lyophilized powder for reconstitution in water for injection, *not* saline. Administer with a conventional syringe and needle.
C. Adrenaline/epinephrine in a disposable autoinjector spring-loaded syringe (EpiPen), boxed and, below, with the plastic covers removed from each end. Press directly onto the skin, and the spring-loaded needle is unsheathed and the drug injected automatically. A similar device, Anapen, has a spring-loaded needle that springs out when a button at the opposite end is pressed. Both deliver 300 micrograms of adrenaline/epinephrine.
D. Adrenaline/epinephrine in Min-I-Jet format. The yellow plastic cover is removed from the back (right-hand end) of the syringe barrel and front of the glass cartridge and the cartridge is screwed into the syringe barrel. Available in two types, with needle fitted (left, recommended) and with luer lock fitting for a conventional needle (slower to use). After removing front cover and fitting needle, if required, use as a conventional syringe. Versions with finer needles for subcutaneous administration are available but the intramuscular route is preferred and the version with the larger 21-gauge needle should be used.
E. Adrenaline/epinephrine as traditional ampoule, ready to inject with a conventional syringe.
F. Chlorphenamine (chlorpheniramine) as traditional ampoule, ready to inject with a conventional syringe.

◆ Why is There No Corticosteroid or Antihistamine in My Dental Emergency Drugs Box, Which is Claimed To Contain the Drugs Recommended for the UK?

The Resuscitation Council UK has published guidance on medical emergencies and resuscitation, revised in May 2008. Its recommendations have been endorsed by the General Dental Council, which states that emergency drugs, listed in Table 3.1, should be available in all dental surgeries in the UK.

The recommended drugs for this case are oxygen and adrenaline/epinephrine, which are required to be kept in every practice. The guidance specifically notes that antihistamines and corticosteroids are not first-line drugs for the treatment of anaphylaxis and that their administration is not expected of dental practitioners in primary care. This is because it is difficult to achieve intravenous access in an individual with reduced circulatory volume and hypotension. Identifying and cannulating a collapsed vein is difficult even for the experienced and is best attempted as soon as adrenaline/epinephrine has taken effect. If competent, the dentist could help later treatment by gaining intravenous access in advance of medical help arriving

TABLE 3.1 Emergency Drugs

Drug	Dose
Glyceryl trinitrate spray	400 micrograms/dose
Salbutamol aerosol inhaler	100 micrograms/puff
Adrenaline/epinephrine injection	1:1000 1 mg/ml
Aspirin dispersible	300 mg
Glucagon injection	1 mg
Oral glucose solution	Gel, tablets or powder
Midazolam	5 mg/ml or 10 mg/ml
Oxygen	

and placing a cannula for later use. This may be made easier by massaging the arm towards the hand to try to inflate the vein.

Maintaining this drug box is a minimum requirement for general practice only. Much more diverse emergency drug boxes are used by those working in hospitals, health clinics and some specialist practices, where dentists may be trained in immediate life support or have other specialist skills through their involvement in conscious sedation or special care dentistry.

The list must also be modified according to circumstances. In remote areas where medical help may not be immediately available, it may be essential to have the additional drugs for longer-term treatment and also for the dentist to be able to gain venous access. These drugs and skills should be within the remit and capabilities of any dental practitioner, with appropriate training.

Dentists must be familiar with the actions and effects of drugs they may need to use, so it is the dentists' responsibility to ensure that they are properly informed about any additional drugs they elect to hold. The General Dental Council also provides guidance that every practice should have available two people trained in medical emergencies whenever such treatment is being carried out. All members of the dental team must practise their skills in simulated emergencies on a regular basis.

Patients with severe allergies may be issued with adrenaline/epinephrine autoinjectors to carry with them at all times, and it is now recommended that they carry two because the dose in one may be insufficient to treat a severe reaction. Patients who carry these devices should be asked to bring them to all dental appointments.

Other Possibilities

◆ If You Discovered That You Had Just Administered a Penicillin Orally To a Patient Known To Be Allergic To Penicillins, What Would You Do?

Absorption of only a very small amount of the penicillin is needed to trigger an allergic response, so there is no point in thinking that inducing vomiting would be helpful. The best thing to do would be to administer chlorphenamine (chlorpheniramine) and steroid immediately if available. As they may well not be, call an ambulance, and prepare the adrenaline/epinephrine injection and oxygen; administer adrenaline/epinephrine immediately if any signs begin to develop. The patient would still have to seek medical care as soon as possible because the late phases of the reaction might still develop even if the immediate phases were prevented.

◆ Suppose the Patient Had Been a Child?

Allergy in children is usually triggered by dietary allergens rather than drugs; however, latex allergy is possible, and children with frequent medical exposure to latex, as in catheters, are at risk. Doses of adrenaline/epinephrine are reduced to 300 micrograms for ages 6–12 years and 150 micrograms for children under 6 years. Giving these doses might prove difficult if you do not have specific paediatric formulations in your emergency drug kit. Autoinjectors provide 300 or 150 micrograms, and Min-I-Jet devices are designed to give a full adult dose. Children with severe allergies may carry autoinjection devices with the correct paediatric dose and should be asked to bring them when they attend for dental treatment.

◆ What Allergens are Important in Dental Surgeries?

Perhaps surprisingly, contact reactions to amalgam and other restorative materials are the most commonly reported, but these are topical, not anaphylactic and not life threatening. The fact that these are now the commonest reported reactions is a result of the systematic exclusion of other more significant allergens from the dental environment over recent decades. Latex causes severe reactions and was previously a significant risk in those sensitized, but natural latex is now completely excluded from gloves, rubber dam and other materials in the UK, although it remains in use elsewhere. Powdered latex gloves are particularly allergenic and cause severe reactions if the powder is inhaled by a sensitized individual. Dental staff members are now more at risk than patients because they regularly handle a range of materials containing acrylates, eugenol and formaldehyde and will have been exposed to latex in the past. In the UK, the most significant risk for a severe anaphylactic reaction probably arises from prescription or administration of a penicillin to a patient allergic to it.

Further Guidance

Anaphylaxis campaign: https://anaphylaxis.org.uk

Use of autoinjectors: https://www.youtube.com/user/AnaphylaxisCampaign

Case 4
Gingival Recession

MANDEEP GHUMAN

Summary

A 30-year-old woman has gingival recession. Assess her condition, and discuss treatment options.

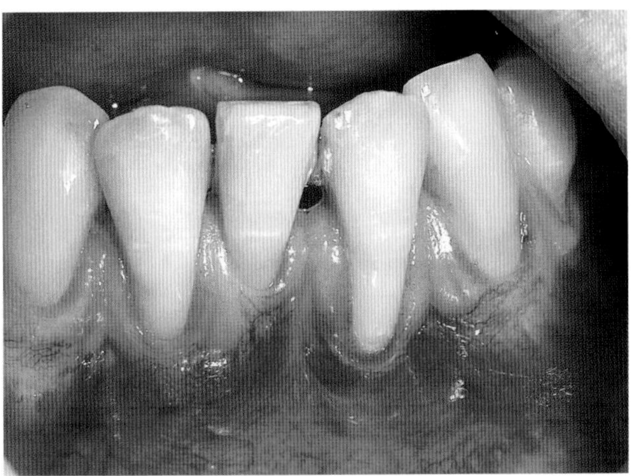

• **Fig. 4.1** The labial view of the lower incisors on presentation.

History

Complaint

The patient is worried about the gingival recession around her lower front teeth, which she feels is worsening.

History of Complaint

She remembers noticing the recession for at least the previous 5 years. She thinks it has worsened over the last 12 months. There has recently been some sensitivity to hot and cold and gingival soreness, most noticeably on toothbrushing or eating ice cream. It is important to document the length of time the patient has been aware of the recession and any period in which it has progressed more rapidly.

Dental History

The person has been a patient of your practice for about 10 years and you have discussed her recession at previous visits and reassured her. She has a low caries rate and generally good oral hygiene. Despite your previous reassurance, it is also important to establish and document why the patient remains concerned. Is she worried about potentially losing the lower teeth, or is the sensitivity the primary concern? Are her concerns related to aesthetics? The latter would be unlikely in this case but certainly could be a factor for upper anterior teeth in individuals with a high smile line and will have implications for management.

Medical History

The patient is a fit and healthy individual and is not a smoker.

◆ What Further Specific Questions Would You Ask To Identify a Possible Cause?

How often does the patient brush her teeth? Some individuals brush excessively in terms of frequency, duration and force used. Trauma from brushing is considered a factor in recession in some patients, and recession may indicate a need to reduce the frequency and duration of cleaning while maintaining its effectiveness. In this instance, the patient has a normal toothbrushing habit, but she should clean no more than twice each day and for a sensible period (2–3 minutes).

Has the patient ever had orthodontic treatment? A lower incisor is missing, suggesting that some intervention may have taken place. Fixed orthodontics in the lower labial segment is associated occasionally with gingival recession in patients with a thin periodontal phenotype – that is, thin buccal gingiva and narrow alveolar processes. There may have been correction of severe crowding previously. Plaque control may be compromised during the wearing of an orthodontic appliance, and even over a relatively short period, this can contribute to the problem. *In this instance, the patient had undergone extraction of the incisor but had not worn an orthodontic appliance.*

Examination

Intraoral Examination

The appearance of the lower incisors is shown in Fig. 4.1. What do you see?

- Missing lower left central incisor
- Unrestored teeth
- No plaque visible except for a small amount at the gingival margin of the lower left lateral incisor
- Gingival recession affecting all lower incisors and, to a lesser extent, the lower canines

- Apart from the abnormal contour, pink and healthy buccal gingivae and normal interdental papillae.
- Reduction in width of keratinized attached gingiva; in places, absent attached gingiva

◆ What Clinical Assessments Would You Make, How Would You Make Them and Why are They Important?

See Table 4.1.

On performing these clinical examinations you find that all probing depths are 1–2 mm, with no bleeding. The width of the keratinized gingiva varies with the degree of recession. The lower left lateral incisor has no attached gingiva, and tension on the lip displaces the gingival margin. No teeth have increased mobility, and no possible occlusal factors are present. There is no reason to suspect loss of vitality, and all teeth respond to testing.

Investigations

◆ What Radiographs are Indicated?

Radiographs would give little additional information. The degree of bone loss on the buccal aspect, including bone dehiscence and fenestrations, is not shown well on radiographs because of superimposition of the roots. Radiographs might help if interdental bone loss is suspected, but intact interdental papillae, together with minimal probing depths, suggest normal interdental bone height. A radiograph would be of value if mobility indicated a need to assess root length and bone height.

Diagnosis

◆ What is Your Diagnosis, and What is the Likely Aetiology?

The patient has gingival recession. In this case, the assessment has not provided a diagnosis any more accurate than that given by the patient, but the features should give some clues to the possible aetiology.

Recession is probably multifactorial in aetiology. The most important factor is probably anatomical variations among patients. Some individuals have very thin gingival tissue buccally, both soft tissue and bone. When the buccal plate of the alveolus is thin, bony dehiscence or fenestrations below the soft tissue are more likely. For these reasons, there is more recession on the teeth that are prominent in the arch and least

TABLE 4.1 Clinical Assessments Carried Out in a Patient with Gingival Recession

Assessment	Method	Importance
Root surface examination	Is the cemento-enamel junction (CEJ) detectable and are there root surface concavities present? Often, the CEJ is not detectable because of cervical tooth wear or caries, or it has been obscured by a cervical restoration.	Needed to establish true degree of recession. Should the care plan include correction of the recession by root coverage surgery, prior reconstruction of the anatomical CEJ (usually with composite resin) is advisable.
Recession	Measure from the gingival margin to the cement–enamel junction.	Provides baseline readings to assess progression.
Probing depths	Perform routine periodontal probing.	Detects associated loss of attachment undermining the reduced width of attached gingiva.
Bleeding on probing	Perform routine recording of bleeding on probing; immediate or delayed.	Indicates the presence of gingival inflammation and poor oral hygiene.
Gingival thickness	Observe whether the probe is visible on insertion in the gingival sulcus of the receded area.	Probe visibility indicates a thinner periodontal phenotype (≤1 mm) and more likelihood of developing recession. The likelihood of completely covering the roots with advanced graft surgery is reduced.
Amount of attached gingiva	Subtract the probing depth recording from the width of keratinized gingiva.	Gives the amount of apparent attached gingiva bound down to bone and, thus, functional. A minimum of 1 mm is desirable but is not necessarily needed if plaque control is optimal.
Presence of functional attached gingiva	Pull gently on the lip or depress the labial sulcus mucosa, placing tension on the attached gingiva or gingival margin.	If the gingival margin is displaced from teeth or is otherwise mobile, there is inadequate functional width of attached gingiva, regardless of its absolute measurement.
Tooth mobility	Try to displace teeth in a bucco-lingual direction using two instrument handles. Fingers are too compressible to do this effectively.	Important if teeth are very mobile, but not a very useful diagnostic or prognostic indicator with small amounts of buccal recession only.
Sensibility testing	Routine methods are electronic pulp tester or hot/cold.	Nonvital teeth are compromised, and this needs to be taken into account in treatment planning.
Occlusion	Perform direct examination of intercuspal position and excursive contacts.	If a traumatic overbite is present, it may cause or exacerbate recession.

on slightly instanding teeth (see the more instanding central incisor in Fig. 4.1). When these predisposing factors are present, other insults become important. The most important is probably traumatic toothbrushing. Plaque-induced marginal inflammation will also destroy the thin tissue at this site relatively quickly. Traumatic occlusion may also contribute.

In this case, the patient is maintaining a very good standard of plaque control, and there is no cervical abrasion, which might be further evidence of toothbrush trauma.

◆ What Advice and Treatment Would You Provide?

- Ensure a sensible, atraumatic but effective brushing regime to remove even the small amount of plaque present, and explain the importance of good oral hygiene in areas of recession. Often, patients will need precise demonstration of how to clean receded areas because the interference of the labial soft tissue limits access to the receded gingival margins. See Table 4.2.
- Reassure the patient that the condition is not necessarily progressive if optimal oral hygiene is established.
- Monitor for progression with the aid of clinical measurements. Clinical photographs and/or study casts are very helpful and should be repeated at intervals.
- Treat the dentine hypersensitivity. Recession alone should not be painful. Ensure that the exposed root surface is suffering neither early caries nor erosion. Check the diet for sugars, acidic drinks and foods. Check the medical history for any possible intrinsic causes. Advise regular use of sensitivity or high fluoride–containing toothpastes. Long-term regular use of these agents show good effectiveness for most patients; if persistent, consider application of topical anti-hypersensitivity agents. However, studies are inconclusive regarding which method is best. Different active agents and modalities are listed below (see Table 4.3).

In this case the patient maintained good plaque control but the recession worsened slowly over a period of several years until there was a lack of functional attached gingiva.

◆ What Other Treatments Might Be Possible? Are They Effective?

Table 4.4 shows alternative treatment options available.

Before carrying out mucogingival surgery, it is important to assess whether patient expectations can be reasonably met. Although free gingival grafts are highly effective, the patient should be made explicitly aware that root coverage is not the intention, whereas increase in keratinized tissue is. The rationale of the proposed mucogingival procedure and potential postoperative symptoms and possible complications need to be clearly communicated and documented. Donor site morbidity for a week or more, especially for free gingival grafts, is not infrequent, and patients should be advised appropriately. If this procedure is carried out in appropriate circumstances, as some studies have shown, these grafts have excellent long-term success rates (25+ years) in patients with good oral hygiene. Occasionally, grafts may need some minor surgical adjustment some months later, depending on how healing proceeds. These studies also show that some treated exposed roots may become partially or fully covered over time after the procedure, a phenomenon termed 'creeping attachment'.

In this case, a free gingival graft was placed, and the result is shown in Fig. 4.2.

Prior to the graft being placed, alternative options, including no treatment, would have been presented to the patient. In this case, because the patient now has good oral

TABLE 4.2 Considerations When Choosing Oral Hygiene Aids for Plaque Control

Oral Hygiene Techniques	Points to Consider
Manual toothbrushing	No worse than powered toothbrushing if done correctly. Areas of current inadequate plaque removal should be addressed by demonstrating an appropriate technique (e.g. Bass) directly in the patient's own mouth such that the patient can subsequently demonstrate correct placement and technique. Toothbrush heads should be compact (not any longer than 2.5 cm), as large ones restrict access. Bristles should be flat and either soft or of medium stiffness. Harder stiffness may exacerbate risk of recession and abrasion.
Powered toothbrushing	Clinical trials show more effective plaque removal than manual toothbrushes; however, differences in effectiveness between different modern types (rotating/oscillating, sonic, vibratory) are negligible. Often used incorrectly, so advice and demonstration should be provided. Most useful for patients with impaired manual dexterity. Additional functions such as timers and pressure sensors are also very useful and can help with compliance. Newer models have smartphone-coupled apps to aid and monitor effectiveness of plaque removal.
Interdental cleaning	Should be done daily, ideally with interdental brushes checked for correct sizes intraorally (normally 2–3 sizes per patient). Floss should be used between teeth where these brushes do not fit.
Mouthwashes	Should only be used as an adjunct to the mechanical plaque removal methods above, and not necessary in themselves in the majority of cases.
Irrigation methods	Evidence of limited effectiveness, and not better than other mechanical methods.

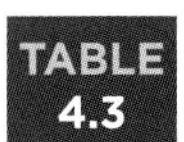

TABLE 4.3 Summary of Evidence for Effectiveness of Self- and Professionally-Applied Desensitising Agents

Agent	Method	Effectiveness
Arginine/calcium carbonate	Toothpaste and prophylaxis paste Mode of action – tubule occlusion reducing fluid flow	More effective than conventional fluoride and potassium toothpaste as immediate and long-term treatment. No good evidence of superiority over other professionally applied agents.
Potassium nitrate/chloride/citrate	Toothpaste, mouthwash and prophylaxis paste Mode of action – raise potassium ion concentration blocking intradental nerve function	Questionable, possibly not effective at all. Less effective than arginine, CSPS, stannous and resin-based formulations.
Amorphous calcium phosphate (ACP) and casein phosphopeptide (CPP)	Prophylaxis paste Mode of action – maintains supersaturated solution of bioavailable calcium and phosphate	Inconclusive. Limited data.
Strontium	Toothpaste Mode of action – tubule occlusion	Strontium acetate salts have similar effectiveness to arginine. Lack of evidence for strontium chloride salts.
Stannous fluoride	Toothpaste Mode of action – tubule occlusion by precipitated calcium fluoride	High-quality evidence showing effectiveness, above that of arginine.
Calcium sodium phosphosilicate (CSPS)	Toothpaste and prophylaxis paste Mode of action – tubule occlusion with bioactive glass	Low-quality evidence suggesting effectiveness as toothpaste, but not when professionally applied.
Oxalates	Mouthwash, prophylaxis paste Mode of action – tubule occlusion by precipitated calcium oxalate	Limited evidence.
Resins	Professionally applied Mode of action – tubule occlusion by hybrid layer formation via HEMA (2-hydroxyethyl methacrylate) Some contain glutaraldehyde causing intratubular protein coagulation	Evidence of effectiveness, but insufficient to recommend other professionally applied treatments
Varnishes	Professionally applied Mode of action – tubule occlusion	Fluoride varnishes have limited or no effectiveness. Other types show some effectiveness but not better than other methods.
Lasers	Professionally applied Mode(s) of action – coagulation of proteins in dentinal fluid reducing permeability, tubule melting	Weak evidence, and strong placebo effect.

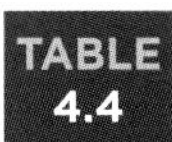

TABLE 4.4 Alternative Treatment Options

Treatment	Effectiveness
Mucogingival surgery to correct the recession, using either coronally advanced or tunnel flaps. A lateral pedicle graft or a double papilla flap are also options. These may be used in conjunction with an interpositional (subepithelial) connective tissue graft in thin periodontal biotypes. These are essentially aesthetic procedures.	May be effective in carefully selected cases. The presence of adjacent interdental papillae and suitable donor sites is essential. Total root coverage is difficult to achieve and unpredictable, especially in the long term.
Mucogingival surgery to provide a wider and functional zone of attached gingiva. This therapeutic procedure provides a zone of thicker tissue that is more resistant to further recession and less prone to soreness with normal brushing. A free gingival graft is the treatment of choice.	Highly effective. Grafting palatal mucosa into the alveolar mucosa prevents the lip pulling the gingiva from the teeth. Even if the gingival margin has little attached gingiva, it can remain healthy if protected from displacement or other trauma.
Provision of a thin acrylic gingival stent or veneer.	Can provide an excellent cosmetic result if well made, but only considered for extensive recession in highly visible areas. The usual indication is to improve the appearance of the upper anterior region following treatment of advanced periodontitis resulting in the loss of papillae

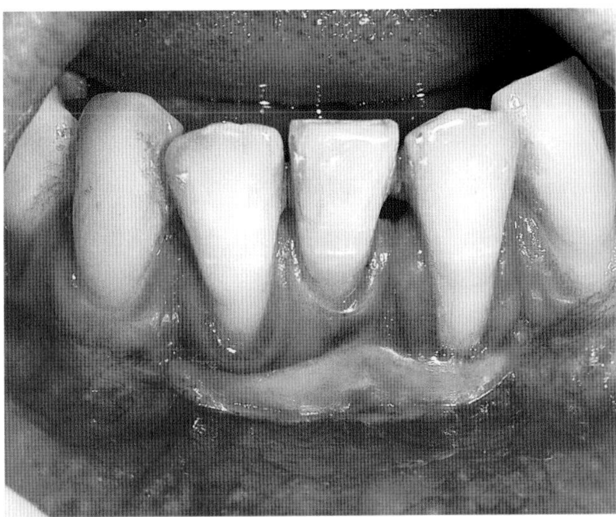

• **Fig. 4.2** Appearance of the free gingival graft 6 months after placement.

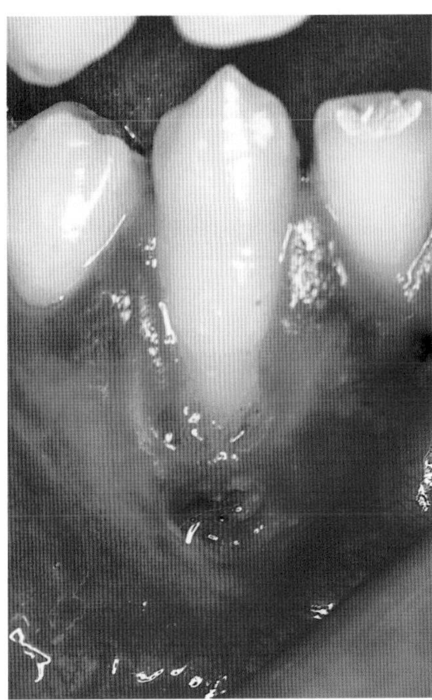

• **Fig. 4.3** A different case with localized labial recession affecting the LR3.

hygiene in the affected region, the recession is unlikely to proceed significantly and could be monitored, so graft placement is a viable long-term option. Should the patient wish to proceed with the procedure, the potential benefits (increased comfort and ease of cleaning the area) and risks (normal postoperative complications, as well as rare ones, such as failure of the graft to take because of infection and numbness of donor site) should also be explained and documented. This should be done in both verbal and written formats some time in advance of the treatment so that the patient has sufficient time to think the options over.

◆ What Do You See; is the Graft Successful?

Yes, the graft appears successful. Palatal connective tissue and overlying epithelium have been placed apical to the lower incisor gingival margin to provide a wider zone of attached keratinized gingiva. Because the palatal connective tissue is transferred, the epithelium retains its keratinized palate structure.

◆ Does the Graft Need To Lie At the Gingival Margin?

No. The graft forms the gingival margin on the lower left lateral incisor, but elsewhere, it lies below the margin. Provided the graft is firmly bound down to the underlying tissue, it will stabilize the gingival margin against displacement on lip movement.

◆ Why Not Place the Graft Over the Root As Well and Correct the Recession?

As noted in Table 4.2, surgical correction of the recession itself is difficult to achieve and the results unpredictable, especially in the long term. The root surface does not provide a nutrient bed on which the free graft can survive. Grafts in this situation would have to be pedicled to ensure their nutrient supply and also need to be placed such that they receive some nutrients from an adjacent exposed connective tissue bed. A more predictable result may be obtained by using an interpositional (subepithelial) connective tissue graft and would be required in cases with thin periodontal biotypes. A free graft is most unlikely to be successful if simply placed over the root surface.

◆ Fig. 4.3 Shows a Different Patient with Recession. What Does the Appearance Tell You?

There is approximately 4 mm of recession buccally on the lower right canine. Apical to the gingival margin there is a hole in the gingival tissue. Plaque and subgingival calculus (formed within a periodontal pocket) are visible, and the tissue is inflamed. The small 'bridge' of tissue at the gingival margin is not attached to the tooth surface and will eventually break down. In this case, the recession is secondary to pocket formation in a plaque-induced periodontitis. Inflammation associated with subgingival calculus has caused loss of much of the buccal bone.

◆ How Would Care of this Patient's Recession Differ?

It would differ only in the early stages. Inflammation must be treated by oral hygiene improvement and subgingival debridement. If, after a period to allow healing, there is resolution of inflammation, the situation is very similar to that in the first case, and assessment and treatment would be identical. There would be no value in attempting to surgically correct the fenestration in the attached gingiva. As discussed above, grafting onto the root surface is technically complex, and success is unpredictable.

Further Reading

Cortellini, P., & Bissada, N. F. (2018 Jun). Mucogingival conditions in the natural dentition: Narrative review, case definitions, and diagnostic considerations. *Journal of Clinical Periodontology, 45*(Suppl. 20), S190–S198.

Case 5

Multiple Missing Anterior Teeth and a Class III Incisor Relationship

DIRK BISTER

Summary

This 12-year-old female patient attends your practice for the first time with missing upper lateral and lower central permanent incisors. The incisor relationship is class III.

History

Presenting Complaint

The patient complains about a 'gappy' appearance of the upper front teeth and mobile lower front teeth and that her bite seems to be the 'the wrong way round'.

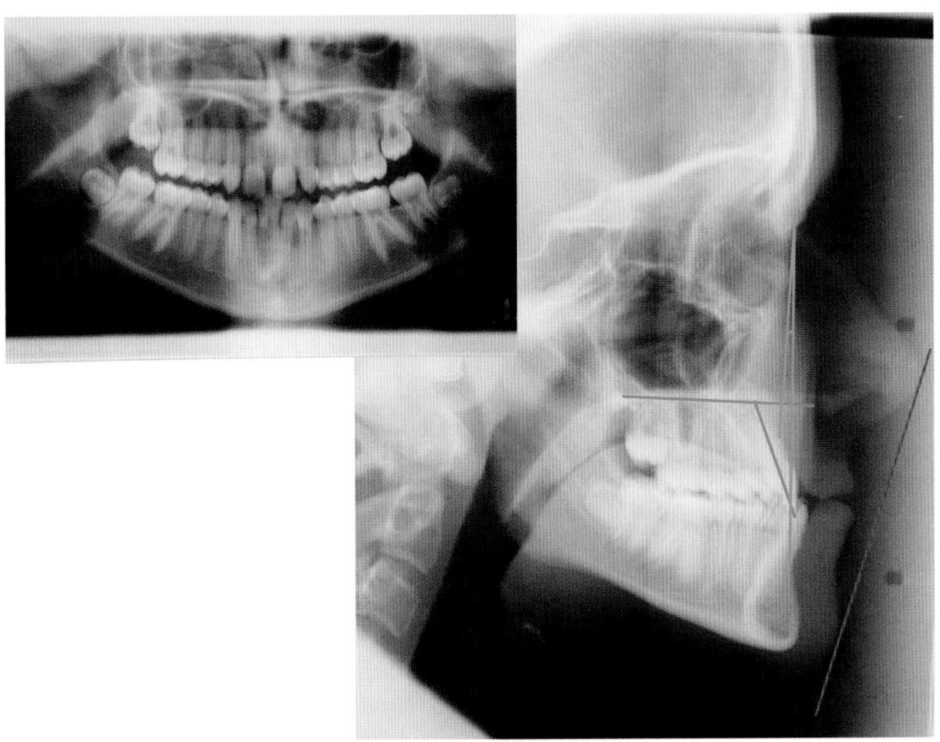

• **Fig. 5.1** Dental panoramic tomogram (DPT) and lateral cephalometric view. The extraoral features of this patient are not consistent with the intraoral malocclusion. One would expect a protruding chin and/or retrusive maxilla in a patient with a significant class III malocclusion. The upper and lower incisors are of normal inclination (108 degrees, green lines). The ANB difference (difference between upper and lower jaw in the horizontal plane, blue lines) is less than 4 degrees; this suggest that the malocclusion can be treated by orthodontics; jaw surgery is not required. Red line is the Aesthetic line (E-line). The DPT shows the presence of all wisdom teeth.

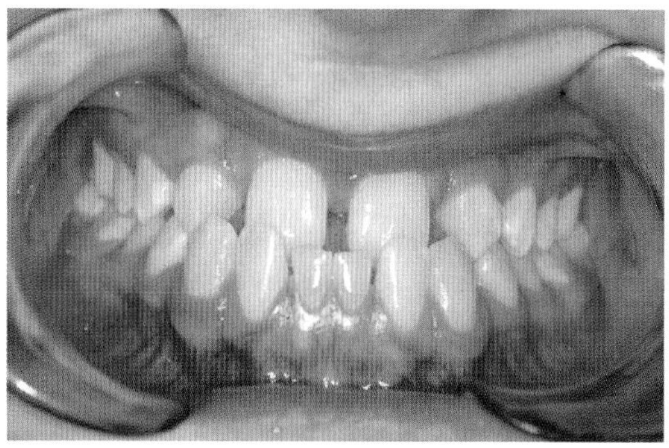

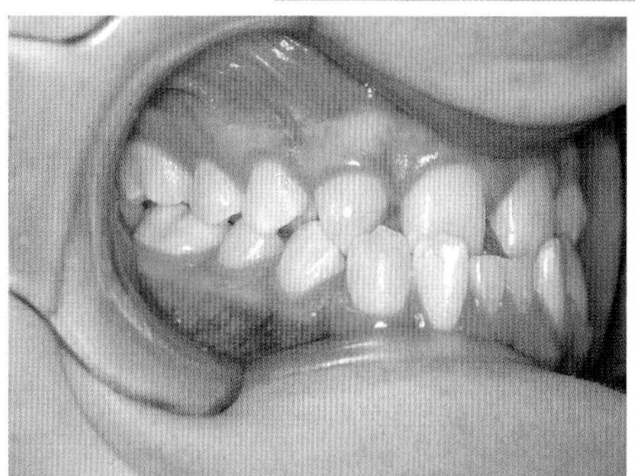

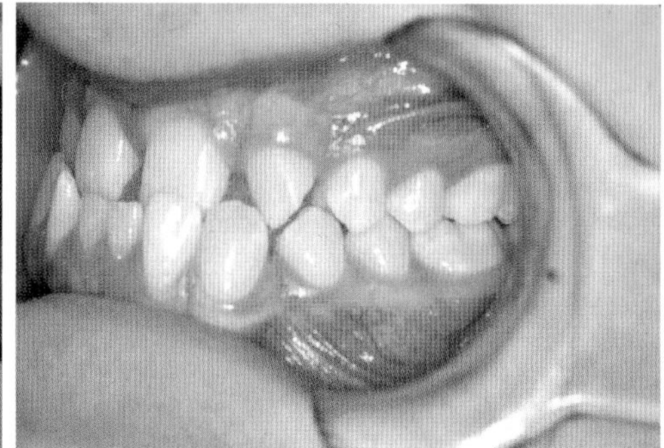

• **Fig. 5.2** Intraoral images of this patient, anterior and lateral occlusal views.

Social History

There is a history of bullying at school because of her dental appearance.

Medical History

The patient is medically fit and well.

Examination

Extraoral Examination

On examination, the facial profile is essentially class I; the extraoral facial features of this patient are balanced; the chin does not protrude, and the maxilla does not appear retroclined clinically. A straightforward way to assess this is by drawing a tangent between the tip of the nose and chin. The vermillion borders of upper and lower lips should lie close to this line (E-line) (Fig. 5.1). There are some signs of ectodermal dysplasia such as thin lips, sparse hair and fair skin.

Intraoral Examination

There is a class III incisor relationship with a reverse overjet.

Teeth present:

76543 1	1 34567
765432A	A234567

Both maxillary permanent lateral incisors as well as both mandibular central incisors are absent clinically. Both lower deciduous central incisors are present and grade 2 mobile. There is an upper midline diastema and rotated upper canines (Fig. 5.2). It is important to assess if there is mandibular shift forwards on final closure; this is known as *displacement*. Clinically, the patient should be asked into go to maximum returned mandibular position: This can be done by asking the patient to roll the tongue to the back of the throat and close the mouth slowly. Manual manipulation can also be tried. Displacement is diagnosed if the incisors meet on closure and the patient has to protrude her mandible to achieve maximum intercuspation. Hallmarks for displacement are signs of attrition on the front teeth. In this patient, there were no signs of displacement.

In summary, the extraoral features (class I) and intraoral features (class III) do not match. Cephalometric analysis will be useful to assess the severity of the class III skeletal base.

◆ What are the Causes for Absent Lateral and Lower Central Incisors and the Class III Incisor Relationship? What Specific Questions Would You Ask the Patient/Parents?

Questions Regarding the Missing Teeth. It may be useful to ask if any teeth were missing in the deciduous dentition. This is unusual but not entirely implausible. It is extremely unlikely that permanent teeth are present if their deciduous predecessors were absent. Permanent teeth may be absent, however, when deciduous teeth are present, as shown in this case for the lower central incisors.

Hypodontia in the permanent dentition is quite common, the prevalence ranges between 0.15% and 16% of the population. It often runs in families, and the family history may reveal this. There are over 300 genes that are related to nonsyndromic hypodontia but *AXIN2*, *MSX1*, *PAX9* and *EDA* are the ones most commonly mentioned in the literature.

Regarding the missing upper lateral incisors, trauma should be excluded.

Questions Regarding the Class III Incisor Relationship. A class III incisor relationship can have a variety of causes, namely, unusual eruption path of the permanent teeth, missing teeth, poor growth of the maxilla and/or excessive growth of the mandible. Class III malocclusion may also run in families and are more common in the Far Eastern populations. The prevalence in Northern Europe is about 3% and is about 13% in the Far East. A positive family history needs careful evaluation and consent by the patient for further unfavourable growth, potentially requiring additional orthodontic or even surgical treatment at a later stage.

Investigations

Radiographs required for orthodontic purposes are a dental panoramic tomogram (DPT) and a lateral cephalometric view (see Fig. 5.1).

The radiographs show the developmental absence of both upper lateral incisors and both lower central incisors.

Diagnosis

The final diagnosis is a class III malocclusion on a class mild III skeletal base, with four missing permanent teeth: upper lateral and lower central incisors.

In the UK, the Index of Orthodontic Treatment Need (IOTN) is used to assess eligibility for treatment free of charge at the point of delivery (https://www.nhs.uk/conditions/Orthodontics/).

The IOTN for this patient was 4 g. More detailed information on IOTN can be found at: https://www.bos.org.uk/Public-Patients/Orthodontics-for-Children-Teens/Fact-File-FAQ/What-Is-The-IOTN.

Care Planning/Treatment

Care planning requires interdisciplinary input with close collaboration between the specialist orthodontist and the general dental practitioner or specialist prosthodontist/restorative dentist.

◆ What Other Diagnostic Tools Can Be Employed To Help Plan the Treatment for This Patient?

The following factors need to be considered before treatment commences:

1. Can the class III incisor relationship be treated by orthodontic camouflage, or will this malocclusion need a surgical (comprehensive) approach?
2. Will the spaces for the missing teeth be closed or opened for prosthodontic replacement of the missing teeth?
3. What kind of prosthodontic replacement will be in the patient's best interests?
4. What will the retention regime be, particularly with a long-term view of the prosthodontic replacement of the missing teeth?

The above radiographs (see Fig. 5.1) can be used to decide question 1:

- The upper incisors are not proclined before start of treatment and the skeletal base is not excessively class III. An ANB difference on the lateral cephalometric radiograph of more than −4 degrees would be considered severe, most likely requiring jaw surgery for comprehensive correction. There is vertical overlap of the incisors, indicating a good prognosis for the orthodontic correction of the incisor relationship. Therefore, orthodontic camouflage can be attempted. There is a small but acceptable risk of unfavourable skeletal growth, which the patient needs to consent to.

To decide question 2, the following issues have to be considered:

- Closing spaces for the missing teeth has the obvious advantage that no prosthodontic replacement will be necessary for replacement in the long term. Modification of the shape and size of the upper canines using resin composite additions needs to be considered because better resemble lateral incisors.
- However, from an orthodontic point of view, biomechanical considerations speak against complete space closure. Space closure mechanics are likely to retrocline the incisors in both the upper and lower arches. This may have undesirable aesthetic consequences. In addition to that, in the lower arch, significant tipping of incisors lingually is associated with the risk of gingival recession. It is also unlikely that a class I incisor relationship can be achieved by retroclining the upper and lower labial segments. In orthodontics, a class III malocclusion can be camouflaged with three lower incisors, and this scenario might work well for the patient. Opening space for the missing upper lateral incisors makes sense because it will lead to proclination of the upper front teeth, thereby achieving a positive overjet and overbite.

Further Diagnostic Tools

A diagnostic set-up can be made to assess whether tooth movement can achieve a satisfactory occlusal outcome (Fig. 5.3).

In this case, the diagnostic set-up should be made in such a way that the position of the posterior dentition is not changed. This reflects the orthodontic anchorage balance; during fixed appliance therapy, the posterior dentition is unlikely to move significantly (the front teeth provide little anchorage and the back teeth provide significant anchorage).

The diagnostic set-up can also be used to answer question 3.

The set-up provided in Fig. 5.3 shows that two upper lateral incisors and one lower central incisor provide a satisfactory occlusal outcome, with a positive overjet and a positive overbite achieved. In other words, the two missing lower incisors will be replaced by one.

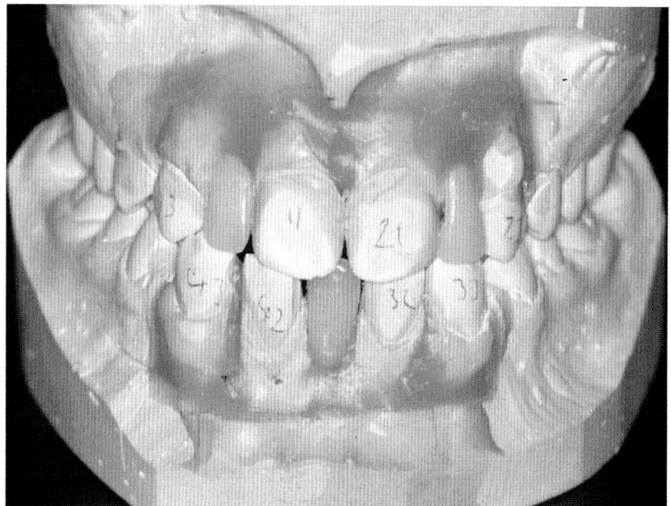

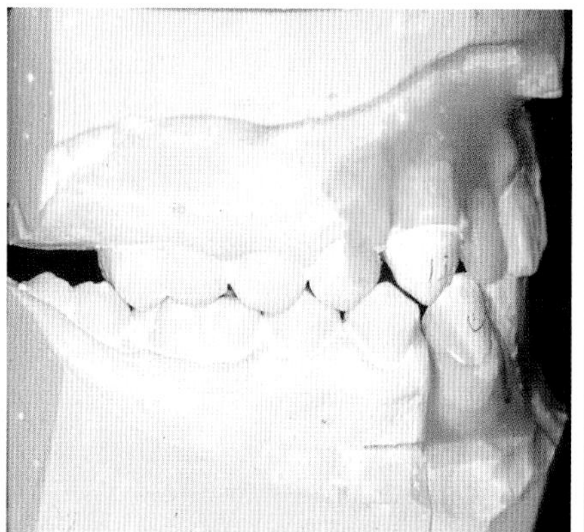

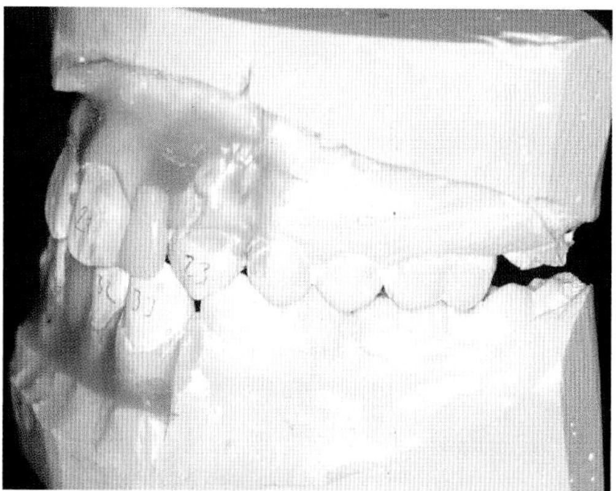

• **Fig. 5.3** Photographs of the diagnostic set-up. Please note that the posterior teeth were not moved; this allows better orthodontic anchorage assessment. The set-up shows that space requirements insufficient for replacing the lateral incisors with implant based restorations. Prosthodontic replacement of the missing teeth with a resin-bonded bridge should be sought. The set-up also demonstrates that space reduction for the two missing lower incisors to one lower incisor will give a satisfactory occlusal outcome.

It also shows that there will be no space for implants to replace the missing upper lateral incisors and the lower incisor. Resin-bonded minimal preparation bridges are the best option for replacing the missing teeth for this patient.

Dental implants, which can be an alternative to resin-bonded bridges, require a minimum amount of bone to be placed successfully. Currently, the smallest commercially available implants are about 3 mm wide. Additional space is needed for gingival margin, and this adds another 1 mm of space or more on either side of the implant at the gingival level. However, narrow implants may not be suitable for all situations, and more space will be required at crown level.

The considerations for question 4 are complex and require input from the general dental practitioner (GDP)/prosthodontist particularly for long-term planning.

The malocclusion was originally also characterized by an upper midline diastema and rotated upper canines. Orthodontic space closure of an upper midline diastema is usually easy to achieve but very difficult to maintain over the long term. Fixed retainers are recommended after space closure of diastemas to avoid relapse.

Resin-bonded bridges replacing upper lateral incisors often use the canines as abutment teeth. The advantage is that the upper canines are darker in appearance compared with the central incisors and are hence not as susceptible to further darkening by palatally bonded attachments of the cantilever abutment.

In this case, it was decided to provide a resin-bonded bridge attached to the central incisors and not the canines. Both upper permanent canines were rotated at the beginning of the orthodontic treatment, and this also is prone to relapse. Fig. 5.4 shows a situation in a different case, where the canine position relapsed and subsequently led to poor alignment of the lateral incisor replacements.

During orthodontics, prosthodontic teeth can be added to the appliance to improve aesthetics (Fig. 5.5). Initial retention was by provided by Hawley retainers. It is important to note that the retainers had 'stops' added adjacent to the replaced teeth. This reduced the chances of relapse if the replacement teeth were to fail. The labial bow was acrylated, and this design was chosen to stop the anterior teeth from rotating and to support the prosthodontic teeth (Fig. 5.6).

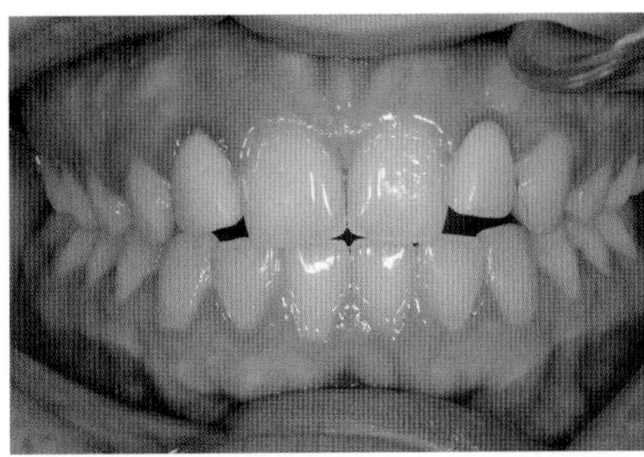
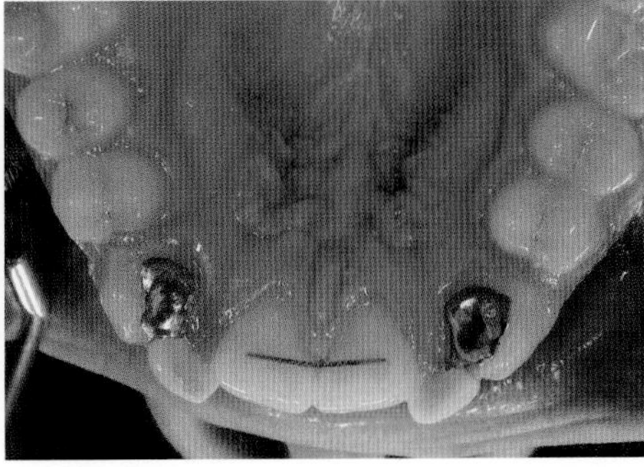

• **Fig. 5.4** This shows a different patient where both canines rotated after orthodontic treatment; the resin-bonded bridges were attached to the canines. The upper midline diastema had been prevented from relapsing by a fixed retainer.

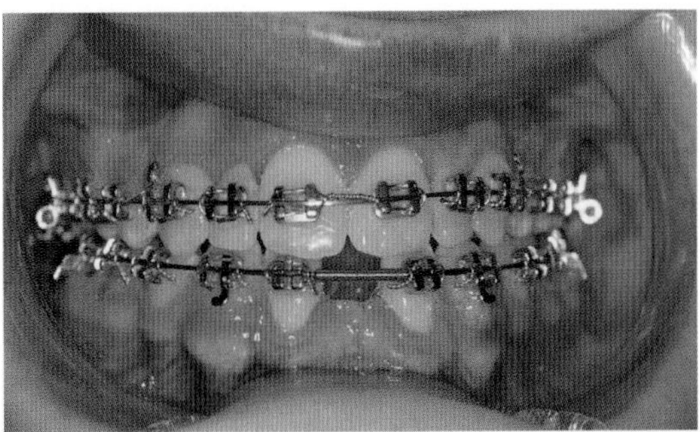
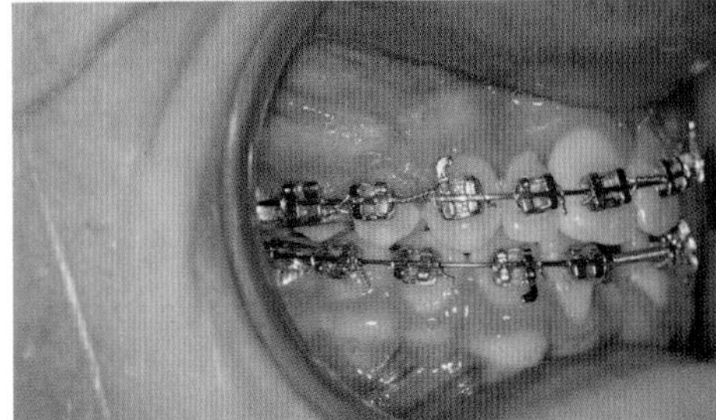
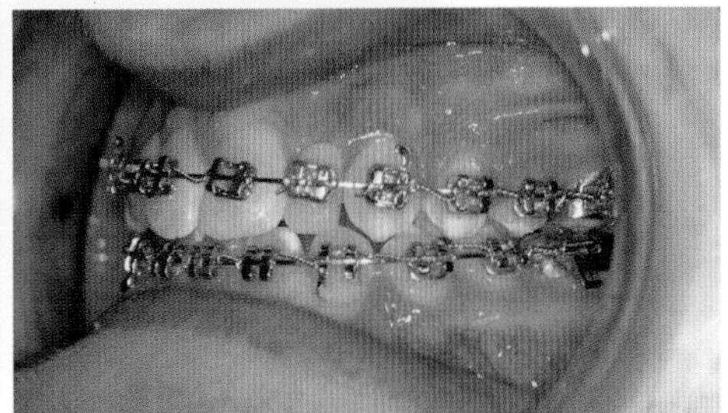

• **Fig. 5.5** Intraoral photographs of the patient during orthodontic treatment. Both upper missing lateral incisors were replaced with prosthodontic teeth that were attached to the fixed appliances; this improves aesthetics during orthodontic treatment.

It is important to provide a new retainer immediately after completion of the restorative treatment (Fig. 5.7). The resin-bonded bridges alone may not be sufficient to prevent unplanned tooth movement, particularly if the restorative work was to fail in the medium to long term.

Consent

Obtaining valid consent is one of the nine principles registered dental professionals must keep to at all times (https://standards.gdc-uk.org/pages/principle3/principle3.aspx).

The patient and her parents/guardian need to be consented by the different teams involved.

This is done in multiple stages. It is paramount to inform the patient that the two treatment phases are likely to take a comparatively long time to complete.

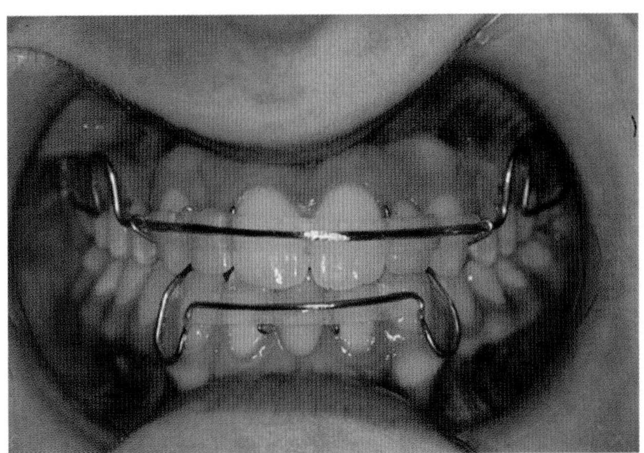

• **Fig. 5.6** Upper and lower Hawley retainers were fitted on the day of debonding the fixed appliances. The retainers contain 'stops' mesial and distal to the missing teeth to avoid tooth movement if the prosthodontic teeth were to fail.

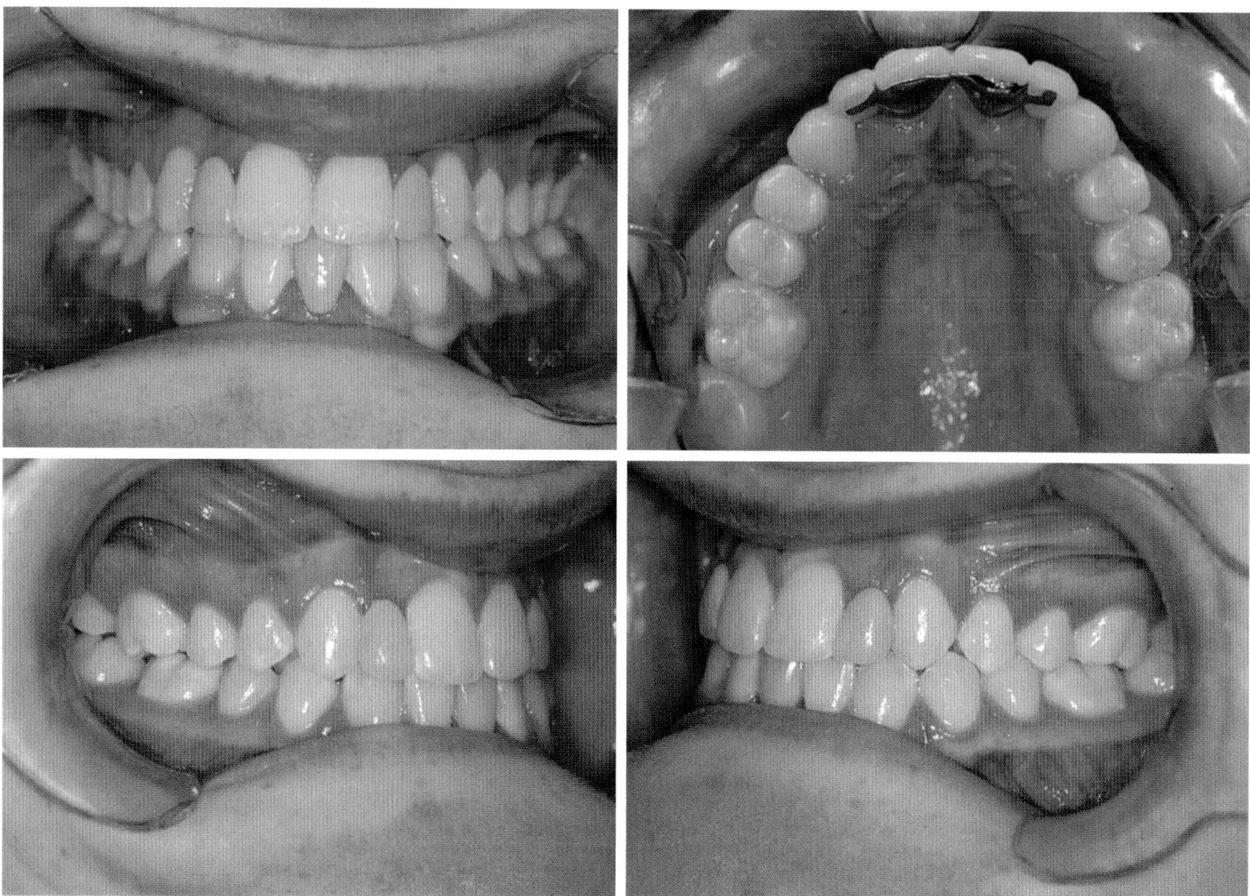

• **Fig. 5.7** Treatment outcome immediately after orthodontic treatment and placement of the resin-bonded bridge. Please note that the upper resin bonded bridge consisted of four units to avoid opening of the upper midline diastema. A removable retainer was also provided in addition to the prosthodontic retention.

Orthodontic Consent

Consent in orthodontics is ideally a two-stage process:

At the first stage, the patient and their parents/legal guardian are handed the relevant written information (often at the stage of orthodontic records: impressions/scan, clinical photographs and radiographs).

Information leaflets for orthodontic treatment are available through the British Orthodontic Society at: https://www.bos.org.uk/Public-Patients/Patient-Information-Leaflets.

On return, the patient and parent/legal guardian sign the consent form. It is important to note that consent is an ongoing process and that changes in the treatment plan that may become necessary need to be documented.

In this particular patient, further unfavourable growth as well as unwanted tooth movement after completion of interceptive treatment should be explicitly mentioned.

It is important to emphasize that retention should ideally continue even after the prosthodontic replacement of the teeth has been undertaken. It should be made clear that aftercare is a shared responsibility of the orthodontist and the dentist. The patient's responsibility in aftercare/maintenance compliance should be clearly discussed and noted.

Under current National Health Services (NHS) England commissioning guidelines, 1 year of retention is provided. Subsequent costs will have to be borne out with NHS agreements. Patients need to be made aware of this and any other such longer-term costs.

However, the patient needs to be informed that it is the responsibility of the dentist, not the orthodontist, to maintain the resin-bonded bridges.

Prosthodontic Consent

This needs to be undertaken separately by the GDP/prosthodontist/restorative dentist. It must be made clear that this is a separate process. Issues such as survival rate and long-term maintenance and costs arising from those issues need to be well documented.

Potential Legal Issues and Pitfalls

Unfavourable growth can be an issue, but a negative family history and a mild class III skeletal base with good vertical overlap will reduce this risk. Consent should be clear about the length of treatment time, as well as the commitments for maintenance and the costs thereof.

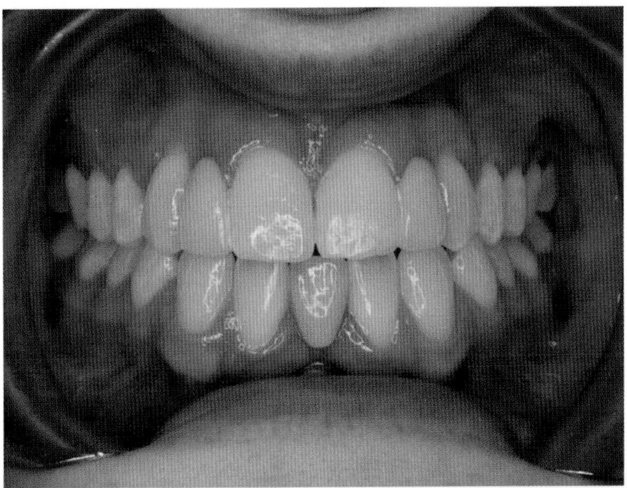

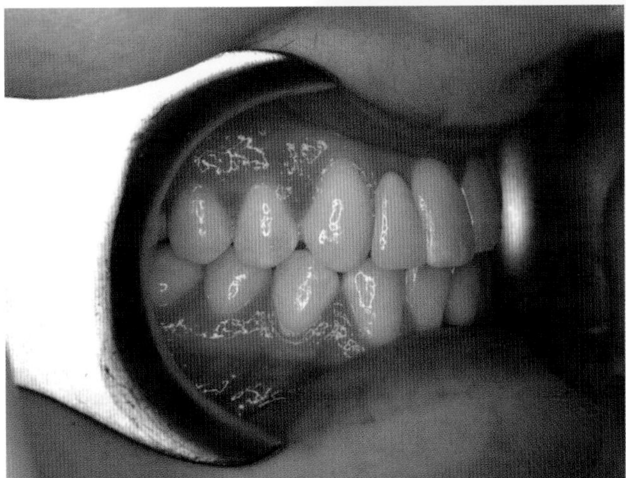

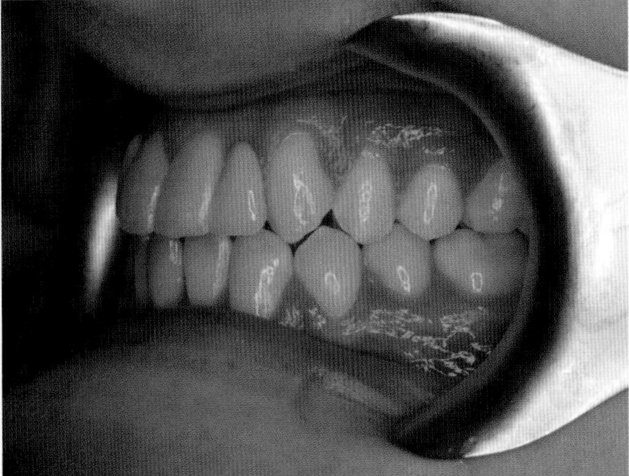

• **Fig. 5.8** Treatment outcome 15 years after debonding. The upper resin-bonded bridges had been replaced to improve aesthetics in the upper jaw. Both upper canines have relapsed and rotated mesio-palatally similar to the original occlusion. Cantilevering the lateral incisors off the canines would have led to compromised aesthetics of the upper labial segment.

Long-Term Outcome

See Fig. 5.8 for the long-term outcome 15 years after debonding. The patient had been provided with a second set of resin-bonded bridges. The upper canines had moved significantly since completion of treatment, but because of the attachment of the cantilevers to the central incisors, this had not resulted in compromised aesthetics. The overjet and the overbite had reduced slightly but remained positive; there was little inadvertent growth. The patient had stopped wearing removable retainers at that stage.

Summary

The case presented was a reasonably complex malocclusion with multiple missing teeth that was resolved by collaboration, input by specialist orthodontist and restorative care. Care planning of cases such as the one presented is often a challenge, and good patient communication is key.

Case 6
An Unsettled Patient

YVONNE M. ROONEY

Summary

A 70-year-old man attends your dental practice for a routine dental check-up accompanied by his wife (Fig. 6.1). He appears confused about why he is here; he had failed to attend his last three appointments.

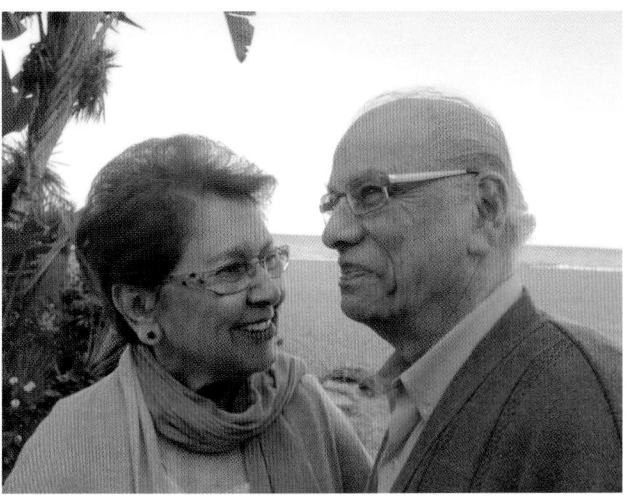

• **Fig. 6.1** The patient and his wife.

History

Complaint

The patient has no dental complaints, but his wife tells you that he has a painful tooth on the top left.

History of Complaint

The patient tells you that he has not had toothache for several months, but his wife interjects to say that the patient complains of toothache every time he eats and is only able to eat on the right side of his mouth.

Medical History

The patient was diagnosed last year with early-stage Alzheimer's disease, for which he is taking donepezil.

Dental History

The patient and his wife have been regular attenders at your practice for the past 20 years. You review his dental records and realize he was due to return for endodontic treatment of the upper left first premolar 1 year ago.

Examination

There is a heavily restored dentition with multiple crowns. The upper left first premolar has unrestorable caries and is tender to percussion. There is generalized periodontitis with moderate attachment loss.

You decide to take a periapical radiograph of the upper left first premolar. As you place the film in the patient's mouth, he becomes restless and agitated. His wife tells you that he has been increasingly irritable in recent months and attributes this to his Alzheimer's disease.

◆ What is Alzheimer's Disease?

Alzheimer's disease is the most common reason for dementia, and its cause is dysfunctional synapses and death of neurones in the cerebral cortex. Its aetiology is protein deposition in the neurofibrillary tangles in the neurone cytoplasm and amyloid plaques between the cells. The key symptom is the inability to remember new information.

◆ How is Dementia Different From Alzheimer's Disease?

Dementia is more broadly defined as a clinical syndrome of progressive neurodegenerative changes characterized by deterioration in memory, learning ability, visuospatial orientation, language, comprehension and judgement.

Dementia affects one in every 14 people over age 65 years, with up to 10% of cases estimated to start at an earlier age. It is estimated that 850 000 people in the UK have dementia, two-thirds of whom are female. Worldwide, it is estimated that 47 million people are living with dementia, with projections that this will almost triple by 2050. Common forms of dementia and their relative prevalence rates are listed in Table 6.1.

◆ What are the Signs and Symptoms of Dementia?

Individual signs and symptoms vary among individuals. Progressive brain damage leads to social and occupational impairments, movement problems and difficulties performing daily activities. There is an increasing dependence on family or formal carers. Behavioural and psychological symptoms affect 90% of patients with dementia at some

TABLE 6.1 Common Forms of Dementia and Their Relative Prevalence Rates

Form of Dementia	Relative Prevalence Rate
Alzheimer's disease	62%
Vascular dementia	17%
Mixed dementia	10%
Dementia with Lewy bodies	4%
Fronto-temporal dementia	2%
Parkinson's dementia	2%
Other	3%

stage of their condition and include agitation, aggression, psychosis, depression and apathy.

◆ What are the Stages of Dementia?

Dementia staging is based on its impact on the person's daily living activities and detailed in Table 6.2. Patients progress through these stages at an unpredictable rate and with differing signs and symptoms.

◆ How is Dementia Typically Managed?

Management of dementia mostly relates to control of symptoms and access to supportive services.

Acetylcholinesterase inhibitors (e.g. donepezil, rivastigmine) are recommended for management of mild to moderate Alzheimer's disease under certain conditions, but many patients are not taking any medications for dementia.

TABLE 6.2 Stages of Dementia

Stage	Clinical Characteristics
No dementia	Occasional forgetfulness.
Mild cognitive impairment	Forgetful of key information normally easily recalled (e.g. dental appointment), or difficulty timing or sequencing a complex task.
Early-stage dementia (mild)	Forgetful of familiar words or unable to recall the right word, problems remembering names, losing or misplacing valuables (e.g. dentures), difficulty with tasks at work. Family or friends start to notice difficulties. Remains independent in daily activities.
Middle-stage dementia (moderate)	Forgetful of own history (e.g. address), frustration at being unable to remember how to do daily tasks (e.g. oral care), change of day–night sleeping patterns, changes in personality and behaviour (e.g. suspiciousness, hallucinations, repetitive habits). Often, this is the longest stage.
Late-stage dementia (severe)	Loss of awareness of surroundings and time, reduced physical abilities (including walking), problems eating and swallowing, weight loss and frailty, difficulty communicating with loss of speech, fully dependent on care, vulnerable to infections (e.g. pneumonia).

◆ Are There Any Medical Conditions Associated with Dementia?

Conditions thought to be linked to the development of dementia include Down's syndrome, Parkinson's disease, type II diabetes mellitus and depression.

You decide to continue your attempt to take a periapical radiograph, but the patient is still agitated.

◆ How Can You Change Your Approach To Increase the Chances of Success?

- Ensure the patient can see your face clearly when you speak.
- Speaking in a calm and clear manner, explain what you are going to do and why a radiograph is necessary.
- Where possible, involve the patient's wife in providing emotional support.

You manage to take the radiograph, and after evaluating it, you decide that removal of the upper left first premolar is necessary. You discuss your plan to extract the tooth, but the patient's wife is concerned that this tooth will be noticeably missing whenever he smiles.

◆ How Would You Respond?

Acknowledge the concerns, and discuss the options for the gap. However, discussions with the patient and his wife should be honest about the future impact of dementia on oral health. The patient will gradually become less able to:

- Understand, identify and communicate the symptoms of dental pain
- Tolerate complex dental treatment and prostheses
- Perform effective oral hygiene
- Provide informed consent.

You check the patient's natural smiling position and state that this will not have a significant impact on his appearance. The patient and his wife are happy to proceed.

◆ How Will You Determine Whether the Patient Can Consent To This Treatment?

Assessing capacity to consent is a two-stage process, as outlined in the Mental Capacity Act 2005 (MCA). The MCA provides a statutory framework to empower and protect vulnerable people in England and Wales who are not able to make their own decisions about treatment. In Scotland, the equivalent legislation is the Adults with Incapacity (Scotland) Act 2000. Common law applies in Northern Ireland. These acts contain guidelines for carers and professionals on making decisions on behalf of people who lack capacity. The Act states that capacity must be assessed at each visit. All decisions should be in the patient's best interests,

TABLE 6.3 Assessment of the Capacity to Consent*

Stage 1	Does the person have an impairment of or disturbance in the functioning of the mind or brain?	Yes, he in the early stages of dementia.
	Is it temporary or permanent?	Permanent.
	Can the decision be delayed?	No, the patient has dental pain. He is at risk of developing an acute infection.
	Does that impairment or disturbance mean that the person is unable to make the decision at the time it needs to be made?	No, he has been able to retain the information for the duration of the appointment
Stage 2	Can the patient understand the information?	Yes, he understands the proposed treatment and has discussed options for the space after tooth extraction.
	Can the patient retain the information?	Yes, he can retain the information, repeat it back and use the information to make a decision.
	Can the patient use the information?	Yes, we have discussed treatment options together.
	Can the patient communicate the decision?	Yes.
	On the balance of probabilities, does the person lack the capacity to make this particular decision at this point in time?	No.

*The patient retains capacity to consent.

and the least restrictive treatment option should be chosen. Table 6.3 describes how you can assess this patient's capacity to consent.

The capacity of patients with dementia tends to fluctuate. There may be better times of the day or days of the week to organize their dental appointment. Compliance does not always decline rapidly with dementia progression. Some people with dementia, who attended the dentist regularly, appear to remember and cope with the normal routine of a dental visit. In the middle to late stages of dementia, patients gradually lose the ability to consent to dental treatment.

You decide that on this occasion, the patient has the capacity to consent. You make an appointment for the removal of the tooth within the following week. At the next appointment, the patient attends with his daughter who has his Lasting Power of Attorney.

◆ What is a Lasting Power of Attorney?

In the UK, a Lasting Power of Attorney is a legal document that gives another person authority to make decisions on a patients' behalf when they lose mental capacity or if they no longer want to make decisions for themselves. There are two different types – one for financial decisions and one for health and social care decisions.

The patient attends for his treatment with his daughter. She asks if she can play classical music from her phone because it helps him to feel more relaxed.

◆ What Other Strategies Might You Also Consider Helpful?

- Communication and reassurance using the approach given above
- Having a relative nearby for emotional support and hand-holding
- Giving the patient something to hold for sensory stimulation, such as a 'sensory/fiddle cushion' or stress ball
- Short appointments – but do not inadvertently put yourself under time pressure
- Remember that it is not what you say but how you make patients feel that affects how they respond

You manage to carry out removal of the upper left first premolar uneventfully, and both the patient and his daughter are pleased.

◆ What are the Important Dental Considerations for Patients with Dementia?

The best time to achieve a stable and healthy mouth is during the early stage of dementia by instituting a preventive regimen, which should include the following:

- Consider verbal reminders about toothbrushing from his wife or a laminated oral health plan on the bathroom wall if forgetfulness is a problem.
- Consider an electric toothbrush or handle adaptation if the patient is unable to perform adequate oral hygiene.
- Consider at what point it would be useful to demonstrate assisted toothbrushing techniques that allow a carer to help.
- Assess caries risk and consider prescription of sodium fluoride 1.1% (5000 parts per million [ppm]) toothpaste to be used twice daily and fluoride varnish applications every 6 months
- Advise limiting sugary foods and drinks to mealtimes. Provide a list of safe snacks.
- Encourage water between meals, and educate on hidden and natural sugars. Dehydration can worsen the symptoms of dementia.

- Stress the importance of living well with dementia and of maintenance of good oral health.

◆ What Additional Measures May Be Necessary in Later Stages?

Depending on their ability to perform activities of daily living, some patients with dementia may not be able to be supported to live in their own home. They may move to residential care or a nursing home. In cases where it is too disruptive for patients to leave their normal environment, domiciliary dental care may be provided. For patients in late-stage dementia who become increasingly frail, management focuses on palliative care, preventing dental pain and oral discomfort. Atraumatic dental techniques are used (e.g. Carisolv for caries removal, glass ionomer restorations and applications of fluoride varnish).

In late-stage dementia, patients become totally reliant on carers to provide their oral care. Toothbrushing may be forgotten amongst other time pressured daily routines. The results of poor oral care and a diet high in sugar can have disastrous consequences, even in as little as 3 months.

◆ How Can Pain of Dental Origin Be Identified in Late Dementia?

In the absence of verbal communication, patients may display changes in behaviour indicating their dental pain, which may include the following:

- Refusing oral care or becoming distressed when toothbrushing
- Waking from sleep displaying pain-related behaviour
- Refusing food, avoiding hard textures or cold foods, or eating on one side of the mouth
- Refusing personal care involving the face (e.g. shaving)
- Changes in normal behaviour (e.g. previously quiet but now distressed)

◆ Do Dentists Have a Role in Recognizing the Signs and Symptoms of Dementia?

Unlike many medical conditions, dementia may not be diagnosed until late in its course. There are multiple barriers to its diagnosis, including stigma and a belief that forgetfulness is a natural part of ageing. The dental team members are well placed to spot subtle changes in behaviour. The following are possible signs and symptoms of early dementia:

- Missed appointments
- Confusion about planned dental treatment
- Difficulty recalling people's names
- Difficulty remembering and finding the right words to describe dental problems
- Anxiety about normal routines such as travel to the practice

If you have concerns, you can suggest patients visit their general medical practitioner (GMP) or, where you feel it may be beneficial, offer to contact their GMP for them.

Also, remember that caring for a patient with dementia has a considerable effect on the carer's health. Ensure the patient's wife is also receiving dental care.

◆ When Might You Consider Referral To Your Local Special Care Dentistry Services?

The role of the general dental practitioner cannot be underestimated. They can successfully support patients through the early stages of dementia by helping patients achieve a healthy, low-maintenance dentition and by implementing preventive advice. Referral should be considered for patients in middle-stage dementia who are finding communication more difficult or displaying more frequent changes in behaviour. The referral should enable effective transition to the next dental team and should include information on medical practitioners, family members/carers and any radiographs.

Further Guidance

Further guidance is available from the Faculty of General Dental Practice UK (https://www.fgdp.org.uk/ and search 'dementia'), the British Society of Gerodontology https://www.gerodontology.com/ and the Alzheimer's Society (https://www.alzheimers.org.uk and search 'dental').

Case 7
A Dry Mouth

PEPE SHIRLAW AND EDWARD ODELL

Summary

A 50-year-old woman presents in your hospital dental department with a complaint of dry mouth. Identify the cause, and plan the treatment.

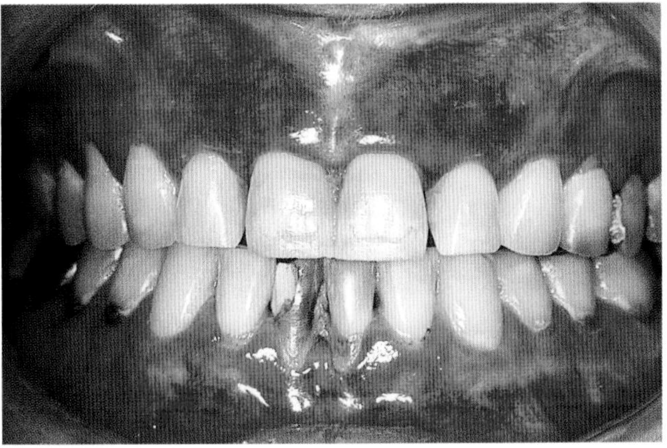

• **Fig. 7.1** Appearance of the patient's anterior teeth.

History

Complaint

The patient complains of dryness of mouth, which makes many aspects of her life a misery. The dryness is both uncomfortable and renders eating and speech difficult. She is forced to keep a bottle of water by her side at all times.

History of Complaint

The patient first noticed the dry mouth about 4 or 5 years ago, although it may have been present for longer. At first, it was only an intermittent problem, but over the last 3 years or so, the dryness has become constant. Recently, the mouth has become sore as well as dry.

Medical History

The patient describes herself as generally fit and well but has had to attend her medical practitioner for poor circulation in her fingers. They blanch rapidly in the cold and are painful on rewarming. She has also used artificial tears for dry eyes for the last 2 years but takes no other medication.

Examination

Extraoral Examination

The patient is a well-looking woman without detectable cervical lymphadenopathy. There is no facial asymmetry or enlargement of the parotid glands, and the submandibular glands appear normal on bimanual palpation. Her eyes and fingers appear normal.

Intraoral Examination

◆ The Appearance of the Patient's Mouth is Shown in Figs 7.1 and 7.2. What Do You See? How Do You Interpret the Findings?

The alveolar mucosa appears 'glazed' and translucent or thin (atrophic), suggesting long-standing xerostomia. Some oral debris is seen adhering between teeth, again suggesting dryness, which causes plaque to be thicker and more tenacious. There are carious lesions and restorations at the cervical margins of the lower anterior teeth, indicating a high caries rate. The tongue is lobulated and fissured. Both features suggest a lack of saliva.

If you were able to examine the patient, you would find that her mouth does feel dry. Gloved fingers and dental mirror stick to the mucosa, making examination uncomfortable for the patient. Parts of the mucosa, especially the palate and dorsal tongue, appear redder than normal. No saliva is

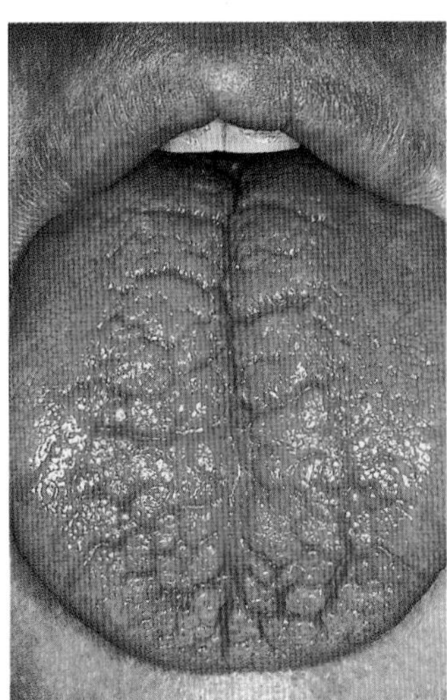

• **Fig. 7.2** Appearance of the patient's tongue.

pooling in the floor of the mouth, and what saliva can be identified is frothy and thick. Small amounts of clear but viscid saliva can be expressed from all four main salivary ducts.

◆ What are the Common and Important Causes of Xerostomia, and How are They Subdivided?

In true xerostomia, the salivary flow is reduced. The term 'false' xerostomia or subjective xerostomia describe the sensation of dryness despite normal salivary output.

Type of Xerostomia	Common Causes
False	Mouth breathing
	Mucosal disease
	Psychological
True	Drugs
	Dehydration
	Sjögren's syndrome
	Irradiation
	Neurological
	Developmental anomaly

◆ On the Basis of the History and Examination, Which Cause is the Most Likely? Why?

Sjögren's syndrome is the most likely cause. It is the commonest single medical disorder causing xerostomia. It also causes dry eyes and predominantly affects female patients of middle age. Sjögren's syndrome is sometimes defined by the presence of dry eyes and dry mouth, with or without an autoimmune/connective tissue disorder. This patient meets these criteria, although they are rather imprecise, and further investigations would be required to confirm the diagnosis.

◆ Which Causes Have You Excluded, and Why?

Drugs are, by far, the commonest cause of true xerostomia, but this patient is not taking any medication.

Dehydration is a common cause in older people who may have a habitual low fluid intake, especially when institutionalized. It also accompanies cardiac or renal failure or use of diuretic drugs. (The combination of drugs and disease probably explains the apparent association of xerostomia with age.) These are not factors in this case.

False or subjective xerostomia is very common. Those who sleep with an open mouth will have xerostomia on waking, compounded by the normal reduction in salivary secretion at night. Diseases causing oral mucosal roughness, such as lichen planus or candidosis, may cause a sensation of dryness, but no such condition is present. False or subjective xerostomia, may be a feature, sometimes a central one, in psychiatric disorders. However, this patient's mouth is genuinely dry; the mucosa is not lubricated, and there is no saliva pooling in the mouth. The history of prolonged and unremitting dryness over a period of years almost always indicates a salivary disorder, and the appearance of the mucosa and the high caries rate indicate true xerostomia.

Neurological and developmental causes such as aplasia of gland or atresia of ducts are very rare and need not be considered further until common causes have been investigated. There is no history of irradiation of the head and neck.

◆ What is Sjögren's Syndrome, and How May the Condition Be Subclassified?

Sjögren's syndrome is an autoimmune disorder in which exocrine glands are destroyed, causing salivary hypofunction. In primary Sjögren's syndrome, the salivary and lacrimal glands are those most affected (although there are often nonspecific systemic signs of autoimmune disease such as Raynaud's phenomenon), and sometimes, there is salivary gland swelling. Other exocrine glands and organs are also affected. In secondary Sjögren's syndrome, there is an accompanying connective tissue disorder such as rheumatoid arthritis, systemic lupus erythematosus, primary biliary cirrhosis or mixed connective tissue disease. Other exocrine glands maybe less severely affected in the secondary form, and the mouth is usually less dry; however, the degree of salivary hypofunction can be quite variable in Sjögren's syndrome.

Investigations

◆ What Simple Test Differentiates False and True Xerostomia?

Measuring the whole salivary flow rate. This may be done by asking the patient to tilt the head forward to allow all saliva to flow into a graduated specimen container for 10 minutes. Although this patient is strongly suspected to have true xerostomia, it would still be a useful test because it provides a baseline reading against which disease severity and progression may be judged.

When you measure the flow, the patient has a whole salivary flow rate of less than 0.1 ml/min.

◆ What Salivary Flow/Objective Rate Would You Consider To Indicate Xerostomia?

Approximately 500 ml of saliva is secreted daily, mostly during eating and drinking, and very little at night. Rates vary greatly among individuals, but less than 2 ml in 10 minutes (0.2 ml/min) unstimulated whole saliva flow is generally considered to indicate xerostomia.

This patient has true xerostomia.

◆ What Further Investigations are Required, and Why is Each Performed?

Although a number of investigations will be required to confirm the diagnosis, the immediate problem is one of soreness. A dry mouth is not usually sore unless there is superimposed candidal infection. A smear sample, a saliva sample or a therapeutic trial of antifungal agent is required to exclude this possibility.

The diagnosis of Sjögren's syndrome is straightforward when the clinical presentation is florid and may then be based on history and the results of physical examination alone. However, numerous investigations are required in most patients with suspected Sjögren's syndrome, in whom there are just a few early signs (Table 7.1). Many investigations are possible, but only the minimum required to make the diagnosis needs to be performed. A selection is usually necessary because every test will be negative in a small proportion of patients, and none is completely specific.

TABLE 7.1 Investigations for Patients with Sjögren's Syndrome

Sample	Test	Relevance
Saliva	Whole salivary flow rate	See above; differentiates false from true xerostomia.
	Culture for candidal count	To exclude superimposed candidosis.
	Stimulated parotid flow	Accurate estimation of maximum possible parotid salivary flow.
Blood	Full blood picture	Mild anaemia is common in all autoimmune conditions and may require treatment.
	Erythrocyte sedimentation rate (ESR)	Relatively nonspecific, but raised in inflammatory conditions, and when there are raised immunoglobulins, especially IgG in Sjögren's syndrome, useful for monitoring their activity after treatment.
	Immunoglobulin (Ig) levels	Often raised in autoimmune disorders and may be markedly raised in primary Sjögren's syndrome.
	Autoantibody screen	Autoantibodies are a frequent finding in autoimmune disease. This appears to be a partly nonspecific effect, and many different autoantibodies may be seen. The exact combination in routine screening varies among centres but usually includes rheumatoid factor, antinuclear, antithyroid, antiparietal cell and antimitochondrial antibodies. Additional autoantibodies that may be seen in Sjögren's syndrome are anti–salivary gland duct antibody and ssA and ssB autoantibodies (anti-Ro and anti-La) directed against extractable nuclear antigens. None of these antibodies is individually helpful in diagnosis, but the presence of more than one is typical. They may aid in the diagnosis of connective tissue disease in secondary Sjögren's syndrome, and ssA and ssB may indicate patients at risk of specific complications. Anti–salivary gland duct antibody is not related to either the periductal infiltrates seen on biopsy or the pathogenesis of the disease.
Urine	Glucose	Occasionally useful to exclude unsuspected diabetes as a cause of dehydration.
Salivary gland	Ultrasonography Sialography	In established disease, ultrasonography almost always shows characteristic changes. Ultrasonography has almost replaced sialography for in investigating Sjögren's syndrome. However, sialography is still useful if salivary stones or strictures are suspected because of additional swelling during eating.
	Other imaging techniques	Pertechnetate scintigraphy is a complex but useful test of secretion from individual glands. It is useful if sialography is not possible but involves a significant dose of radiation. Magnetic resonance imaging is useful to delineate the extent of salivary gland swelling, if present.
	Minor salivary gland biopsy	The histological appearances of salivary glands are characteristic in established disease. Biopsy of major glands is difficult, but the same changes may be seen in the minor glands of the lips and cheeks, provided a sufficient sample is removed (6–8 glands).
	Parotid gland biopsy	Biopsy of the tail of the parotid is possible without significant risk to the branches of the facial nerve. It provides an excellent sample and may be useful when other techniques have failed or when other conditions need to be excluded. It may also be helpful in the diagnosis of lymphoma in swollen parotid glands. Core biopsy taken under imaging guidance is performed more easily compared with an open biopsy, which is rarely undertaken unless indicated for clarifying whether another disease such as IgG4 disease or a lymphoma is present.
Eye	Schirmer test	This measures lacrimal secretion. Narrow filter paper strips are placed with one end under the lower eyelid and the length wetted is recorded after 5 minutes. In practice, the test is not very reproducible. (It is also uncomfortable and may cause corneal abrasions when the eye is very dry and, for this reason, is no longer recommended.) Ophthalmological examination is preferable, but the Schirmer test remains widely used.
	Ophthalmological examination	An ophthalmologist uses a slit lamp to detect conjunctival splits and Lissamine Green staining identifies dried tear secretion on the front of the eye. Although these changes are rarely helpful in diagnosis, examination and follow-up are required to prevent long-term complications of dry eyes.

The results of this patient's investigations are given below:

Salivary culture	10 000 colony-forming units (cfu) *Candida* sp./ml
Smear for *Candida*	Hyphae present
Red blood cell indices	Normal
White blood cell count/ differential count	Normal
Platelets	Normal
Erythrocyte sedimentation rate	20 mm/hour
Immunoglobulin levels	Normal
Autoantibodies	
Rheumatoid factor	Negative
Antinuclear	Weak positive
Antithyroid	Negative
ssA	Positive
ssB	Positive
Urinary glucose	Normal

◆ The Parotid Ultrasound is Shown in Fig. 7.3. What Do You See? What is Your Interpretation?

The top of the image shows the skin surface, and the vertical scales indicate tissue depth in centimetres. The parotid gland lies between 5 mm and 2 cm deep. In this region, the tissue shows heterogeneous consistency and many round or oval, dark, hypoechoic areas that are likely to be cystic dilatation of ducts. The small cystic spaces are best seen on the left image. These appearances are in keeping with Sjögren's syndrome.

◆ The Minor Salivary Gland Biopsy Specimen is Shown in Figs 7.4 and 7.5. What Do You See?

The low-power view shows several minor salivary glands. A minimum of 6–8 glands is required for reliable diagnosis, and this sample is sufficient. Even at this low magnification, dark foci of inflammatory cells are visible (although they cannot be identified as such), and it is evident that the lobular structure of the glands is largely intact.

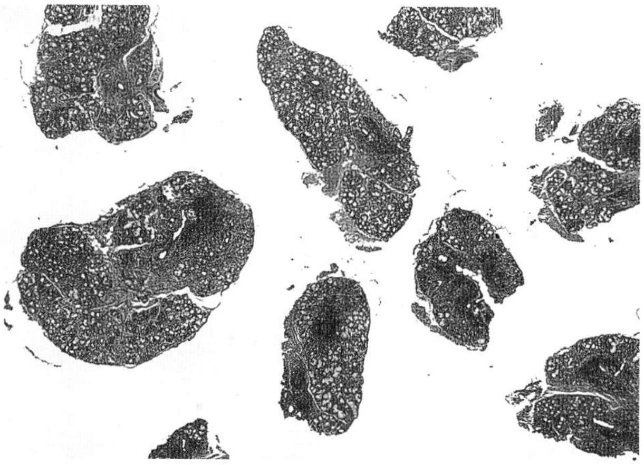

• **Fig. 7.4** Minor salivary gland biopsy; low power.

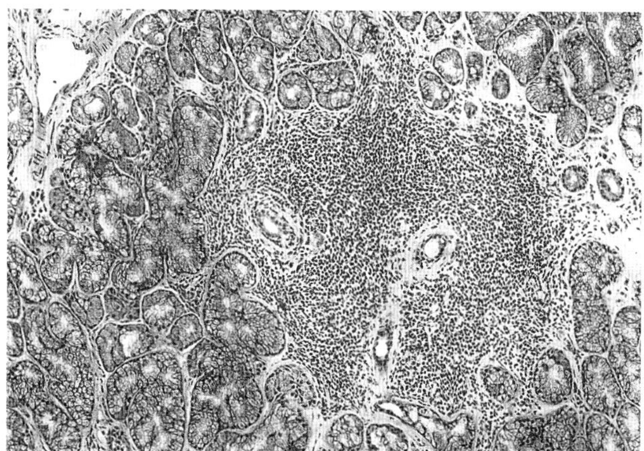

• **Fig. 7.5** Minor salivary gland biopsy; high power.

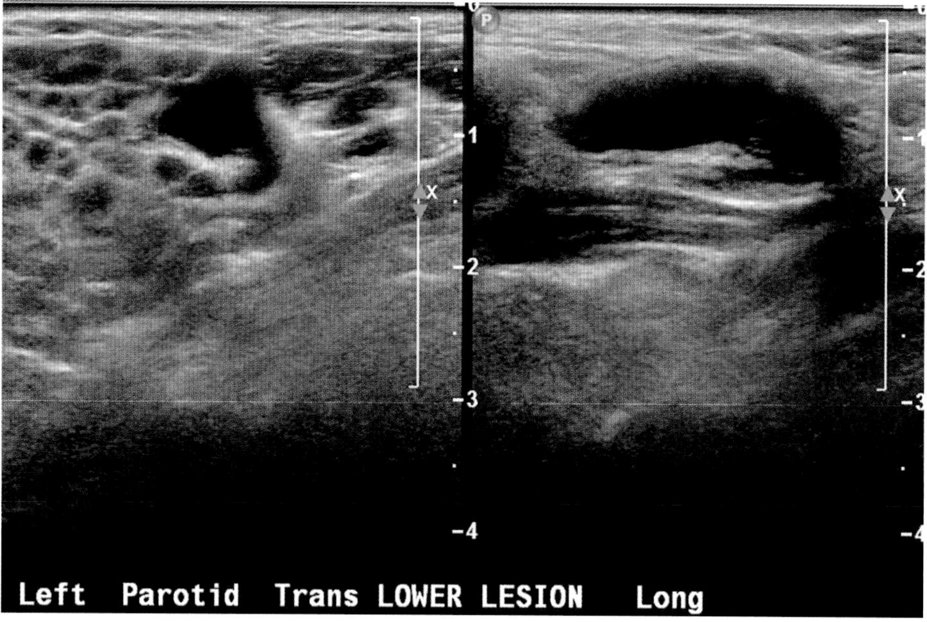

• **Fig. 7.3** Parotid ultrasound. *Long,* longitudinal; *Trans,* transverse.

The high-power view shows one gland lobule. Centrally, there are three small ducts surrounded by a dense lymphocytic infiltrate. The infiltrate is sharply defined, and within the lymphocytic focus, there is complete loss of acinar cells (acinar atrophy). Around the lymphocytes, there is a zone of essentially normal uninflamed mucous salivary gland.

◆ How Do You Interpret These Histological Appearances?

Focal lymphocytic sialadenitis centred on ducts and concentric, sharply defined zones of acinar atrophy surrounded by normal acini are characteristic of Sjögren's syndrome.

Diagnosis

◆ What is Your Final Diagnosis?

The patient has primary Sjögren's syndrome. The diagnosis was suspected on the basis of history and the results of physical examination and was confirmed by the characteristic findings on sialography and biopsy analysis. The primary form of Sjögren's syndrome is indicated by the lack of autoimmune/connective tissue disease and the positivity for ssA and ssB autoantibodies. The presence of Raynaud's phenomenon, the severity of the xerostomia and the dryness of the eyes are also more consistent with the primary form. In addition, the patient has candidosis, which is the probable cause of the soreness.

Treatment

◆ How Could You Contribute To the Management of This Patient?

Control of the underlying disease is not possible but the patient requires treatment for complications and continued follow-up:

- Treat the candidosis, and follow up regularly for recurrence.
- Help preserve what salivary secretion remains; saliva is more effective than saliva substitutes. Instruct the patient as follows:
  - Sip water rather than drinking it, so as to expand remaining saliva and not wash it from the mouth. At night, use simple oils such as coconut or olive oil to lubricate the mouth instead of water.
  - Whenever possible, avoid drugs that cause xerostomia.
  - Maintain fluid intake.
  - Stimulate residual salivary flow by using chewing gum (sugar-free).
  - Take pilocarpine if the condition is severe (although side effects and an appropriate dosing regimen can be problematic).
- Prevent and treat dental caries.
  - Have the patient avoid sweets or overuse of citrus fruit to stimulate salivary flow.
  - Prescribe high-fluoride toothpaste (5000 parts per million [ppm]) for a period.
  - Provide appropriate dietary analysis and preventive advice.
  - Treat caries.
- Consider prescribing saliva substitutes, although these are generally unsatisfactory and not liked by patients.
  - Carboxymethyl-cellulose and similar starch-based liquids may be prescribed.
  - Mucin-based preparations are more effective and generally better tolerated.
- Warn the patient about, and follow up for, attacks of acute bacterial ascending sialadenitis in the major glands, which destroy residual gland function. Treat aggressively if it develops.
- Warn the patient, and follow up for, development of persistent salivary gland swelling.
- Provide continued reassurance and care to patients with this distressing condition.
- Medications such as pilocarpine can be used to stimulate saliva production and to relieve the dry mouth symptoms. In some patients, the antirheumatic drug hydroxychloroquine has been beneficial in decreasing fatigue and joint pain.
- Disease-modifying agents such as the tumour necrosis factor-alpha inhibitors infliximab and etanercept have been investigated, but neither has been found to improve disease outcomes. Rituximab, an anti-CD20 antibody that depletes B cells, has been evaluated in several trials with mixed results.
- Transcutaneous electrical nerve stimulation (TENS), a nonpharmacological technique, has shown encouraging results in increasing salivary secretion without side effects but is not widely available. Acupuncture has been tried in patients with Sjögren's syndrome but has weak evidence, and further research is necessary.

◆ What is the Significance of the Development of Salivary Gland Swelling?

This is usually the first sign of lymphoma development; 10% or more of patients with primary Sjögren's syndrome eventually develop lymphoma, and in some cases, gland swelling is the presenting sign. The lymphoma is usually a form of low grade B-cell lymphoma (mucosa-associated lymphoid tissue [MALT] type), which has a slow indolent growth pattern, remains localized to the salivary glands for a long period and initially responds well to treatment. However, high-grade lymphoma may also develop. Persistent gland swelling would be an indication for biopsy.

Less common complications might occur in various organs, causing pneumonia or bronchitis in the lungs and hepatitis or cirrhosis in the liver and might lead to problems in kidney function. In some patients, peripheral neuropathy develops, causing numbness, tingling and burning in the hands and feet.

Further Guidance

The Sjögren's Syndrome Foundation clinical practice guidelines can be recommended to patients as a source for further information (https://www.sjogrens.org/home/research-programs/clinical-practice-guidelines).

Case 8
Painful Trismus

RODHRI DAVIES AND LUKE CASCARINI

Summary

A 27-year-old woman is unable to open her mouth normally. What is the diagnosis, and how should she be managed?

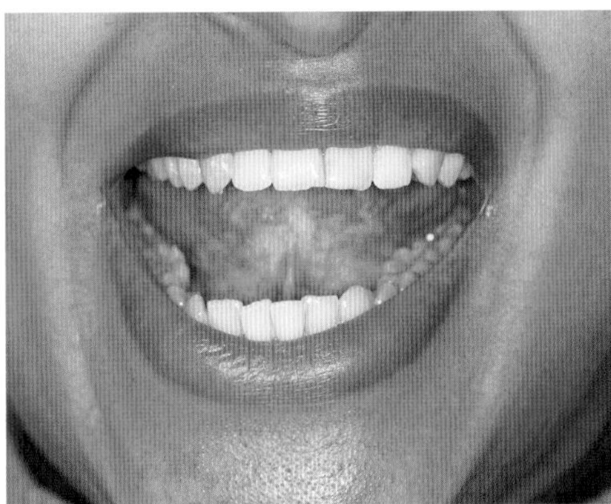

• **Fig. 8.1** The appearance of the patient's mouth on maximal opening.

History

Complaint

The patient reports a sudden inability to fully open her mouth.

History of Complaint

The patient reports that 3 days ago she was chewing a tough piece of meat and felt a sudden pain in front of her right ear. Since then, she has not been able to open her mouth more than halfway. She reports an approximately 10-year history of intermittent painless clicking of her right jaw joint. Over the last few months, the clicking has become painful and seems to be louder. She has experienced some hesitancy in mouth opening just at the position where the clicking is usually felt. She has not felt unwell at any point and does not report any symptoms indicative of infection. There is no history of trauma, recent dental work or toothache.

Medical History

The patient is otherwise well and, other than occasional paracetamol or ibuprofen, takes no regular medication. In her 20s, she suffered from a few episodes of knee pain when she exercised. The rheumatologist had diagnosed 'generalized hypermobility' of her joints.

Social History

She works at a marketing company and is a nonsmoker. As a teenager, she was a successful gymnast.

Family History

When directly questioned, she denies any family history of rheumatoid arthritis or psoriasis.

Examination

Extraoral Examination

The patient appears clinically well and is apyrexial. Her facial appearance appears symmetrical, and she does not seem to be in acute discomfort. The skin overlying her preauricular regions is of normal colour and without swelling. On palpation, there is tenderness over the right mandibular condyle and generalized bilateral tenderness of the muscles of mastication on the right – the masseter, lateral pterygoid and temporalis. Neurological examination of her trigeminal nerve reveals no abnormalities. Examination of her fingers, wrists and elbows shows an increased range of movement, but no tenderness or swelling.

Intraoral Examination

◆ The Patient's Appearance is Shown in Fig. 8.1. She is Trying To Open Her Mouth To the Maximum Extent. What Do You See?

When the patient is asked to open her mouth as wide as she can, she has noticeably reduced mouth opening. When measured between the tips of the incisors, opening is 23 mm, with a marked deviation to the right. When asked to move her jaw from side to side, lateral excursion to the right is reduced at 1 mm compared with 8 mm on the left. She is able to bring her teeth into maximal intercuspation, and she reports that this occlusion feels normal.

Differential Diagnosis

◆ The Patient Has Trismus. What is Trismus?

True trismus is defined as reduced mouth opening caused by spasm of the muscles supplied by the trigeminal nerve. It was traditionally used to refer to the 'lockjaw' seen in tetanus, which is an infection with the toxin-producing anaerobe *Clostridium tetani*, but is more commonly used to refer to reduced mouth opening of any cause. Trismus can be

TABLE 8.1 Causes of Trismus

Intra-Articular Causes	
	Internal derangement of the joint
	Fracture of the mandibular condyle
	Traumatic synovitis
	Avascular necrosis and bone necrosis in sickle cell crisis
	Septic arthritis
	Osteoarthrosis
	Inflammatory arthritis such as rheumatoid or psoriatic arthritis
	Ankylosis – bony or fibrous (secondary to trauma or infection)
	Lesions of the condylar head such as osteochondroma
Extra-Articular Causes	
	Trauma such as a fractured mandible not involving the condyle
	Postoperative removal of impacted lower third molar or recent prolonged dental treatment/misplaced inferior dental nerve block
	Acute infections of the oral tissues especially involving the cheeks or the muscles of mastication, usually odontogenic in origin
	Muscle spasm of masticatory muscles, as in myofascial pain
	Disease of masticatory muscles, such as myositis ossificans or neoplasms
	Scarring of muscles, skin or mucosa, as in submucous fibrosis or scleroderma or after radiotherapy
	Inflammatory conditions of the oral mucosa, such as painful ulcers or other forms of stomatitis
	Rare causes such as tetanus, Gaucher's disease; rare syndromes such as trismus–pseudocamptodactyly syndrome; and central causes such as suprabulbar paresis, neonatal misoprostol exposure.

permanent or temporary, but most causes of true trismus are temporary.

◆ What are the Causes of Trismus?

The causes of trismus are often divided into intra-articular causes and extra-articular causes, which are described in Table 8.1.

◆ What are the Common Causes of Pain in the Temporomandibular Joint?

Pain in the temporomandibular joint (TMJ) is a common complaint, but much of that pain is referred to the joint rather than originating in it. Many of the above causes of trismus are painful, but most disease of the joint is asymptomatic. The pathogenesis of painful TMJ disorders is poorly understood, and causes are notoriously hard to classify. Here are three common causes:

Osteoarthrosis (noninflammatory degenerative changes) in the TMJ. These are similar to arthritic changes, but occur in the absence of severe inflammation. The cause has commonly been put down to 'wear and tear' but is probably multifactorial, with a genetic predisposition and abnormal cartilage repair. The severity of the process may be compounded by occlusal malalignment, ligament laxity and dysfunctional muscle contraction causing torsional loading. It is hypothesized that this causes mild trauma and persistent mild inflammation. Clinically, the disease is characterized by clicking, locking, chronic pain, stiffness, reduction in range of movement and crepitus. This is associated with anatomical and radiographic changes to the joint architecture, such as destruction of cartilage, resorption of subchondral bone, synovitis and osseous remodelling.

Internal derangement of the TMJ is a description of a situation in which the biomechanics of the joint have become dysfunctional as a result of displacement of the articular disc on the mandibular condyle. Anterior displacement of the disc is most common, but it can occur laterally, medially or, rarely, posteriorly. Patients with internal derangement will often report an audible clicking or popping sound on opening the jaw. The condition is classified on the basis of the position of the disc, whether it returns to a normal position (is it reduced?) and whether there is associated reduction in mouth opening or locking.

Temporomandibular joint disorder with myofascial pain is part of a group of TMJ disorders in which masticatory muscle pain predominates. The classification and nomenclature is contentious and complex, and the spectrum includes overlapping conditions from local to generalized myalgia. It is an extra-articular condition, and the joint is anatomically normal. This condition is often called *temporomandibular joint pain–dysfunction syndrome*, inappropriately suggesting that the condition is one of the joint. The patient reports a dull, heavy, diffuse ache over the side of the face, and the pain tends to vary in severity. Classically, one of two pain patterns is seen: pain being worst in the morning and slowly easing or pain that worsens progressively during the day. The masticatory muscles are often tense and tender to palpation, and joint movements are often painful. The causes are multifactorial and poorly understood. However, it seems that muscle tension/spasm, local and central pain processing and psychological response to stress all play a part.

◆ Why Do Temporomandibular Joints Click?

The TMJ is a ginglymo arthroidal joint – that is, the condyle both slides and rotates. Anatomically, it is composed of the condylar head of the mandible, which articulates with the mandibular fossa of the temporal bone. Unlike most other joints of the body, these surfaces are lined with fibrous connective tissue rather than hyaline cartilage. In between, sits a biconcave fibrous disc held in place posteriorly by the superior and inferior retrodiscal laminae and anteriorly by collagenous fibres and the lateral pterygoid. The structure creates superior and inferior joint cavities filled by synovial fluid, allowing for both hinging and translational movement.

In normal mouth opening, the initial opening results from a hinging movement that occurs predominantly in the lower compartment. As the mouth is opened further, translation occurs in the upper joint cavity and the disc, and the condyle slides forward. The thin part of the disc consistently lies in between the condyle and the temporal eminence. If the disc is anteriorly displaced, for example, because of laxity of the retrodiscal ligaments, then the thicker posterior part may restrict translation. When this is overcome, the disc snaps back with a click and mouth opening can continue – this is known as an 'opening click'. On closing of the mouth, the condyle can be rapidly repositioned posteriorly, stretching the lax retrodiscal ligaments and forcing the disc anteriorly again. This creates an audible click or clunk and is known as the 'closing click'. If opening and closing clicks occur in sequence, the patient is said to have reciprocal clicking. The mechanisms of clicks are shown in Fig. 8.2.

◆ Why Do Joints Lock in Internal Derangement?

Inability to open the jaw indicates obstruction of the condyle during forward sliding/translational movement. The most common internal derangement to cause this is a grossly anteriorly displaced disc resulting from overstretched or ruptured posterior retrodiscal ligaments. The disc becomes fixed in the anterior fornix of the joint space and mechanically obstructs anterior translation of the condyle.

Locking of the joint in internal derangement is rarely complete. It most often occurs after the initial hinge/rotational movement of the condyle. The patient will complain of being able to partly open the mouth but finds that it locks when the mouth is about half-open. This is called 'closed lock' despite the fact that the patient can usually open and close a little. It is uncommon for the patient to be completely unable to open the mouth. Closed lock can be acute but usually follows a long history of reciprocal clicking.

'Open lock' causes a TMJ to be 'locked open' and usually results from anterior subluxation or dislocation of the joint. The movements of the TMJ and the mechanisms of closed lock and open lock are shown in Fig. 8.2.

◆ Does This Patient Have an Intra-Articular or Extra-Articular Cause for the Locking? Explain Why

The cause in this case is almost certainly intra-articular.

In extra-articular causes, the joint itself is normal, and thus, although opening can be restricted, translation occurs, and the lateral and protrusive movements are usually unaffected.

In intra-articular causes, the joint is abnormal and translation of the condyle is usually the movement initially affected. Translation occurs in the upper joint space, which is where opening, protrusion and lateral excursion take place. As a result, if the cause is intra-articular, then movement is restricted in all directions. Because there is both deviation on opening (indicating unilaterally reduced translation) and restricted lateral excursion in this case, the cause is more likely to be intra-articular. Movements possible in intra- and extra-articular trismus and locking are shown in Fig. 8.3.

◆ What is the Most Likely Cause?

The patient is young, and both her social history and physical examination results indicate a degree of joint hypermobility. She reports no history of trauma or surgery and shows no signs indicative of septic arthritis, odontogenic infection or inflammatory arthritis. She gives a history of a chronic progression of painless clicking to rapid-onset intra-articular trismus, typical of internal derangement involving the articular disc and anterior displacement causing a closed lock. On examination, the mandible is found to be deviated to the right, indicating that condylar translation is intact on the left but restricted on the right. Lateral excursion is reduced on the right but unaffected on the left. The most likely cause is internal derangement with an anteriorly displaced disc in the right TMJ.

Synovitis is an appropriate differential diagnosis but the history is usually of slowly progressive pain and all, rather than just some, joint movements are painful.

Investigations

◆ What Investigations May Help?

Laboratory tests: In this case, it would be expected that all laboratory test results would be within the normal range. Blood tests such as a complete blood count, Cross-reactive protein level, erythrocyte sedimentation rate, rheumatoid factor, anticyclical citrullinated peptide (anti-CCP) and an autoantibody screen can help rule out other possible causes such as septic or rheumatoid arthritis.

Plain radiography: The structure of the joint is unaffected in this condition so that, other than the abnormal po-

Temporomandibular joint

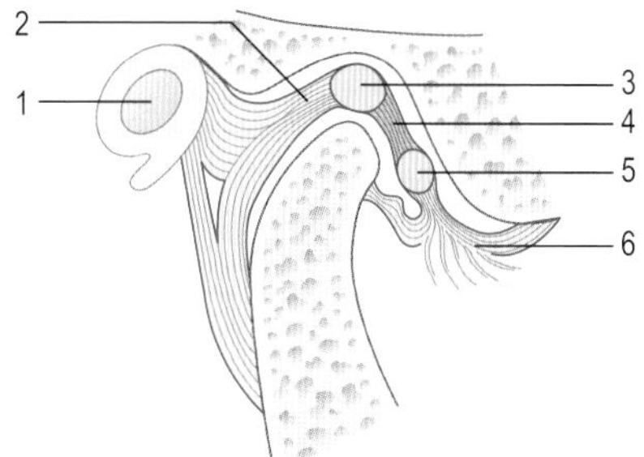

Normal

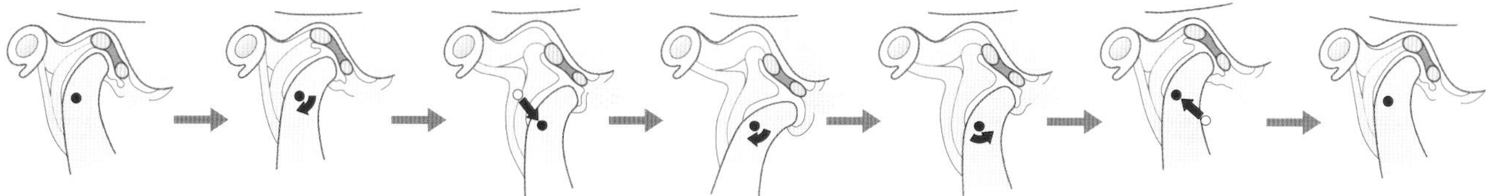

Reciprocal clicks (anterior displacement with reduction)

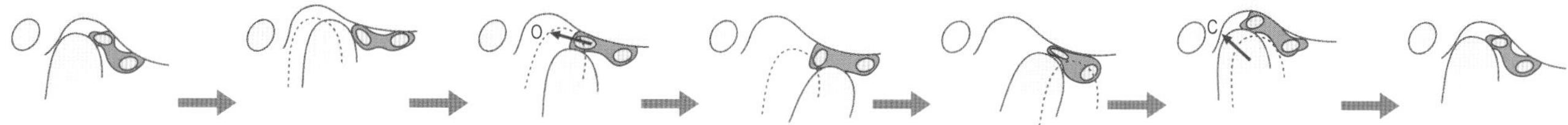

Closed lock (anterior displacement without reduction)

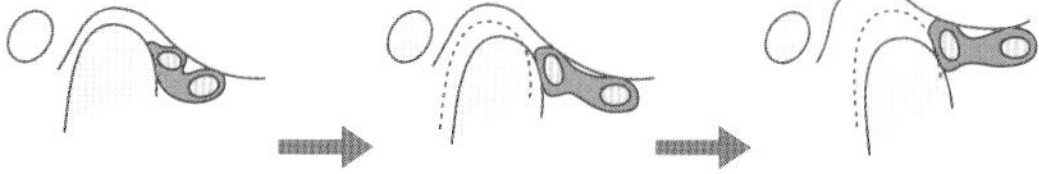

Open

Closed　　Closed

• **Fig. 8.2** The top image shows the anatomy of a normal temporomandibular jaw (TMJ): 1, External auditory meatus; 2, bilaminar region of disc; 3, posterior band of disc; 4, intermediate zone of disc; 5, anterior band of disc; 6, insertion of lateral pterygoid. Below are a series of three images that highlight the position of the disc during normal movement, contrasting with reciprocal clicking and closed lock. The first row shows the normal opening-and-closing cycle. Rotation occurs in the lower joint compartment and translation in the upper. The mechanism of reciprocal clicking is shown in the middle row, with arrows indicating the sudden movements of the disc and condyle that cause opening (O) and closing (C) clicks, respectively. The bottom row shows partial opening in a patient with closed lock as a result of anterior displacement of the disc with reduced translation and opening.

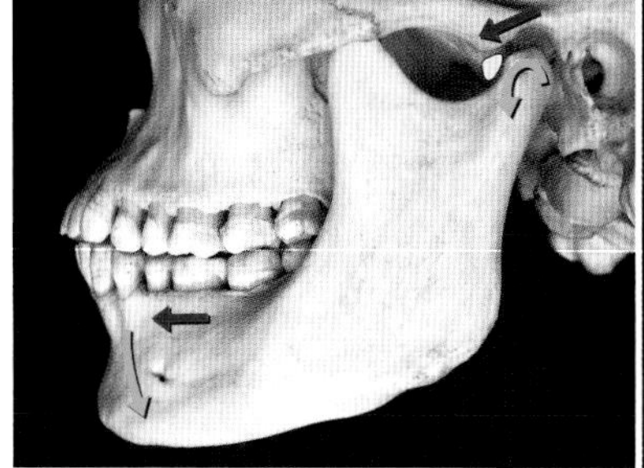
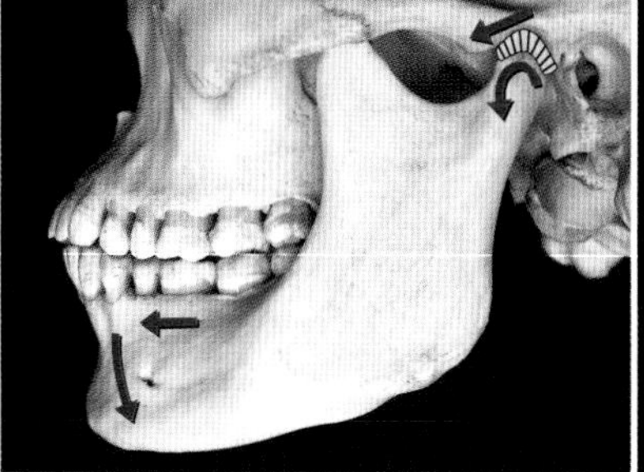
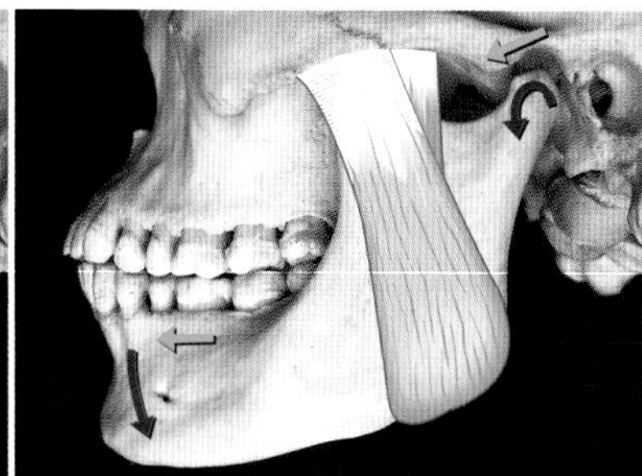

• **Fig. 8.3** Images showing the movements possible in intra- and extra-articular trismus. Green arrows indicate movements that are possible, and red arrows indicate those that are impossible. Left, intra-articular trismus: closed lock caused by an anteriorly displaced disc (yellow). Middle, intra-articular trismus: ankylosis (red). Right, extra-articular trismus: spasm or fibrosis of masseter muscle (red).

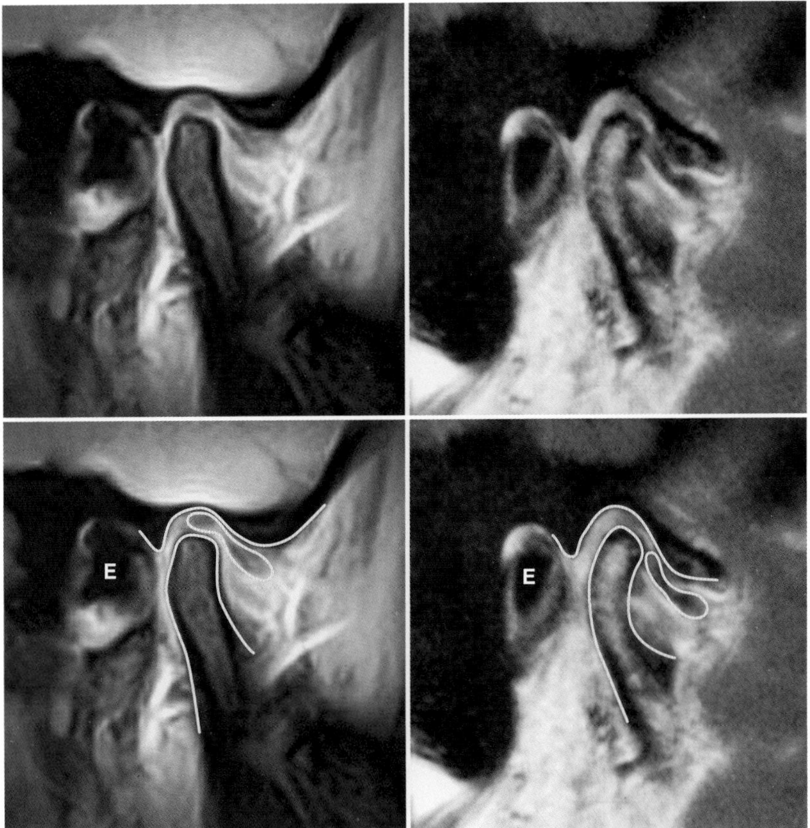

• **Fig. 8.4** A series of images from a T1-weighted magnetic resonance imaging scan of the right temporomandibular joint (TMJ). A normal joint is shown on the left, and the patient's TMJ is shown on the right. The external auditory meatus is labelled E. In this technique, air, dense cortical bone and the disc all appear dark. In the lower panels the condyle, temporal bone and disc are outlined. Note the anterior position of the disc in the lower right image.

sition of the condyle, plain radiography is unlikely to show any abnormality. Plain radiography is useful if joint disease is suspected, and dental panoramic tomograms (DPTs) with specific TMJ projections (transpharyngeal or transcranial) are usually favoured initially. If further information is required, then spiral or cone beam computed tomography (CBCT), at higher radiation dose, provide additional information.

Ultrasonography: Recently, the supplementary use of high-resolution static and dynamic ultrasonographic scanning of the TMJ has been highlighted as a non-invasive radiological adjunct used in clinical decision making. The position, size, shape and movements of the disc can be seen.

Magnetic resonance imaging (MRI) is probably the most useful investigation for this case because it will show the position of the disc as well as the surrounding structures. Scanning can be performed with functional movement to produce a series of dynamic images. Common indications for MRI include severe pain or clinically abnormal locking, previous TMJ surgery or any anatomical abnormalities unclear on the DPT. Furthermore, extensive MRI scanning may be undertaken if other diseases are suspected. MRI images from this patient are shown in Fig. 8.4.

Arthrography: A radiograph with contrast medium injected into the joint space. Once a commonly used technique, it has largely been replaced by noninvasive techniques such as MRI.

Diagnostic aspiration: Unlikely to be used in this case, but would be necessary if septic arthritis were suspected. The resulting aspirate would be sent for microscopy, culture and sensitivity testing.

Treatment

◆ How Should This Condition Be Managed?

The majority of cases with closed lock related to internal derangement and an intact anteriorly displaced disc resolve spontaneously. It is generally accepted that a conservative approach with appropriate review for 3–6 months is appropriate. This should be combined with targeted education and counselling, if needed. Acute adjunctive management may involve simple oral analgesia (paracetamol or nonsteroidal anti-inflammatory drugs [NSAIDs]), warm or cold compresses and gentle mobilization, as tolerated. The use of short courses of low-dose oral steroids and benzodiazepines is controversial but may have a place in select cases. Rehabilitation programs have been shown to reduce the time to resolution of symptoms and decrease the likelihood of recurrence. Programs often include targeted physiotherapy, joint mobilization, home exercise, use of passive joint-motion machines and the construction of an intraoral orthotic (splint). Current evidence indicates that forced manipulation or manipulation under anaesthesia provides no benefit over conservative management. There is a growing body of evidence suggesting that there is a complex interplay between the biomechanics of the TMJ and the surrounding musculature, with underlying mental illness or psychological impairment. A psychological component may be added to the rehabilitation, such as a formal psychological assessment, assessment of maladaptive oral habits and cognitive–behavioural therapy.

◆ Suppose There is No Improvement After 6 Months?

In selected cases where mouth opening does not improve, patients may be considered for TMJ arthrocentesis or 'lysis and lavage'. Under local or general anaesthesia, sterile saline or Hartman's solution is injected into the joint, either blindly or under arthroscopic/fluoroscopic guidance, and the fluid allowed to exit through a second needle or port. The process is intended to flush the joint spaces, removing inflammatory mediators and toxins and breaking down adhesions. The inflation of the joint space can also encourage the disc to assume a more normal position. At the time of the procedure, additional medications such as sodium hyaluronate can be injected. When this procedure is not effective, the patient may be considered for arthroscopic or open joint surgery. Procedures generally aim to reposition the disc but may require meniscectomy, retrodiscal shortening or disc replacement.

Long-term MRI studies have shown that an anteriorly positioned disc is compatible with normal function and that the condyle and disc can remodel. Therefore, these more invasive treatments, which have a weak evidence base, are restricted to carefully selected cases.

◆ Should Treatment Be Undertaken in Primary or Secondary Care?

TMJ disorders can be challenging for both the patient and the clinician. Like other conditions with vague or poorly defined signs and symptoms, a multifactorial aetiology and a chronic course, explaining these factors to patients can be difficult. Treatment is commonly prolonged and can often have a less than satisfactory outcome. Sensitive communication, including a realistic and clear description of expectations, is essential for success.

The complex aetiology and the need for investigations mean that TMJ disorders can be best treated in a specialist centre. Examples of criteria for immediate referral include limited or progressively limited mouth opening, inability to maintain a normal diet and associated joint disease such as rheumatoid arthritis. In primary care, assessment and diagnosis should be undertaken, and appropriate habit modification, simple analgesic advice and bite splints can be appropriate treatments. If the symptoms remain problematic after approximately 6 months, then referral to a specialist should be considered.

Guidance on management in primary care can be found at https://www.rcseng.ac.uk/-/media/files/rcs/fds/publications/temporomandibular-disorders-2013.pdf.

Evidence supporting TMJ treatments is of relatively low level, and following accepted guidelines is prudent because invasive treatment is a medico-legal minefield. Accurate and detailed clinical note taking is paramount.

Another Possibility

◆ Is There Any Significance in the History of Joint Hypermobility?

Possibly. Being genetically predisposed to generalized joint hypermobility or suffering from a disease such as Ehlers-Danlos or Marfan's syndrome would make the patient much more likely to suffer from TMJ internal derangement. However, internal derangement is one of the most common TMJ disorders, and only a tiny fraction of patients have an underlying hypermobility disorder. Of note, joint hypermobility would not have been caused by this patient's childhood involvement in gymnastics but likely indicates that she performed well in this field.

Case 9
A Deep Carious Lesion

AVIJIT BANERJEE

Summary

How will you deal with a deep, cavitated carious lesion in a permanent maxillary molar tooth?

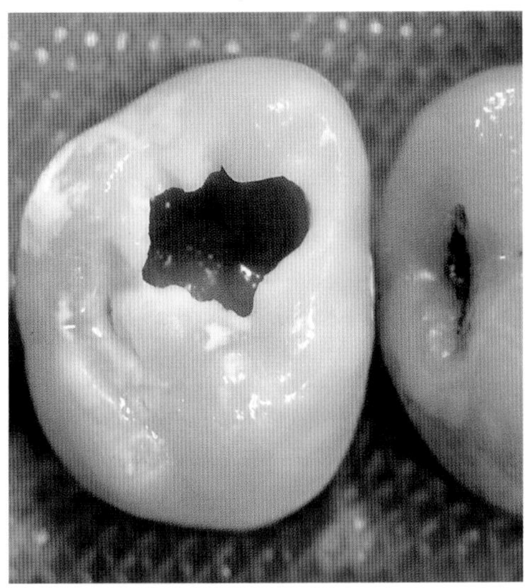

• **Fig. 9.1** The patient's maxillary right second molar on presentation.

History

Complaint

A 30-year-old patient complains of severe attacks of pain, each of a few seconds duration and fading slowly, but she cannot identify which tooth is responsible. Hot, cold or sweet foods and cold air on the upper right jaw make the pain worse.

History of Complaint

The pain has been present intermittently for several months but has only recently become severe. There is no pain on biting.

Dental History

The patient attends on a casual basis for dental treatment. Despite the fact that this carious lesion is very large, perhaps surprisingly, it is the only lesion in an otherwise intact arch, and there have been no other lesions noted in the last 3 years. The patient is, therefore, classified as having a low risk for dental caries.

Medical History

The patient is fit and well.

Examination

Extraoral Examination

The extraoral examination reveals no significant abnormality.

Intraoral Examination

There is no tenderness or swelling over the buccal or palatal roots.

◆ The Maxillary Right Second Molar is Shown in Fig. 9.1. What Do You See and How Do You Assess the Problem So Far?

The classic history of acute pulpitis and repeated attacks of pain – as opposed to continuous severe pain – probably indicates that the pulp can be preserved if the caries is treated. The fact that there is no pain on biting and no tenderness over the roots also suggests a reversible pulpitis and helps exclude periapical periodontitis.

There is a deep, cavitated lesion on the occlusal surface, with extensive exposed carious dentine. Opaque white demineralization of the marginal, unsupported enamel indicates that it is demineralized despite not having fractured off during function. The slightly darker appearance of the tooth distally suggests that caries undermines enamel somewhat distally and that it possibly involves the dentine supporting the enamel of the mesial proximal surface.

This is a relatively small upper second molar. Females have slightly smaller teeth, and when second molars are this small, the third molar may not have developed. This may influence the decision to restore or extract the tooth.

Investigations

◆ What Investigations Would You Carry Out?

A test of tooth sensibility (vitality) is required, even though the symptoms suggest a vital pulp. This is a large cavity in a molar, and partial pulp sensibility is a distinct possibility.

Radiography is required for a variety of reasons. The proximity of the lesion to the pulp and its lateral extension, undermining cusps and the proximal enamel will all affect the overall restorability of the tooth. Pulp size reduction by tertiary, reactionary dentine will also be visible, depending on the chronic nature of the caries process

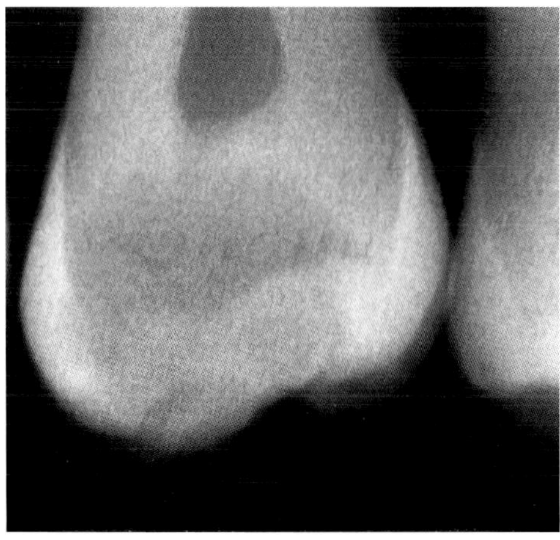

• **Fig. 9.2** Radiograph of the tooth.

in this tooth. It may also be possible to see evidence of periapical periodontitis, widening of the periodontal ligament and loss of the lamina dura. The ideal views would be a periapical or bitewings, depending on your suspicions about pulp sensibility or caries in other teeth. If symptoms were of an irreversible, chronic pulpitis, and there was potential indication for root canal therapy, cone beam computed tomography (CBCT) could also be considered. This imaging modality would give a much clearer indication of periapical pathological and anatomical changes with regard to radiolucencies, bone resorption, proximity to the sinus floor and the root canal apices that might be affected.

When you perform these investigations, the tooth responds quickly and strongly to ethyl chloride (cold), indicating a hypersensitive pulp, although the proximity of the pulp to the cavity may also contribute to this strong response.

◆ The Radiograph is Shown in Fig. 9.2. What Do You See?

The coronal radiolucency indicates that the carious lesion is extensive. It reaches the inner third of the dentine close to the pulp. There appears to be a bridge of intact dentine between the lesion and the pulp chamber. Caries has undermined most of the occlusal enamel and also the distal enamel, but there are no separate proximal lesions or cavitation present. The coronal pulp chamber is rounded and reduced in size, with the pulp horns obliterated by reactionary ('tertiary') dentine.

There is slight radicular cervical 'burn-out' of the dentine immediately above and below the mesial and distal amelo-dentinal junction. This could be mistaken for caries extending from the crown into the distal root, but the shape and site of the relative radiolucency do not suggest caries. If other radiographs are taken (e.g. bitewings), often the cervical burn-out can be observed on other teeth in a similar anatomical location. Of course, findings on radiography must be reconfirmed by further careful clinical examination of the particular area concerned.

Diagnosis

◆ What is Your Diagnosis?

Acute pulpitis in the maxillary second molar caused by extensive occlusal caries. The pulp appears vital, and there is no evidence of periapical periodontitis. The pulp does not appear exposed radiographically.

Treatment

◆ Is This Tooth Restorable?

Yes. The prognosis may be guarded because the pulp may still lose sensibility over time, as a result of either the caries process or restoration placement. There is no indication for immediate endodontic treatment. There is also sufficient supragingival tooth tissue available to support the restoration.

◆ What Will You Do First?

The patient is in pain, and the immediate management response must be to relieve it. Pulpitis does not respond to analgesic drugs, and the appropriate treatment is suitable caries excavation and then restoration.

If a definitive restoration cannot be placed immediately, a provisional dressing could be placed following the selective excavation of carious tissues. This would help relieve pain by removing the stimulus (bacterial products and acid penetrating dentine) and by insulating the inflamed pulp from any triggering stimuli. Eugenol-containing temporary restorative materials have an obtundent effect on the pulp, thus reducing pain. However, it must be noted that eugenol-containing materials must not be used if the definitive restoration to be placed is an adhesive resin composite as the eugenol affects adversely the bond/resin polymerization process. A second alternative might be to place a longer-term provisional restoration with indirect therapeutic pulp protection, as required, in an attempt to induce further reactionary dentine formation in the pulp. However, the carious lesion does not appear to be in imminent danger of breaching the pulp. Indeed, a growing body of evidence argues that indirect pulp protection is not necessary or beneficial because many of the modern adhesive biointeractive materials exhibit the desired properties of pulp protection materials (see later).

Removal of caries will leave a weakened crown, more susceptible to fracture under normal occlusal loading. An immediate definitive restoration is the best course of action.

Subsequently, the patient needs a full caries risk/susceptibility assessment and an intensive preventive regime that may include topical fluorides if other lesions are found or develop. Further details and discussion can be found in Case 1.

◆ Why Not Extract This Tooth?

Such a large lesion in a casual dental patient might well lead to extraction if that were the patient's wish. However, this is a young patient, and she may not have a third molar or, if present, it may not erupt spontaneously after extraction of the second molar. Even though the prognosis may be guarded, there is a good chance that this tooth could be retained for many years, with careful maintenance by the patient, aided by recall consultations with the oral healthcare team. This would be the better immediate option because the condition of the rest of the dentition has not yet been fully assessed.

Minimally Invasive Operative Treatment

◆ How Will You Provide Analgesia?

Buccal infiltration of a local anaesthetic, including a vasoconstrictor, should be sufficient. There is no continuous pulpal pain to suggest that obtaining analgesia will be a problem. If this fails, palatal infiltration or intraligamentary injection would be an appropriate next step.

◆ Is a Rubber Dam Essential for This Restoration?

Yes, it is required. There is a risk of pulp exposure. Although the exposure is small, contamination of the cavity by oral bacteria could reduce the chances of success of subsequent endodontic treatment.

The lesion is extensive, and some carious tissue will have to be retained (selective caries removal). The marginal seal of the restoration will be critical to its final success. An adhesive restoration will require a controllable, dry field to achieve the best seal. A rubber dam will also help by controlling soft tissues, thus improving visibility and access. The final quality of restorations placed under the rubber dam is considered to be higher than those placed without a rubber dam.

◆ How Do You Gain Access To the Lesion? How Much Enamel Will You Remove?

The lesion is already open/cavitated, making access to dentine straightforward, but much of the peripheral occlusal enamel is demineralized, unsupported and weakened. Ideally, enamel at the cavity margins should be completely sound to ensure that etching and adhesion are most effective. Unfortunately, this is not always easy to assess clinically. All frosted, demineralized, unsupported and friable enamel must be removed. Pressure with a hand instrument (e.g. enamel chisel or excavator) will fracture off unsupported enamel, if the operator is unsure. Compromises might have to be made to conserve the cusp enamel. Once the enamel joining the cusps and marginal ridges, that form the thick outer perimeter of the occlusal surface, is lost, much of the intrinsic structural strength of the crown is lost. A tungsten carbide or diamond bur in an air-turbine handpiece or hand instruments may be used to remove the enamel and introduce a slight bevel, if required (Fig. 9.3).

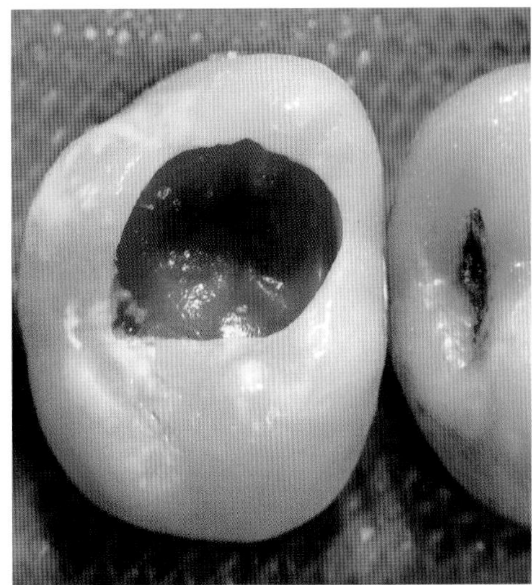

• **Fig. 9.3** The cavitated lesion after unsupported enamel removal.

TABLE 9.1 Techniques for Excavation of Carious Dentine

Technique	Mechanism/Advantages
Burs (carbon-steel, plastic)	Mechanical, rotary
Hand excavators	Mechanical, nonrotary
Air-abrasion (alumina/bioglass), ultrasonics, sono-abrasion, air polishing	Mechanical, nonrotary
Caridex, Carisolv gel, enzyme-based gels	Chemomechanical
Lasers	Ablative
Photoactive disinfection (PAD), ozone	Oxidative destruction and bacterial killing

◆ How Should You Remove the Carious Dentine?

Conventionally, carious dentine is removed with large, slowly revolving, rose-head, carbon-steel burs and hand excavators. Possible alternative techniques are shown in Table 9.1.

No method is completely guaranteed to remove only the necessary amount of carious dentine. The best methods are those that give the most tactile feedback to the operator because assessment of tissue softening and texture is critical to remove the optimal amount of dentine. These include the mechanical and chemomechanical methods.

◆ How Much Carious Dentine Needs To Be Removed?

The 'correct' amount to remove is the minimum required to restore the tooth successfully, allow the dentine–pulp complex to stimulate healing and prevent further disease progression. To achieve this, it is necessary to understand the structure of different parts of a carious lesion.

There is a continuous histological spectrum of degrees of dentine destruction in caries. At the advancing front (at the depth of the lesion closest to the pulp), there is demineralization (and remineralization during reversal). Behind that, the

TABLE 9.2 Histological Layers of Carious Dentine

Location	Dentine Caries Zones		Features
Superficial (closest to enamel)	Destruction/contaminated	Infected	Irreversibly denatured and demineralized, highly infected, 'necrotic' dentine with little residual tubular structure and lateral clefts. Loss of odontoblast processes.
Middle	Bacterial penetration/contaminated	Infected	Bacteria penetrate along tubules widened by demineralization. But there is less damage to the tubular structure. Loss of odontoblast processes, less loss of mineral and collagen breakdown.
Deepest (closest to pulp)	Demineralization	Affected	Tubules widened by acid diffusing ahead of the advancing bacteria, dentine softened but structurally intact. Loss of odontoblast processes. Some bacteria also present in this zone, but significantly less than in the infected zones more superficially.

TABLE 9.3 Pulp–Dentine Complex Responses to Dentine Caries

Reaction/Change	Effect
Peritubular reactionary dentine	Forms on the inner wall of tubules where odontoblast processes remain alive. Gradually obliterates tubules around the sides of the carious lesion and between it and the pulp. Occlusion of the tubules makes the dentine translucent and more radio-dense. This is known as the *translucent zone* (not to be confused with the translucent zone in enamel caries, which is quite different). The circumpulpal dentine has the largest tubule diameter and is softer and more porous than dentine further from the pulp. Peri-/intratubular sclerosis is, therefore, a very useful reaction in the deepest layers.
Regular reactionary dentine ('tertiary' dentine)	Forms in the pulp below the lesion, obliterating pulp horns and increasing the amount of dentine between caries and the pulp. Only slowly formed reactionary dentine is regular, and it forms a good barrier to caries, even though it does not always form at the most useful sites.
Irregular reactionary dentine ('tertiary' dentine)	A rapidly formed reactionary dentine in the pulp below caries. As regular reactionary dentine, but forms a less well-organized, more permeable and less effective barrier.

tubules are widened by demineralization and can be more easily penetrated by bacteria. Between this layer and the surface is progressive destruction of dentine by both demineralization and proteolysis induced by bacteria. The dentine structure is destroyed, and numerous bacteria live within it.

This continuous spectrum of destruction is divided conventionally into zones to aid understanding, but it must be appreciated that this is an artificial concept and that the boundaries of the zones are based loosely on histological examination findings, not clinical appearance.

Carious dentine can be divided into zones of destruction, bacterial penetration and demineralization, or caries-infected (bacterially contaminated) and affected (demineralized) zones. The features of the zones are shown in Table 9.2.

In addition, there are changes in dentine caused by reactions of the pulp–dentine complex. These are not exclusive to the caries process (they may be induced by trauma, attrition or age, for example) but are present to some degree in carious but vital teeth and form an integral part of the overall picture. The pulp–dentine defence reactions are shown in Table 9.3.

During carious tissue removal, the aim should be to remove all dentine that contains bacteria and where the collagen structure is denatured (contaminated/caries-infected dentine). Dentine that is only softened by acid can partially remineralize and be repaired and thus may be retained, especially when in close proximity to the pulp. Thus, it will be necessary to identify the layer or zone of the lesion that clinically corresponds to the level of the red line in Fig. 9.4.

◆ How Can You Recognize This Excavation Endpoint Clinically?

This is difficult to do with clinical accuracy. The relatively smooth lines marking the edges of the zones in Fig. 9.4 do not reflect the irregularly shaped advancing front and the small tongues of bacteria that penetrate tubules in advance of the main lesion. Again, it must be emphasized that these zones are not histologically distinct but blend into each other with diffuse clinical boundaries.

It is accepted universally that not all bacteria have to be removed during excavation. Those that are sealed from the oral environment, the primary source of their substrate, will either die or become dormant. Provided the restoration provides a good seal, the retained bacteria will not be sufficient to allow the caries process to progress below the restoration. Excavation of grossly contaminated/infected dentine is relatively

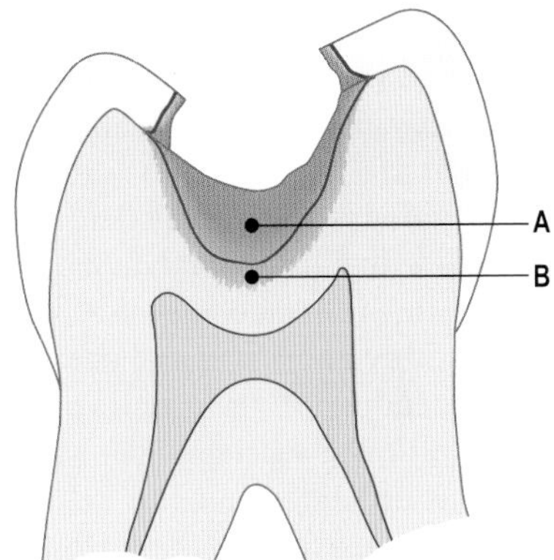

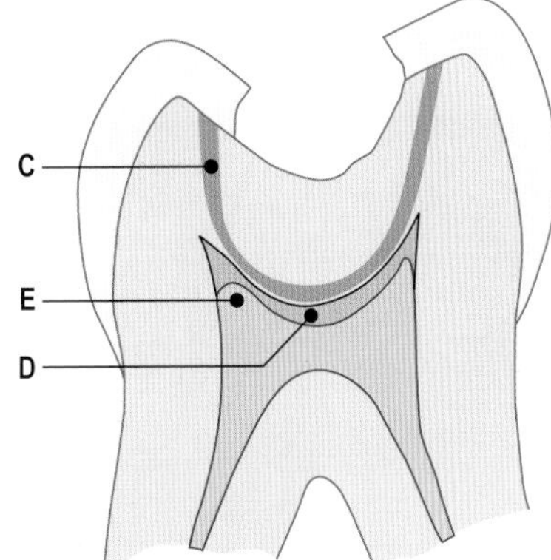

• **Fig. 9.4** The zones of carious dentine and pulp–dentine defence reactions. Left panel, zones of caries: (A) Contaminated (infected) dentine (including the zones of dentine destruction and bacterial penetration along intact tubules); (B) affected, demineralized dentine. Right panel, pulp defence reactions: (C) translucent zone formed by peri-/intratubular sclerosis surrounds the lesion; (D) regular and/or irregular reactionary ('tertiary') dentine that has reduced the size of the pulp; (E) pulpitis, an immunological and inflammatory reaction triggered by odontoblast damage, but not helpful in resisting the advance of caries.

straightforward. All superficial, very soft, wet (often more darkly stained) dentine is highly contaminated and is readily removed.

Whether the underlying demineralized caries-affected dentine, which can potentially be repaired by the dentine–pulp complex, may be spared is a decision that must be made on a case-by-case basis. It is usually preserved in the cavity depths to protect the pulp but cleared from around the enamel–dentine junction to ensure that the peripheral seal is most effective.

Demineralized (caries-affected) dentine is often stained and is softer than the surrounding healthy dentine. A possible clinical indicator that the boundary zone between infected and affected dentine has been reached is that the cavity surface is both scratchy and sticky to a sharp dental probe (sometimes termed *leathery*). Unfortunately, this sensation cannot be appreciated in the words from a textbook and requires first-hand experience of the sensation!

◆ Can Caries Detector Dyes Help Identify the Zones in Carious Dentine?

The original caries detector dyes, developed in the 1970s and based on propylene glycol solutions, were claimed to stain collagen that had become denatured by the caries process. However, they tended to penetrate too far into porous dentine and stain acid-denatured collagen, thus staining both infected and affected zones and even sound dentine. Removing all dye-stained dentine, therefore, risked excessive and unnecessary dentine removal.

New caries indicators that are still being developed detect bacterial metabolism and have the potential to identify the contaminated/infected zone more accurately in future.

◆ The Appearance After Initial Caries Removal is Shown in Fig. 9.5. What Do You See?

The dentine surface is still friable and flakes parallel with the surface, along clefts that are the result of bacteria breaking out of the tubules. The base of the cavity must still be in the contaminated/infected zone. It is just starting to feel scratchy with a probe. Further caries should be removed.

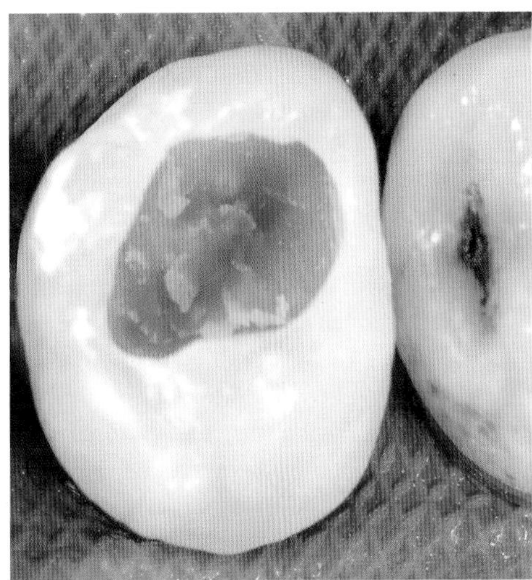

• **Fig. 9.5** Initial removal of grossly infected dentine.

◆ The Final Extent of Excavation is Shown in Fig. 9.6. What Do You See?

Further dentine has been removed around the cavity periphery. Affected dentine over the pulp has been retained. It does not show the gross flaking seen in Fig. 9.5 but is still stained, but dry and appearing matt. It is still noticeably soft but distinctly scratchy with a sharp probe. Consideration must be given to the relative hardness of the dentine retained at the base of the final cavity. If it is too soft, there is a risk that cohesive failure could occur within the dentine itself on shrinkage of an adhesive restorative material. This decision must also take into account relative pulp proximity. Unnecessary exposure of a still vital pulp will significantly reduce the medium-/long-term success of maintaining pulp sensibility and should be avoided.

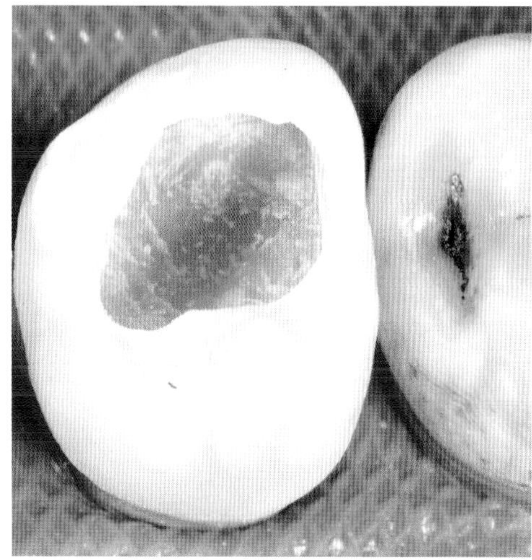

• **Fig. 9.6** Final caries excavation.

◆ Should This Restoration Have a Mesial Box?

The amelo-dentinal junction is visible in Fig. 9.6, and both mesial and distal enamel have lost all, or most, of their support. There is an argument that the unsupported enamel will fracture, leading to failure of the restoration. If amalgam were being used, then both mesial and distal boxes would definitely be required.

Conversely, removing the mesial or distal enamel would seriously compromise the strength of the remaining crown and predispose to cuspal fracture, particularly buccally. Modern adhesive materials have good compressive strength and adhesion to the whole of the dentine and enamel inner surface of the cavity and will provide some support for enamel. It must be accepted that leaving this enamel does incur a small risk of failure, but the potential benefit of a more conservative approach outweighs the risk. Proximal caries, adverse occlusion or the possibility that the patient might not return immediately if the tooth fractured would influence this decision.

◆ Surely Caries Has Been Left Under This Restoration, and It Will Fail?

In the past, this cavity preparation would have been considered inadequate, with soft and stained dentine remaining on the cavity floor. There are certainly bacteria remaining in dentine. If this cavity were to be restored with a modern high-copper-alloy amalgam, with its inherently poor marginal seal, the restoration might fail fairly quickly. However, the principles of carious dentine removal have been revolutionized, partly by the advent of adhesive biointeractive restorations, which seal effectively, and partly by recognition that carious dentine can remineralize biologically and the caries process can arrest.

There is a risk that this more conservative, minimally invasive (MI) approach will lead to failure if the quality of the overlying restoration is suboptimal. Leaving more carious tissue than was accepted in the past does carry a risk, but the affected dentine has been left behind for specific, justifiable reasons. This MI approach will require continued monitoring for success and, as with all operative dentistry, good patient behavioural adherence to oral hygiene regimens.

Annual review will permit any visual changes to the restoration and its seal to be noticed. Early in its life, the restoration may develop some staining along sections of the margin but this does not constitute failure of the seal. However, if staining is accompanied by roughness/gap formation detectable with a ball-ended dental explorer (not accounted for by fracture of resin composite 'flash'), this might indicate the seal has been breached and the restoration would require repair, depending on the extent of the breakdown (see Case 68). The ultimate success of the MI operative management protocol is dependent on case selection, appropriate selective (MI) caries removal protocol, appropriate handling/placement technique of the adhesive, biointeractive restorative material and patients' ability to maintain adequate preventive care in the long term.

◆ What is Stepwise Excavation?

A technique in which carious tissue is removed in increments to allow the dentine–pulp complex to heal the deeper layers of caries-affected dentine. Superficial infected dentine is removed and a provisional restoration placed to seal in the remaining tissue. Over a period of months, the deepest affected dentine remineralizes and develops an appearance similar to arrested carious dentine: darker, harder and drier than previously. Peritubular and reactionary dentine is also laid down around the lesion and at the pulp–dentine interface during this period.

If this technique were to be followed, the restoration would be removed after approximately 6–9 months, further carious dentine excavated and a definitive restoration placed. Current evidence suggests that this second intervention is clinically unnecessary and can lead to cavity overpreparation. The peripheral seal of modern adhesive restorations is now good enough that lesion arrest and remineralization are predictable outcomes. Thus, the two-stage stepwise complete excavation protocol essentially becomes redundant.

The notes might record that this tooth has been excavated conservatively and repeat restoration can be delayed until either the restoration peripheral seal fails or, perhaps, some unsupported enamel fractures off. At that stage a decision can be made about further excavation. After removal of the failed restoration, if the cavity floor is hard and dry, no further dentine removal may be necessary.

◆ Does the Cavity Require a 'Lining' for Pulp Protection?

The purposes of cavity 'linings' are:

1. to protect the pulp from the bacterial infection and diffusion of bacterial acid and toxins
2. to seal, impregnate and mechanically reinforce any layer of caries-affected dentine that may have been retained
3. to stimulate the dentine–pulp complex to lay down tertiary dentine as a defence response, usually when using calcium hydroxide–based linings
4. to protect the pulp from thermal, electrical and mechanical stimuli transmitted through the overlying restoration.

Many adhesive restorative materials and adhesives carry out all these functions and so the value of a separate 'lining'

TABLE 9.4 Potential Direct Restorative Materials for This Tooth

Material	Advantages	Disadvantages
Resin composite	Good appearance, favourable wear characteristics and mechanical properties, intact enamel margins.	Technique sensitivity (moisture control, multiple increments), high volumetric polymerization shrinkage and shrinkage stress (could be minimized with the use of bulk-fill composites).
Glass ionomer cement	Less technique sensitive (more moisture tolerant than resins), bulk fill possible, fluoride released, dynamic chemical exchange, bonds to both enamel and dentine.	Good initial, but poorer long-term, appearance and mechanical properties than composite (brittle fracture and abrasion resistance lower after initial set).
Adhesive layered restoration ('sandwich' or laminate) of resin composite and glass ionomer cement (GIC)	Most useful for very deep cavities with margins primarily in dentine. Good mechanical properties with GIC as dentine replacement, composite replacing enamel. Good appearance and long-lasting. No base or pulp protection required.	Technique sensitivity as for composite, choice between using GIC or resin-modified GIC as the dentine replacement, and their poor resistance to acid-etch, bulk GIC required for strength and durability.
Amalgam (consider phase down, after Minamata Treaty 2017)	Least technique sensitive, good mechanical properties, longevity.	Poor appearance, risk of overpreparation to provide macro-retention (may possibly be partly overcome with bonded amalgams).

is nowadays debatable and, indeed, may compromise the final seal and adhesion of the material to the tooth structure.

◆ What Materials Could You Use To Restore the Cavity?

The choice of restorative material will be a balance between physicochemical properties, the skill of the dentist placing the restoration and the ability of the patient to maintain it. Choices for this cavity are shown in Table 9.4.

◆ Which is the Most Appropriate Choice for This Cavity?

There is no absolutely correct answer. In this case, the decision was made to use resin composite. Resin composite would adhere well to the extensive supragingival enamel margins, supporting the surrounding tooth structure because of its adhesive and mechanical properties. One disadvantage of resin composite alone is the need to place the restoration in small increments to reduce shrinkage stress on the cavity margin. This is especially important in this case, where there is considerable poorly supported enamel, but can be overcome by using the latest low-shrink bulk-fill resin composite materials (for which less than 0.9% shrinkage by volume is claimed).

The final restoration is shown in Fig. 9.7. It was finished using composite finishing burs and polishing discs and pastes to improve the final lustre of the restoration surface. This will improve the aesthetics.

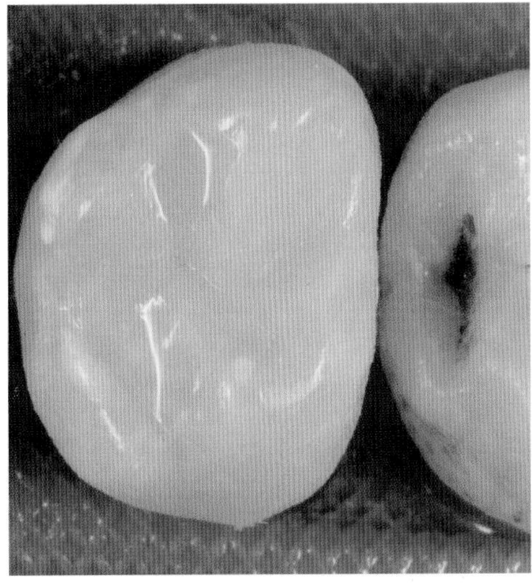

• **Fig. 9.7** The final restoration.

◆ Are There Any Medico-Legal Considerations To Consider When Practising This MI Operative Approach?

It is imperative that good-quality, contemporaneous notes are maintained. Patients should be included in the decision-making journey, with all options and material risks discussed. Intraoral photography is a sensible addition to the records that could be kept, showing the original situation along with a midtreatment and final outcome image. Suitable consent would be required for these. Medico-legally, there is significant clinical and scientific evidence that the MI approach is a valid alternative to the conventional complete excavation protocols. The onus is on the oral healthcare practitioner to offer this option as an alternative to the traditional approach. Ignorance and lack of clinical knowledge or skill is not a defence in a court of law. This MI approach is being taught and can be referenced in many textbooks.

Case 10
A Lump On the Gingiva

ANWAR R. TAPPUNI

Summary

A 48-year-old man presents with a gingival swelling. What is the cause, and what would you do?

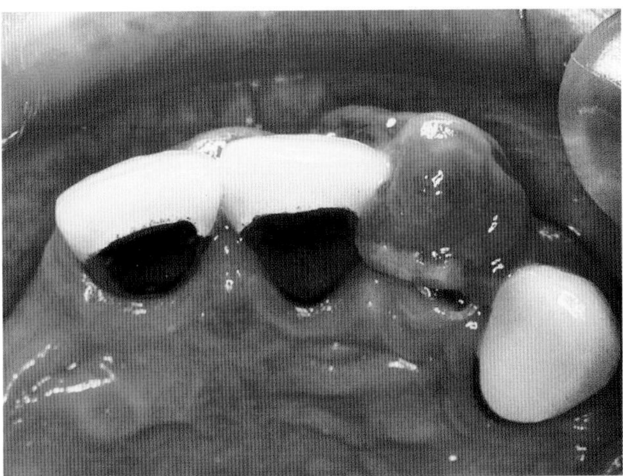

• **Fig. 10.1** Appearance of the swelling.

History

Complaint

The patient complains of a lump on the gum at the front of his mouth on the left side. It bleeds sometimes, usually after brushing or eating hard food, but it is not painful.

History of Complaint

The swelling has been present for 4 months and has grown slowly during this period. It was never painful but now looks unsightly. The patient gives no history of other mucosal or skin lesions.

Medical History

The patient has hypertension, controlled with atenolol 50 mg daily.

Examination

Extraoral Examination

The patient is healthy looking but slightly overweight. There are no palpable cervical lymph nodes.

Intraoral Examination

The patient is partially dentate and has relatively few and extensively restored teeth. He wears an upper partial denture. The root of the upper lateral incisor is present, and its carious surface lies at the level of the alveolar ridge. The teeth on each side of the lesion are restored with metal–ceramic crowns.

There is a mild degree of marginal gingivitis. Most of the interdental papillae are rounded and marginal inflammation is present around the crowns. Flecks of subgingival calculus are visible.

◆ The Appearance of the Lesion is Shown in Fig. 10.1. Describe Its Features

Feature	Appearance
Site	Appears to arise from the gingival margin of the lateral incisor root or the interdental papilla mesially.
Size	Approximately 10 × 7 mm.
Shape and contour	Irregular rounded nodule. It is not possible to say whether it is pedunculated or sessile, although from its size and the fact that it overlies the lateral incisor root, it is probably pedunculated.
Colour	Patchy red and pink, with a thin grey translucent sheen. The surface is almost certainly ulcerated.

If you were able to palpate the lesion, you would find that it is fleshy and soft and attached by a thin base to the gingival margin. It bleeds readily from the area between the tooth and the lesion when pressed with an instrument, but it is not tender.

◆ On the Basis of the Information From the History and Examination So Far, What is Your Differential Diagnosis?

Likely:

- Pyogenic granuloma (if the patient had been female, pregnancy epulis might have been considered)
- Fibrous epulis

Less likely:

- Peripheral giant cell granuloma

- Sinus papilla (parulis)

Unlikely:

- Papilloma
- Benign hamartoma or neoplasm
- Malignant neoplasm

◆ Justify Your Differential Diagnosis

A very wide range of lesions may affect the gingiva, and many possible causes cannot be excluded on the basis of the information given so far. However, the gingiva is the site of predilection for a number of inflammatory hyperplastic lesions comprising fibrous tissue and epithelium. All are associated with poor oral hygiene, and the lesion is almost certainly of this type on statistical grounds.

Pyogenic granuloma is a localized proliferation of granulation tissue or very vascular fibrous tissue. It arises in association with local irritants such as poor oral hygiene, calculus or the margin of a restoration. The present lesion has many features of the pyogenic granuloma: it is asymptomatic, soft and vascular, bleeds readily, and has an ulcerated surface. If it were a female patient, a pregnancy epulis (a variant of pyogenic granuloma arising during pregnancy) would have been a possible diagnosis.

Fibrous epulis (gingival fibroepithelial polyp/nodule) is a nodule of more fibrous hyperplastic tissue. It is not usually ulcerated, is firmer on palpation and does not bleed so readily. Some fibrous epulides develop from pyogenic granulomas through maturation of the fibrous tissue, and some arise de novo. They are usually associated with a local irritant in the same manner as pyogenic granulomas. The current lesion could well be a fibrous epulis, although its vascularity and red colour are more suggestive of pyogenic granuloma. These two terms are really no more than convenient labels for lesions at the opposite ends of a spectrum ranging from granulation tissue to dense fibrous tissue. All are hyperplastic.

Peripheral giant cell granuloma is another hyperplastic lesion that seems to develop in response to a local irritant. Clinically, it may have a deep red, maroon or blue colour but is otherwise indistinguishable from pyogenic granuloma or fibrous epulis. However, histologically, it is distinctive, containing numerous multinucleate osteoclast-like giant cells lying in a very cellular vascular stroma. Giant cell epulis is commoner in children, although it can arise in an adult. Although it cannot be excluded, it is a less likely diagnosis for the present lesion.

Sinus papilla (parulis) is essentially a pyogenic granuloma developing at the opening of a sinus. Infection and inflammation are the stimuli inducing hyperplasia. If the sinus heals, the sinus papilla may disappear, or it may mature and shrink into a small fibrous nodule. The usual site is on the alveolar mucosa and the lesion is usually no more than 4 or 5 mm across. This is an unlikely cause of the lesion in this case.

Papillomas are lesions of proliferating epithelium. Their exact cause is not always clear although it is generally considered that most are caused by human papilloma virus infection. Others do not appear to contain the virus and may be benign neoplasms. Papillomas may arise at any site in the oral cavity but are often seen at the gingival margin and lips. Sometimes, patients have warts on their fingers as well. Papillomas usually have a white spiky or frond-covered surface or a smoother cauliflower-like surface, and neither is seen in the present lesion. Papillomas do not bleed easily, so this seems an unlikely diagnosis.

It would not be useful to list the many other possible causes, but a few groups of lesions may also be considered.

Hamartomas and benign neoplasms can arise at all sites. If this were such a lesion, a haemangioma would be likely in view of the vascularity. A haemangioma could appear very similar to a pyogenic granuloma.

Odontogenic tumours can occasionally arise extraosseously in the gingiva but usually form uninflamed sessile nodules.

Malignant neoplasms occasionally present in the gingiva. Metastatic deposits are commoner than primary lesions, and leukaemia is the most likely cause. Kaposi's sarcoma might also be considered in an individual with human immunodeficiency virus infection. Both these lesions are vascular, may bleed on pressure and ulcerate.

Further Examination and Investigations

◆ What Further Examinations and Investigations Would You Perform? Explain Why

The definitive diagnosis will require a biopsy, and excision is indicated as this swelling will not regress spontaneously. However, a number of other investigations (Table 10.1) need to be performed to identify possible causes. If the cause is left untreated the lesion may recur after excision. The results of these further examinations are shown in Table 10.1.

Differential Diagnosis

◆ What is the Most Likely Diagnosis?

On the basis of the clinical appearance and the results of the tests in Table 10.1, the lesion is almost certainly a pyogenic granuloma or fibrous epulis.

Treatment

◆ What Treatment Would You Provide?

- Excision biopsy
- Removal of causative factors (i.e. plaque and calculus)
- Provide treatment for the generalized periodontitis
- Extract or restore the lateral incisor root

◆ Would You Perform This Biopsy in General Dental Practice? What Complications Might Develop?

Yes, this amounts to no more than the removal of a flap of gingiva, and ideally this would be performed in general practice. The only significant complication may be bleeding because this is a highly vascular lesion. However, haemostasis should not prove a problem because pressure can be readily applied to the gingival margin.

The steps to be taken after removal are shown in Table 10.2.

TABLE 10.1 Investigations and Findings

Test	Reason	Findings in This Patient
Periodontal examination	To assess pocketing around the lesion and detect subgingival calculus, a common cause	There is generalized chronic adult periodontitis with loss of attachment of 3–4 mm. There is a 5-mm probing depth adjacent to the lesion, most of which is false pocket below the lesion. This pocket and others contain subgingival calculus
Tests of vitality of the adjacent incisor and canine	To determine whether the cause could be irritation from a periapical infection draining into the pocket	Both teeth are vital on electric pulp testing
Periapical view of the incisor and canine	Not useful for diagnosis but might be indicated on the basis of probing or vitality tests	Not indicated

TABLE 10.2 Carrying Out a Biopsy and Obtaining a Pathology Report

Aim	Procedure
Avoid distortion or crushing of specimen	If a suture has been placed through the lesion to hold it and prevent it being lost in the vacuum, do not remove it. Cut the thread 1 cm or so from the lesion.
Ensure rapid and efficient fixation	Place immediately in 10 times the tissue volume of 10% formol saline (available in biopsy containers from pharmacies, hospital suppliers and some pathology departments). In the absence of fixative, postpone the biopsy, if possible. Spirits and other solutions used in dental surgeries are ineffective. An unfixed specimen will autolyse (rot) on the way to the laboratory.
Provide the pathologist with sufficient clinical information to enable diagnosis	Fill in a request form or write a letter, including the patient's name, age and gender; a complete clinical description of the lesion; the differential diagnosis; and medical history. Include any details of previous lesions or lesions elsewhere in the mouth. Do not forget to include your own name and practice address and phone number.
Protect those handling the specimen in transit	Package the specimen according to the post office regulations for sending hazardous materials through the post. Make sure the container is labelled with a hazard sticker identifying the contents as formalin. Place the specimen container in either an unbreakable second container or a box with padding. Include enough absorbent material (e.g. tissue) to soak up all the formalin in the pack in the event of breakage. Label the package 'Pathology specimen – handle with care' and send by first-class post.

◆ How Would You Obtain a Report On the Biopsy Specimen?

Most histopathology departments, either specialized oral pathology departments associated with dental schools or departments in district general or other hospitals, provide postal or courier services for sending pathology reports to dentists and/or medical practitioners in their area Reports may also be sent electronically according to local and national patient information governance policies.

Diagnosis

◆The Microscopic Appearances of the Biopsy Specimen are Shown in Figs 10.2 and 10.3. What Do You See, and How Do You Interpret Them?

The surface is ulcerated and covered by a slough of fibrin containing nuclei of inflammatory cells. At higher power, you would be able to identify these as neutrophils. Below the surface is pale-stained tissue in which the endothelial lining of numerous small blood vessels stands out. The vessels have a radiating pattern and point towards the surface, reflecting a pattern of growth outwards from the centre. Between the vessels, there is a little fibrin, and the tissue is oedematous, myxoid or both. More deeply, there is a cluster of inflammatory cells, and collagen bundles are more prominent between the vessels.

The lesion is a nodule of ulcerated maturing granulation and fibrous tissue.

◆ What is the Diagnosis?

Pyogenic granuloma.

Other Possibilities

◆ Is a More Conservative Approach To Treatment Ever Justified?

Yes, elimination of the causative factors may induce considerable resolution. However, the degree of resolution varies; softer

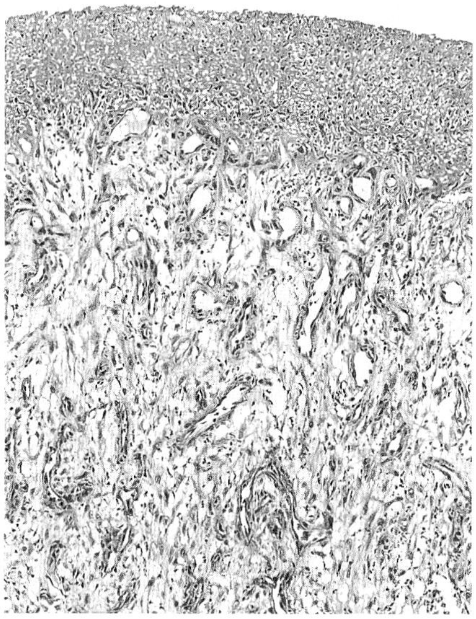

• **Fig. 10.2** Histological appearance of the surface layers of the excision specimen.

more vascular lesions shrink most and firmer more fibrous lesions hardly at all. Removal of calculus and improved oral hygiene may cause partial resolution and reduce the size of the lesion, which is then easier to excise and bleeds much less. Such a course of action is often appropriate for the treatment of pregnancy epulis, both because of the wish to avoid the procedure during pregnancy and because excision during pregnancy carries a risk of recurrence. Definitive excision may then be delayed until after parturition. Only very occasionally is resolution so complete that no further treatment is required.

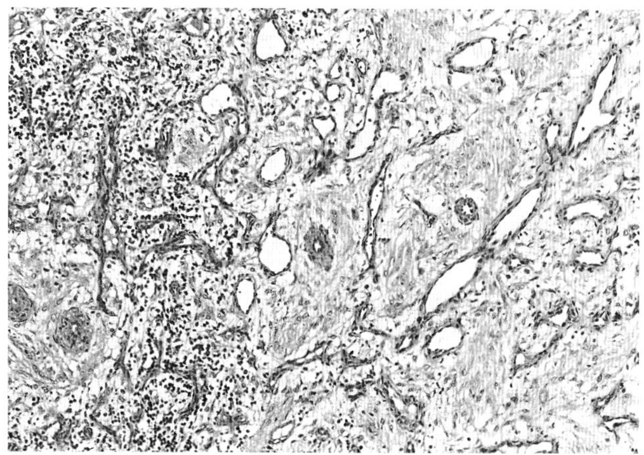

• **Fig. 10.3** The deeper tissue of the specimen.

◆ If, On Removing the Lesion, You Felt Bone Within It, What Would This Signify?

Woven and lamellar bone, sometimes quite large pieces, can lie within fibrous epulides and pyogenic granulomas. Bone may be noted on excision or on histological examination. Sometimes, such lesions are referred to as mineralizing epulides (or peripheral ossifying fibroma in the USA). The presence of bone seems to be of no great significance, and it may indicate that such lesions arise by proliferation of the deep fibrous tissue of the periosteum. Some consider lesions that contain bone more likely to recur than those that do not, but there is no good evidence to support this belief.

Case 11
Pain On Biting

FRANCESCO MANNOCCI

Summary

A 64-year-old man presents with intermittent pain on biting. Identify the cause, and discuss the treatment options.

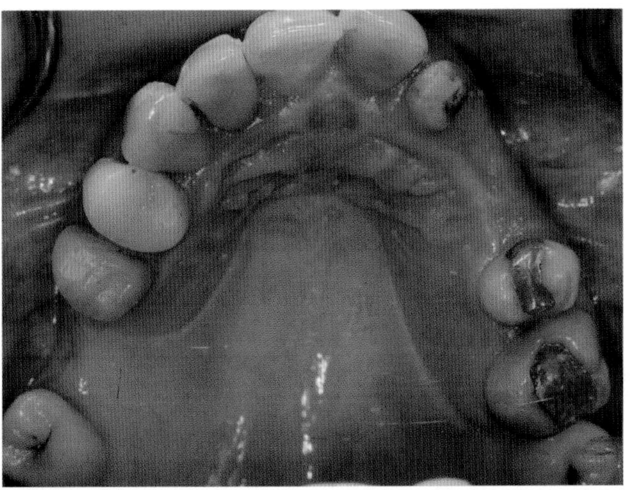

• **Fig. 11.1** A mirrored occlusal view of the teeth in the upper right and left quadrants; the upper right quadrant is the source of pain.

History

Complaint

The patient complains of pain on biting; the pain is unpredictable, extremely painful and sharp but poorly localized. It originates in the upper right quadrant and lasts a very short time, only as long as the teeth are in contact, and it is so painful that he has become accustomed to eating on the right side. The pain only arises on biting hard foods or deliberately clenching his teeth. Apart from this sharp electric shock–like pain, he has no other symptoms.

History of Complaint

The pain is a recent phenomenon, having been first noticed a month or two ago. At first, it was frequent, but it has become less of a problem now that he has learnt to avoid triggering the pain. He has not noticed the pain being provoked by hot or cold foods.

Dental History

The patient has been an irregular attender at another practice since childhood. At his last appointment, 2 years ago, the dentist had placed an amalgam restoration in the upper right first molar.

◆ On the Basis of What You Know Already, What are the Likely Causes? Explain Why

Pulpal pain is the most likely cause because the pain appears to originate in a tooth and is poorly localized. Pain of periodontal ligament origin should be well localized. However, pulpitis does not appear to be present because there is no sensitivity to hot or cold foods. Pulpitis caused by placement of the recent amalgams, and pain caused by caries or exposed dentine can be excluded for the same reasons.

A crack in the tooth and electro-galvanic pain are possible causes suggested by pain on biting. Both are triggered by tooth–tooth contact.

Trigeminal neuralgia should be considered as an unlikely nondental cause. It causes paroxysmal stabbing or electric shock–like facial pain in distributions of the trigeminal nerve and may be initiated by touching or moving trigger zones. It usually affects middle-aged or older adults. Pain on biting almost certainly has a dental cause, but it can be difficult to exclude trigeminal neuralgia in some patients, particularly when trigger zones lie in the mouth or attacks are triggered by eating. If no dental cause is found, the possibility of trigeminal neuralgia may need further investigation.

Acute periodontitis caused by an occlusal high spot on the recently placed amalgam needs to be considered. However, although this could cause significant tenderness on biting, it would be expected that the pain from the bruised periodontium would be present at other times as well. Also, such a periodontally triggered pain would be well localized to the specific tooth in most circumstances.

◆ What Additional Questions Would You Ask? Why?

The patient should be asked about clenching, grinding or bruxing of teeth because the additional occlusal load can cause fracture, and this information will help determine treatment options.

This patient describes a habit of nocturnal bruxism, with some tenderness of masticatory muscles at times of stress.

Please note that partners can often be a source of useful diagnostic information because patients may not be aware of nocturnal parafunctional dental habits.

Examination

Extraoral Examination

There is a suspicion of hypertrophy/enlargement of the masseter muscles on clenching.

Intraoral Examination

The incisal edges of the lower anterior teeth are worn, and dentine is exposed. The cusps of the posterior teeth are slightly flattened or rounded, consistent with mild attrition. There is no evidence of any loss of attachment or gingival recession.

The appearance of the teeth in the upper right quadrant is shown in Fig. 11.1. The upper right first molar and premolar contain moderate-sized class II amalgam restorations.

◆ What Features of the Restorations Would You Note Particularly?

The restorations should be inspected for occlusal high spots, indicated by a burnished mark on the occlusal surface. Premature occlusal contacts could be confirmed by using articulating paper, and relieving the area might cure the pain indicating the aetiology of the problem.

Although they are unlikely causes for this particular pain, marginal caries, poor marginal adaptation or a cracked restoration should be investigated.

Differential Diagnosis

◆ What is Your Differential Diagnosis? Why?

The pain is almost certainly caused by a cracked cusp or crown. The presence of masseteric hypertrophy and attrition on the occlusal surfaces of the teeth would suggest a parafunctional habit that could predispose to cracked tooth syndrome.

Galvanic pain may be excluded because there are no occluding restorations of dissimilar metals.

◆ Which Tooth Would You Suspect? Why?

The upper first molar appears the most likely to be cracked. It should be investigated first because the pain seems to have started shortly after restoration. The risk of cracking is associated with the size of restorations. The upper teeth have restorations that are limited to fissures and mesial and distal surfaces. In the upper molar, the ridge of enamel joining the disto-buccal and mesio-palatal cusps is not intact, so the cusps may be undermined.

Intact teeth can also crack, although usually only in association with an increased occlusal load. The most susceptible teeth are the premolars because moderately sized amalgams undermine the lingual and palatal cusps in the small crowns. Upper first molars are also prone to cracking because they tend to contain the largest restorations in the mouth.

Root-filled teeth are prone to cracking but obviously could not cause pulpitic pain. Symptoms would then only be produced if the periodontal ligament were involved, and the pain would be well localized.

Investigations

◆ What Tests and Further Examinations Would You Perform To Identify the Causative Tooth? What Do the Results Tell You?

The investigations are described in Table 11.1.

On performing these tests, you discover that all the teeth in the quadrant are vital. Biting on cotton wool on the upper first molar provokes pain that the patient identifies as the same as that on biting. No particular cusp can be identified, and no crack can be found.

Treatment

◆ What Would You Do Next? Explain Why

The path of the crack must be defined as far as possible because this will determine the treatment options. The restoration(s) in the tooth should be removed and a further attempt made to find the crack by using transillumination and dye as described in Table 11.1. If the crack appears to enter the pulp or is directed towards it, root treatment will be required.

After investigation, the crack is found to run across the mesio-palatal cusp and disappear subgingivally. It does not appear to enter the pulp.

◆ What are the Treatment Options for Restoring Cracked Teeth? What are Their Advantages and Disadvantages?

These are listed in Table 11.2.

◆ If, At Presentation, the Cracked Portion is Seen To Have Already Broken Off and the Pulp is Not Involved, What Restoration Options are Open To You?

Assuming no second crack were present, this would present a simple choice. One of the methods described in Table 11.2 could be used, and this would have the advantage of preventing further cracks. In view of the history of bruxism, this may be an appropriate option.

However, most cracks are single, and it would also be possible to adopt a more conservative approach and restore the tooth with a resin composite and a dentine bonding agent or a 'sandwich' restoration. The latter uses a high viscosity glass–ionomer cement to replace dentine and a resin composite to replace enamel. An amalgam restoration is also simple and highly effective, but with the shift to minimally invasive dentistry and the global phase-down of amalgam use in dentistry, it is less frequently indicated. Both approaches would require the cusp to be reduced in height to reduce the occlusal load.

TABLE 11.1 Identifying the Causative Tooth

Investigation	Significance
Tests of sensibility of all teeth in the upper right quadrant should be performed, either with an electric pulp tester or a cold stimulus.	The pain must originate from a vital tooth. It is also possible that the cracked tooth might be hypersensitive. This could aid diagnosis though hypersensitivity to testing would not be expected in the absence of pain on eating hot and cold foods. Vitality might also affect the choice of treatment.
Close examination with a good light (bright fiberoptic light is especially useful for transillumination). A soluble dye such as a disclosing agent may be painted onto the crown. After the excess is washed off, small amounts may remain in the crack, rendering it visible.	May reveal a crack.
Attempts to stimulate the pain by pressing the handle of an instrument against each cusp, preferably from more than one direction.	Pain indicates a cracked cusp, and the causative cusp is identified.
Asking the patient to bite hard on a soft object such as a cotton wool roll.	This transmits pressure to the whole occlusal surface and forces the cusps slightly apart. Pain on biting suggests a cracked tooth.
Placing a wooden wedge/tooth sleuth against each cusp in turn and asking the patient to bite on each.	This is a more selective test to identify the cusp or cusps which are cracked. By placing the wedge on different surfaces of the cusp, it may be possible to tell in which direction the crack runs. There may be pain on biting, but pain that is worse on release of pressure is said to be characteristic.
Radiography	To exclude the possibility of caries and to assess the feasibility of root filling, the tooth should it be necessary. Radiography is unlikely to be of direct help in diagnosis and may not be necessary if other investigations successfully identify the cracked cusp.

TABLE 11.2 Restoration Options for Cracked Teeth/Cusps

Option	Advantages and Disadvantages
No treatment	This is not an option, even if the patient is willing to put up with the pain. Cracks may propagate into the pulp, allow bacterial contamination and devitalize the tooth.
Removal of the cracked portion, followed by restoration	This is unsafe. Levering of the cracked portion risks a catastrophic fracture with pulpal communication. Many cracks are incomplete and leverage may propagate them in unpredictable directions. Occasionally, the fragment will be limited to the enamel and dentine of the crown, particularly where the tooth already contains a large restoration undermining the cusp, but even then a deliberate fracture is not recommended.
Full- or partial-coverage indirect gold restoration	This is the treatment of choice. The preparation should finish supragingivally, wherever possible. Gold is malleable and allows some plastic deformation, which is not possible with ceramics or composites, which are more brittle. Full occlusal coverage is needed to protect the tooth from further damage, and a casting can provide some splinting, reducing the potential for further cracks.
Full-coverage bonded porcelain crown	Full coverage with porcelain bonded to metal has the advantage of better appearance, but the ceramic is brittle. This disadvantage may be offset by using an adhesive to lute the crown. There is then the potential for the crack to be sealed by the infiltrating cement.
Adhesive restoration	In theory, an adhesive restoration would cement the crack and prevent movement of the two fragments. However, on curing, adhesive materials undergo polymerization shrinkage, which places further stress on the crack and may propagate it further. Modern adhesive restorative materials undergo significantly less shrinkage, so this option may be indicated.
Porcelain inlay/onlay	These have the same disadvantages of metal-fused-to-porcelain crowns.

◆ Suppose You Had Been Unable To Identify the Causative Tooth By Using the Methods Described Above. What Would You Try Next?

Sometimes, it is difficult to identify a crack. The pain is poorly localized, and the first step would be to repeat the whole procedure on the upper molars and premolars in case the patient has incorrectly localized the pain.

If no crack is identified, the restorations must be removed from other teeth that appear to be likely causes. Finally, the most suspect tooth may have a tight-fitting copper band or orthodontic band cemented around it. This can be left in situ for several weeks to see whether the pain is abolished and is a particularly useful test when the pain is felt infrequently. If the pain is persistent after 3–4 weeks, root canal treatment may be indicated, as suggested in the 2008 guidelines from the American Association of Endodontology; cuspal coverage with a cast restoration is then indicated, followed by a 1-year clinical and radiographic review (periapical radiography).

Case 12

CAD/CAM Fixed Prosthodontics

RUPERT AUSTIN AND DEBORAH BOMFIM

Summary

A 38-year-old man presents with a missing anterior tooth. Discuss the fixed prosthodontic management options, including the role of CAD/CAM (computer-aided design/computer-aided manufacturing) in providing indirect restorative options in this case.

Complaint

The presenting patient complains of a missing front tooth, which he felt was impacting on his ability to smile and speak confidently.

History of Complaint

The patient reports having been punched in the face 6 months ago during a fight, resulting in the fracturing of the entire crown of his upper right central incisor. The patient attended a hospital's accident and emergency department at the time, and there, it was confirmed that there were no head or maxillo-facial injuries. However, the patient also sustained injuries to his adjacent teeth and, therefore, underwent root canal treatment of the left maxillary central incisor in an emergency dental clinic. He was advised to follow up with a local dentist; however, as the affected teeth were asymptomatic, he did not seek treatment sooner.

Dental History

The patient was previously a regular attender before he moved to your area 2 years ago and has only recently managed to see a dentist. He appears motivated to improve his oral health and would prefer a fixed option for replacing the missing tooth. Five years ago, while abroad, he suffered a trauma, which resulted in crown fractures of his mandibular central incisors; his injured teeth were crowned in a practice there, and he has not had any issues since.

Medical History

The patient is fit and well. He has been smoking filtered roll-ups, 20 a day, for over 20 years. He also reports increased alcohol consumption: 25–35 units per week.

Examination

Extraoral Examination

No submandibular or cervical lymph nodes are palpable. The muscles of mastication are not tender to palpation, and the temporomandibular joints (TMJs) are normal.

Intraoral Examination

The patient has an extensively restored dentition, and there are clinically evident broken teeth, carious lesions and generalized discoloration/staining. As shown in Fig. 12.1, the maxillary right central incisor crown is missing. However, there is a root palpable in the labial sulcus. The root-filled maxillary left central incisor has an enamel–dentine crown fracture, with no mobility or tenderness. The mandibular central incisors have been restored with linked single crowns, and the mandibular right lateral incisor is missing, space closed. The mandibular right first molar has lost a restoration and is severely broken, with evident caries (Fig. 12.2). The general condition of the patient's teeth shows heavy staining and presence of generalized moderate tooth wear, consistent with the appearance of attrition, erosion and abrasion in combination. The gingival tissues are inflamed and erythematous, with generalized supra- and subgingival plaque and deposits. The generalized pocket probing depths range between 2 and 4 mm.

Investigations

◆ What Investigations Would You Carry Out?

See Table 12.1 and Fig. 12.3.

Diagnosis

◆ What are Your Provisional Diagnoses?

- Generalized gingivitis
- Generalized moderate tooth wear, consistent in appearance with erosion, abrasion and attrition, noncarious bucco-cervical lesions – UL6,5,4/UR5/LL5,6
- Generalized tooth discoloration/staining
- Caries – UL7 MO/LR6/UL5/UR4
- Retained root – UR1
- Nonvital UR2, with associated chronic apical periodontitis

- Crown fracture – UL1/UL2/LR6
- Asymptomatic chronic apical periodontitis/granuloma – LL1.

Treatment

◆ What is the Priority in the Management of This Case Before a Fixed Restoration Can Be Provided to Replace the Missing Anterior Tooth?

Reduction of the risk factors for primary disease (i.e. caries, periodontal disease, erosive tooth wear and oral cancer) to control the primary disease and reduce the risk factors for recurrence. Provide the following education to the patient:

- High caries susceptibility
  - Brush twice daily, with a prescribed 5000 parts per million (ppm) fluoride toothpaste.
  - Brush last thing at night and at least on one other occasion.
  - Spit, and do not rinse after brushing.

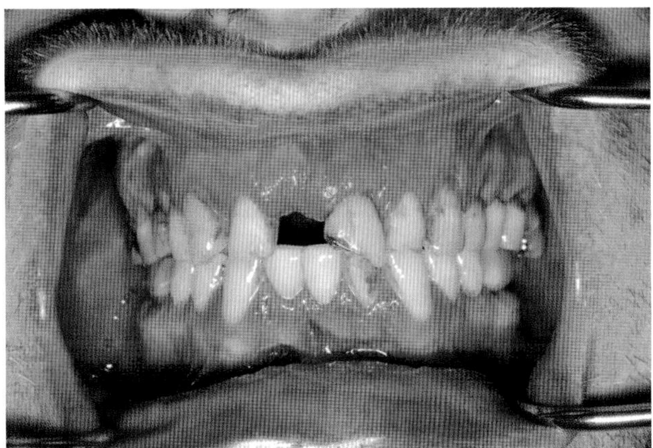

• **Fig. 12.1** Anterior view of patient's dentition in maximum intercuspation at presentation.

  - Investigate diet and patient adherence to advice given
  - Use fluoride mouth rinse (0.05% sodium fluoride [NaF]) at a time different to brushing.
  - Follow oral hygiene advice regarding careful interproximal cleaning.
- Mild periodontal disease susceptibility
  - Remove plaque effectively as shown by the oral healthcare team.
  - Brush gum line and each tooth twice a day.
  - Use a powered brush, with small tooth brush head, medium texture.
  - Follow advice regarding interdental plaque control (flossing and use of interdental brushes).
- Moderate erosive tooth wear susceptibility
  - Undergo oral hygiene and dietary assessment, and follow advice regarding routine maintenance and observation.
- Moderate oral cancer susceptibility
  - Follow smoking cessation advice and referral to a smoking cessation team if considering quitting.
  - Reduce alcohol consumption to no more than 14 units a week.

Following a prevention and stabilization phase, the plaque scores reduced to 12%, and the periodontal condition improved. The patient sought treatment for gastro-oesophageal reflux and reduced the frequency of intake of cariogenic and erosive foods and drinks. All carious lesions were stabilized with resin composite restorations (the early lesions evident radiographically – UL5 – were managed with nonoperative prevention, as outlined above), and endodontic treatment of the upper right lateral incisor was provided successfully. An Every-type provisional partial denture was provided, and on reassessment, the patient was considered a suitable candidate for a fixed prosthodontic solution to replace the missing upper right central incisor.

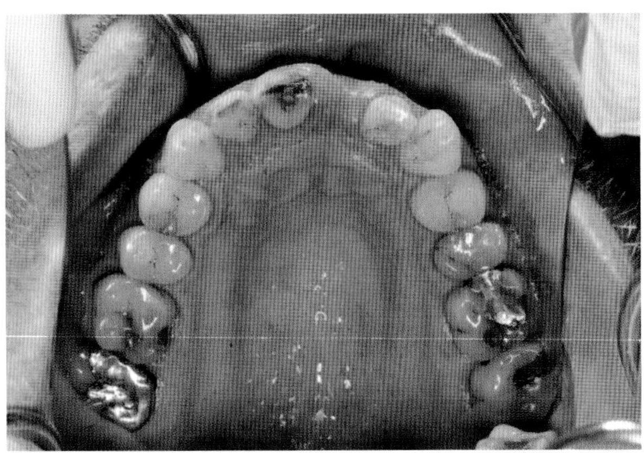

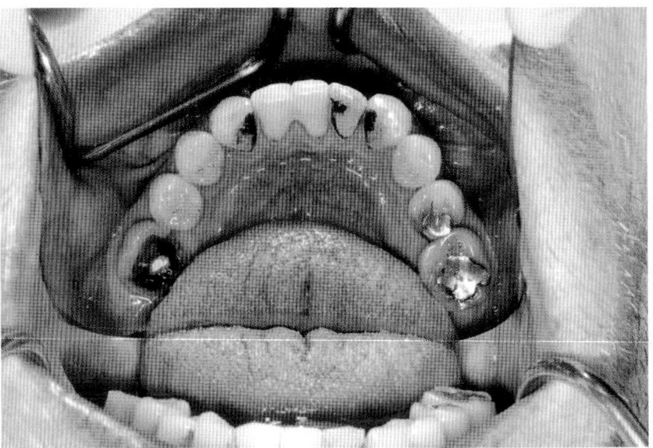

• **Fig. 12.2** Clinical intraoral photographs showing the occlusal views of **(a)** the maxillary and **(b)** the mandibular dentition.

TABLE 12.1 **Investigations To Be Carried Out, Justification of Investigation and Outcome in This Case**

Investigation	Reason	Outcome
Plaque and bleeding scores	To ascertain the level of supragingival plaque control. Ideally no fixed prosthodontic restorations should be provided until the plaque and bleeding scores are below 10% signifying good plaque control and periodontal health.	Initial plaque score was 76% and bleeding score 66%.
Diet analysis and advice	The patient is showing signs of erosive tooth wear; therefore, it is important to ascertain the correct cause of this, especially in terms of dietary acids.	The patient does not frequently consume dietary acids and does experience symptoms of heartburn and indigestion, for which he is willing to visit his general medical practitioner for investigations and treatment for possible gastroesophageal reflux disease.
Sensibility testing	All heavily restored and traumatized teeth require sensibility testing to establish if there is any pulp involvement.	All teeth respond normally to electric pulp and thermal testing, except for the upper right lateral incisor.
Clinical photographs and study casts (either digital or conventional)	Clinical photographs record the baseline shade and colour of teeth and enable a digital smile design to simulate the replacement and restoration of teeth in the aesthetic zone. Also useful for dento-legal purposes as a baseline record on presentation. Study casts record the occlusion and provide a baseline for future assessment of tooth wear as well as provide diagnostic wax-ups. An alternative to conventional gypsum study casts would be intraoral scans for a digital wax-up and three-dimensional (3D) printed resin models.	As shown in Figs 12.1 and 12.2 below, the dentition displayed generalized extrinsic staining (most likely nicotine related) and the baseline shade was A4. The digital smile design is shown in Fig. 12.4 below. Study casts show generalized faceting consistent in appearance with attrition possibly as a result of parafunctional bruxism.
Long cone periapical radiographs and bitewing radiographs of all teeth with restorations	To detect carious lesions, assess bone levels and to determine if there is any pulp/periapical pathology as well as the quality of any existing endodontic treatments. To determine the pulp canal morphology in case root canal (re-) treatment is required or the root morphology, in case extraction is necessary.	As shown in Fig. 12.3 below: Caries – caries associated with restorations/sealants (CARS – recurrent caries): UL7 MO; caries LR6, UR4 MO, DO; early lesions UL5 • Overhanging restoration – UR6 • Retained root – UR1 • Generalized mild horizontal bone loss – UR2, with periapical radiolucency with loss of lamina dura • Root canal fillings – UR5, UL1, LR1 and LL1 of reasonable taper, condensation and length and no signs of associated periapical pathology, except for the lower left central incisor which has a well-defined radiolucency and loss of lamina dura

◆ What are the Definitive Replacement Options for the Missing UR1?

A conventional cantilever bridge, with use of the central incisor as the abutment, is a possibility. Minimal preparation bridgework is not an option here because the central incisor is fractured (thus reducing the surface area of enamel for bonding), and both potential abutments are root filled. A minimal-preparation adhesive bridge, with use of the lateral incisor as the abutment, to replace the central incisor is generally contraindicated because of the reduced enamel surface area palatally for bonding, as well as the presence of generalized faceting and attritional wear, suggesting possible parafunctional bruxism.

A conventional fixed–fixed bridge, with use of the upper left central incisor and the upper right lateral incisor, is a more predictable option. Clinical research evidence supports greater longevity for conventional fixed–fixed bridgework in comparison with conventional (or minimal-preparation) cantilever bridge work. Additionally, because the patient has a history of both repeated dental trauma and parafunctional activity, a fixed–fixed bridge design is likely to be more robust and provide a predictable and maintainable outcome. Using endodontically treated teeth as bridge abutments is less ideal. However, in this case, there was evidence that the endodontic treatment has been successful, and because the teeth were already restored, there

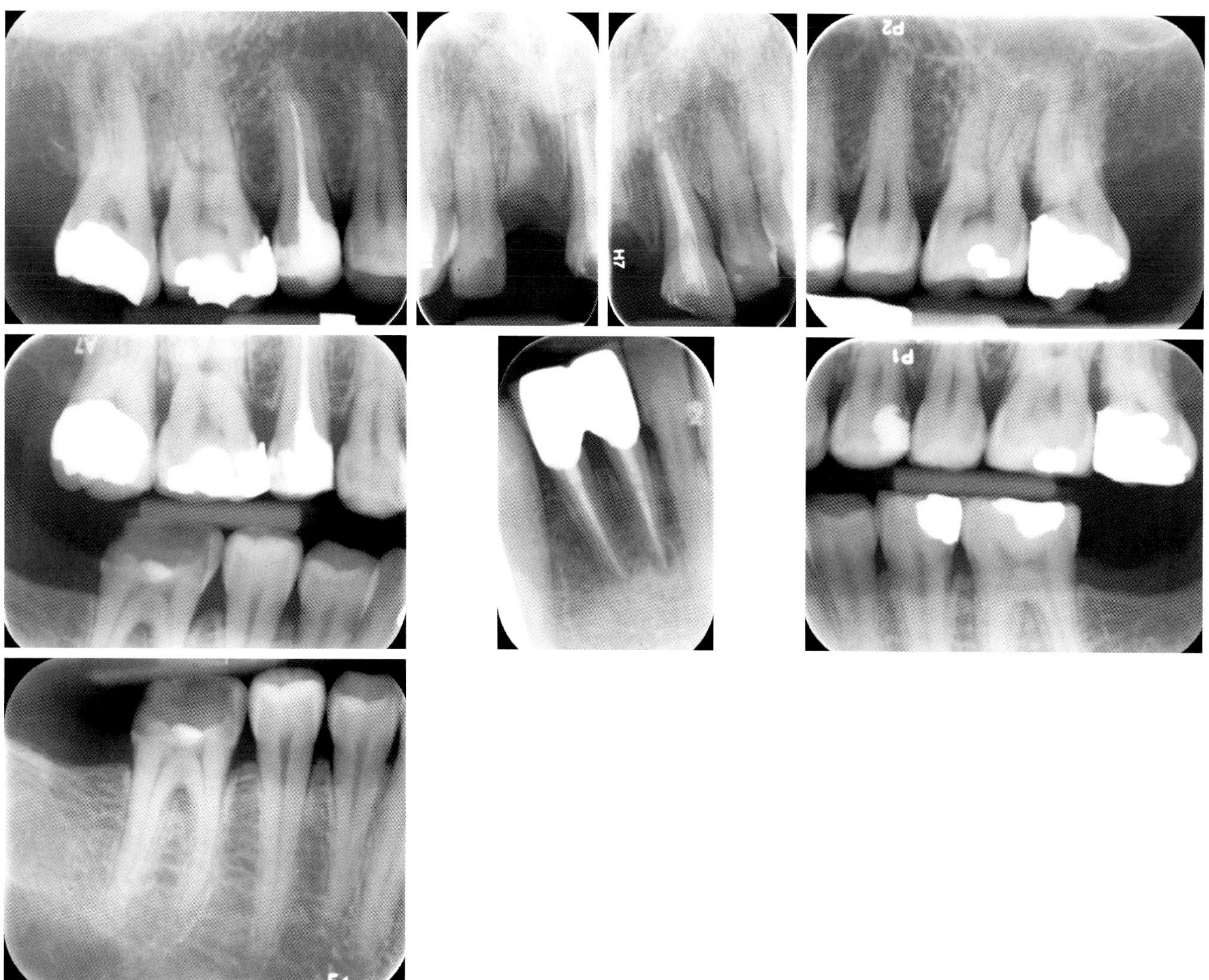

• **Fig. 12.3** Intraoral radiographs (long cone periapicals and bitewings) of teeth on presentation.

would be less removal of natural sound tooth structure, justifying the more invasive restorative option in this case.

A single tooth implant–retained crown is the alternative option; however, the patient would need to stop smoking, and the retained root would need to be removed. The patient expressed an interest in implants; however, he was not interested in stopping smoking. Therefore, the root was left in situ for the time being, to preserve alveolar bone and ridge morphology and, thus, facilitating future implant therapy.

After additional diagnostic and care planning, the definitive restorative care included provision of direct resin composite restorations to recontour the buccal aspect of the maxillary canines, an indirect lithium disilicate veneer restoring UL2 and a conventional fixed–fixed conventional metal–ceramic bridge to replace the missing UR1 by using full coverage crown retainers on the UL1 and UR2 abutments. A fully digital workflow was followed, with use of intraoral scanning and CAD-CAM for design and construction of both the provisional and definitive restorations.

◆ What are the Potential Benefits of a Digital Workflow for Each of the Clinical Stages Involved in the Provision of Indirect Fixed Prosthodontics in This Case?

See Table 12.2 and Figs 12.4–12.7.

◆ What is the Step-by-Step Digital Workflow Using CAD/CAM to Design and Manufacture Restorations?

1. Full face and intraoral digital photography and shade taking, digital smile design
2. Preoperative intraoral scans, three-dimensional (3D) diagnostic wax-up guided by digital smile design
3. Printing of 3D design and construction of vacuum-formed or silicone indices for preparation guides and chairside provisional restorations
4. Intraoral scan of prepared teeth, intraoral scan of the opposing teeth and intraoral scan of the dentition in occlusion; assessment of preparations and interocclusal space to ensure that there is sufficient space for the restorations
5. CAD of the provisional restorations
   a. Marking margins of restorations
   b. Superimposition of preoperative scan onto prep scan

TABLE 12.2 Benefits of CAD-CAM in the Stages of Prosthodontic Rehabilitation of This Case

Stage	Reason	Role of CAD/CAM
Study casts, diagnostic wax-up and smile design	To ensure that the anterior guidance is distributed evenly, a wax-up on a semiadjustable articulator is essential when providing multiple anterior restorations. In this case, the upper left lateral incisor was also planned to receive a veneer to restore aesthetics and provide even anterior guidance in protrusion. A digital smile design can help with visualizing the result of restoring teeth in the aesthetic zone.	Intraoral scanning and virtual articulation can allow for digital analysis of the occlusion, including transfer of a facebow record and three-dimensional (3D) facial scanning into the software. A digital smile design can be used to analyze the aesthetic zone and plan the optimal height/width ratio and shape/size of new anterior restorations, as shown in Fig. 12.4. This two-dimensional (2D) digital smile design can then be superimposed onto a 3D digital diagnostic wax-up to design the optimal aesthetics and function of the restorations. 3D resin models can then be printed to provide an index for a preparation guide and to fabricate a chairside provisional restoration.
Tooth preparation	Appropriate preparation is required for either all-ceramic restorations or metal–ceramic restorations. An index of the diagnostic wax-up can construct a bis-acryl provisional restoration, which can also be checked prior to refining the preparations. For a fixed–fixed bridge, the preparations need to have a common path of insertion to allow the bridge to be seated. Once the preparations have been optimized and the chairside temporary constructed, an impression can be taken for a laboratory-made provisional restoration.	During the preparations, intraoral scans of the prepared teeth can be examined to determine if the preparations are optimal, as shown in Fig. 12.5. This allows for digital measurement of the tooth reductions while the patient is still in the dental chair and guide further refinement of the preparations, where indicated by the software. When preparing fixed–fixed bridgework, the path of the insertion of the preparations can be assessed as shown in Fig. 12.5b and any undercut quickly removed.
Design and manufacture of provisional restorations	Providing well-made provisional restorations are important when restoring multiple anterior teeth. These are usually laboratory made from composite or acrylic resin so that they can be adjusted to optimize aesthetics, phonetics and occlusion. An impression of the provisional restorations in situ can be used to guide the design of the definitive restorations.	Intraoral scanning and chairside CAD software can allow same-visit in-surgery milling of provisional (composite or acrylic resin) or definitive (lithium disilicate ceramic) bridgework during a single visit. This saves time and provides clinicians with greater control over the design. The diagnostic wax-up can be scanned prior to tooth preparation to superimpose the design onto the scan of the prepared teeth (Fig. 12.6) to construct provisional restorations (Fig. 12.7)
Design and manufacture of definitive restorations	The options of material for the definitive restoration are either metal–ceramic (conventional manufacture) or all-ceramic restorations (pressed or CAD/CAM). All-ceramic restorations can be milled by using CAD/CAM or pressed by using a lost-wax technique; however, they require more preparation and smooth, rounded transition lines. Metal–ceramic restorations have greater longevity, more conservative preparation, narrower connectors that are more aesthetic and more strength compared with ceramic.	Intraoral scanning allows the clinician to ensure that the preparations are suitable for an all ceramic restoration. All-ceramic restorations can be designed and milled in a single visit; however, there are special design considerations, especially with regard to material thickness (1.5+ mm), margin (shoulder), preparation shape (rounded and smooth) and finally connector thickness (less than 9 mm^2 anteriorly and 15 mm^2 posteriorly). As shown in Fig. 12.6, intraoral scanning of the provisional restorations aids in the design of the definitive restorations.
Maintenance of restorations	A stable and maintainable long-term outcome depends on prevention of wear of teeth and restorations and periodontal disease and caries. Once the final restorations have been fitted, impressions or scans can record the final occlusion, allow for construction of occlusal guard and provide a baseline for future assessment of tooth wear.	Intraoral scans of the fitted definitive restorations can be a useful reference for future comparison, especially with regard to future tooth wear. Wearing a hard occlusal mouthguard will protect teeth and restorations from wear.

CAD/CAM, computer-aided design/computer-aided manufacturing.

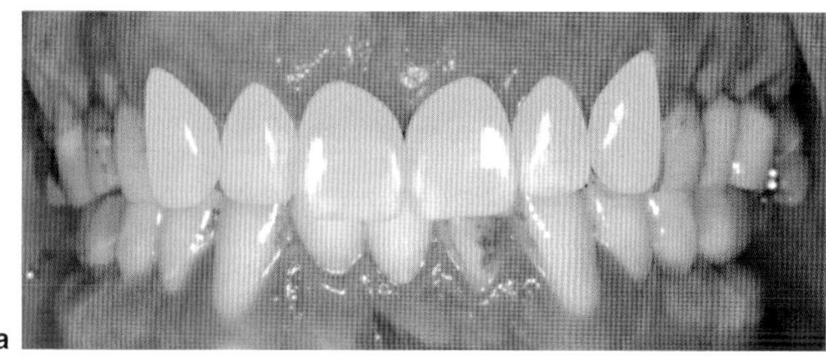

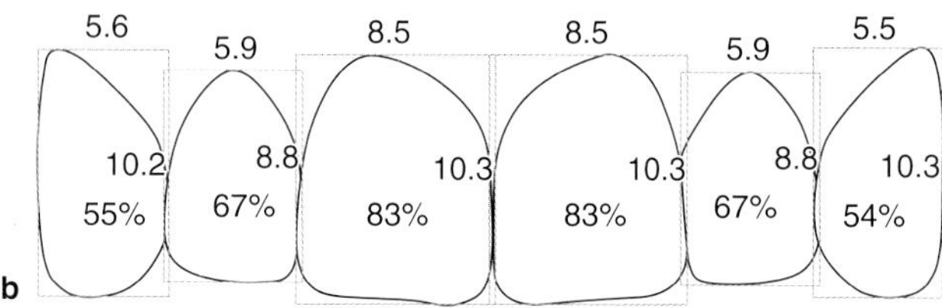

• **Fig. 12.4** Digital smile design showing proposed aesthetic outcome of the restorations and smile design silhouette showing the gingival line/contour, golden proportion height to width ratios (%) and width of teeth (mm).

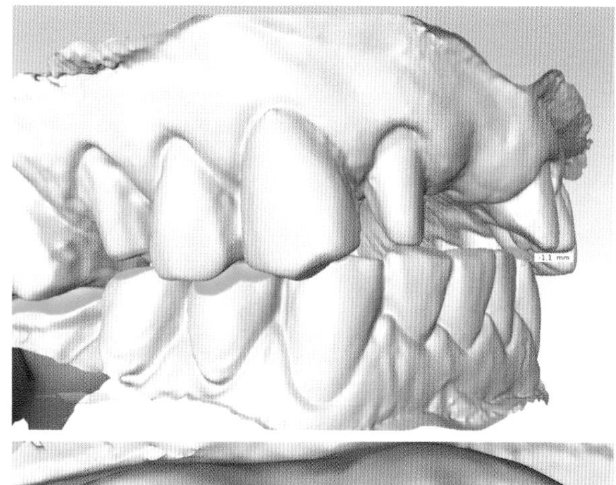

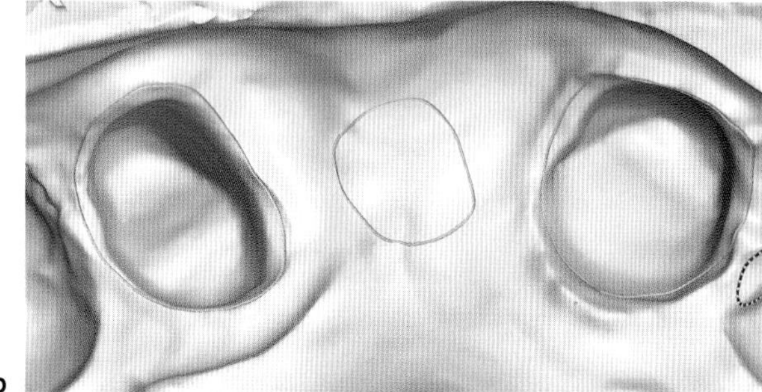

• **Fig. 12.5 a,** Articulated intraoral scans of the preparations showing adequate 1.1 mm of interocclusal space, which is sufficient for metal occlusal surface of the restorations. **b,** Assessing the parallelism of the preparations. Marking the margin of the restorations (including the pontic), as shown in blue, helps identify any undercut. Note the undercut of UL1, where more buccal preparation will be required, and UR2 disto-palatally, where more preparation will be required.

   c. Designing restorations, including designing connector that links pontic to retainers if a bridge is being constructed
6. CAM of the provisional restorations using a chairside mill
   a. Selection of the appropriate CAD/CAM material block size and shade

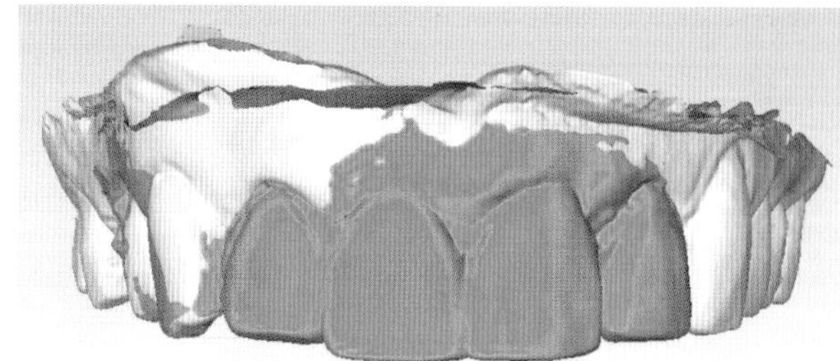

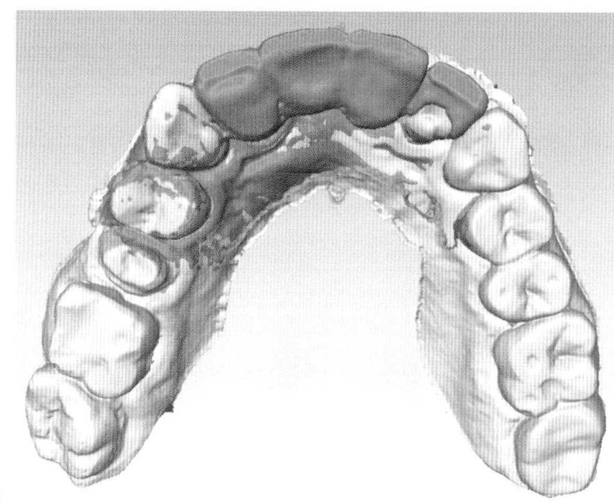

• **Fig. 12.6** Computer-aided design (CAD) of the provisional restorations. Superimposition of the scan of the diagnostic wax-up (orange) onto the intraoral scan of the prepared teeth (white) for construction of same-visit chairside CAD/CAM indirect provisional restorations.

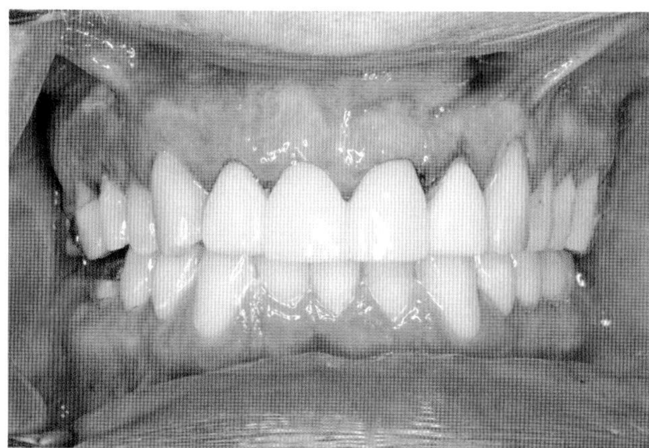

• **Fig. 12.7** Chairside milled provisional restorations fitted on the same day as the preparation.

   b. Positioning sprue position in thickest portion of restoration away from interproximal contacts
   c. Sending design to mill, loading block and closing mill to start milling
   d. Chairside milling of restoration
   e. Removal of block and separation of milled restoration from remainder of block by sectioning sprue
7. Intraoral try-in of restorations, checking aesthetics, occlusion, contact points and margin
8. Finishing and polishing restoration, which may involve placing milled restorations in a furnace to crystallize, if

TABLE 12.3 Key Features of Intraoral Scanning Systems

Optical Principles	Light Source	Imaging Type	≈ Weight of Wand	≈ Wand Tip Dimensions	Powder
Video Scanning Technology	Pulsating blue light	3D video	≈ 200 g	14.4 × 16.2 mm	Light powdering required to facilitate image stitching
Laser Scanning Technology	Red or blue Laser	Still images	≈ 280 g up to 1.5 kg	16 × 16 mm up to 30 × 23 mm	Not required

3D, three-dimensional.

milled in a partially crystallized state (This is especially the case if using lithium disilicate ceramic restorations, which are milled in their partially crystallized state and then firing in the furnace converts the material from lithium metasilicate crystals [Li_2SiO_3] to lithium disilicate crystals [$Li_2Si_2O_5$], which has a higher flexural strength once fully crystallized.)

9. Checking final fit of restoration
10. Adhesive cementation of restoration
11. Immediate postoperative periapical radiographs scans and photographs and construction of hard occlusal splints
12. Follow-up examinations, imaging and radiography.

An intraoral scanner is a device to acquire digital impressions of teeth, soft tissues and occlusion. Intraoral scanners utilize optical principles such as stereoscopic photogrammetry or laser scanning to acquire thousands of individual images, which are stitched together to generate a 3D model of the entire arch.

◆ What are the Key Features of Intraoral Scanners (Table 12.3)?

All scanners comprise an acquisition device (scanner), hardware (laptop or tablet) and software (scanning only or scanning and chairside CAD-CAM). Some scanners are also linked to chairside CAD/CAM software or other software, including implant planning and surgical guide design, digital smile design, orthodontic planning software and removable partial denture design software. In addition, scanners can be linked to chairside mills for single-visit restorations, or scans can be sent to the laboratory for conventional indirect design and fabrication of restorations.

All intraoral scanners apply an optical pattern to the tooth, so the scanner can trace its contours. There are two main ways to apply these patterns: video scanning technology and laser scanning technology. Video scanning requires a powder to apply a pattern to the tooth, whereas the laser scanning pattern originates from a laser beam projected on the tooth surface. By using a scanning powder spray, the pattern on the tooth is fixed, providing more consistently accurate scans compared with those from laser scanners. This technology is similar to that used by 'motion capture' movie effects; however, it does require application of an optically active powder to the teeth, and this is an additional process that affects the ability to overlay high-resolution true colour images for shade matching and improved margin marking detail.

◆ How Do Digital Intraoral Scans Compare with Conventional Impressions?

Table 12.4 below lists the main applications of intraoral scanning in comparison with conventional impressions:

The main advantages in comparison with conventional impressions include the following:

- Ability to link to a chairside CAD/CAM system for single-visit restorations
- Patient preference because of no taste, smell or gagging sensation
- Ease of telemedicine by transferring the files to any laboratory worldwide instantaneously
- Improved patient communication because patients can observe and appreciate the scan and design and manufacture of the restorations
- In a model-free workflow, environmental benefits because there is no need for disposal of conventional impressions, chemical disinfectants, gypsum models and casting investment materials
- Ability to save intraoral scans indefinitely, with no need for physical storage, thus assisting future recall and comparison.

The main disadvantages in comparison with conventional impressions include the following:

- Because of the optical stitching processes, artefacts can arise and can result in inferior full arch accuracy in comparison with a printed model of the intraoral scan.
- Because of the limitations of the milling process, preparations may need to be reduced more than cast restorations, to compensate for the limitations of the dimensions of the burs needed to mill the restoration.
- CAD/CAM materials are usually constructed from monochromatic blocks; therefore, the aesthetics of the milled CAD/CAM materials can be less than those of pressed or hand-layered ceramics.

TABLE 12.4 The Main Applications of Intraoral Scanning in Comparison with Conventional Impressions

	Digital Intraoral Scans		Conventional Impressions
Single-unit crowns	Chairside design and milling of CAD ceramic, acrylic, hybrid composite-ceramic restorations	Laboratory manufacture of pressed ceramic, metal ceramic and all-metal restorations	All laboratory CAD/CAM options via laboratory scanning Conventional analogue options
2–4 unit bridges	Chairside design and milling of CAD ceramic, acrylic, hybrid composite-ceramic restorations	Laboratory manufacture of pressed ceramic, metal ceramic and all-metal restorations	All laboratory CAD/CAM options via laboratory scanning Conventional analogue options
Long-span fixed restorations	Contraindicated because of issues with full arch accuracy of intraoral scanning		All laboratory CAD/CAM options via laboratory scanning
Removable prostheses	Tooth and tissue supported prostheses for bounded saddles only		Mucosa-borne complete and extensive partial dentures with free-end saddles
Implant impressions	Single unit restorations and removable prostheses supported by nonlinked implants only Multiple crown units, small- and large-span bridgework contraindicated because of issues with full arch accuracy of intraoral scanning		Single and multiple crown units, small span and full arch bridgework, removable implant prostheses
Orthodontic planning	Digital Kesling set-up and virtual orthodontic movements for clear aligners		Conventional case assessment and planning or digital planning via laboratory scanning
Study and master cast production	Stereolithography/3D printing		Gypsum cast production
Articulation	Digital facebows and articulation		Conventional physical mounting of casts and articulation

3D, three-dimensional; *CAD/CAM,* computer-aided design/computer-aided manufacturing.

- As the scans can be retained indefinitely, clinicians may need to consider the possibility of future medico-legal claims; for example, claims regarding crown and bridgework may result in the preparations being analyzed for possible flaws or inadequacies in the tooth preparations, diagnosis and care planning.

◆ Are There Any Medico-Legal Issues with Intraoral Scanning and Chairside CAD/CAM and Any Guidelines That Can Help Guide Their Adoption?

As with adoption of all new technologies, detailed training, knowledge of the properties and safe handling and strict adherence to the manufacturer's instructions are recommended. In addition, careful case selection is essential to ensure that the right treatment methodology is selected for the right patient. This is especially the case with technology with high capital costs, where clinicians may be tempted to prescribe more indirect restorations to amortize the cost of the equipment. Minimally invasive protocols must still be followed and direct restorations conserving tooth structure prescribed, where appropriate.

In addition, the manufacturer's instructions and guidelines need to be followed when preparing CAD/CAM restorations. All-ceramic restorations require specific preparation depths and cementation protocols, and not following them may lead to premature facture or decementation of the restoration. Intraoral scanning makes this medico-legally more difficult to defend because the intraoral scan can be analyzed precisely for the correct preparation features. This may result in more challenging medico-legal scenarios, especially because the cost of these types of restorations can be higher than that of conventional restorations.

Intraoral scans can also be used diagnostically to analyze and record occlusion, aesthetics, restoration integrity and tooth wear. As with all diagnostic processes, medico-legal issues can be raised as a result of underdiagnosis, where issues apparent on scans were not picked up as soon as they should be, or because scans were used to overprescribe invasive treatments, for example, providing multiple indirect restorations in cases of minor nonprogressing tooth wear. Therefore, when adopting digital CAD/CAM technology, it is important to follow existing good practice guidance and, when in doubt, to seek second opinions and specialist expert advice to ensure that the technology is used optimally in the patient's best interests.

Case 13
Sudden Collapse

EMILY SHERWIN

Summary

A 55-year-old male patient suddenly collapses in your general dental practice. What is the cause, and what would you do?

History

Complaint

The patient has attended for a routine dental appointment to receive some simple restorative work under local anaesthesia. He is a regular attender but dislikes injections.

Twenty minutes after injection of the local anaesthetic, he suddenly becomes anxious and complains of a pain in his chest. He is breathless. When your nurse asks the patient if he is all right, there is no response.

Medical History

Having checked the medical history before starting treatment, you are aware that the patient has well-controlled diabetes. He is overweight and suffers from hypertension, for which he takes enalapril (Innovace) 20 mg daily. He smokes 20 cigarettes a day and describes himself as a 'social drinker', consuming 30 units of alcohol each week.

◆ What Would You Do Immediately?

Check to see whether the patient is conscious. Make a determined effort to rouse him by shaking him and asking loudly, in both ears, whether he can hear you.

◆ The Patient Does Not Respond. What Causes of Sudden Loss of Consciousness Might Affect a Patient Undergoing Dental Treatment?

The important causes of unexpected loss of consciousness are:

- vasovagal attack (faint)
- hypoglycaemia
- cardiac arrest
- steroid crisis.

Loss of consciousness may also follow several other emergencies, including respiratory obstruction or respiratory failure, epilepsy, stroke or anaphylactic shock, in which the cause is likely to be evident.

◆ How May These Causes of Loss of Consciousness Be Differentiated?

See Table 13.1 for common causes of loss of consciousness and the different associated signs and symptoms.

◆ Which is the Most Likely Cause in This Case? Why?

In this case, the cause is very likely to be cardiac arrest. The symptom of pain in the chest radiating to the neck and arm is characteristic of myocardial infarction, the commonest cause of cardiac arrest, and is not seen in the other causes of collapse. Diabetes, hypertension and a high alcohol intake are all risk factors for atheromatous arterial disease and its complication myocardial infarction.

◆ Does Cardiac Arrest Always Follow Myocardial Infarction?

No. The heart may continue to pump unless a large area of the myocardium or conducting tissue is damaged. Cardiac arrest may also follow hypoxia or respiratory obstruction.

◆ How Will You Confirm Your Provisional Diagnosis?

For a diagnosis of cardiac arrest the patient must be:

- unconscious
- not breathing or have abnormal breathing (infrequent noisy gasps).

Examination

You place a hand on the patient's forehead. His skin feels cold and clammy. Even though it is only half a minute since he lost consciousness, the patient already looks grey and he is beginning to look cyanosed. He is not breathing.

◆ What is the Current Protocol for Assessing and Managing Sudden Collapse?

It is critically important to start Basic Life Support (BLS) procedures immediately without further consideration of possible causes. The current 2015 Resuscitation Council guidelines (Resuscitation Council (UK) (2015)) for adult basic life support (https://www.resus.org.uk/resuscitation-guidelines/adult-basic-life-support-and-automated-external-defibrillation/)

TABLE 13.1 Causes, Signs and Symptoms of Loss of Consciousness

Cause	Signs and Symptoms
Vasovagal attack (faint)	Often associated with anxiety. Usually, although not always, some premonitory symptoms of faintness before losing consciousness. Cold clammy skin, pallor, initially bradycardia and low pulse volume followed by tachycardia and a full pulse. Rapid recovery on placing supine or slightly head down (maximum recommended inclination 10 degrees).
Hypoglycaemia	Seen in starved patients or those with diabetes experiencing relative insulin overdose caused by starvation or stress. Rapid recovery on administering oral glucose or, if unconscious, glucagon followed by oral glucose on regaining consciousness.
Steroid crisis	Seen in patients taking systemic steroids in relative insufficiency as a result of stress.
Cardiac arrest	No central pulse. Usually, history of angina, coronary arterial disease, hypertension or other risk factors.

for the management of respiratory and/or cardiac arrest in an adult are:

1. Check the area for danger to yourself and victim
2. Assess responsiveness by shaking shoulders and shouting
3. Shout for help (do not call 999 (UK) yet)
4. Open the airway (tilt head and lift chin or jaw thrust)
5. Check mouth for vomit/debris, and remove with finger scoops
6. Assess breathing – listen and feel for breathing while observing chest movements. Take no more than 10 seconds
7. If breathing is abnormal (infrequent noisy gasps) or absent, call emergency service on 999; you may have to leave the patient to do this
8. Perform 30 chest compressions of 5–6 cm at 100–120 per minute; correct hand position is the middle of the lower half of the sternum
9. Give two ventilations with airway adjuncts such as a pocket mask
10. Send for an automated external defibrillator; as soon as it arrives, switch it on, and follow instructions
11. Continue compressions (30) and ventilations (2) until help arrives, the patient shows signs of life or until you are physically exhausted and unable to carry on.

◆ What are Basic, Immediate and Advanced Life Support?

Basic Life Support (BLS) is the diagnosis and immediate management of cardiac arrest (of whatever aetiology) with the use of basic equipment. Dental teams should have immediate access to airway adjuncts such as a pocket mask or two-person self-inflating bag-valve-mask, which avoids the need for mouth-to-mouth ventilation. BLS represents the minimum standard of resuscitation skills that all dentists, dental hygienists and dental nurses must acquire and maintain on a regular basis.

Immediate Life Support (ILS) includes the recognition and treatment of an unwell patient by using the systematic approach of ABCDE (Airway, Breathing, Circulation, Disability and Exposure) to prevent cardiac arrest along with immediate cardiopulmonary resuscitation and defibrillation as required.

Advanced Life Support (ALS) is concerned with the restoration of spontaneous circulation and stabilization of the cardiovascular system. Techniques include electrocardiography (ECG) assessment of shockable and nonshockable rhythms, administration of drugs, treatment of underlying causes and postresuscitation care.

◆ What is the Aim of Basic Life Support?

To protect the brain from irreversible hypoxic damage. This develops within 3–4 minutes of cardiac arrest in a previously healthy and well-oxygenated individual, and BLS aims to delay the rate of deterioration of cerebral function. Effective and continuous chest compressions along with early defibrillation increase the chances of survival.

◆ Why Not Dial '999' in the UK As Soon As the Patient Loses Consciousness?

The most common cause of sudden loss of consciousness in the dental chair is a vasovagal attack (faint), which does not require attendance by the emergency services. The call for help in step 3 is intended to summon local helpers such as dental nurses or receptionist.

◆ What is the Most Common Cause of Failure or Difficulty with BLS?

Airway obstruction in the unconscious patient is the commonest problem and is usually caused by the relaxed tongue falling back to obliterate the airway in the oropharynx. This may be overcome by measures that pull the tongue forward, such as head tilt, chin lift and jaw thrust. Blood, vomit or other foreign materials, including poorly fitting or broken dentures, may also obstruct the airway.

◆ Should Dentures Be Removed During BLS?

Only if they are loose or broken. Well-fitting dentures usually facilitate a good oral seal during expired air ventilation.

◆ Having Dialled 999, What Information Should Your Helper Give the Operator?

- Your name
- Address (with directions)
- Your telephone number
- That a patient has collapsed with a suspected cardiac arrest.

Although this sounds simple, hurried calls may omit essential information. Response to cardiac arrest is usually provided at highest priority by a specialized team and is not a routine ambulance call. Failure to provide your telephone number leaves the emergency services unable to return your call.

Prognosis

◆ Is It Likely That Your Patient Will Recover Spontaneously?

Unfortunately, no. Even with prompt life support from a specialist team, the chances of survival are 50%. In this case, the patient recovered after ALS care provided by a specialist ambulance team that arrived at the practice 8 minutes after the 999 call was placed – a very rapid response.

◆ How Long Would You Continue To Provide BLS?

Until help arrives, the patient shows signs of life or you are exhausted.

◆ How Can You Increase Your Chances of Providing Effective Basic Life Support?

By regular practical instruction and testing the competence of yourself and your practice team. BLS cannot be learned from a book.

◆ What are the Medico-Legal Considerations After Providing BLS?

Although the priority is to provide efficient life support and immediate care to the unconscious patient, it is also important to document the events that took place as soon as possible. This should include a timeline detailing observations and vital signs, treatment provided and any drugs administered. Having accurate records are important because further investigation into the incident may be carried out.

Case 14
A Difficult Young Child

WENDY BELLIS

Summary

A mother brings her nervous 4-year-old daughter for treatment. How will you approach examining her and defining a treatment plan?

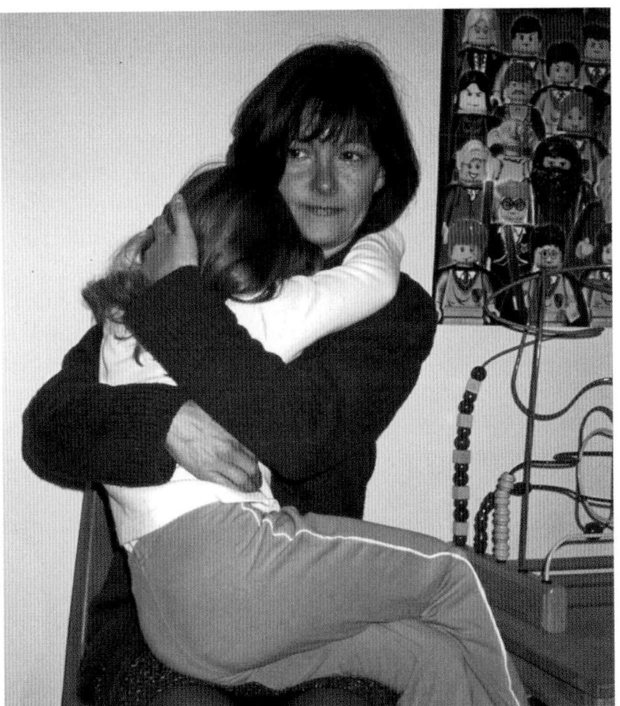

• **Fig. 14.1** The child and mother in your surgery.

History

The nurse in your practice shows the child and mother into the surgery. The child is clinging tightly to her mother and will not look at you or acknowledge you (Fig. 14.1).

Complaint

The child has no complaint, but her mother has noticed holes in the child's posterior teeth.

History of Complaint

The mother first noticed the holes 6 months ago, and there has never been any toothache.

Dental History

The child has never had a dental examination or treatment before. She was taken to another dentist but became hysterical in the waiting room and refused to go in. She is in your surgery only because she has been bribed with a chocolate bar.

Medical History

The child is fit and well.

◆ This is Not Looking Hopeful. What Must You Do Before You Can Attempt To Examine the Child?

You need to encourage the child to feel safe and engender feelings of trust. To do this, you must take the time to establish a rapport with the child. Without some form of rapport, little progress is possible.

◆ The Child Appears Frightened. What Fears Would You Expect in a 4-Year-Old in a Dental Setting?

A typical 4-year-old is usually scared of:

- the unknown
- pain
- new environments
- new people.

◆ What Further Questions Would You Ask, and Why?

Does the Child Attend a Nursery or Playgroup Full Time or Part Time? If So, for How Long Has She Attended? A child attending nursery should be more used to dealing with people outside her home and consequently have greater coping skills, be more socially developed and be used to being separated from the mother. The child should also understand the concept of rules that have to be followed. You can be more confident of successfully managing the behaviour of such a child.

How Does the Mother Feel About Going To the Dentist? Maternal anxiety is a strong influence on the young child's reaction to dentistry. If the mother is nervous at this appointment, the child will already have sensed this. Indeed, if the mother is severely anxious, it may be better to elect for another trusted adult to accompany the child. A mother who is herself very nervous may not be able to support you or her child later on if things get difficult.

How is the Child's Behaviour Away From the Dental Surgery? Here, you are trying to find out if the child is generally anxious or shy in other nondental situations such as going to see her medical practitioner or social situations. This would indicate a more generalized problem that will be more difficult for you to address.

As there are different parenting styles, it important to identify which approach is used in the family. Some parents adopt an authoritarian approach and others a permissive approach, depending on social and cultural factors. Both approaches can be a challenge to the successful dental management of any child.

The authoritative approach is the most desirable, in which the parent attempts to direct the child's activities in a rational, issue-oriented manner. It is known that dental stress tolerance and coping skills of children are best when the home environment is structured, parents are responsive and self-assured and parents set limits, providing both ample rewards and appropriate punishments.

Limit setting is considered good parenting practice. If the child is used to having limits set to her behaviour, she will be much easier to direct in the dental setting. In the case of an only child, the parents may lack experience. Others may lack role models or have their parenting strategies thwarted by relatives.

Is the Child Genuinely Nervous or Just Playing Up? Your strategies for managing fear, shyness and naughtiness would be very different. However, this is difficult to assess without observing the child's behaviour for some time and getting to know the child. You may not be able to make an immediate decision, and of course, it is quite possible that there are many contributing factors.

You discover that the patient is an only child. She has just started part-time nursery and has settled well there. The child is generally good at home, and like most children, she likes to have her own way. However, she responds well to direction and is not allowed to have her own way all the time. Her mother attends the dentist but is rather nervous about her child's treatment. From this, you can see that in addition to allaying the anxiety of both child and mother, you will also have to teach the child what behaviour is appropriate at the dentist's clinic.

◆ What Can the Average 4-Year-Old Child Be Expected To Do? How Does This Knowledge Help?

Some of the developmental milestones for a 4-year-old child are shown below.

MILESTONE
• Usually separates well from mother • Names four primary colours • Can state own age and address • Listens intently to stories • Understands turn-taking • Starts to understand concept of obeying rules • Washes and dries own hands • Understands yesterday, today and tomorrow, simple past and future • Blows nose reliably

Talking about these abilities with the mother allows you to develop a rapport with her and may alert you to any educational difficulties that the child may have. Not all parents are completely forthcoming about any problems with their child's development. You need to know if there are issues because your approach will be slower and more considered if the child has learning difficulties. Some children may be small or tall for their age, and hence appear younger or older. This child is tall for her age, and so it is important not to overestimate her ability to cope with the experience.

You discover that the child appears to have reached the normal developmental milestones for her age and is not usually anxious in other situations. You suspect, therefore, that shyness may be contributing to her behaviour, rather than fear.

◆ Now That You Have a Better Appreciation of the Background, How Will You Develop a Rapport with the Child?

Dispel Fear of the Unknown. Tell the child that all you want to do today is talk to her and her mother, count her teeth and check that 'mummy has brushed them properly'. Stress that you are going to do nothing else. Continually check back with the child to involve her, and ensure that she understands the limits of the planned dental experience.

Use Nonverbal Communication. Young children generally respond better to nonverbal communication, particularly touching and smiling. A pat or a stroke of the hand or hair is valued much more by a young child than a comment such as 'good girl' or 'well done'.

Be Aware of Body Language. Children are very sensitive to nonverbal communication. Watch the child, and be aware of your own body language. Are you being defensive, or are you welcoming and friendly?

Make Eye Contact. You may catch the child's attention while talking over the previous points with the parent and already be interacting with her in some way or other. If not, you must now direct all your attention to the child. Start with a compliment about the child's clothes, toys, hair or a similar topic, and catch her eye.

Talk To the Child in Appropriate Language. You must be able to converse at the level of a 4-year-old, and this takes knowledge and practice. Always use the child's first name and child-friendly language, and avoid potentially fear-promoting words. This is often called speaking 'childrenese', and examples are referring to your dental suction as a 'hoover' and the operating light as 'sunshine'. Ask open-ended questions that cannot be answered with a simple yes or no to promote responses. Knowledge of some current children's television characters is always useful and will provide plenty of topics of conversation.

Consider Engaging Through Play. Children learn through play, so consider the use of familiar toys or puppets. Perhaps she would like to show you how she brushes her teddy bear's teeth? However, remember that toys and play alone are only a means to an end and are not a substitute for good behaviour management. The dental assistant may be able to help considerably with the use of this approach.

With use of these strategies, you are able to open a conversation, although the child does not separate voluntarily from her mother. Ideally, you would examine the child at this visit to assess the treatment needs. As the child is not in pain, you could delay examination until the next visit, at which time you and the surgery will be more familiar to her. However, the mother is worried and would prefer that you would examine the child today.

Examination

◆ Would You Try To Use the Dental Chair for This First Examination?

Not necessarily. The child may be examined initially on the mother's lap, on an ordinary chair, or standing between the mother's knees, all of which are more familiar to her than the dental chair. Place the mother where your dental light can be used if the child will tolerate it. If the child does not allow her teeth to be examined in these positions, then you must consider an examination under more controlled conditions.

◆ How Could You Safely Examine the Child Without Frightening Her Further?

If you decide to perform a full examination on a reluctant child, it must be done in a controlled, caring and confident manner, with experienced nursing support and with the consent and cooperation of the mother. You must explain to the mother exactly what you are going to do, seek verbal consent and repeat to the child that you are just going to count her teeth. It is often helpful to explain both approaches to the parent before he or she sits in the dental chair so that everyone is prepared and the transition to the second approach, if required, is seamless. Then:

- Align the chair in a fairly upright position
- Ask the mother to sit in the chair as if she is being examined – the child will probably come with her
- Ask the child to sit on the mother's lap with her back on her mother's chest, facing away from the mother.

Explain to the child what you are going to do possibly by using something familiar such as a toothbrush; you may be able to examine the child's teeth in this position; if the child will not allow an examination in this position, it is time to adopt another approach.

- Ask the mother to turn the child so that she is sitting across the mother's lap, with her head at the 10 o'clock position
- Ask the mother to control the child's arms and hands
- Have your nurse gently control the child's feet
- Slowly and calmly lower the child's shoulders and head onto your lap, explaining what you are doing; it is helpful to have a pillow on your lap or a folded blanket on which to rest the child's head (Fig. 14.2).

This position is useful not only in uncooperative children but also in young disabled children. Understandably, the child sometimes cries, but not always. Although not ideal, crying often allows good access to the mouth. If the child will not open the mouth, having your nurse tickle the child's stomach will usually have the required effect. Your nurse will need to position the operating light carefully because shining a light directly in the eyes often upsets children.

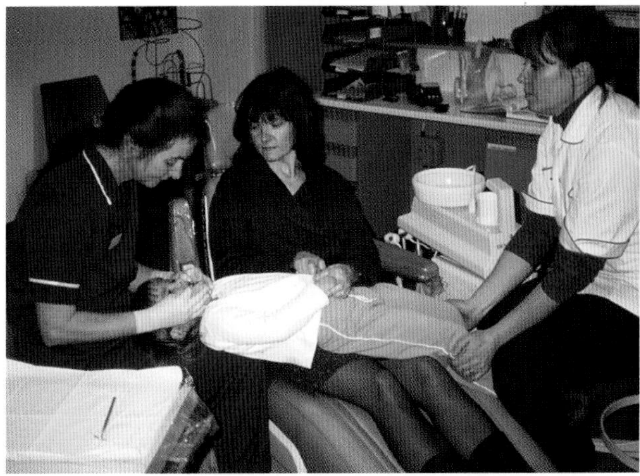

• **Fig. 14.2** Controlled examination technique.

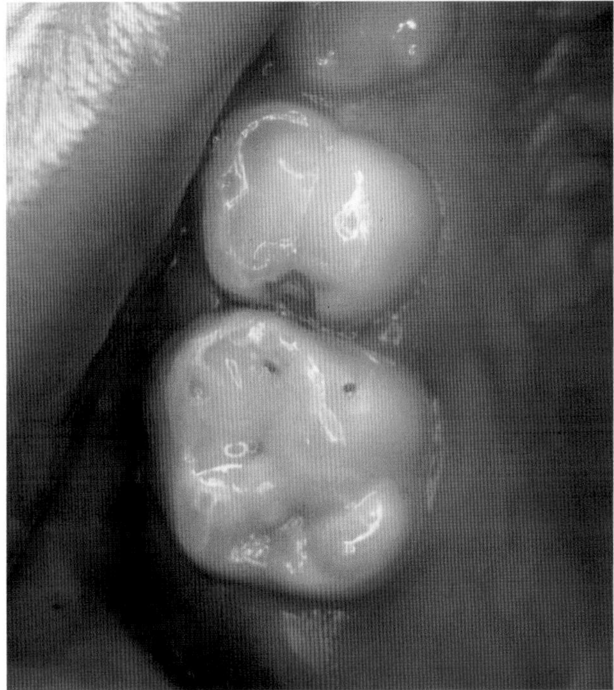

• **Fig. 14.3** Appearances on examination.

Keep the examination short, and immediately afterwards, whether the child is upset or not, reward her with words (a 'soft' reward) and a sticker or balloon (a 'hard' reward). This will encourage the child to allow examination at the next visit.

It is important to explain the different approaches before the mother sits in the dental chair so that you can move, if necessary, from one technique to another quickly and confidently. This approach also ensures that everyone is aware of his or her respective role in the process.

In your brief examination, you see the appearances shown in Fig. 14.3.

◆ The Appearances On Examination are Shown in Fig. 14.3. What Do You See, and What Do the Appearances Indicate?

- Caries in the occlusal pits and fissures of the second primary molar
- Caries in the distal of the first primary molar, the marginal ridge has collapsed
- Reasonable gingival condition with some interdental marginal inflammation.

The management of caries in primary teeth should be approached in accordance with the relevant guidelines based on good clinical evidence on this subject.

For this child, a key feature is the collapse of the marginal ridge of the first primary molar. However, you do not have any radiographs at this point, and so you are unable to assess the depth of the lesion and the likelihood of pulpal compromise. Depending on the radiographic appearance, this tooth may require pulp therapy and definitive restoration with a preformed metal crown restoration. However, provided the criteria governing their use are met, a Hall crown may be appropriate in this situation. Such a restoration has the advantage that local anaesthesia and tooth preparation are not required, which obviously is easier for all concerned and better tolerated by the child.

It is also important to consider that for an anxious child and limited cooperation, it might be appropriate to stabilize the lesion with a temporary intracoronal restoration and delay the definitive restoration for a few months whilst the child's confidence is increased.

◆ What Would You Do Next At This Appointment?

Nothing further is to be gained from this first visit. However, it is essential that you prepare the child for the next visit. Ask her to bring her toothbrush next time, and introduce the concept of future visits and a radiograph ('photograph'). Perhaps tell her you are going to polish her teeth with a special electric toothbrush next time which is fun and tickles! Giving the child a plastic mirror to practise with at home may also be useful and will engage the parents.

Discuss your findings and proposed approach, possible treatment needs and preventive advice with the mother, including use of a 3-day diet diary.

During this period, your nurse should take the initiative to talk informally with the child, introduce the dental chair and equipment in a play-like manner and allow the child to take the lead in exploring the surgery. Some children respond very well to this indirect approach by a second person.

◆ How Will You Plan Treatment Taking the Child's Nervousness Into Account?

The child may require treatments ranging from oral hygiene instruction to a pulpotomy and a preformed metal crown. You must teach the child to accept the more complex treatment by leading her along a graded pathway of increasing challenge.

If treatments are listed in order of increasing difficulty for any child, the challenge scale would look something like Fig. 14.4.

The speed at which you progress along the scale will depend on the individual child's ability to cope with each procedure. You need to monitor the child's reactions continually to check that you are not progressing too fast.

Items in the treatment plan should be arranged as far as possible in order of increasing challenge. A child may accept a challenging treatment when in pain but subsequently might only accept a lower rated treatment.

◆ What Behaviour Management Strategies, Tips and Tricks Might You Use During Examination and Treatment of Nervous Children?

A range of methods are given in Table 14.1. All may be appropriate at various times.

◆ Are There Strategies You Should Avoid?

Yes, the following will almost certainly make the situation worse. Try not to:

- use bribes or coercion – these do not work in the long term and reinforce bad behaviour rather than good behaviour.
- use bland reassurance such as 'Well done' or 'That's fine'. Be more specific, tell the child what was helpful and she will usually try to help again in most instances.
- belittle the child or tell her she is behaving like a baby. This lowers her self-esteem, and poor self-esteem is often linked to anxiety in children.

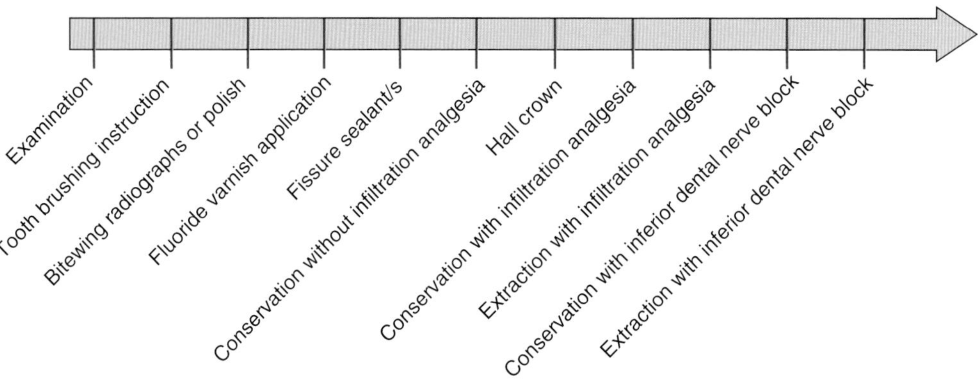

• **Fig. 14.4** Treatments in order of increasing difficulty.

TABLE 14.1 Behaviour Management Strategies

Technique	Comments
Tell–show–do	An important part of shaping the child's behaviour, effective for many children and widely taught. Explain what you are going to do, show the patient how you will do it and only then do it.
Behaviour shaping	Introducing the child to new experiences in a number of small stages or increments ('approximations'). This involves using tell–show–do. Backtrack if the desired behaviour is not forthcoming and only progress to next behavioural challenge after the child has accepted each previous stage. Use prevention to get started and work along the scale of challenge above.
Voice control	Consider repeating an instruction in a slightly different way if you sense that the child is not responding, perhaps with a different tone of voice, eye contact, facial expression or touch.
Use of empathy	Question to elicit the patient's feelings, for instance: 'Is that OK?', 'How is that feeling?', 'Is that better now?'. This is one of the most useful tools in child management; empathic statements have been shown to reliably lessen anxiety in children. They make children feel that you are genuinely concerned about them. In contrast, reassurance is much less effective. Comments such as 'It will be all right', 'That's fine', 'You are doing well' are frequently used, but it would be much better to make an empathic statement.
Provide sense of control	A child who feels helpless will feel anxious. Minimize this by establishing a sense of control for the child. Arrange stop signals, and give the child choices. Stop signals are particularly effective. Tell the child to raise a hand if she wants to tell you something or if something is worrying her (but watch out for children who abuse this power). Limit unpleasant treatment such as use of the air rotor to short bursts of defined length, and count out loud as you use up the time. Agree the number of seconds that is acceptable counting down from 10 to 1 with the child and gradually extend the period.
Specific reinforcement	Use specific reinforcement for any behaviour; tell children what they are doing well and also what you find to be unhelpful behaviour.
Soft rewards	Keep rewarding the child verbally throughout; most children like to be told how clever they are. Say how well the child is trying and reward her for doing her best.
Hard rewards	These are items such as stickers or balloons. Rewards work best when they are consistent, immediate and relevant to the child. They need to be matched to the child's age and gender.
Modelling	Using another child of similar age, perhaps an older sibling or a video, to demonstrate good behaviour can sometimes be helpful, but it is of limited use in young anxious children.

- send the parent of a child this age outside. Removing the main source of security for a young child is counterproductive.
- lose your cool or raise your voice. Treating anxious children can be stressful, and you need to recognize this.

◆ If These Strategies Fail, What Other Options Might Be Open To You?

With skilled behaviour management, many anxious children can accept restorative treatment. However, sometimes, when a child is too anxious and unable to cope, alternatives may need to be considered. If a child is not showing the desired behaviour by the second or third visit, you should consider referral to a specialist paediatric dentist or the use of nitrous oxide inhalation sedation.

Inhalation sedation usually works best in children 5 years of age and older, although some younger children are receptive, depending on their emotional maturity and ability to cooperate. Intravenous sedation is unpredictable in children and not recommended. If all else fails, treatment under general anaesthesia is the last resort, but this must be carefully planned, definitive and completed in one visit to avoid the need for further episodes of general anaesthesia.

If the child is older, the use of cognitive behavioural therapy can be considered to help address anxiety.

◆ How Could You Have Made the First Appointment Easier?

If you had known that the new patient was a nervous child, you could have used a preappointment questionnaire to obtain much useful information such as likes and fears, personality, previous experiences, nicknames, preventive habits and the names of favourite toys or pets. The form could also give information to the parent on your approach to children's dental care and the concept of introducing the child to dentistry in a measured way through prevention. This allays maternal anxiety.

Administering a questionnaire beforehand helps address unrealistic expectations in the parent, perhaps avoiding the situation where the mother asks why you are not going to do a filling at the first visit. It can also stress the need to manage the child through a preventive and measured approach.

You would also have greeted the child and parent in the waiting room, reception area or office, rather than in the surgery, because this helps reduce anxiety in children. You also need to maintain a child-friendly environment with comics, computer games, toys or music and videos. These confirm to both the parent and the child that they are at a caring and understanding practice.

Are You At a Disadvantage Dealing with Nervous Children if You are Male?

There is no good evidence that children prefer female dentists. However, many preschool or nursery children are more familiar with female carers and may take more time to settle with a male dentist. However, there is no need to refer small children to female dentists.

Some male dentists feel uncomfortable about the use of touch as part of their nonverbal communication approach; indeed, some consider it culturally unacceptable. This could be a handicap in treating very young children. If you are male and are worried that touching children may be misconstrued by the parent, it is important to touch only the head and the hands and always in the presence of a chaperone.

Case 15

Pain After Extraction

TARA RENTON

Summary

A 36-year-old lady presents with severe pain a few days after tooth extraction. What is the cause, and what can be done?

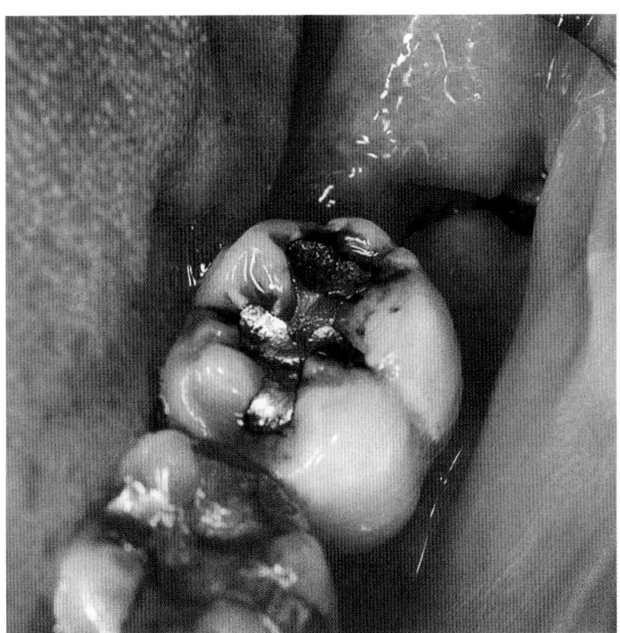

• **Fig. 15.1** The appearance of the socket.

History

Complaint

The patient complains of a distressingly severe pain in an extraction socket on the left side of her mandible. The pain is localized to the extraction socket and is not sensitive to hot or cold. It is a constant, dull, boring pain, unrelieved by aspirin or paracetamol preparations. It prevents the patient from performing any normal activity, and it kept her awake last night.

History of Complaint

The patient underwent surgical removal of the lower left third molar tooth at her dentist 4 days ago. The extraction had proved more difficult than expected and involved repeated attempts at elevation and a small amount of bone removal with the use of a bur. After the extraction, bleeding had stopped normally. The extraction site had been tender but apparently was healing slowly until the pain started yesterday. Since then, the patient has also noticed halitosis and a bad taste in her mouth.

Medical History

The patient is otherwise fit and well. She is taking an oral contraceptive, and no other positive findings were revealed by the medical history.

Examination

Extraoral Examination

The patient has moderate extraoral swelling of the facial soft tissues overlying the extraction socket and some early discolouration of the skin as a result of ecchymosis. There is trismus, and she is able to open her mouth to only 22 mm interincisal clearance. There are no palpable lymph nodes in the deep cervical chain or submandibular triangle.

Intraoral Examination

Halitosis is noticeable. The appearance of the socket is shown in Fig. 15.1. The lower left third molar socket contains no tissue, only food debris. The surrounding soft tissues are slightly swollen but not significantly inflamed as judged by the redness.

Diagnosis

◆ On the Basis of What You Know Already, What is the Most Likely Diagnosis?

The diagnosis is most likely to be dry socket (alveolar osteitis). The history of severe and persistent pain localized to the tooth socket appearing 3–5 days after extraction, particularly a traumatic one, is characteristic. The lack of local inflammation or enlarged lymph nodes is compatible with this diagnosis and argues against postextraction infection either in bone or soft tissue.

The diagnosis is confirmed by the examination, which shows that the blood clot has disappeared from the socket. In severe cases, the bone of the socket may be exposed, and the bone of the distal lip of the socket can be seen (see Fig. 15.1).

Halitosis is the result of food debris in the socket being degraded by partially anaerobic bacterial flora. The trismus is almost certainly related to the surgical trauma of extraction.

◆ What Other Causes of Postextraction Pain are There? Are They Likely in This Case?

Pain from surgical trauma to tissues should be considered when extraction is difficult. However, pain starts immediately after sensation is regained in the area and responds to analgesics. Tenderness is characteristic, rather than spontaneous pain.

Osteomyelitis is rare but should be considered because of its severity and difficulty of treatment, especially if diagnosed late. It causes a deep, boring pain, not dissimilar from dry socket, but is poorly localized. Osteomyelitis is almost exclusively seen in patients who are immunocompromised or have sclerosis of the jaw bones. It usually takes several weeks to become evident.

Osteoradionecrosis is rare and only associated with previous radiotherapy in the field of surgery.

Medication-related osteonecrosis (MRONJ) resulting in persistent symptoms should be considered if the patient has a history of osteoporosis treated with oral bisphosphonates or metastatic cancer treated with intravenous bisphosphonates or antiangiogenic agents (see Case 23, pages 127–134). However, this is not the case here.

Fractured mandible is a very rare complication of extraction. It might be considered if swelling and bruising appeared out of proportion to dental extraction. Fracture is usually evident clinically if it is displaced.

Retained root fragments are surprisingly rarely a cause of long-term pain, although the surgical trauma of the failed extraction may cause pain. Root fragments are almost never found in dry socket.

None of these alternative causes matches the patient's symptoms or signs as well as dry socket.

◆ What Investigations Would You Carry Out?

At this stage, the history and examination are completely compatible with the diagnosis, and no investigations are indicated. If there were features of infection, culture of pus and antibiotic sensitivity would be necessary and the temperature would have to be taken. Radiographs are not useful unless a root fragment is suspected but cannot be seen or palpated. Even if osteomyelitis is suspected, radiographs would not provide useful information because there has been insufficient time for the characteristic radiographic changes to develop.

◆ What is Dry Socket?

Dry socket results when blood clot in the socket is lost before it can become stabilized by ingrowth of granulation tissue. The exposed bone surface becomes colonized by anaerobic bacteria and spirochaetes and is partially and superficially devitalized. Loss of blood clot is thought to be the result of excessive fibrinolysis caused by bacterial, local tissue or salivary factors. In the absence of a blood clot, healing is delayed because soft tissue must grow from the gingival margin to cover bone and fill the socket.

◆ What Factors Predispose To Dry Socket?

The risk factors associated with development of dry socket are given in Table 15.1.

TABLE 15.1 Risk Factors for Dry Socket

- Surgical or traumatic extraction
- Mandibular extraction, especially third molar
- Female gender, especially if patient is on contraceptive medication
- Smoking
- Infection or recent infection at site
- Periodontal disease or acute necrotizing ulcerative gingivitis elsewhere in the mouth
- Local bone disease or sclerosis reducing blood supply for clot formation, as in Paget's disease, cemento-osseous dysplasia or after radiotherapy
- Excessive use of local anaesthetic; vasoconstrictor in excess around the socket may prevent formation of blood clot
- History of previous dry socket
- Being young adult or middle-aged patient

◆ How Would You Treat This Patient?

Reassure the patient that although extremely painful, this condition does not signify any serious consequence of the extraction. Inform her that the socket will heal normally but more slowly than usual and that during the healing period, treatment can be provided to relieve the pain, although she may have to return for several sessions of treatment.

Local treatment to the socket is the most effective measure. Irrigate the socket gently with warm saline. Place a dressing into the mouth of the socket to prevent further impaction of food. Many proprietary dressings are available, including resorbable materials, antiseptic preparations and analgesic formulations. In practice, almost all are satisfactory, provided they are used appropriately and replaced as required. Care should be taken not to pack the socket too much with the dressing because this would prevent it from filling up with granulation tissue as healing progresses.

Effective socket cleansing and socket hygiene are more important than the type of dressing used, and the patient should come back every 2 days for retreatment, if necessary. In severe cases, a daily dressing may be appropriate initially, and as the socket heals and pain is reduce, the period between dressings may be extended. The trismus should be monitored and should reduce.

◆ What Drugs Might You Prescribe?

Antibiotics should not be prescribed because they are ineffective. Analgesics are also largely ineffective in the absence of local measures. A nonsteroidal anti-inflammatory drug should be adequate in most cases. The pain of dry socket is notorious for its severity, and in the past, controlled drugs have been prescribed. This is only occasionally justified but may need to be considered.

◆ How Quickly Will the Pain Be Relieved?

Improvement of symptoms will usually be noted within minutes or in up to an hour and more quickly if the dressing contains a local anaesthetic agent. Pain may start again a day or two after dressing, gradually increasing in severity. After a few days, the pain will reduce and redressing may not be necessary. After about 10 days, the socket should be filled with tissue, and it will probably be asymptomatic for the last few days of healing.

◆ What if the Condition Persists for Longer Than This or Appears To Be Worsening?

Failure to resolve in the longer term usually indicates the presence of small sequestra of devitalized lamina dura or root fragments. These are normal sequelae of extraction and are usually resorbed in the remodelling process during healing. Larger pieces may delay healing and sometimes sequestrate through the alveolar ridge mucosa many weeks after extraction, although they are not usually associated with significant pain. Occasionally, larger sequestra of lamina dura may be seen on periapical radiographs. If the sequestra are associated with symptoms and are not shed, surgical removal may become necessary. In practice, this intervention is extremely rarely required, and sequestra are usually small and lost without being noticed. The diagnosis will have to be reviewed, and radiographs are also useful to exclude other causes for the pain. The possibility of osteomyelitis should be considered and thoroughly investigated if the nature of the pain has changed or if the patient suffers any condition predisposing to this condition (local bone sclerosis, pathological or therapeutic immunosuppression, bisphosphonate drugs).

Case 16
A Numb Lip

NICHOLAS M. GOODGER

Summary

A 68-year-old man presents to you at your general dental practice complaining that his lower lip has become numb. How would you investigate and manage this symptom?

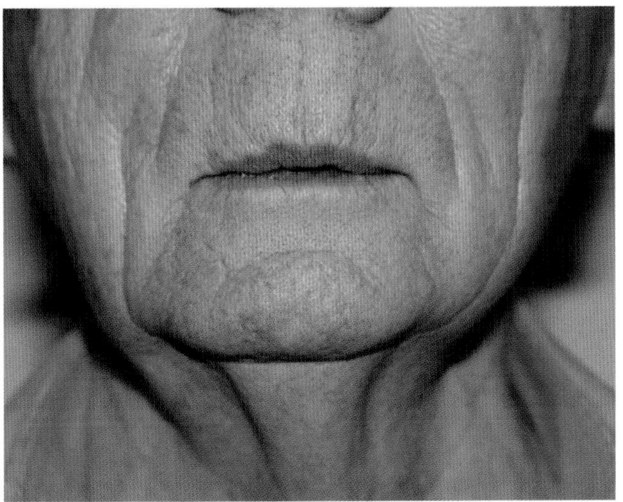

• **Fig. 16.1** The patient on presentation.

History

Complaint

The patient complains of sudden onset of numbness of the lower right lip. It feels cold, as if he had had an injection for dental treatment (Fig. 16.1).

History of Complaint

The patient noticed the numbness immediately after he woke up the previous morning. His jaw has been aching for some months, and he has noticed some tingling in the lip, which he ascribes to recent dental treatment.

Dental History

You are seeing the patient at an emergency appointment. He is normally under the care of one of your colleagues, and the patient's records and radiographs are available.

A series of appointments over the last few months have addressed pain in the lower right quadrant of the patient's mouth. The tingling in the lip was noted 3 months ago. The lower right first molar had been considered as the cause. Your colleague had placed a root filling 4 months ago, but the pain did not resolve completely. Three weeks ago, the lower right second premolar was extracted as it was thought to be a likely cause of the pain. However, the patient's discomfort continued.

Medical History

The patient reports that he is fit and well. He takes 50 mg atenolol daily for mild hypertension. In the past, he had suffered from depression and had been treated with antidepressants.

◆ What is the Sensory Nerve Supply To the Lip?

The sensory nerve supply to the face is shown in Fig. 16.2. The three divisions of the trigeminal nerve supply most of the face. The greater auricular nerve is formed by the ventral rami of the cervical nerves C2 and C3.

The lower lip is supplied by the mental nerve.

◆ What is the Course of the Nerve Supply?

The trigeminal nerve starts in the pons, where its sensory and motor roots arise. The ophthalmic and maxillary branches leave the skull via the superior orbital fissure and the foramen rotundum, respectively. The mandibular branch leaves the skull at the foramen ovale to enter the infratemporal fossa, where it divides into an anterior group of mostly motor branches and a posterior group of sensory branches.

The anterior group of branches includes the nerves to lateral pterygoid, deep temporal nerves to masseter and the sensory long buccal nerve. There are three posterior branches, including the auriculotemporal nerve, which

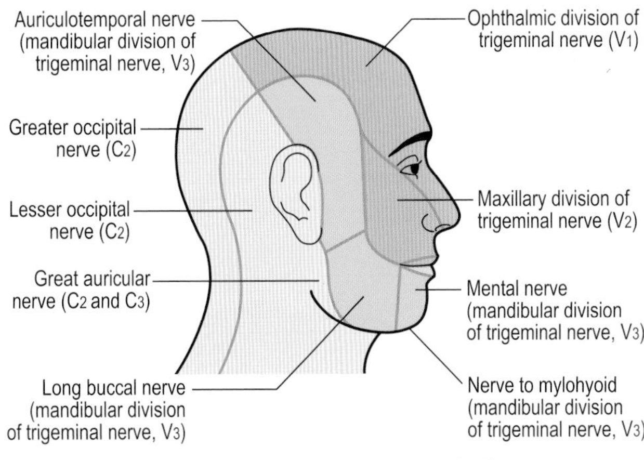

• **Fig. 16.2** Sensory nerve supply to the face.

TABLE 16.1 Major and More Frequent Causes of Numb Lip

Infection	Osteomyelitis Periapical periodontitis causing pressure on nerve in mandibular canal
Tumour	Primary malignant neoplasm of bone such as osteosarcoma Primary malignant neoplasm of mucosa invading bone such as oral squamous cell carcinoma Primary malignant neoplasm of brain or tissues along path of nerve Metastatic malignant neoplasm to brain or tissues along path of nerve Benign tumour such as meningioma or schwannoma
Trauma	Mandibular fracture Direct trauma to nerve at mental foramen
Autoimmune	Peripheral neuropathy Multiple sclerosis
Vascular	Vascular compression of nerve root
Psychological	Tetany from hyperventilation
Metabolic	Tetany from alkalosis
Iatrogenic causes	Intraneural injection of local anaesthetic Direct trauma to the inferior dental nerve at the lingula or mental foramen from dental injection Trauma to the inferior dental bundle from dental extraction (particularly third molars), apicectomy or implant placement Injury to the mental nerve during surgical extractions/apicectomy Injury to the inferior alveolar nerve by extruded root filling material or caustic endodontic agents

is given off almost immediately. This passes backwards to innervate the side of the scalp and part of the ear. The main nerve then divides into the lingual nerve, which passes to the tongue along the lateral pterygoid, and the inferior alveolar nerve, which gives off the small motor branch to mylohyoid and then enters the mandibular foramen in the mandibular ramus. It emerges from the mental foramen to provide sensation to the lip.

Unlike many other areas of sensory innervation, those on the face are well defined and sharply delineated. Although there is some slight variation among individuals, there is little overlap of the areas supplied by different nerves.

◆ What are the Causes of Numbness of the Lip?

Numbness may be constant or temporary/intermittent, depending on the cause. The main causes are shown in Table 16.1, and each may affect the nerve at different parts along its course.

Examination

Extraoral Examination

The appearance of the patient is shown in Fig. 16.1. He appears normal; the lip is of normal colour and shows no distortion or drooping to suggest a motor nerve lesion.

When you examine him, you find that there is only a very mild swelling of the posterior right lower jaw. There is no detectable mass, but the patient reports tenderness in the right submandibular area. There is normal movement of the lip.

◆ How Will You Test for Sensation? Why is This Necessary?

A sensation of numbness may be central in origin, denote damage to the peripheral nerve or be psychosomatic. Only by testing sensation can the exact area affected be defined, and this will help define the cause.

Tests of sensation may include light touch (with a wisp of cotton wool or a Von Frey hair – fine filaments of calibrated rigidity for testing touch), pain (with a sharp and blunt point), vibration, temperature and two-point discrimination. A cotton wool fibre and a sharp point such as a hypodermic needle are usually sufficient for a dental setting. Outline the area affected, making sure that hand movements cannot be seen by the patient so that the results are objective. Test and retest if the results are unclear.

If the results are abnormal, it will be necessary to test the other cranial nerves because these may be affected if a lesion is present in the brain or along the common paths of the cranial nerves.

◆ How Will You Test Cranial Nerve Function?

The main head and neck functions of cranial nerves may be tested as described in Table 16.2.

When you do this, the skin of the patient's lip is found to be almost completely without light touch and pain sensations in the area below the vermilion border and on its mucosal surface. There is a sharp cut-off in the midline, and the skin below the chin has normal sensation.

◆ How Do You Interpret the Findings So Far?

The extraoral findings are relatively subtle. There is mild swelling of the mandible, which suggests a local mandibular cause. The tenderness in the right submandibular area might represent infection or reactive lymphadenopathy.

The fact that the area of anaesthesia is sharply delineated suggests a peripheral nerve cause. It also almost excludes a

TABLE 16.2 Methods To Test the Functions of Cranial Nerves in the Head and Neck

Cranial Nerve	Test	Comment
I. Olfactory	Check each nostril individually with easily recognized nonpungent smells.	If the smell is pungent or irritant it will trigger a pain response via the trigeminal nerve as well.
II. Optic	Check pupil reactivity to light and visual acuity.	Test each eye separately.
III. Oculomotor IV. Trochlear VI. Abducens	Check eye movement in each gaze (up/down/lateral/medial and each oblique gaze), asking the patient to follow a finger with the eyes – the finger should be 25 cm from the patient's eyes.	Check both eyes together and individually.
V. Trigeminal	Check sensation in each division by touch, comparing each side. The ophthalmic division can also be tested with corneal reflex. Check motor component of mandibular division by asking the patient to clench teeth.	
VII. Facial	Ask the patient to raise the eyebrows, tightly shut the eyes, smile and purse the lips.	Compare left and right sides for asymmetry.
VIII. Auditory	Check to see if the patient can hear fingers being rubbed together close to the ear, a ticking watch or whispering.	The distance from the ear is important.
IX. Glossopharyngeal X. Vagus	Ask the patient to say 'aaah', and look for symmetrical movement of the soft palate.	Functions of cranial nerves IX and X in the head and neck region are intermingled, so these nerves are effectively tested together.
X. Vagus	Check vocal cord movement/hoarseness.	
XI. Accessory	Ask the patient to press the chin downwards on to your hand, and the bulk/power of the sternomastoid and trapezius muscles can be compared. Then, ask the patient to turn the head against your hand. Finally, ask the patient to shrug the shoulders.	Weakness is demonstrated in the muscle opposite the direction of head turning.
XII. Hypoglossal	Ask the patient to stick out the tongue.	The tongue deviates to the affected side.

psychosomatic origin, as psychosomatic sensations do not tend to follow neurological or vascular distributions. The fact that lip movement is normal indicates normal facial nerve function. As the roots and paths through the base of skull of the trigeminal and facial nerves are close, this would suggest that a central or base-of-skull lesion is not the cause.

The distribution on the skin of the lower lip suggests injury or compression of the inferior alveolar nerve. The normal sensation under the chin is significant. This area is supplied by the nerve to mylohyoid, given off the inferior alveolar nerve just above the lingula, to supply a thumb-print-sized patch of skin under the chin. Therefore, the cause must lie between the start of the inferior dental canal and the lip.

Intraoral Examination

The oral mucosa is healthy, apart from the lower right second premolar extraction site. The socket opening is swollen and filled with granulation tissue that is growing out slightly above the alveolus. There are no sequestra and no sinus or pus at the socket mouth. The remaining teeth appear healthy, and none is tender to percussion.

◆ How Should a Healing Socket Appear 3 Weeks After Extraction? Is This Socket Normal?

The initial clot starts to be replaced by granulation tissue growing in from the periphery a few days after extraction. By 8–10 days, even a large molar socket should be filled with granulation tissue. At 2–3 weeks, there should be an intact layer of epithelium over the granulation tissue for a large socket. *This socket is not epithelialized. The granulation tissue growing out from the socket indicates a process of hindered healing, which could have many causes. This socket has failed to heal.*

◆ What are the Causes of Failed or Delayed Socket Healing?

General causes

- Age
- Diabetes
- Drugs
  - Steroids and other immunosuppressants
  - Bisphosphonates
  - Denosumab
  - Antiangiogenic or tyrosine kinase inhibitor therapy
- Malnutrition
- Cancer chemotherapy

Local causes

- Impacted food debris
- Foreign bodies – bony sequestra, root fragments
- Dry socket
- Infection, including tuberculosis
- Oroantral fistula formation
- Previous radiotherapy to the site
- Sarcoidosis
- Local malignancy

◆ How Do You Interpret the Findings Now?

There would appear to be a local cause in the body of the mandible causing compression or injury to the inferior alveolar nerve. Inflammation or infection from nonvital teeth or the nonhealing socket could involve the nerve. Alternatively, another process may cause both nerve injury and may have prevented socket healing. The fact that a malignant neoplasm might be the cause is a concern.

Investigations

◆ What Investigations Should You Perform?

The remaining teeth in the affected quadrant should be tested for vitality.

A radiograph is required to assess the extraction socket, the adjacent teeth, the whole height of the slightly expanded mandible and the full length of the inferior dental canal. Either a dental panoramic or an oblique lateral radiograph would be an appropriate view.

The lower first molar is root filled. The second molar is vital, but the lower right incisors, canine and first premolar appear nonvital.

◆ The Panoramic Tomograph is Shown in Fig. 16.3. What Does It Show?

Several teeth have been heavily restored. The lower first molar is root filled, and there is a poorly defined radiolucency about 2 cm in length extending from the distal root of the second molar to the premolar socket. The cortical bone outline of the inferior dental canal cannot be seen in this region. The recent extraction socket still has the lamina dura present, although it appears slightly more indistinct than normal, consistent with infection or another process causing resorption. No sequestra or root fragments are present in the socket, although a plain periapical view would have been a better view to assess this particular point because it provides higher resolution.

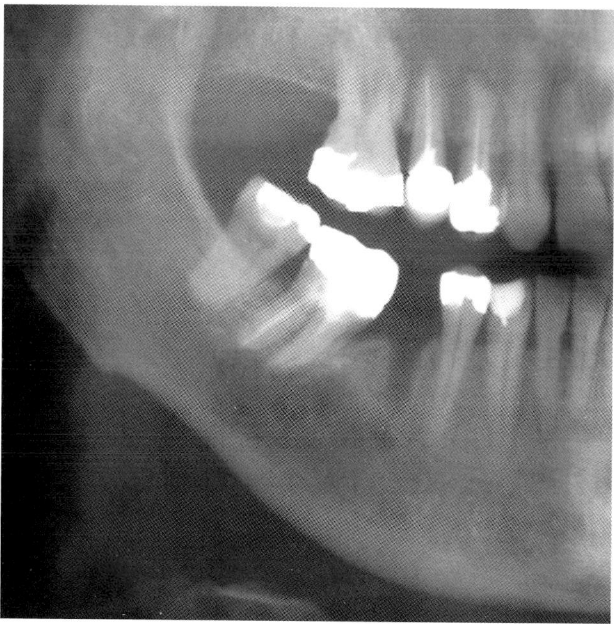

• **Fig. 16.3** The panoramic tomograph.

Differential Diagnosis

◆ What is Your Differential Diagnosis? Justify Each Possible Diagnosis

Chronic osteomyelitis. There is a history of dental infection, extraction with a nonhealing socket and tenderness at the site. This would be a statistically likely cause and should be considered first. However, some features do not fit. Chronic osteomyelitis is usually associated with a predisposing cause. Besides this patient's age, none is present. There is no definite lymphadenopathy and no discharge of pus from the socket or any sinuses. The radiological features are partly consistent, but osteomyelitis is usually a more patchy radiolucency with zones of sclerosis. Peripheral bone sclerosis and sequestra seen radiographically or in the socket would also be expected. The radiological features of osteomyelitis take several weeks to develop, but the symptoms started several months ago.

Acute osteomyelitis is not suspected. There are no systemic symptoms of infection, and the delay since extraction is rather long. Acute osteomyelitis tends to affect younger patients, and the pain is deep and throbbing. Onset was soon after extraction, and there are no radiological signs.

Malignant neoplasm. The patient is an older adult, and there is a long history of vague pain and paraesthesia, suggesting a long-standing lesion. The dental extractions may have been performed for valid reasons or as a result of the misdiagnosis of the cause of pain. The nonhealing socket could well be caused by malignancy, and the radiological features are suggestive; the lesion is poorly defined and purely destructive. Although this is the statistically less likely option, it is the best match to the findings.

◆ What Malignant Neoplasms are the Most Likely Causes?

Jaw malignancy may be primary or secondary (metastatic). The main options are as follows:

Primary

- Osteosarcoma
- Odontogenic carcinomas and sarcoma
- Primary intraosseous squamous cell carcinoma

Secondary

- Breast carcinoma
- Bronchogenic carcinoma (lung)
- Renal carcinoma
- Prostate carcinoma
- Thyroid carcinoma

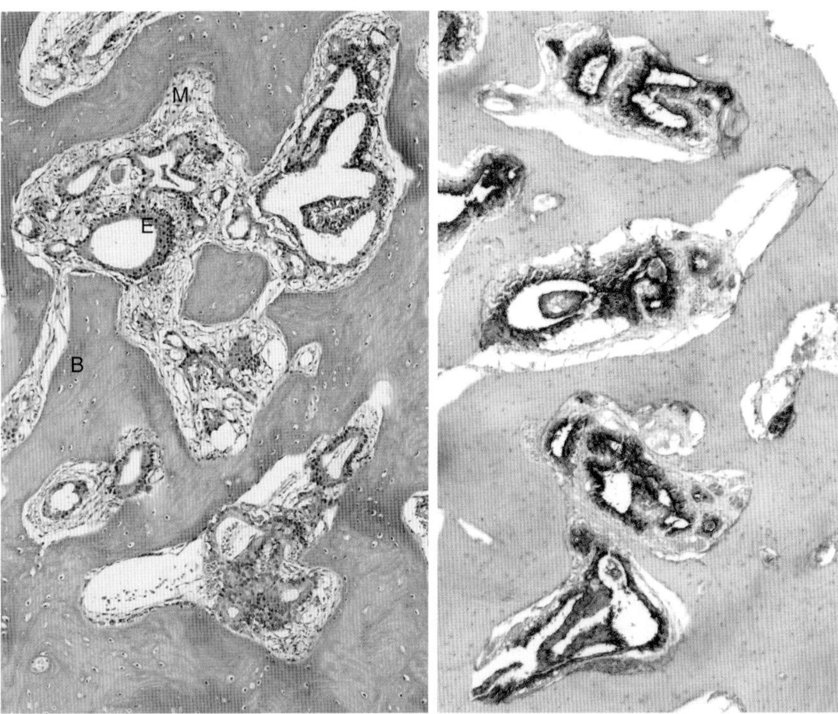

• **Fig. 16.4** Histological appearances of the socket curettings.

• Other less common sources

All the primary neoplasms are relatively rare in the jaw.

Metastasis the most likely malignant cause. Carcinoma of the breast would be very unlikely, although not impossible, in a male. All the other options need to be considered. Although those listed above are the commonest jaw metastases, almost any malignancy can spread to the jaws.

Breast and prostate metastases are unusual in that they sometimes cause bone formation at the site, producing a sclerotic or mixed radiolucency rather than the more typical pure 'moth-eaten' poorly defined radiolucency. In this case, the lesion is purely destructive, and any of the common options could be the cause.

◆ What Further Investigation is Required?

Biopsy of the socket is required to establish the diagnosis. This may be performed under local or general anaesthesia but must be representative of the lesion. It will, therefore, need to include tissue from the socket and the underlying radiolucency. Some of the sample must be fixed in formalin for histological examination, and a portion must be kept fresh to send for microbiological culture and sensitivity in case the diagnosis turns out to be osteomyelitis.

This biopsy would be best performed in a specialist unit or local cancer centre, not in a general practice, because malignancy is strongly suspected.

◆ The Biopsy is Shown in Fig. 16.4. What Do You See?

The left panel shows the bone curettings from the socket composed of normal lamellar bone (B) with several marrow spaces (M). These would normally be filled by fatty marrow in a patient of this age.

However, they contain rings of epithelium (E), recognized by its darker staining pattern and the fact that it surrounds duct or gland-like spaces. The overall pattern is that of a glandular tissue. No glands are present in the normal mandibular marrow – this must be metastatic adenocarcinoma.

Because the biopsy shows adenocarcinoma, lungs, kidneys, gastrointestinal tract and the prostate gland will be the most likely primary sites of carcinoma because these tissues give rise to adenocarcinomas.

◆ How Can the Primary Cancer Be Identified?

Start again with a more detailed medical history, and refer the patient for medical examination. The diagnosis may already be known because metastasis to the jaw is usually a feature of late-stage disease. In other cases, jaw lesions may be the presenting sign.

Some of the most likely primary sites can be investigated by relatively simple techniques such as physical examination, ultrasonography, chest radiography and blood tests for circulating prostate-specific antigen (PSA). If no primary cancer is suggested, imaging would be the next step.

Often, it is possible to determine the primary site on the basis of the biopsy results. Cells in malignant neoplasms often retain some characteristics of their tissue of origin, and in this case, the glands have a resemblance to normal prostate gland, although metastatic adenocarcinoma from other sites would also be possible.

It is often possible to detect specific marker proteins of the tissue of origin by using immunohistochemistry. The right-hand panel of Fig. 16.4 shows the biopsy specimen stained with antibodies to PSA. PSA is an enzyme secreted by prostate cells and expressed in their cytoplasm. Although not completely specific to the prostate gland, there are few other tissues that express high levels. The presence of PSA is indicated by positive staining (brown colour) around all the glands in bone marrow.

Histopathology suggests strongly that this is metastasis of prostate carcinoma. A blood test reveals high levels of circulating PSA. No mass can be detected in the prostate gland on clinical examination, but prostate ultrasonography reveals a small nodule, and needle biopsy and histopathological analysis reveal prostate carcinoma.

Diagnosis

The diagnosis is metastatic prostate carcinoma.

◆ What is the Prognosis?

In general, metastases to the jaws carry a poor prognosis because they indicate advanced disseminated malignancy, often malignant disease that has become refractory to treatment. In many cases, palliative care is all that can be offered, and patients with breast, colon or lung metastases are likely to die within a year. When bony metastases are in sites that risk significant morbidity, such as vertebrae, they may be treated surgically or with radiotherapy, but this is rarely indicated in the jaw unless there is severe pain.

Some prostate carcinomas can respond to hormone treatment. Although the cancer remains sensitive to these treatments, it may progress only very slowly. This may be so even when there are widespread bone metastases and the course of disease may be significantly extended.

◆ Might There Be Implications for This Patient's Future Dentistry?

Yes, patients with multiple bone lesions of myeloma or metastatic breast or prostate carcinoma are often treated with intravenous bisphosphonates or denosumab (a monoclonal antibody that inhibits osteoclasts) to slow bone destruction and prevent spinal cord damage, pathological fracture and bone pain.

Bisphosphonates such as zoledronic acid and monoclonal agents such as denosumab prevent bone turnover and reduce bone viability. There is a small but significant risk of developing the unusual pattern of medication-related osteonecrosis of the jaws (MRONJ) associated with these drugs.

Case 17
A Loose Anterior Tooth

RUPERT AUSTIN AND DEBORAH BOMFIM

Summary

A 25-year-old man presents at your general dental practice with a loose anterior tooth. Identify the cause, and summarize the treatment options.

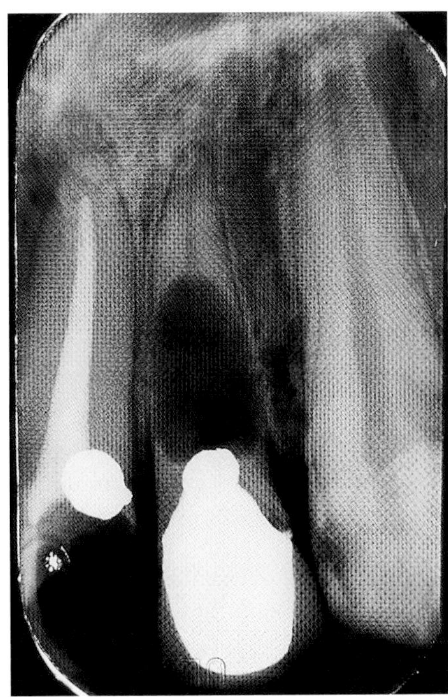

• **Fig. 17.1** Periapical radiograph of the mobile maxillary left lateral incisor.

History

Complaint

The patient complains of a loose tooth and points to his upper left lateral incisor which is crowned. He says it is uncomfortable when it moves and has become so mobile that he is concerned that it may fall out.

History of Complaint

The patient has noticed that the tooth has become progressively looser over the last few months and would like a replacement. There has been no pain associated with the tooth, but he is aware of an unpleasant taste that appears to emanate intermittently from his upper front teeth.

Dental History

The patient had been a regular attender at another dental practice for many years until he recently moved to your area. He is motivated and does not wish to lose any teeth.

Four years previously, the lateral and central incisors had been fractured in an accident at work. Both teeth sustained enamel–dentine coronal fractures with no pulp involvement but were initially left untreated. Several months later, another dental practitioner provided a root canal treatment on the upper central incisor and some direct resin composite restorations on both teeth, and shortly afterwards the patient asked for the lateral incisor to be crowned because he was unhappy with its appearance.

Medical History

The patient has insulin-controlled diabetes. Otherwise he is fit and well.

Examination

Extraoral Examination

No submandibular or cervical lymph nodes are palpable.

Intraoral Examination

The patient has an extensively restored dentition, with a metal ceramic crown on the upper left lateral incisor and a large resin composite restoration on the upper left central incisor. There is no evidence of caries on any teeth, and generally the periodontal condition is good, with generalized pocket probing depths of 2–4 mm. There is supra- and subgingival plaque associated with the crown margin of the upper left lateral incisor and localized erythema and delayed bleeding on probing around the gingival margin. The crown is grade II mobile; however, there are no increased probing depths associated with the upper left lateral incisor. The adjacent teeth are firm. No sinuses are present to explain the bad taste, and no swelling or pus is detected on periodontal probing or palpation.

◆ What Additional Questions Might You Ask?

What Was the Nature of the Previous Trauma? Different patterns of dental trauma (e.g. crown fractures, crown and root fractures, root fractures, luxations, avulsion, etc.) have varying sequelae requiring a wide variety of management strategies. The history of the initial trauma suggests that the patient's teeth suffered crown fractures only without any luxation injury or pulp/root involvement; however, the delayed provision of endodontic treatment suggests that possibly the root canal and/or the periodontal ligament may also have been affected by the trauma.

Did You Recently Notice the Mobility Suddenly Increase or Hear a Crack From the Tooth? The increased mobility without evidence of periodontitis suggests a recent root fracture, which may be secondary to the provision of the restorations and/or endodontic treatment. *The patient did not notice any movement of the teeth at the time of the injury and is not sure why the root canal treatment was needed. The patient did not notice any sudden increase in mobility or hear a recent crack from the tooth.*

◆ How Would You Clinically Assess the Possibility of Root Fracture?

By determining the axis of rotation of the mobile crown. Apply digital pressure forwards and backwards to identify how far down the root the axis of rotation appears to be. If when moving the crown bubbles of saliva are produced at the gingival margin, this would be an indicator of a root fracture communicating with a periodontal pocket or the gingival crevice.

When you palpate the crown, you find that the crown appears to rotate bucco-cervically about a point 2–3 mm below the gingival margin. No such bubbles are seen at the crown margin.

◆ On the Basis of What You Know So Far, What are the Likely Causes?

Having excluded mobility caused by periodontitis and coronal bone loss, the two possibilities that remain the most likely are resorption or root fracture. The mobile tooth is rotating about a point just below the gingival margin, so either process must affect the coronal part of the root.

Resorption of the apical half of the root would move the axis of rotation of the remaining tooth coronally. There would have to be extensive resorption to cause this degree of mobility and raise the axis of rotation so far. Resorption is a recognized complication of trauma to teeth, and so this would be the most likely cause.

Root fracture is possible. No fracture was noted but the marked mobility would be consistent with the root fracture of the coronal part of the root. If there is a root fracture it would appear to be independent of the original trauma. Teeth that suffer coronal fractures do not usually suffer root fractures as well because most of the energy is absorbed by fracturing the crown. However, if a root fracture had been present for the last 4 years, it might have triggered slow resorption, combining both possible causative factors.

An unsuspected lesion may have destroyed the bone and/or the tooth root apically, leaving support only coronally. The tooth would then be mobile, whereas the periodontal ligament would remain intact in the mid- and coronal-third. The commonest lesion to do this would be a radicular cyst arising on a nonvital tooth.

Finally, **a neoplastic lesion** remains a remote possibility. However, this seems most unlikely because there is no expansion and the adjacent teeth are not displaced or mobile.

Investigations

◆ What Investigations Would You Carry out? Why? Any Problems with Interpreting These Results?

See Table 17.1.

On performing the tests of tooth sensibility, you find that it is impossible to obtain a response from both the upper left central and lateral incisors. All other anterior teeth respond normally to sensibility testing.

◆ The Periapical Radiograph is Shown in Fig. 17.1. What Do You See?

The left lateral incisor is crowned. The core material appears to communicate with the pulp chamber/coronal one-third of the root canal; however, no root canal filling is evident. The middle third of the root shows a large oval radiolucency, which appears to fill the entire middle third of the root canal and extends laterally to replace the full width of the root dentine and communicate with the periodontal ligament. The margins of the defect are smooth and sharply defined. The lamina dura around the apex appears intact. The bone level mesially and distally is coronal to the defect, and there is no evidence of either horizontal or vertical bone loss. Very little root dentine remains below the crown and gingival margin.

The upper left central incisor is root filled, with an apparently radiolucent restoration. The root filling appears well condensed and extends very close to the ideal level apically; however the gutta percha is close to the pulp chamber coronally which may suggest a poor coronal seal. The root appears to have a curve at the apex. There is a poorly defined radiolucency around the apex mostly on its mesial side, where the lamina dura is missing.

The canine has a mesial radiolucency, indicative of caries, and its apical lamina dura is indistinct. However, no obvious periapical radiolucency is present.

◆ What is Wrong with the Radiograph in Fig. 17.1?

This radiograph is of suboptimal quality because of positioning issues, in that not all of the central and lateral incisors are visible, as well as issues with film processing artefact. A regular pattern is superimposed over the whole film, suggesting that this is not a digital radiograph. This artefact may be caused by some wet film processors that use woven nylon bands to transport the film between solutions during development of the film. If these bands are dirty or worn, their surface texture transfers an imprint onto the film. A less marked example of the same artefact is shown in Fig. 35.3.

TABLE 17.1 Investigations To Be Carried Out

Test	Reason	Problems
Sensibility testing	To check the sensibility of all four upper and lower incisors and canines (excluding any known root-filled teeth), either thermal (usually cold testing) or electrical stimuli may be used. Late loss of sensibility is a complication of trauma and any one of these teeth could have periapical infection and be the cause of the bad taste. The sensibility of the lateral incisor needs to be known, to plan treatment once the diagnosis is established.	Electric pulp tests are notoriously difficult to perform on crowned teeth and the results must be interpreted with caution. The lateral incisor has a metal ceramic bonded crown and the ceramic will insulate the tooth while the metal layer will diffuse the applied voltage and conduct the stimulus to the gingiva. The patient may mistake a gingival sensation for a vitality response. Thermal pulp testing is also unreliable on teeth with indirect restorations involving ceramic, as the thermal conductivity of ceramic is poor.
Long cone periapical radiography	To detect the possible causes and assess bone levels around the teeth. To determine the pulp canal morphology in case root canal treatment is required, and the root morphology in case extraction is necessary.	Root fractures may be difficult to identify if the fragments are not separated. A second view at a slightly different angle (e.g. upper standard occlusal or bisecting angle periapical) may allow detection of a root fracture, which is invisible in the first. Alternatively 3D radiography in the form of small-volume, high-resolution CBCT may help identify fractures, resorption and extent of any periapical pathology.

Another uniform artefactual pattern results from exposing the wrong side of an intraoral conventional film packet to the beam. The embossed metal backing foil casts a patterned shadow onto the film, and the shielding causes an additional underexposure, differentiating this artefact from the one illustrated.

Digital radiography helps prevent this type of artefact from occurring. However, digital radiographs can result in other types of artefacts, for example, those related to the type of sensor (phosphor plate or charge-coupled device).

Diagnosis

◆ What are Your Provisional Diagnoses?

Extensive internal resorption of the maxillary left lateral incisor. The central incisor has a failed root filling with a periapical granuloma or abscess, possibly associated with microleakage resulting from a poor coronal seal. The cause of the taste could be intermittent drainage of pus from this periapical lesion, plaque trapped in the resorption defect or caries on the mesial surface of the upper left canine.

◆ What Types of Dental Resorption are There? What are Their Characteristic Features?

Resorption is the process of removal of dental hard tissues by osteoclasts. There is usually some form of repair by either reactionary dentine or bone. This repair may lead to ankylosis. All resorption is identical in its basic process, but it is convenient to subdivide resorption into clinically relevant types. Resorption may be classified by location (i.e. internal or external), as well as by aetiology (i.e. inflammatory or replacement). All types may be transient or progressive.

Internal root resorption starts on the pulpal aspect of dentine. It typically affects the middle third of the root and forms a well-demarcated defect with a smooth symmetrical shape. Internal resorption indicates that the pulp is vital and that, provided the lesion has not perforated the root, the process will be halted by root canal treatment.

External root resorption starts on the surface of the tooth, usually on the root but occasionally on the crown of unerupted teeth. A microscopic degree of superficial external root resorption can occur normally and is usually repaired by cementum. Greater apical root resorption may be seen radiographically, most commonly on teeth that have been moved orthodontically. Extensive apical resorption may accompany periapical inflammation or infection on nonvital teeth. A nonvital pulp may trigger external resorption of the middle or coronal one-third of the root by producing noxious byproducts, which diffuse outwards to the periodontal ligament along the dentine tubules. External cervical root resorption usually starts just below the gingival margin and may affect one or many teeth that may be otherwise healthy and vital. Radiographically, the early stages may mimic the appearance of an infra bony periodontal pocket. All types of external resorption are irregular in outline, and extensive lesions often spare a thin layer of dentine around the pulp so that the pulp can remain vital until a late stage, even if the defect communicates with a periodontal pocket.

Inflammatory root resorption is associated with detectable inflammation and may be internal or external. This may be evident radiographically, as radiolucency in the adjacent bone, or clinically as redness. The inflammatory type of resorption has the positive aspect that removal of the cause of the inflammation (i.e. infected necrotic tissue) may halt the resorption.

Unfortunately, this is not entirely predictable. Many cases of so-called inflammatory resorption, both internal and external, are not associated with significant inflammation clinically or histologically and are perhaps better regarded as idiopathic.

Replacement root resorption is root resorption starting externally accompanied by progressive replacement of the tooth by bone. It is often associated with ankylosis and is a complication of luxation injuries, particularly intrusion and avulsion. Inflammation is absent; therefore, treatment must be directed at removing the resorptive tissue itself, which has a less predictable outcome. Internally, the pulp canal space may be filled with tertiary dentine, which is known as *pulp canal obliteration*, and is not a true form of resorption.

◆ What Causes Resorption?

Resorption and repair may be physiological or pathological processes on both the external surface of the root and internally. Internally pulpal surface resorption is pathological; however, repair is one of the pulp's natural responses to injury, as in the case of tertiary dentine formation. External resorption is known to follow damage to the cementum layer or loss of vitality of cementum, which triggers osteoclastic activity, which is why external resorption is very common after an avulsion injury. External cervical root resorption is assumed to be primarily inflammatory in aetiology, caused by the periodontal flora, though this does not explain cases where multiple lesions affect several otherwise healthy teeth.

Internal resorption may follow loss of the predentine layer separating pulp from dentine, but the causes of this loss are unknown. A degree of pulp inflammation and increased pulp pressure are thought to be possible trigger factors.

◆ What are the Features of Resorption?

- Asymptomatic (unless an inflammatory cause is symptomatic)
- Internal resorption occurs in vital or partially vital teeth
- External resorption may develop on vital or nonvital teeth
- Resorption itself does not compromise vitality until the pulp communicates with the oral environment
- Usually slow and intermittent, occasionally very rapid
- Mobility or pathological fracture
- External cervical root resorption and extensive internal resorption appears as a 'pink spot', which is pulp/granulation tissue visible through the crown
- Ankylosis (continuity of tooth and bone) is the sequelae of replacement resorption
- Radiolucency and loss of tooth substance are the radiographic signs.

◆ What are the Signs of Ankylosis?

- Lack of normal mobility
- High pitched metallic percussive sound
- Infraocclusion (submerging tooth in the growing jaw)
- Sometimes identifiable radiographically as a bridged periodontal ligament
- Patchy 'moth-eaten' root surface/lamina dura.

◆ What are Your Definitive Diagnoses in This Case?

The maxillary lateral incisor has internal resorption, probably as a late sequela of the previous trauma or restoration of teeth. Resorption is advanced, and the root has suffered a pathological fracture making the coronal fragment mobile.

The maxillary central incisor has a persistent periapical periodontitis despite root canal treatment, suggesting a lack of an efficient coronal seal. In addition, the restorative prognosis of the tooth is questionable, depending on whether a ferrule is present.

There is a carious lesion present on the upper left canine.

Treatment

◆ How Would You Manage the Lateral Incisor in the Short Term and the Long Term?

The prognosis for the lateral incisor is poor, and it requires extraction. It cannot be restored because the resorption has involved the periodontal ligament around much of the tooth circumference. A tooth with a more localized perforation might be repaired surgically. However, in combination with the necessary root canal treatment, this would be heroic treatment with an unpredictable chance of success at best. Surgical repair is more suitable for external cervical resorption, as opposed to middle third internal root resorption.

Postextraction alveolar bone healing and remodelling will need to occur prior to definitive replacement; therefore, a provisional restoration will be required.

◆ What are the Immediate Replacement Options for the Lateral Incisor?

- A vacuum-formed clear Essix retainer with an acrylic tooth in the lateral incisor position
- An acrylic removable partial denture, Every-type or spoon design major connector
- A minimal preparation bridge of a cantilever design with a resin composite pontic for ease of adjustment after extraction
- The existing crown could be splinted to the adjacent teeth using a fibre-reinforced resin composite splint.

◆ What are the Definitive Replacement Options?

Minimal preparation adhesive bridge replacing the lateral incisor, of a cantilever design with a retainer on the canine. This would require the carious lesion in the canine to be small and for there to be sufficient occlusal clearance for the retainer.

A conventional cantilever bridge using the canine as the abutment, is a possibility; however, this is a more invasive option than a minimal preparation bridge. Either all-ceramic or metal-ceramic materials could potentially be used, each with advantages and disadvantages.

A conventional cantilever bridge using the upper left central incisor as the abutment would be a less predictable option. The failed root filling in the central incisor would require retreatment, which would have a less certain outcome than de novo endodontics. Initially an investigation of the restorability of the tooth would involve removal of the pre-existing restoration and assessment of the amount of remaining tooth structure to ascertain if there was sufficient tooth tissue for at least a 2-mm ferrule. If there was less than 4 mm of coronal dentine, then a post would be required to provide additional retention for the crown retainer. This would require a parallel-sided, cast or preformed post and core to support a single cantilever pontic replacing the lateral incisor. Using a post crowned tooth as a bridge retainer has a relatively high failure rate; indeed, post retention is best avoided in all bridge designs. If an orthograde repeat root canal treatment is not successful in healing the periapical infection, then an apicectomy will have to be considered for this tooth; and if it is performed, the root length available for a post will be reduced. Therefore, considering these complicating factors together with the time necessary to ensure apical healing (up to 4 years), this suggests that the central incisor is probably not suitable as a bridge abutment in this scenario.

A single tooth implant crown would be possible; however, the patient's diabetes would ideally need to be well controlled to ensure a predictable outcome. Diabetes is not an absolute contraindication for implant provision, but the possibility of delayed healing in diabetes, in the maxillary site (where implants have a reduced survival rate), means that an implant might not be recommended. Further discussion of anterior single tooth implants will be found in Case 35.

When managing trauma cases, comprehensive note keeping and documentation are essential to support optimal decision making and communication with the patient and clinical colleagues and also in the event of medico-legal scenarios. Depending on the nature and severity of the trauma, legal proceedings may be entered into, and clinical record keeping may form a part of the legal case. Therefore, the history of the trauma should be recorded as completely as possible. In addition, with regard to complex clinical scenarios such as this, effective liaison with specialist colleagues may be required, especially if three-dimensional (3D) cone beam computed tomography (CBCT) or endodontic surgery may be required. Adjunctive clinical photography with suitable consent forms signed would also be a sensible option in cases such as these.

For this case, a specialist endodontic option was sought, and the outcome was that both the central and lateral incisors had a poor prognosis and were not amenable to endodontic treatment. Therefore, following discussion with the patient regarding the replacement options, the teeth were extracted and replaced with two separate cantilever-design minimal preparation bridges, by using the upper right central incisor as the abutment to replace the upper left central incisor and the upper left canine as the abutment to replace the upper left lateral incisor.

Case 18
Oroantral Fistula

TARA RENTON

Summary

A 42-year-old man presents with pain following extraction of an upper first molar. What is the cause, and how will you treat him?

History

Complaint

The patient is suffering dull throbbing pain in his upper jaw and face on the left side only. Pressure below his eye is painful, and all his upper teeth on the left are tender on biting. He has a nasal discharge and blocked nose on the left.

History of Complaint

The patient has had the pain for 2 weeks following extraction of the upper left first molar by his dentist. The extraction was difficult, and the roots required surgical removal. There was little pain immediately afterwards, but pain has slowly developed so that it is now preventing him from sleeping. The pain is constant.

Medical History

The patient gives a history of smoking 20 cigarettes a day for 18 years but considers himself fit and healthy.

Examination

Extraoral Examination

He is a healthy-looking man with no facial swelling or lymphadenopathy. There is a lightly blood-stained discharge from the left nares, and halitosis.

Intraoral Examination

◆ **The Appearances on Presentation are Shown in Fig. 18.1. What Do You See, and How Do You Interpret the Features?**

There is a large defect in the alveolus at the site of the first molar socket; the socket appears empty and the oral mucosa has grown to line the visible sides of the socket. After 2 weeks, the oral epithelium should have proliferated to cover the socket mouth, but there must have been a failure of clot formation and/or organization. One possibility is that the patient has dry socket (see Case 15). No bone is visible in the socket, but it could be exposed further apically. However, dry socket is rare in the maxilla, and it is more likely that the socket is communicating with the maxillary antrum.

Differential Diagnosis

◆ **What Causes for This Pain are Possible, and Why?**

Sinusitis Secondary To Oroantral Fistula. An oroantral communication itself causes little or no discomfort but usually induces a degree of sinusitis. The nature and distribution of pain and presence of nasal discharge are typical of sinusitis. This seems the most likely diagnosis. Fistula formation is most commonly associated with the extraction of maxillary first and second molars.

Dental Pain. Before jumping to conclusions, it is worth considering whether the wrong tooth may have been removed. If the extraction was performed for pulpitis (which is often poorly localized), it is possible that at least some of the symptoms may arise from the adjacent teeth. You will need to check whether additional symptoms suggest pain of dental origin.

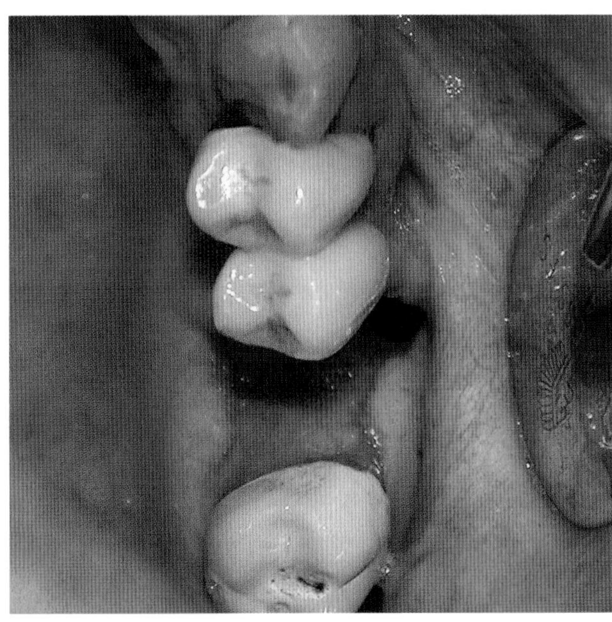

• **Fig. 18.1** The extraction socket on presentation.

◆ What is an Oroantral Fistula?

An oroantral fistula is a persistent epithelialized communication between the maxillary antrum and the mouth, present for more than 48 hours. The epithelial lining of the fistula grows from the gingival epithelium, periodontal pocket lining or the antral lining, and it may take up to 7 days for the epithelium to completely line the walls of the communication. If the tract is not lined by epithelium, it is known as an *oroantral communication* or *perforation*. Oroantral communications either close spontaneously or become epithelialized and persist as fistulae.

◆ What is the Aetiology of Oroantral Fistula?

The vast majority of OAF result from dental extraction. Up to 10% of upper molar extractions may create oroantral communications, but very few, only 0.5%, persist to become fistulae. Other causes include malignant neoplasms arising in the oral cavity or in the antrum.

◆ What Factors Predispose to Formation of Oroantral Fistulae After Extraction of Teeth?

- Proximity of roots to maxillary antrum, large sinus
- Difficult extraction, unfavourable root morphology
- Periapical lesions such as apical granulomas or cysts
- Bone loss caused by periodontitis or periodontal–endodontic lesion
- Hypercementosis
- Displaced root fragment
- Local infection or sequestrum
- Predisposition to infection (e.g. diabetes)
- Dry socket or other poor healing
- Advanced age
- Pre-existing diseases in the sinus, although this is probably not a very significant factor.

◆ What are the Signs and Symptoms of Oroantral Fistula?

The symptoms depend on the size of the fistula. Initially, there may be persistent pain localized to the tooth socket but later, when inflammation has subsided, the fistula will be painless. If pain is a prominent symptom, some additional element such as infection must be suspected. The socket may present as an empty cavity or as a prolapse of antral lining through the socket into the mouth. The most characteristic symptoms are the escape of fluids from the mouth into the nose on eating, or air or fluid into the mouth on blowing the nose. Passage of saliva, food and bacteria into the antrum causes sinusitis and the symptoms experienced will depend on its severity. Unilateral nasal obstruction, a feeling of fullness, pain over the maxilla and tenderness on pressure are typical.

Investigations

◆ What Investigations Would You Carry Out, How and Why?

Investigations need to be performed to confirm the communication with the antrum, to check for associated complications and to exclude the possibility that a malignant neoplasm is the cause of either the antral communication itself or the failure of the socket to heal. Investigations are summarized in Table 18.1.

TABLE 18.1 Summary of Investigations

Aim of Investigation	Methods
To demonstrate communication between antrum and mouth, the definitive test for oroantral fistula if there is no history of fluid or air passing between sinus and mouth.	If the fistula is large it may be possible to see into the antrum or pass a probe or large gutta percha point through into the antrum. If not, the patient can be asked to blow air into the nose with the anterior nares pinched closed and keeping the mouth open. You may see air bubbles, hear a hissing noise or detect air movement with a wisp of cotton wool at the socket opening.
To detect retained root fragments or sequestra in the socket.	Radiographs of the socket, ideally a periapical view, possibly also a panoramic tomograph.
To exclude the possibility of other lesions such as malignant neoplasms.	
To detect root fragments displaced into the antrum and exclude other antral disease.	Radiographs of antrum, usually a panoramic tomograph or standard occipito-mental view is sufficient. However, it is difficult to visualize the whole antrum in any one view without superimposition of other structures. Cone beam computed tomography (CBCT) is the best modality to examine the sinus if a root fragment is suspected but cannot be detected on other views. However, it requires a higher x-ray dose, and a plain film should be taken first.
To eliminate dental causes for any pain.	Vitality tests (thermal and/or electric) and examination for mobility of adjacent teeth.
To exclude malignancy or identify other causes for impaired socket healing.	Biopsy. Not usually required but if there is a worrying radiographic appearance or solid tissue in the socket, biopsy is indicated.

◆ The Periapical Radiograph of the Socket is Shown in Fig. 18.2. What Do You See?

The first molar socket is indistinct. The lamina dura has been resorbed, probably as a result of inflammation or infection. The tract of a fistula is not visible. This is usually the case because the cortex is intact buccally and palatally,

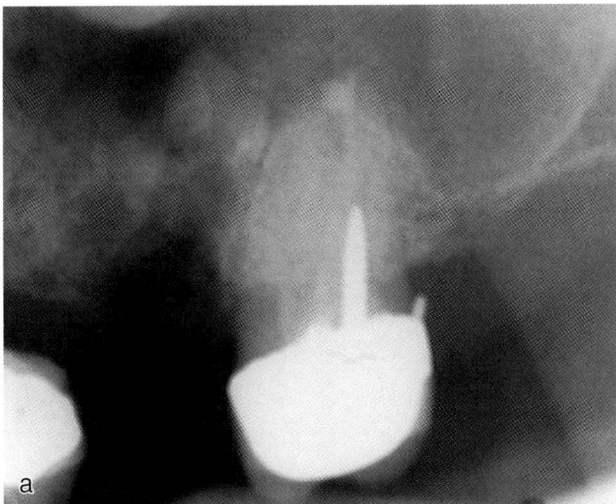

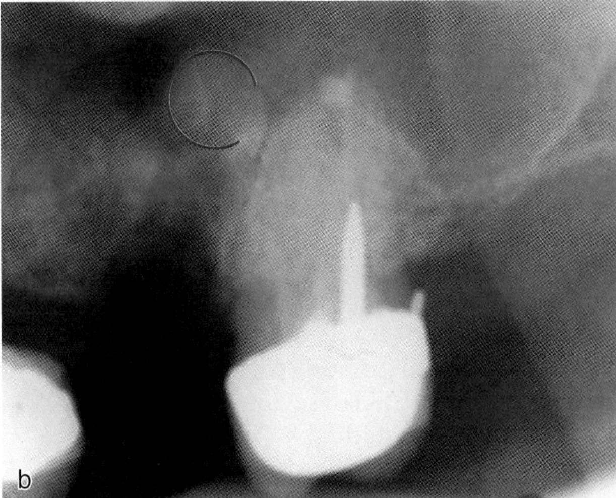

• **Fig. 18.2** a and b, Periapical view of the socket on presentation.

providing most of the radiodensity of the socket. The floor of the antrum is just visible, and a root fragment, approximately 3 mm long, lies on the sinus floor (outlined as a partial red circle in the lower figure). The second molar has had an inadequate root canal treatment, probably associated with loss of apical lamina dura and a small periapical radiolucency. A pin has perforated the distal root.

◆ What Else Do You Need to Know About the Root Fragment?

Whether it is loose in the antrum or trapped under the sinus lining or in granulation tissue. The root will have to be removed and if it is under the lining or trapped, it should be possible to remove it through the socket. If it is loose in the antrum, removal in this way may prove impossible, necessitating a later elective surgical procedure such as the Caldwell–Luc approach.

◆ How Will You Decide Where the Root is and Whether It is Mobile?

If the fistula opening is large you might try to visualize the fragment directly. If not, a second radiograph at right angles to the periapical, such as an occipito-mental view, would help localize it. A further view with the patient's head tilted would reveal whether or not the root moves.

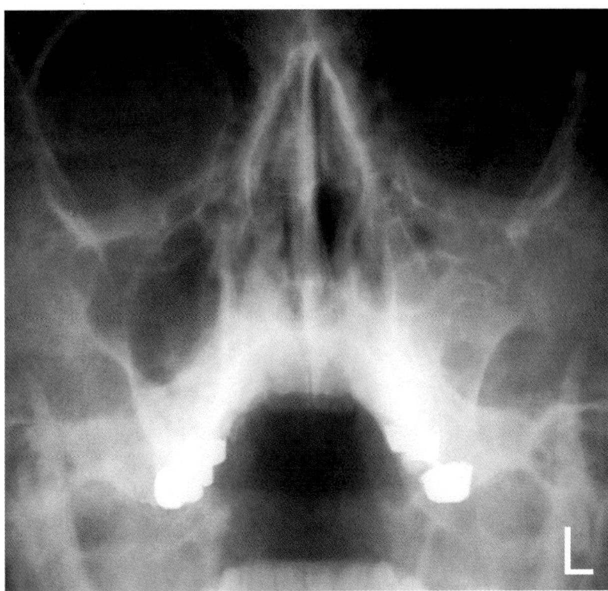

• **Fig. 18.3** Part of the occipito-mental view.

◆ A Section of the Occipito-Mental View is Shown in Fig. 18.3. What Do You See, and How Do You Interpret the Appearances?

The sinuses and facial bones are symmetrical, and there is no expansion of the maxillary antrum. However, the sinus on the left is much more radiopaque than that on the right, indicating oedema and thickening of the sinus lining or exudates within it. There is no fluid level visible. The root fragment is not visible because it lies on the sinus floor and is obscured by the superimposed alveolus.

Diagnosis

◆ What is Your Final Diagnosis?

Sinusitis secondary to oroantral fistula caused by extraction of the upper first molar. A root fragment has been displaced into the sinus. Apical periodontitis of the second molar may also contribute to the sinusitis, but this is a chronic problem and a lower priority for treatment.

Treatment

◆ How Would You Treat This Patient?

- If pus is present in the fistula or if symptoms are severe, consider treating the sinusitis first and closing the fistula later after the sinusitis has partially resolved (it will not resolve completely until the fistula is closed). If there is long-standing infective sinusitis, this must be treated prior to surgical closure otherwise healing will be compromised.
- Excise the fistula, otherwise remnants of the epithelial lining may proliferate to reform the tract.
- Remove the root fragment from the sinus.
- Close the oroantral communication surgically.

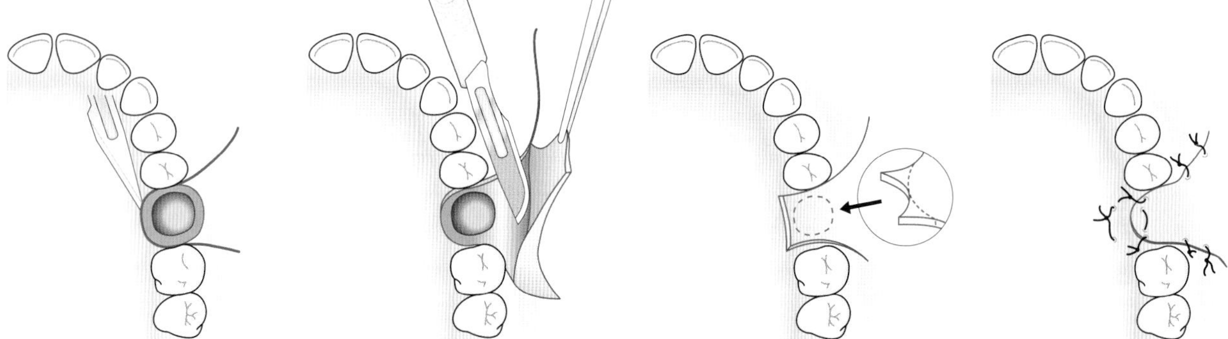

• **Fig. 18.4** The buccal advancement flap. Note how the relieving incisions buccally flare widely, shallow incision of the periosteum, trimming of the flap apex to ensure a good fit palatally and the rim of palatal bone on which it lies.

◆ Would You Treat This Patient in General Practice?

Provided you are confident of your ability to remove the root fragment, there is no reason why this cannot be dealt with in a general practice. However, if the root is mobile in the antrum, the patient should be referred to hospital.

◆ How Would You Excise the Fistula and Remove the Root?

Under local anaesthesia, incise around the edge of the socket from gingiva right down into the antrum, removing all the soft tissue in the socket as a cylinder or cone-shaped piece, and draw it into the mouth. Depending on the size of the bony defect and the amount of bone resorption (usually greater in long-standing fistulae), this opens up a large hole into the sinus. With suction, good light and direct vision, try to identify the root fragment, and remove it with fine forceps, sucker tip or other instrument. Take care not to displace it into the sinus. If it becomes displaced, it may be possible to wash it out by flushing saline into the sinus. Alternatively, better surgical access to the sinus may be achieved by using the Caldwell—Luc approach under general anaesthesia. This is the main reason for referring patients with mobile fragments to hospital.

Send the excised tract for histopathological examination in case of unexpected underlying lesions.

◆ How Will You Close the Defect?

The buccal mucoperiosteal flap with advancement (buccal advancement flap) is the most commonly used technique, and it has more than a 90% success rate. The technique is shown in Fig. 18.4. After excising the fistula, as above, proceed as follows:

Make two incisions buccally, anterior and posterior to the socket, passing parallel up the attached gingiva and then splaying to provide a wider base to ensure a good blood supply for the flap. The line of the incisions must be compatible with the flap sliding palatally to cover the defect in the alveolus.

Elevate the mucoperiosteal flap you have outlined by lifting the soft tissues in the plane beneath the periosteum.

Advance the flap. The flap cannot yet be pulled across the defect because the periosteum cannot be stretched. Fold the flap back to expose its periosteal surface and make several shallow parallel incisions across the flap that penetrate only the periosteum (about 0.25–0.5 mm in depth). This must be done very carefully with the flap under slight tension. As the periosteum is incised the flap will be felt to stretch. Do not perforate the flap, or it will either be cut off or have a compromised blood supply. Make sufficient incisions to lengthen the flap so that it can reach across to the palatal side of the defect with minimal tension.

Prepare the palatal aspect of the alveolar defect. Refresh the margin of the palatal side to expose a narrow bony rim at least 1 mm wide, preferably 2 mm. The flap must be sutured into place at a site that has bony support.

Suture the flap in place using slowly resorbable sutures (e.g. 3/0 vicryl) or nonresorbable sutures. Place several sutures around the apex of the flap (mesial, distal and central) and buccally. The flap must not be under tension, and sufficient sutures must be placed to ensure an airtight and watertight seal supported by underlying bone. Ensure haemostasis. The sutures must remain in place for 10–14 days.

◆ What Alternative Flap Designs are Possible?

The buccal advancement flap may not be possible when the bony defect is very large or when a previous attempt at repair has failed.

A number of other flaps are possible, including the palatal island flap, submucosal palatal island flap, combined buccal and palatal flaps and even pedicled grafts from the tongue. However, most of these techniques are complex and have been superseded by the buccal fat pad technique. The buccal fat pad technique, the second most commonly used method, is shown in Fig. 18.5. Alternative methods to close oroantral fistulae are noted in Table 18.2.

◆ What Postoperative Instructions are Required?

In addition to the routine instructions given after extraction, the patient must be placed on an antral regime to reduce inflammation and prevent a rise in air pressure in the antrum.

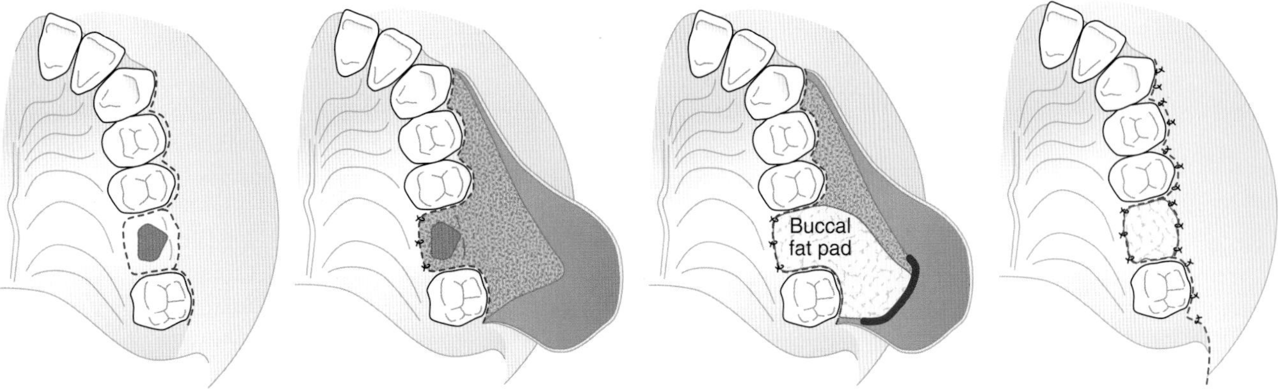

• **Fig. 18.5** The buccal fat pad technique. Note how the flap has double layered closure with pedicled fat and advanced mucosa sutured into place. The exposed fat will granulate and re-epithelilialize. There is no need for a pack during healing.

TABLE 18.2 Local Flap Design

Local Flap Design	Indications/Advantages	Contraindications/Disadvantages
Buccal advancement flap (see Fig. 18.4).	Relatively simple, no flap donor site to heal, suitable for local analgesia.	Not ideal for large defect, advancing the flap reduces the depth of the residual buccal sulcus. Alveolar rather than masticatory mucosa advanced onto the ridge. Flap may break down if under tension.
Buccal fat pad technique. As above, and the buccal fat pad is dissected from under the buccal flap on a pedicle and secure in the socket (see Fig. 18.5).	As above, able to fill a larger defect.	General anaesthesia is required for fat pad dissection, sulcus loss.
Palatal flap.	Possible when buccal flap has failed or would have insufficient length to cover a palatally placed bone defect. Covers the defect with masticatory mucosa.	The flap is of thick tissue and is difficult to mobilize. The donor site is left to granulate and this is painful until healed.

The upper first molar is situated in the lowest point of the maxillary sinus. Persistent infection or inflammation will induce exudates that will drain to this point and cause breakdown of the clot. Increased air pressure in the sinus, for instance, from sneezing or blowing the nose, will force air or exudate through the alveolar defect as well as physically disrupting the clot and flap. Decongestants maintain the patency of the opening of the sinus to favour drainage to the nose.

A suitable antral regime would be:

- an absolute ban on blowing the nose for 48 hours
- sneeze allowing pressure to escape through the mouth
- nasal decongestant (e.g. ephedrine nasal spray 0.5%)
- decongestant inhalant.

In addition, chlorhexidine mouthwash should be given. The repair will fail if there is leakage of saliva and bacteria past the flap from the oral aspect. No rinsing should be performed for 18 hours.

Other Considerations

◆ How Might Formation of Oroantral Communication Be Prevented?

The risk of oroantral communication should be assessed routinely on a radiograph before extraction of upper molars. If the risk is high, an experienced surgeon should remove the tooth. Surgical extraction, possibly with elective sectioning of the tooth, reduces the chances of disrupting the maxillary floor.

◆ The Preoperative Radiograph is Shown in Fig. 18.6. What Do You See?

Several features in the list of risk factors above are evident. There is a low antral floor in contact with the roots, there is little alveolar bone height, and there is loss of lamina dura around the tooth root apices.

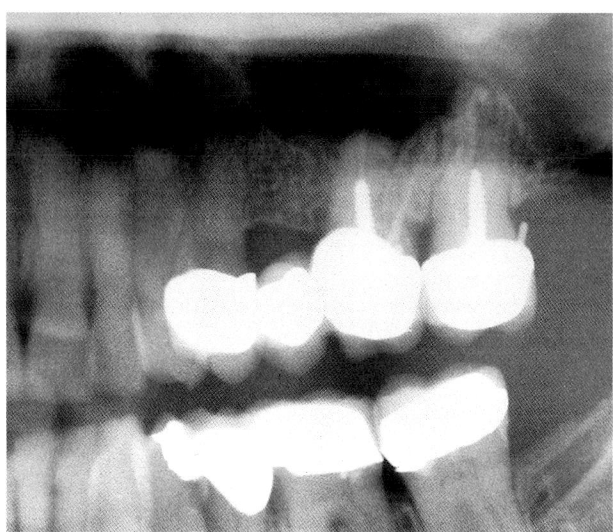

• **Fig. 18.6** Preoperative radiograph.

◆ How Could an Oroantral Communication Be Confirmed At the Time of Extraction? How Might This Help?

If an antral communication is present, an echoing 'wind tunnel sound' will be heard if a small suction tip is held in the socket, the result of air being sucked from the antrum as well as the mouth. If the communication is large, you may be able to see into the antrum or identify nasal regurgitation of your irrigation fluids or blood from the extraction site. Do not ask patient to blow through their nose while holding it. The sinus lining may still be intact but would be burst by the pressure and a small communication might be enlarged.

If a communication is suspected, stabilization of the clot, closure of the socket with resorbable sutures and appropriate warnings to the patient about blowing the nose should prevent a fistula developing. This is likely to be effective if the diameter of the communication is 4 mm or less. If it is larger, it should be repaired immediately using a suitable flap technique to avoid sinusitis and infection.

Case 19

Troublesome Mouth Ulcers

PEPE SHIRLAW AND SHALINI NAYEE

Summary

A 38-year-old woman with mouth ulcers has noticed a recent exacerbation in severity. You need to make a diagnosis and decide on suitable investigations and treatment.

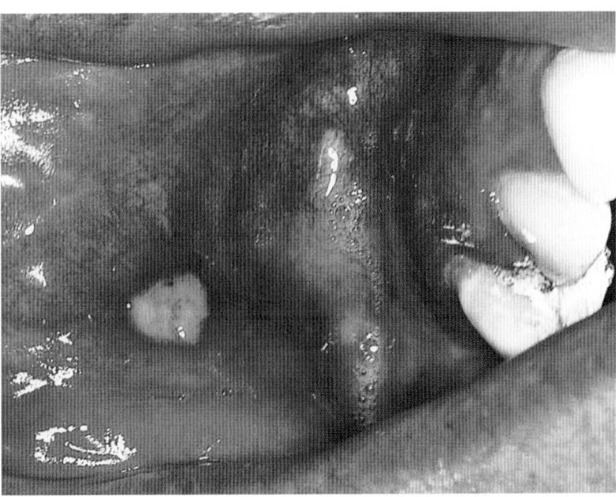

• **Fig. 19.1** Right buccal mucosa.

History

Complaint

The patient complains of mouth ulcers that have become more troublesome recently.

History of Complaint

The patient has experienced occasional mouth ulcers for approximately 25 years. Usually, she has one ulcer at a time, but recently she has experienced 3–4 ulcers at a time, and the ulcers have become more frequent. She has tried some over-the-counter mouth ulcer products, but because she was attending your surgery for a filling, she wonders whether you can suggest any other treatments.

Medical History

The patient does not have any known medical conditions.

◆ The Patient Has Already Provided Several Pieces of Information of Value for Differential Diagnosis. How Do You Assess Her Ulcers On the Basis of the Information Available?

The patient has reported recurrent attacks of oral ulceration since her teenage years, with a mixture of single ulcers and small crops of ulcers. There are many causes of oral ulceration but these ulcers appear to be **recurrent**, appearing periodically and healing completely between attacks.

◆ What are the Common or Important Causes of Recurrent Oral Ulceration?

These can be considered by using a surgical sieve.

- Idiopathic
  - Recurrent aphthous stomatitis (RAS)
    - Minor type
    - Major type
    - Herpetiform type
- Hypersensitivity
  - Erythema multiforme
- Nutritional
  - Haematinic deficiency (iron, vitamin B_{12}, folate), coeliac disease
- Traumatic
  - Intraoral appliances, parafunction

◆ How Will You Differentiate Among These Conditions?

The history is the most important factor in differentiating among the types of recurrent ulcers. Findings from clinical examination, blood tests and biopsy may also be of assistance.

◆ What Features of the Ulcers Would You Ask About To Determine the Diagnosis? Explain Why for Each.

See Table 19.1. This patient's answers are shown in the right-hand column.

◆ How are Major and Minor Recurrent Aphthous Stomatitis Differentiated?

By severity, rather than by any one feature alone. RAS may be labelled as major because of the size of the ulcers, their long duration or because they cause scarring on healing.

TABLE 19.1 Features of Ulcers

Feature	Details	This Patient's Ulcers ...
Site of ulcer	Recurrent aphthous stomatitis (RAS): Typically nonkeratinized mucosa. Erythema multiforme: Vermilion border of lip, buccal and labial mucosa. Traumatic ulceration: Usually recurs at the same site, often close to a sharp tooth. Crohn's disease: Typically affects buccal sulcus.	*... affect the labial mucosa and buccal mucosa. They never occur on the dorsal tongue or palate.*
Size of ulcer	Minor RAS: 3–8 mm in diameter. Major RAS: greater than 1 cm in diameter (up to 3–4 cm). Herpetiform RAS: 0.2–3 mm in diameter.	*... are usually 3–5 mm in diameter.*
Duration of each ulcer	Minor RAS: 7–10 days. Major RAS: May take weeks to months. Ulcers heal with scarring. Herpetiform RAS: 7–10 days. Erythema multiforme: Variable (10–21 days).	*... last 1 week.*
Number of ulcers	Minor RAS: Single ulcers or small crops of 2–5 ulcers Major RAS: One or two ulcers at a time. Herpetiform RAS: 30–100 ulcers at a time, which can coalesce such that it becomes difficult to count individual ulcers.	*... are normally single. Occasionally 3–4 develop at once.*
Frequency of attacks	RAS: Variable frequency; some patients may have ulcers continuously, whilst others experience ulcers just once per year. Erythema multiforme: Ulcers may recur at 6–8 week intervals in severe cases; other patients experience one-two attacks per year. Nutritional deficiencies/inflammatory conditions: Patients may have continuous ulceration.	*... are usually confined to one or two attacks a year. However, she has had three outbreaks of ulceration in the last 4 months.*
Shape of ulcer	RAS: Usually round/oval and sharply defined; may become more irregular with healing. Herpetiform ulcers coalesce to form irregular shapes. Erythema multiforme: Irregular and ragged, merging with inflamed surrounding mucosa. Those on the lips are often covered by bloody fibrin sloughs.	*... are round or oval.*
Are the ulcers preceded by vesicles?	The presence of vesicles indicates possible viral infection or immunobullous disease. This fact may be helpful in the differential diagnosis of herpetiform ulcers, which resemble viral ulcers but are not preceded by vesicles.	*... have not been preceded by any vesicles.*
Age of onset	RAS: Usually before or around adolescence. Erythema multiforme/inflammatory bowel disease: Typically second or third decade. Immunobullous disease: Typically, fourth decade onwards.	*... started with occasional ulcers in childhood and have continued into adulthood.*
Family history	RAS: May have family history of ulceration. Coeliac disease/inflammatory bowel disease: May have positive family history. Erythema multiforme: Typically no family history. Traumatic ulceration: No family history.	*... appear to be sporadic. Her parents and siblings do not experience mouth ulcers. However, her 7-year-old son occasionally has ulcers.*
Exacerbating or relieving factors	Ulcers can develop at a site of minor trauma in both RAS and immunobullous disease. Stress and menstruation can precipitate attacks of RAS. Erythema multiforme may be triggered by a drug, viral or other infection, although often no trigger is identified.	*... occasionally develop where she bites herself or knocks her mucosa with a toothbrush.*

◆ What is the Most Likely Diagnosis Based On This Patient's History?

The history is suggestive of RAS minor, which has recently increased in severity.

Examination

Intraoral Examination

◆ The Appearance of One Ulcer is Shown in Fig. 19.1. What Do You See?

There is an obvious ulcer on the anterior buccal mucosa. It is shallow, a few millimetres in diameter and has a slightly irregular but well-defined margin. There is a halo of erythema around the ulcer, but the surrounding mucosa is otherwise unremarkable. There is a temporary restoration in the upper right first premolar, and the ulcer would lie in approximately this region at rest.

When you examine the patient, you find two more ulcers. One is 2 mm in diameter and lies in the lower labial mucosa adjacent to the lower right canine. A third ulcer, also 3 mm in diameter, lies on the upper left buccal mucosa anterior to the parotid papilla. They appear to be identical to the ulcer shown.

◆ What Can You Deduce From These Appearances?

The appearance alone is not particularly helpful in differential diagnosis but is typical of minor recurrent aphthous stomatitis. The slightly irregular, rather than smooth, outline suggests early healing. The ulcers are not at all suggestive of erythema multiforme, which would cause more extensive, irregular ulceration of the anterior oral mucosa. They do not suggest immunobullous diseases, which cause ragged mucosal ulcers.

If you were able to examine the patient, you would find no evidence of scarring, supporting the diagnosis of recurrent aphthous stomatitis minor, as opposed to recurrent aphthous stomatitis major.

Diagnosis

◆ What is Your Diagnosis, and What Would You Do Next?

The history and examination findings indicate recurrent aphthous stomatitis minor (RAS minor). However, it is necessary to consider whether there is an underlying predisposing condition that could account for the recent change in the pattern of ulceration.

◆ What Features of the Ulcers Might Indicate the Presence of an Underlying Predisposing Condition?

Any feature in the history or examination that is atypical for RAS minor should raise suspicion of an underlying condition. In particular, the following should trigger a search for underlying predisposing causes:

- Onset after the second decade
- Significant increase in ulcer size, duration, symptoms or severity

◆ Which Underlying Predisposing Conditions and Lifestyle Factors Should Be Considered for This Patient?

- Haematinic (iron, vitamin B_{12}, folate) deficiency
- Gastrointestinal disease (e.g. coeliac disease, Crohn's disease, ulcerative colitis)
- Behçet's disease
- Smoking cessation
- Medications

◆ How Do You Assess and Investigate These Underlying Conditions?

Iron deficiency is relatively common, particularly amongst females of child-bearing age. Check for a history of anaemia and its cause. Ask about common causes of iron deficiency anaemia include menorrhagia and upper or lower gastrointestinal bleeding (nonsteroidal anti-inflammatory drug [NSAID] use, excessive alcohol use, peptic ulcer disease, inflammatory bowel disease, haemorrhoids and colorectal cancer). Dietary deficiency should be considered in patients who follow a restrictive diet. Coordination with the patient's general medical practitioner is required. Patients should undergo blood tests for microcytic anaemia (reduced haemoglobin, reduced mean cell volume [MCV] and serum ferritin levels. Ulcers may be associated with minor degrees of iron deficiency insufficient to cause overt anaemia. Any evidence of iron deficiency anaemia should be followed by thorough investigation and treatment of the underlying cause.

Other vitamin deficiencies associated with oral ulceration are typically folate or B_{12}. Check whether the patient follows a restrictive diet, particularly a strict vegetarian diet, or has high levels of alcohol consumption. Both can result in vitamin B deficiency. Ask about any previous diagnosis of the autoimmune condition pernicious anaemia (B_{12} deficiency). Consider undiagnosed pernicious anaemia in patients who have a history of vitiligo, hypothyroidism or Addison's disease, as these conditions are related. Consider the possibility of gastrointestinal disease (see below). Patients with suspected B_{12}/folate deficiency should undergo blood tests (full blood count [FBC], folate, B_{12}) with their general practitioner. These would show macrocytic anaemia (reduced haemoglobin levels and elevated MCV).

Gastrointestinal disease can cause reduced absorption of iron, folate and B_{12}, all of which cause recurrent oral ulceration. Ask about diarrhoea, constipation, abdominal cramps, weight loss and blood in the stools. Enquire about any family history of gastrointestinal disease. Patients with gastrointestinal disease may also experience recurrent oral ulceration in the absence of haematinic deficiency, reflecting their underlying inflammatory disease state. Pyostomatitis vegetans may occur in ulcerative colitis, linear ulcers of the buccal sulcus in Crohn's disease and herpetiform-type ulcers in coeliac disease.

Behçet's disease is a rare autoinflammatory condition that can present with oral ulcers as the most significant problem. Patients may suffer from a broad spectrum of signs and symptoms and should be questioned about any history of genital ulcers, rashes including erythema nodosum or skin pustules, arthritis of large and small joints and history of venous thrombosis. Ocular signs including uveitis are found in a minority of patients, as well as central nervous system symptoms. There are no specific tests for Behçet's disease (although human leucocyte antigen [HLA] typing may help identify those at risk from ocular disease). A biopsy of an oral ulcer may be helpful because it can demonstrate underlying vasculitis.

Smoking cessation should be excluded by questioning. Ulceration related to smoking cessation can be difficult to manage, often not responding well to topical therapies, and may be sufficiently troublesome that the patient will recommence smoking. This does not usually induce remission of ulcers.

Medications must be considered as a potential cause for oral ulceration. Review the medication history to ensure that nothing has been missed. Check for medication side effects in the British National Formulary (BNF) and assess whether the ulcer history coincides with recent prescription of a new medication, or a change in the dose of an existing medication. Medication causes of oral ulceration include nicorandil, used for management of angina, and methotrexate, which is used for such conditions as rheumatoid arthritis. However, these do not follow the pattern of typical recurrent oral ulcers seen in RAS.

Treatment

◆ What Treatments are Available, and Which Would You Suggest?

Many treatments are available, but none is highly effective in all patients and treatment must be selected to suit individual cases. Treatments may be topical or systemic, and sometimes both are used. Reassurance is an important part of treatment in RAS minor so that patient information leaflets can be provided. Specifically, inform the patient that:

- RAS is very common and is a 'nuisance' condition rather than one that is harmful to health.
- Although many treatments are available, none will 'cure' the ulcers. Rather, the goal of treatment is to reduce the duration and frequency of oral ulceration.

Treatments available are shown in Table 19.2.

For this patient, the most important initial step is to exclude an underlying cause, which may account for the recent change in the pattern of the oral ulceration. The overall history and examination findings are consistent with a diagnosis of RAS minor. The recent worsening ulceration is likely to represent a concurrent underlying problem, such as iron deficiency anaemia, and it would be advisable for this patient to see her general medical practitioner for blood tests. Treatment of the underlying cause of this exacerbation should reduce the ulcer severity to the previous pattern of occasional, solitary ulcers. In the meantime, a mouthwash such as benzydamine hydrochloride may improve the patient's comfort. Prescription of hydrocortisone pellets could also be considered.

◆ The Patient Asks Whether the Buccal Ulcer Could Be Caused By the Temporary Restoration in the Adjacent Tooth. What is Your Opinion?

No, this is very unlikely to be the primary cause. The history of RAS is so typical that the diagnosis is not in doubt. Reactions to dental materials are not associated with ulcers of this type. Remember that aphthae often develop at the sites of minor trauma. Mucosal trauma during restoration placement, from a sharp edge on the restoration, or from biting while the mucosa was anaesthetized might well explain the location of this particular ulcer.

TABLE 19.2 Treatments for Minor Recurrent Aphthous Stomatitis (RAS)

Treatment	Description and Indications
Lifestyle advice	Simple advice may help to make ulcers more manageable: Avoid spicy foods, acidic fruit juices and carbonated drinks; consider drinking with a straw when ulcers are present; avoid sharp foods such as crisps, and astringent toothpastes.
Covering agents (e.g. Orabase)	Good for infrequent, solitary ulcers anteriorly in the buccal and labial mucosa. Use is difficult and the patient must be capable of some dexterity.
Analgesic mouthwash (e.g. benzydamine) Antiseptic mouthwash (e.g. chlorhexidine)	Both types of mouthwash are useful when ulcers affect a range of oral mucosal sites not accessible to covering pastes. These are symptomatic treatments, which do not have any impact on ulcer duration or frequency. Popular with most patients.
Low potency topical steroid pellets such as hydrocortisone (Corlan)	Ulcers must be at sites where the pellet can be left to dissolve, usually in the sulci. Useful first-line treatments if the ulcer-free period is longer than 1 month. May reduce ulcer frequency in some patients.
Steroid mouthwashes (e.g. betamethasone)	Bethamethasone soluble tablets are available for prescription by dentists in primary care in the UK. Used when ulcers affect a range of oral mucosal sites. Patients must dissolve tablets to make a rinse, which is held in the mouth and then expectorated. Patients may experience less frequent ulceration with regular use.
Steroid aerosols (e.g. fluticasone, beclomethasone)	Beclomethasone pressurised inhaler is available for prescription by dentists in primary care in the UK. Sometimes used for solitary ulcers. May be useful in patients who cannot expectorate steroid mouthrinses, such as children.
Systemic therapies (steroids, colchicine, azathioprine, thalidomide)	Not available for prescription by dentists in primary care in the UK. Indicated for severe cases, recalcitrant to topical therapies. Long-term steroid therapy should not be used to manage oral ulceration.

Case 20
A Lump in the Neck

NICHOLAS M. GOODGER AND SELVAM THAVARAJ

Summary

A 55-year-old man presents to your oral and maxillofacial surgery department clinic with a lump on the left side of the neck. You must make a diagnosis.

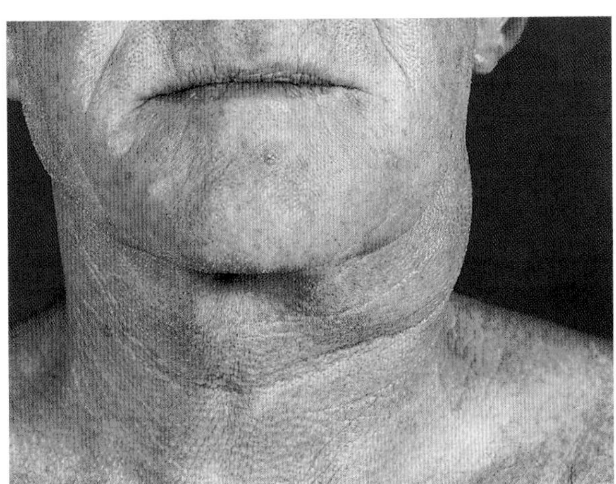

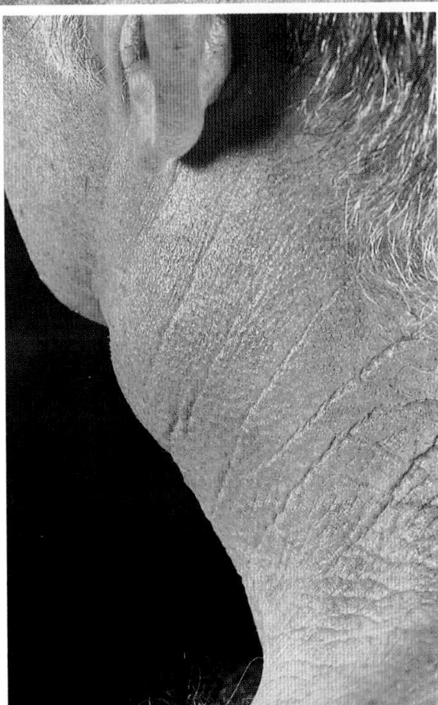

• **Fig. 20.1** a and b, The appearance of the swelling.

History

Complaint

The patient complains of the lump and has noticed some discomfort on swallowing, as if something is stuck in his throat. He assumes the lump is the cause.

History of Present Complaint

He thinks he first noticed the lump about 3 months ago. It has always been painless and is slowly enlarging. The discomfort on swallowing is of recent onset.

Medical History

The patient is otherwise fit and well. He has never smoked and drinks 10 units of alcohol (beer) each week.

Examination

Extraoral Examination

The appearance of the swelling is shown in Fig. 20.1.

◆ What Do You See? What is the Likely Origin of the Mass?

There is a swelling just anterior to the anterior border of the sternomastoid muscle and below and behind the angle of the mandible. It is several centimetres in diameter and extends forwards below the angle of the mandible towards the submandibular region. The overlying skin does not appear to be inflamed.

The swelling lies over the deep cervical lymph node chain and could well arise from a cervical lymph node. It is too low and too far posterior to be arising from the submandibular gland and too low to have arisen in the lower pole of the parotid gland. Other soft tissues of the neck could be the origin, but a lymph node is the most likely cause.

If you could palpate the lesion, you would find that it is approximately 8 × 6 cm in size and feels very soft on palpation, making its edges difficult to localize. It is possibly fluctuant and seems cyst-like. It is mobile, not fixed to the overlying skin or deep structures. The patient has not noticed any tenderness on palpation. There are no other swellings or enlarged lymph nodes palpable on either side of the neck.

Intraoral Examination

The submandibular glands are palpable bimanually and appear symmetrical. Both are mobile and clearly separate from the swelling, which lies posterior to the gland.

The patient's mouth has been well restored in the past but suffers from recent neglect, and several carious cavities are visible. There is no significant periodontal disease, with most probing depths less than 5 mm, and no mobile teeth. The lower left first permanent molar has lost a large restoration and has extensive caries. There is no soft tissue swelling, sinus or tenderness in the sulcus adjacent to the apices of the roots. The tooth is not tender to percussion. The oral mucosa appears normal, and the tonsils appear to be symmetrical.

Differential Diagnosis

◆ What are the Most Likely Causes of the Lump, and Why?

Metastatic malignancy appears likely, and this lesion is so typical of a cervical lymph node metastasis that it must be considered to be malignant until proven otherwise. The combination of features suggestive of metastasis is the patient's age (should be considered a possible cause in any patient older than 45 years of age), the site (consistent with a cervical lymph node) and lack of tenderness. Fixation to the skin or other structures would be almost conclusive of malignancy but is a late sign. The one feature that seems to point away from a metastasis is the soft cystic consistency of the swelling. Metastases from oral, skin or salivary gland cancers, lymphoma or melanoma are typically firm or hard. However, some carcinomas such as those arising in the tonsil characteristically produce a cystic metastasis. Occasionally, a metastasis from carcinomas of the oral cavity, salivary glands or thyroid gland may be full of cystic spaces.

Branchial or lymphoepithelial cysts develop at this site and, given the soft, fluctuant consistency, need to be considered. However, branchial cysts usually present in childhood or early adulthood. Lymphoepithelial cysts arise in developmental epithelial rests in upper cervical lymph nodes and present just like this in a middle-aged or older population. However, cystic metastatic carcinoma is such an important diagnosis that investigation must exclude this before considering these benign possibilities.

Tuberculosis may present as a soft and painless neck lump and needs to be considered both as a possible diagnosis and as a factor affecting management. Most patients with cervical lymph node enlargement caused by tuberculosis have reactivation ('secondary' or postprimary) tuberculosis, in which a previous quiescent infection becomes reactivated. This localized infection may or may not be accompanied by pulmonary disease, although there may be radiological evidence of past tuberculosis on chest radiograph. Cervical tuberculous lymphadenitis is common in those from the Indian subcontinent.

◆ Which Additional, But Less Likely, Causes Need To Be Considered Whenever a Patient Complains of an Enlargement At This Site? Why are They Unlikely Causes in This Case?

Numerous lesions could arise at this site, and it is not useful to list them all. A number of possible causes (Table 20.1) merit consideration because they are common, easily excluded or cause significant morbidity.

Investigations

◆ What is the Most Important Investigation? Which Methods Might Be Used, and What are Their Advantages and Disadvantages?

The critical requirement when malignancy is suspected is to obtain tissue speedily for microscopic diagnosis. All other investigations are less important at this stage. Three techniques are in common use; fine-needle aspiration biopsy, core biopsy and the surgical incisional biopsy (Table 20.2).

◆ What Other Investigations Might Be Performed, Either Now or At a Later Date? Why?

See Table 20.3.

In this case, a suitable combination of investigations would be fine-needle aspiration, dental radiography, vitality tests and possibly ultrasonography. Sialography would have been performed if a salivary origin remained a possibility after clinical examination.

The lower first molar was nonvital and a periapical radiograph revealed apical radiolucency. Fine-needle aspiration of the mass was performed, but in this instance, there was insufficient cellular yield to reach a definitive diagnosis. A core biopsy was therefore performed under ultrasound guidance. The core biopsy specimen is shown in Fig. 20.2.

◆ What Does the Core Biopsy Show, and How Do You Interpret the Appearances?

The image on the left is taken at low magnification. A cohesive sheet of epithelial cells is present on the left and these have a similar morphology to basal and lower prickle squamous epithelial cells. Occasional darkly stained (hyperchromatic) cells and variation in nuclear size (anisonucleosis) can be appreciated even at low magnification. Many normal lymphocytes are present towards the right of the image (around the yellow asterisk). There should be no epithelium in a lymph node; this indicates metastatic carcinoma to a lymph node. The image on the right is at higher magnification and highlights cells with pleomorphic nuclei (yellow arrow). An abnormal tripolar mitosis is indicated by the black arrow. These features also indicate malignancy. Although no keratinization is present, the basal and lower prickle morphology and cohesive sheets of epithelium suggest that this is squamous cell carcinoma, as opposed to adenocarcinoma or lymphoma.

Diagnosis

◆ What is Your Diagnosis?

The patient has metastatic squamous cell carcinoma in a cervical lymph node.

Further Investigations

◆ What is the Next Step in Diagnosis? How Can This Be Achieved?

To determine the primary site of this carcinoma. No oral carcinoma has been noted on examination. The primary

TABLE 20.1 Further Possible Causes of the Enlargement

Cause		Reasons
Infectious causes	HIV infection	Should always be considered in chronic lymph node enlargement but causes generalized lymphadenopathy. May be accompanied by signs of immunosuppression. A most unlikely diagnosis for this presentation. Nodes feel firm or rubbery.
	Cat scratch disease	A less likely cause of lymphadenitis is cat scratch disease because it may present with a single markedly enlarged node. There may be a history of exposure to cats or other pets or history of a primary skin infection at the site of a scratch. Diagnosis of cat scratch disease is confirmed by serological tests.
Inflammatory causes	Lymphadenitis	This is a common result to a local cause and so must be considered. However, there is no tenderness on palpation to suggest an inflammatory cause. If this were a reactive inflammatory enlargement, the most likely source of infection would be a dental, pharyngeal or skin infection. The patient has a potential source of dental infection in the lower left first permanent molar but the tooth is neither tender to percussion nor associated with overt infection, making it an unlikely cause.
	Sarcoidosis	Another cause of generalized lymphadenopathy or enlargement of a group of nodes. More common in the 20- to 40-year age group. African American, West Indian and Irish immigrants to the UK are at particular risk. Usually accompanied by other signs that aid diagnosis. An unlikely cause for this patient's swelling as sarcoid usually presents as multiple firm and rubbery nodes.
Benign neoplasms	Salivary gland neoplasm	The tail of the parotid gland extends low into the neck, to just below and behind the angle of the mandible. This lesion does not appear to be in the correct site for a parotid gland origin but the possibility of a benign salivary neoplasm might be considered. Of the benign salivary neoplasms, only Warthin's tumour seems likely because these are typically soft and cystic. A metastasis from a malignant salivary neoplasm would usually feel firm or hard.
	Carotid body tumour (paraganglioma)	These arise from the carotid body at the carotid bifurcation and cause a swelling just in front of the sternomastoid muscle but slightly higher than the present swelling. They are rare, affect the 30- to 60-year-old age group and are sometimes bilateral. Although an unusual cervical swelling, the accompanying pulsation, thrill or bruit from the carotid blood supply aids diagnosis. The lesion is mobile horizontally but not vertically because it is attached to the carotid artery. An unlikely cause for this patient's swelling.
	Other benign soft tissue neoplasms	Many are possible, arising from muscle, nerve, fat or fibrous tissue. None merits being singled out as a possible cause in this case. Only lipoma feels very soft.
Other primary malignant neoplasms	Lymphoma	An enlarged lymph node in the deep cervical lymph chain could be the first presentation of lymphoma. Non–Hodgkin's lymphoma would be the most likely type in a patient of this age. However, enlarged lymph nodes in lymphoma are almost always multiple and feel rubbery. The presence of such a large discrete lesion without other enlarged lymph nodes almost completely excludes lymphoma.

TABLE 20.2 Techniques for Obtaining Tissue

Investigation	Advantages	Disadvantages
Fine-needle aspiration biopsy/cytology (FNAB or FNAC)	The least invasive procedure which can provide a sample of the lesional tissue. Fine-needle aspiration does not risk seeding tumour or tuberculosis into the tissues of the neck. Rapid. Readily repeated if it fails. Leaves no scar.	It is possible to miss the lesion when inserting the needle. If this is likely to be a problem, the procedure can be performed under ultrasound or radiological guidance. For cysts, as here, it is important to sample the wall, not the lumen. Provides only a small sample and definitive diagnosis on cytology may not be possible (although a sufficiently accurate diagnosis to plan treatment may be provided).

Continued

TABLE 20.2 Techniques for Obtaining Tissue—cont'd

Investigation	Advantages	Disadvantages
Core biopsy	Easy to perform, providing a core of tissue for histological analysis. Minimal scarring.	It is possible to miss the mass, and if this is likely to be a problem this procedure can be performed under ultrasound guidance. This also minimizes the risk of damage to adjacent structures especially the major vessels. If the lesion is cystic, the biopsy may be of poor quality. Core biopsy also has an advantage over fine-needle aspiration by providing more tissue if ancillary tests (e.g. immunohistochemistry) are required. There is a very small theoretical risk of tracking of tumour along the needle track.
Incisional biopsy	Readily performed and provides a large tissue sample that will almost certainly be sufficient for diagnosis. In lymphoma, a lymph node is usually required for classification of disease. (However, the neck is not the favoured site for the resulting scar and another node would probably be sampled).	If the lesion were malignant, it would probably spread into the tissues of the neck, making subsequent surgical treatment very difficult, if not impossible. This complication can be minimized by taking the biopsy from an area which would later be excised. However, spread into the tissue planes of the neck cannot be reliably prevented. Surgical risk to adjacent structures in the neck.

TABLE 20.3 Other Investigations

Investigation	Reason
Vitality tests	To search for dental causes of infection.
Radiography of teeth on left side	To search for a dental infectious cause and provide information to plan necessary dental treatment.
Sialography	To determine whether the mass is within the submandibular or parotid glands, unlikely in this case.
Chest radiography	To search for metastasis in lungs or for evidence of tuberculosis.
Serology	Viral titres and specific tests to determine potential infectious causes such as cat disease.
Ultrasonography	To determine the lesion's relationship to the salivary glands; determine its extent, and whether it is cystic; to find out whether other masses or enlarged lymph nodes are present.
Computed tomography/magnetic resonance imaging scan/positron emission tomography	To localize the lesion and its relationships to normal tissues. Unnecessary at this stage. May be required later to plan treatment when diagnosis is established.

carcinoma could be small or located in deep tissues. It might even be in the chest or abdomen, although this is unlikely, as discussed below.

The primary site can be sought in several ways. The biopsy specimen already taken can be subjected to further laboratory tests that may indicate the site or, at least, narrow down the possibilities. Imaging of the head and neck with computed tomography (CT) or magnetic resonance imaging (MRI) may reveal the primary. A more complete examination of the upper aerodigestive tract can be undertaken with endoscopy, and any suspicious sites subjected to biopsy. If the primary is visible endoscopically, this is the definitive investigation. However, it will require general anaesthesia and is best deferred until the biopsy investigations and imaging have been completed, as these may provide additional useful information on where to look.

◆ What are the Likely Primary Sites for This Metastasis?

The site must be in the drainage area of the lymph node, and it must contain epithelium, probably squamous cell epithelium. The likely sites, therefore, are:

- Oral mucosa, particularly ventrolateral tongue, floor of mouth, soft palate or retromolar mucosa
- Oropharynx (including tonsil and base of tongue) or nasopharynx
- Maxillary sinus
- Larynx
- Facial skin and scalp.

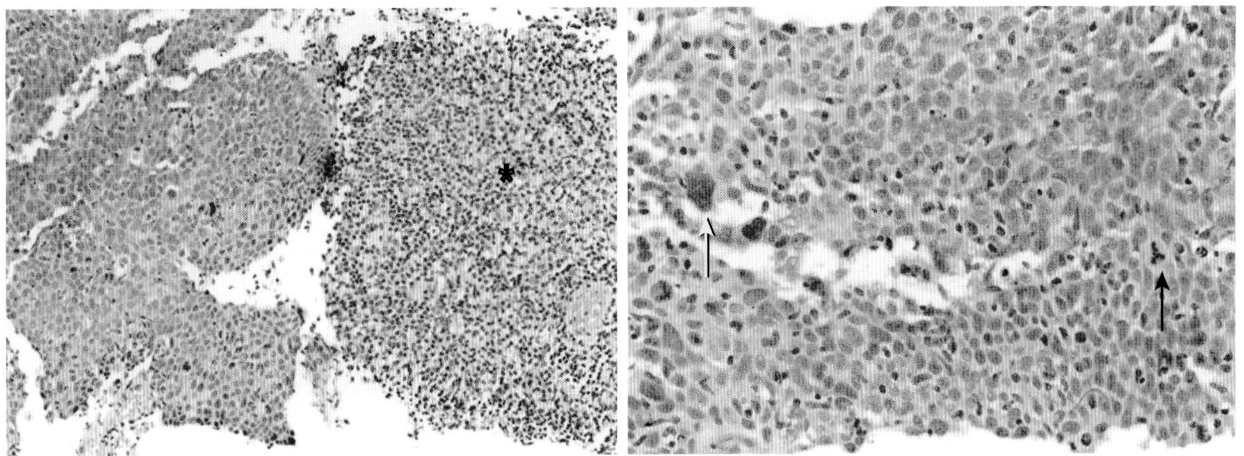

• **Fig. 20.2** **a** and **b**, Core biopsy of the lesion.

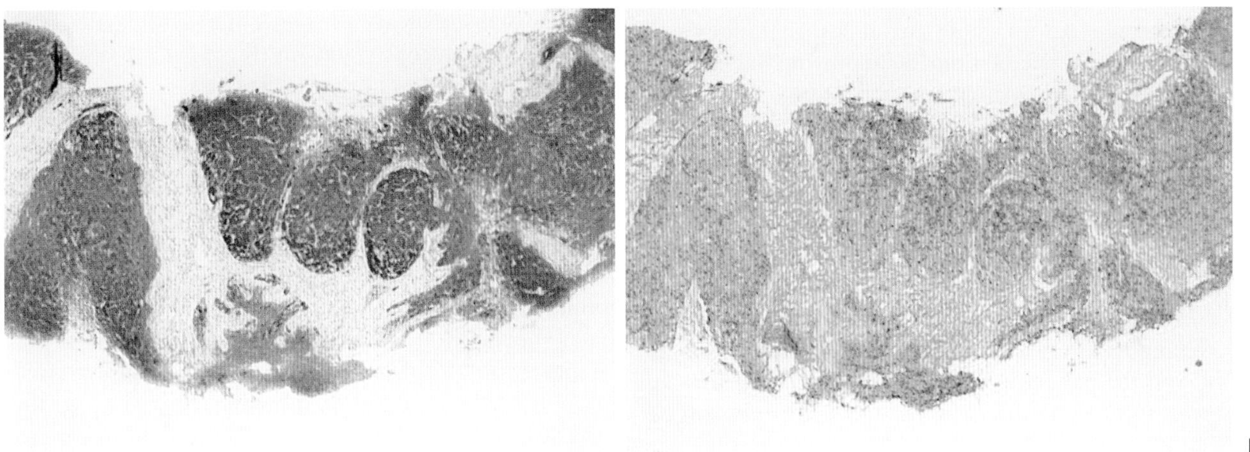

• **Fig. 20.3** Immunohistochemical stain for the p16 protein (**a**) DNA in situ hybridisation for high-risk human papillomavirus (HPV) DNA (**b**).

◆ What Further Investigations On the Biopsy Specimen May Be Useful?

It is possible to confirm the squamous differentiation of the carcinoma cells by immunohistochemistry. These stains detect cytoskeletal proteins or cell cycle control proteins that are normally only expressed in squamous epithelium, using antibodies that bind to them. In this case, the morphological appearances are typical of squamous cell carcinoma and immunohistochemical confirmation was not necessary.

Once the squamous cell differentiation is confirmed, current guidelines recommend testing the tissue for high-risk human papillomavirus (HPV) and Epstein-Barr virus (EBV) if no primary is known. This is because HPV and EBV are the causes of many oropharyngeal and most nasopharyngeal carcinomas, respectively. These carcinomas often present with metastasis, and the primary tumour can be very small, so these tests are particularly helpful in directing imaging and further biopsy to either the oropharynx or nasopharynx.

The biopsy was stained immunohistochemically for the p16 protein and by DNA in situ hybridization for HPV DNA of the high risk subtypes. The results are shown in Fig. 20.3.

◆ How Do You Interpret the Results of These Extra Investigations?

When high-risk HPV infects a cell, one of the first proteins it synthesises, called E7, interferes with the cell cycle, putting the cell into continuous cell division to favour viral replication. The cell overexpresses the p16 cell cycle control protein as a result. In the left panel of Fig. 20.3, an antibody against p16 has been applied to the tissue where it has bound to the p16 protein. A brown reaction has then been produced to indicate the site of the p16 protein. The islands of carcinoma stain strongly and diffusely for p16. This makes it highly likely that they are infected with HPV and also shows that the virus has deregulated cell division. To prove the presence of the virus, DNA in situ hybridization must be undertaken. This uses DNA probes complementary to the viral DNA sequence and hybridization is shown by the blue staining. Note how the positive reaction stains only the carcinoma, in the same distribution as the p16 stain.

Together these investigations demonstrate that the carcinoma is caused by HPV. There is a very strong likelihood that the primary carcinoma is located in the tonsil or base of tongue because HPV carcinomas start in tonsil crypt epithelium of the major or minor tonsils.

The soft cystic nature of the mass and its site at level 2 or 3 in the neck are highly consistent with metastasis from an HPV associated carcinoma of the oropharynx. This presentation is unlike most other head and neck carcinomas because the primary carcinoma is usually very small, and the metastasis is often large and cystic. HPV associated oropharyngeal squamous cell carcinoma also more commonly arise in nonsmokers.

◆ What is the Next Step?

Imaging and biopsy can now target the oropharynx and an endoscopy arranged. Co-localized positron emission tomography and CT (PET/CT) is the best imaging modality because it shows both anatomical alterations and the high metabolic rate of a cancer, improving the chances of finding even a very small primary carcinoma.

◆ What Would You Do if a Primary Carcinoma is Not Found?

If no abnormal tissue is seen on endoscopy, bilateral tonsillectomy and a large mucosal excision (mucosectomy) of the base of tongue are performed because these are the most common sites for HPV associated squamous cell carcinoma. Very occasionally, no primary lesion is found, and the patient is said to have an 'occult primary'. However, even if no primary were found, it would still be almost certain that it lay in the oropharynx, nasopharynx or other head and neck tonsil site because of the presence of HPV. It would simply be that the primary is too small to be found.

In this case, a carcinoma 10 mm in diameter was found in the base of the tongue on biopsy during endoscopy. It was invisible on imaging.

Treatment and Prognosis

◆ What are the Treatment Options, Assuming a Primary is Identified in the Oropharynx?

Most patients with tonsillar, tongue base and pharyngeal tumours are offered radiotherapy or chemoradiotherapy as primary treatment. Surgical options, including robotic resection of the primary tumour and neck dissection involving lymph nodes from the deep cervical chain, are also offered in some centres.

◆ What is This Patient's Overall Prognosis?

Patients with HPV-positive oropharyngeal squamous cell carcinoma have a significantly better overall survival compared with patients with HPV-negative head and neck cancers. The reasons for improved survival are complex but may be explained, in part, by increased sensitivity to radiotherapy.

Another Possibility

◆ If the Fine-Needle Aspirate Had Shown Adenocarcinoma, Which Possible Primary Sites Would Then Have Required Investigation?

Adenocarcinomas are carcinomas that show glandular differentiation and would have arisen in a gland or mucosa in the drainage area of the node. The thyroid, salivary glands and minor mucous glands in the upper aerodigestive tract would be the most likely primary sites.

However, adenocarcinoma is much more common in the breast, lung or prostate gland. Although a solitary metastasis high in the neck would be unusual, it is not unknown, and these sites should be considered. A metastasis to the neck from these sites would be likely to be one of many disseminated metastases, although these might be as yet undiagnosed.

The stomach and the oesophagus are further possible sources and a low (supraclavicular) cervical metastasis on the left side is a recognized presentation. However, in this case, the swelling is too high in the neck for the metastasis to have arisen from the stomach.

◆ Why Does a Gastrointestinal Carcinoma Sometimes Metastasize To the Left Side of the Neck?

Lymph from the oesophagus and the upper part of the stomach drains upwards in the thoracic duct, which enters the lower end of the internal jugular vein. There is a rather variable anatomy at the site, and often the subclavian and internal jugular lymph trunks join the thoracic duct rather than the internal jugular vein. In this situation, malignant cells draining up the thoracic duct can be carried a short distance into the lymphatics of the neck by retrograde flow (because the lymphatics are at a low and fluctuating pressure). Such cells can seed metastases in the lymph nodes just above the clavicle, the presentation known as *Virchow's node.*

Case 21
Trauma Causing Displacement of an Upper Central Incisor

SERPIL DJEMAL AND RAVI CHAUHAN

Summary

A 33-year-old male presents with displacement of his upper left central incisor after falling over at a party where he had been drinking.

History

Complaint

The patient presents complaining of a displaced upper left central incisor (UL1 or 21).

History of Complaint

The patient was under the influence of alcohol and was playing around with friends when he tripped and knocked his mouth on the floor.

He did not lose consciousness and was taken to the local hospital Accident and Emergency (A&E) department, where a head injury was ruled out and a laceration below his lower lip was sutured. He was then advised to see a dentist to manage his upper left central incisor. He presented for management of his displaced tooth 5 days after the injury had occurred.

No other injuries were sustained.

Medical History

The patient was medically fit and healthy, with no known allergies.

Dental History

The patient was an irregular dental attendee.

◆ What Additional Questions Would You Ask the Patient, and Why?

Have You Suffered Trauma Previously? Previous trauma to these teeth, depending on the age at which the trauma was sustained, could have resulted in arrested root development, disturbed crown formation, pulp necrosis or pulp canal obliteration.

Such changes could affect treatment.

In this case no previous trauma could be recalled.

Can You Bring Your Back Teeth Together? If a patient is unable to bring the posterior teeth into maximum intercuspation, it may suggest displacement of a tooth.

In this case, the patient had a class III incisor relationship, so the palatal displacement of the upper left central incisor resulted in a cross-bite, allowing him to bring his posterior teeth into maximum intercuspation (Fig. 21.1).

In patients with a class I or II incisor relationship, presenting with a palatally displaced tooth, an occlusal disturbance would be seen preventing the patient from bringing the posterior teeth into normal intercuspation.

Do You Smoke? This may influence healing and the health of the dento-alveolar and periodontal supporting tissues.

Examination

Extraoral Examination

The patient was not particularly distressed but complained of a 'pressure' feeling in the upper left central incisor (UL1 or 21).

There was a sutured laceration below his lower lip in the midline.

Intraoral Examination

◆ The Appearance of the Tooth is Shown in Fig. 21.1. What Do You See?

The following clinical features were noted:

1. There was a sutured laceration below the lower lip at the midline.
2. The overall oral hygiene was suboptimal.
3. There was marginal inflammation of the soft tissues.
4. There was generalized recession of 1–2 mm.
5. There was a small fracture affecting the mesial corner of the upper right central incisor.
6. The patient was able to bring his posterior together into maximum intercuspation.
7. The upper left central incisor was firm, and no discolouration was observed.

◆ The Palatal Appearance of the Tooth is Shown in Fig. 21.2. What Do You See?

The following features were noted from the palatal view:

1. Palatal displacement of the upper left central incisor (UL1 or 21) by approximately 7 mm (measured with a Williams periodontal probe or clinical endodontic ruler)
2. Bunching up of the palatal mucosa around the gingival margin associated with the UL1 (21)

◆ What Additional Examination(s) Would You Perform?

Injuries to the adjacent teeth and the lower teeth should be investigated. Any mobility or tenderness to touch should be noted.

The teeth should not be percussed and should not be tested for loss of vitality at this stage. Sensibility tests have been shown to give false-negative results for the first 3 months after trauma.

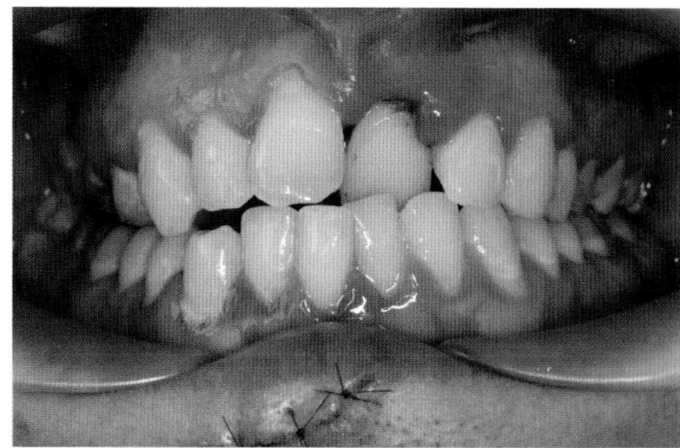

• **Fig. 21.1** Labial view of the patient's dentition on presentation showing the displaced upper lateral incisor (UL1) and associated soft tissue trauma. © Serpil Djemal.

Investigations

◆ What Investigations Would You Perform? Justify Each Option

Percussion Sounds of Teeth. Traumatized teeth should not be tapped to check the percussion sound because it is too distressing for patients and yields very little value at the acute stage of management.

Sensibility Testing. These may be thermal tests (e.g. cold test using Endo-Frost at −50 degrees) or electric pulp testing and are useful to help assess pulpal viability.

These tests have been shown to give **false-negative** results for up to **3** months after acute trauma and so will not provide any useful information and can make patients more anxious.

Radiography is required to visualize displaced teeth and the adjacent teeth.

Periapical views should be taken of all upper incisors. Changes in the periodontal ligament space will be indicative of displacement. The periapical view is shown in Fig. 21.3.

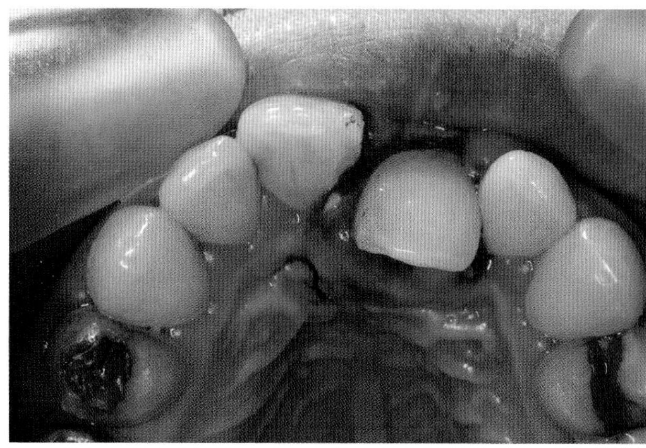

• **Fig. 21.2** Palatal view of the patient's dentition on presentation showing the displaced upper lateral incisor (UL1). © Serpil Djemal.

◆ What Does the Periapical Radiograph Show?

The radiograph shows:

1. Good alveolar bone levels
2. The incisal edge of the upper left central incisor appearing apical to the upper right central incisor
3. Socket outline visible of the upper left central incisor
4. Transportation of the apex of the upper left central incisor away from the socket outline
5. Even periodontal ligament space in the upper right central incisor
6. Small volume loss of coronal tooth tissue in the upper left central incisor
7. Loss of coronal tooth tissue at the mesial incisal edge of the upper right central incisor (as seen clinically).

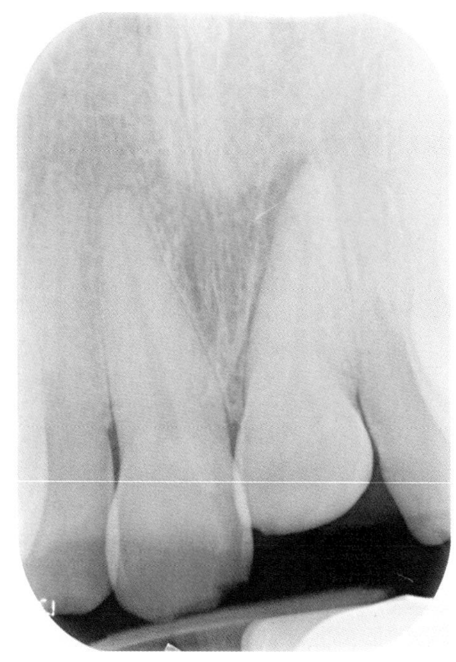

• **Fig. 21.3** Preoperative periapical radiograph of the maxillary incisors. © Serpil Djemal.

◆ What are Your Differential Diagnoses?

There are two main possibilities with regard to the upper left central incisor.

It may be an extrusion or a lateral luxation. In the former, the tooth would be mobile clinically. Because the tooth was firm and 'locked' into position, extrusion was ruled out. A lateral luxation injury is often associated with a dento-alveolar fracture with the apex of the tooth being locked into the fracture line, resulting in the tooth being firm and immobile.

◆ What are Your Final Diagnoses?

The following diagnoses were made:

1. Enamel fractures of the upper left and right central incisors
2. Lateral luxation of the upper left central incisor associated with a dento-alveolar fracture

Treatment

◆ Should the Upper Left Central Incisor Be Repositioned After the 5-Day Delay in Presentation?

It is advisable to reposition the upper left central incisor as soon as possible to prevent the tooth healing in the displaced position.

After repositioning, the tooth should be should be held in place by a flexible splint (e.g. wire and resin composite) for **4 weeks** (see table below).

Sequence of the Treatment Required

1. After explaining the treatment and gaining written consent, the patient should be anaesthetized with a local anaesthetic by using buccal and palatal infiltrations.
2. The UL1 should then be repositioned digitally first by applying buccal pressure in the region of the apex to disengage the apex (which has been locked in front of the dento-alveolar fracture) and then by moving the crown of the tooth labial with digital pressure.
3. Check that the patient can then bring the posterior teeth together.
4. The upper left central incisor can be held in place temporarily with a light cured acrylic material such as TRIAD or a sausage of resin composite placed onto the incisal edges **without** etching.
5. A verification radiograph should then be taken to ensure optimal positioning has taken place (Fig. 21.4).
6. Once this is achieved, the tooth should be splinted to the adjacent teeth, one either side, using a flexible wire (018 stainless steel) with resin composite as seen in the 4-week follow-up appointment (Fig. 21.5).
7. Labial splints are preferred because they are easy to place and remove, give good control of the teeth and do not interfere with the occlusion. Some patients may request a palatal splint, but these should be avoided because they are more difficult to place and remove and do not stabilize the teeth as well as a labial splint can. Most importantly, a palatal splint may interfere with occlusion.
8. If there is time, enamel fractures in both upper central incisors should be built up with resin composite, but this can be deferred until the splint is removed.
9. Oral hygiene instruction should be given and the patient advised not to bite on the splinted teeth for 4 weeks.

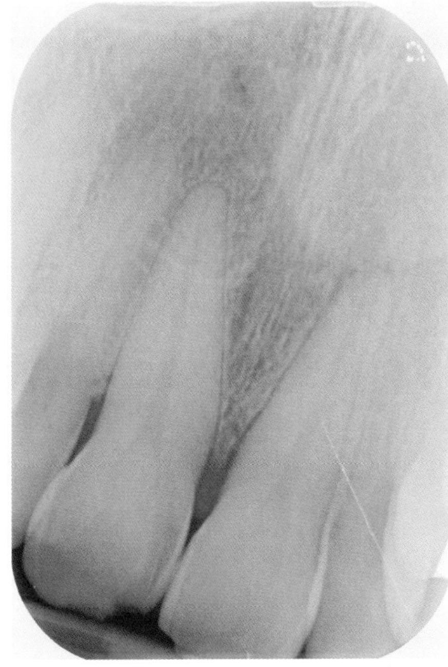

• **Fig. 21.4** Postoperative periapical radiograph showing the apex of the upper left central incisor back in position in the socket. © Serpil Djemal.

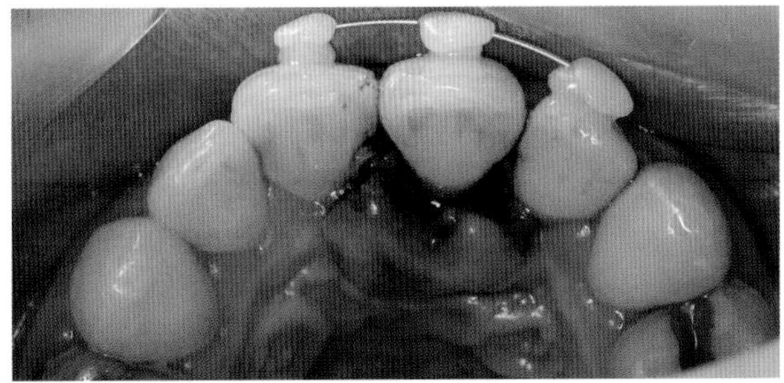

• **Fig. 21.5** Palatal view of repositioned tooth with labial flexible wire and resin composite splint in situ. © Serpil Djemal.

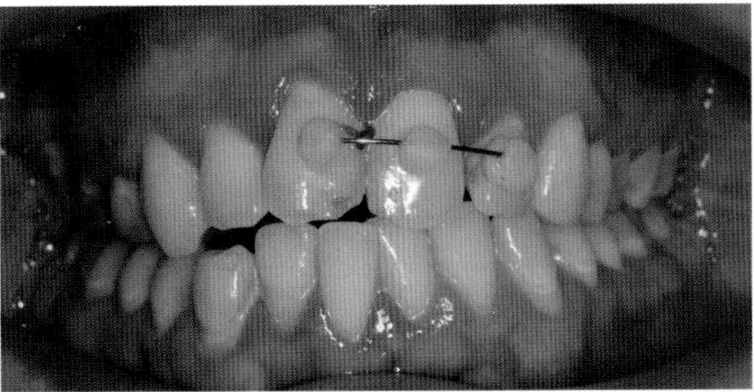

• **Fig. 21.6** Anterior view of repositioned tooth with flexible labially positioned splint in situ 4 weeks later. © Serpil Djemal.

TABLE 21.1 Tissue Injuries and Their Complications

Injury	Complication
Crushing of the cementum on the palatal aspect of the root	Loss of the surface cementum renders the root susceptible to replacement root resorption with the possibility of ankylosis in the longer term. If bacterial invasion takes place, inflammatory root resorption may result.
Dento-alveolar fracture	Severance of the apical neurovascular bundle at the apex of the tooth.
Severance of the apical neurovascular bundle at the apex of the tooth	Loss of pulp sensibility/vitality.

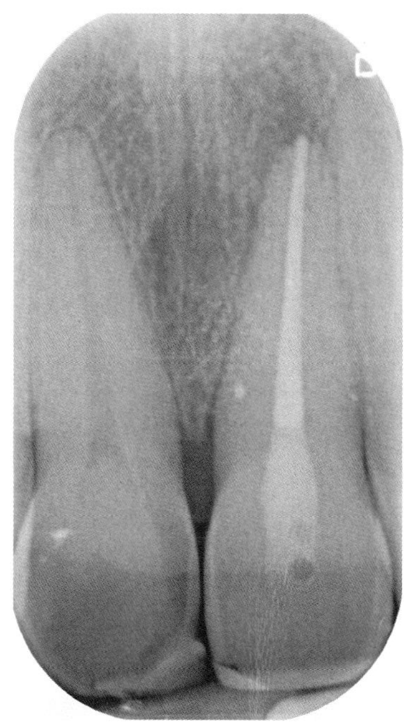

• **Fig. 21.7** Periapical radiograph of the maxillary central incisors taken 6 months after root canal treatment of the upper left central incisor. © Serpil Djemal.

◆ What Types of Tissue Injury Result From Lateral Luxation, and What are Their Complications?

See Table 21.1.

There is no indication to prescribe antibiotics in this case.

◆ What Follow-Up Should You Arrange?

The patient should be seen after 4 weeks for splint removal when baseline sensibility testing should be recorded. The follow-up protocol is 3 months, 6 months and then annually.

Each follow-up visit should include the following:

- An enquiry into any symptoms experienced since the repositioning
- A clinical examination to look for any discolouration, mobility, tenderness to percussion and palpation and the presence of a sinus
- Periapical radiography to assess for any apical radiolucency or widening of the periodontal ligament space
- Sensibility testing using cold and electric pulp testing.

The aim of the follow-up assessment is to monitor for any signs or symptoms of pulp necrosis or root resorption.

Root canal treatment should only be initiated if there are **two or more** signs and/or symptoms of pulp necrosis.

Because of the severance of the neurovascular tissues at the apex resulting from the dento-alveolar fracture, there is a high chance that a laterally luxated tooth will become necrotic and require root canal treatment in the future (Fig. 21.7). This must be clearly explained to the patient and the patient's expectations managed and documented in the notes. As for all cases, any investigations, including radiography, should be justified, graded and fully reported on, and this communicated to the patient. If a patient understands and appreciates the consequences of the treatment offered with a two-way open dialogue between the patient and the oral healthcare team, misunderstandings and eventual litigation risk can be minimized.

TABLE 21.2 Splinting Times for Other Luxation Injuries

Type of Luxation Injury	Splinting Time
Subluxation	2 weeks, if needed
Extrusion	2 weeks
Lateral luxation	4 weeks
Intrusion	4 weeks
Avulsion (extraoral dry time less than 60 minutes)	2 weeks
Avulsion (extraoral dry time greater than 60 minutes)	4 weeks
Apical one-third root fracture	4 weeks
Middle third root fracture	4 weeks
Cervical one-third root fracture	4 months

Throughout this period, the need for maintaining good oral hygiene should be reinforced.

◆ What are the Splinting Times for Other Luxation Injuries?

See Table 21.2.

Websites for Further Information

www.iadt-dentaltrauma.org/
www.dentaltrauma.co.uk

Further Reading

Diangelis, A. J., Andreasen, J. O., Ebeleseder, K. A., Kenny, D. J., Trope, M., and Sigurdsson, A. et al. (2012). International Association of Dental Traumatology Guidelines: *Fractures and Luxations of Permanent Teeth*. *29*(1), 2–12.

Djemal, S., Singh, P., Polycarpou, N., Tomson, R., & Kelleher, M. (2016). Dental trauma. Part 2 – Acute management of fracture injuries. *Dental Update*, *43*(10), 916–918, 920–922, 924–926.

Djemal, S., Singh, P., Tomson, R., & Kelleher, M. (2016). Dental trauma. Part 1 – Acute management of luxation/displacement injuries. *Dental Update*, *43*(9), 812–814, 817–818, 820–822, 823.

Case 22

Hypoglycaemia

BARBARA CAREY AND MICHAEL ESCUDIER

Summary

A 55-year-old man collapses in your general dental surgery. What is the cause, and how would you manage this patient?

History

Problem

At the end of the treatment session, the patient becomes sweaty and has a slight tremor of the extremities. He is unable to respond rationally to questions.

Medical History

Having rechecked the medical history before commencing treatment, you are aware that he has insulin-dependent diabetes. He has had diabetes mellitus for 40 years and is currently taking long-acting insulin 20 IU in the morning and 15 IU at night. In addition, he has peripheral vascular disease, resulting in intermittent claudication and angina, for which he takes glyceryl trinitrate (GTN) spray, when necessary.

Dental History

The patient has been a regular attendee for a number of years. On this occasion, he has an appointment for endodontic treatment during his lunch hour.

◆ What is the Likely Diagnosis?

Hypoglycaemia.

◆ Why Was This Particular Patient with Diabetes At Risk for Hypoglycaemia?

The patient has insulin-dependent diabetes. This type, or class, of diabetes usually results from autoimmune destruction of insulin-producing beta cells of the pancreas, leading to absolute insulin deficiency. The patient requires exogenous insulin to control his blood glucose. Hypoglycaemia results if insulin or oral hypoglycaemic drug levels exceed physiological needs. Thus, hypoglycaemia is a consequence of drug therapy for diabetes, not the underlying disease process.

◆ What are the Underlying Events Leading To the Clinical Presentation?

The patient took his insulin as normal. This has mobilized glucose from blood into tissues, reducing the blood glucose level. The patient must eat to replenish his blood glucose; otherwise, the level will continue to fall. The brain relies almost exclusively on glucose as fuel, and hypoglycaemia starves the brain and causes abnormal brain activity. This may present as cognitive impairment, behavioural changes, psychomotor abnormalities, and, at very low plasma glucose concentrations, seizure and coma.

◆ What Would You Do Immediately?

- Reassure the patient
- Assess vital signs, blood pressure, pulse and respiratory rate.

Examination

The patient is conscious. However, he is becoming increasingly confused and restless and has tachycardia.

◆ What Other Symptoms and Signs Might You Expect?

Autonomic symptoms may accompany hypoglycaemia as the body tries to mobilize glucose. The symptoms include tremor, palpitations, anxiety, arousal, sweating, hunger and paraesthesias. The patient may be tachycardic.

Neuropathy and vascular disease are common complications of diabetes and may prevent signs of sympathetic activation being apparent until at a late stage. It is important not to waste time looking for other signs to confirm your diagnosis for the following reasons:

- the condition can worsen quickly
- the history of diabetes and presentation are diagnostic
- treatment cannot cause any significant adverse effects – raising blood glucose in the short term is safe.

Treatment

◆ What Treatment Would You Provide?

Give a glucose drink (20 g of glucose) quickly because otherwise the patient may become unconscious in minutes. Alternatively, the equivalent amount of glucose gel, sugar lumps or a proprietary glucose drink may be used. Measure blood glucose levels by using glucose monitors (glucometers) or finger stick testing. The patient should return to a normal state rapidly (within about 5–10 minutes). If necessary, a glucose drink may be repeated in 10–15 minutes. The patient should then be given long-acting

TABLE 22.1 Causes, Symptoms and Signs of Hypoglycaemia

Cause	Symptoms and Signs
Vasovagal attack (faint)	The commonest cause of collapse and often associated with emotional stress. There are usually premonitory symptoms before loss of consciousness. Cold, clammy skin, pallor, sweating, nausea, initial bradycardia and low volume pulse, followed by tachycardia and a full pulse. Rapid recovery on being placed supine; and in the absence of associated breathlessness, raise legs to improve cerebral circulation. Loosen any tight clothes around neck, and once consciousness is regained, give a glucose drink.
Postural hypotension	This can be a consequence of rising abruptly or standing for too long. Antihypertensive drugs predispose to this. Management is as for a vasovagal attack.
Steroid crisis	Usually only seen in patients taking, or who have recently taken, systemic corticosteroids or with a background of Addison's disease. Arises as a result of relative insufficiency during periods of stress.
Cardiac arrest	Usually a history of cardiovascular disease in the form of angina, hypertension or previous myocardial infarction. No central pulse.

carbohydrate, such as two biscuits, a slice of bread or 200–300 ml milk.

Unfortunately, there is a delay finding and dissolving the glucose, and the patient lapses into unconsciousness before he is able to drink it.

◆ How May This Cause of Loss of Consciousness Be Distinguished From Other Similar Causes?

See Table 22.1.

◆ What Treatment Would You Now Commence?

Hypoglycaemia which causes unconsciousness is an emergency. In this situation, there are three options:

Give 1 mg of glucagon intramuscularly. This will mobilize glucose from the remaining stores of glycogen in the patient's liver, sufficient for him to regain consciousness. It is not a definitive treatment, but a way of producing a conscious patient who can swallow oral glucose. Glucagon works for about 15 minutes and is easy and safe to administer. As soon as the patient is alert and able to swallow, oral glucose should be given. Without this further treatment, the patient will lapse back into a hypoglycaemic coma, and a second dose of glucagon will be ineffective because all the liver glycogen will have been metabolized. Glucagon may take 15 minutes to work and may be ineffective in undernourished patients and in severe liver disease.

Or give 100 ml of 20% glucose intravenously. This requires venous access. Care is required because this concentration is an irritant, especially if extravasation occurs. Glucose 10% infusion may also be used but larger volumes are needed.

Or give 50 ml of 50% glucose intravenously. This treatment is not recommended. Glucose 50% infusion is like thick syrup and very difficult to inject. It is also a very strong irritant, will irreversibly damage the vein into which it is injected and is associated with higher risk of extravasation injury.

The presentations of drugs useful in the treatment of hypoglycaemia are shown in Fig. 22.1.

◆ How Would You Proceed Once the Patient Has Recovered?

- Abandon dental treatment
- Monitor blood glucose
- Continue to monitor the vital signs
- Arrange transfer of the patient to an appropriate secondary care facility
- Advise the patient of the need for formal review of his diabetic control
- Establish the cause of the episode (e.g. missed meal, dosage error, increased exercise, alcohol excess, deliberate overdose).

Other Possibilities

◆ Can This Happen To a Patient with Non–Insulin-Dependent Diabetes Mellitus?

Yes. Non–insulin-dependent diabetes mellitus (NIDDM) is managed by diet control, oral hypoglycaemic drugs, insulin or a combination of these. Both oral hypoglycaemic drugs and insulin could potentiate hypoglycaemia if there is a relative deficiency of glucose, for instance, if the patient does not eat despite having taken the normal dose of medication. Patients with hypoglycaemia caused by an oral hypoglycaemic drug should be transferred to hospital because the hypoglycaemic effects of these drugs may persist for many hours.

◆ What Could Have Been Done To Minimize the Risk of Such an Event?

The scheduling of the appointment should have taken account of the patient's need for avoiding disturbances in the normal daily routine. Routine treatment under local anaesthesia should be undertaken at a time that allows for completion of the procedure and recovery before the next food intake is due. In this way, the possibility of a hypoglycaemic episode can be minimized. It is also advisable to avoid appointment times at the end of the day when medical assistance may be less readily available in the event of a complication. In general, morning appointments are advisable because endogenous cortisol

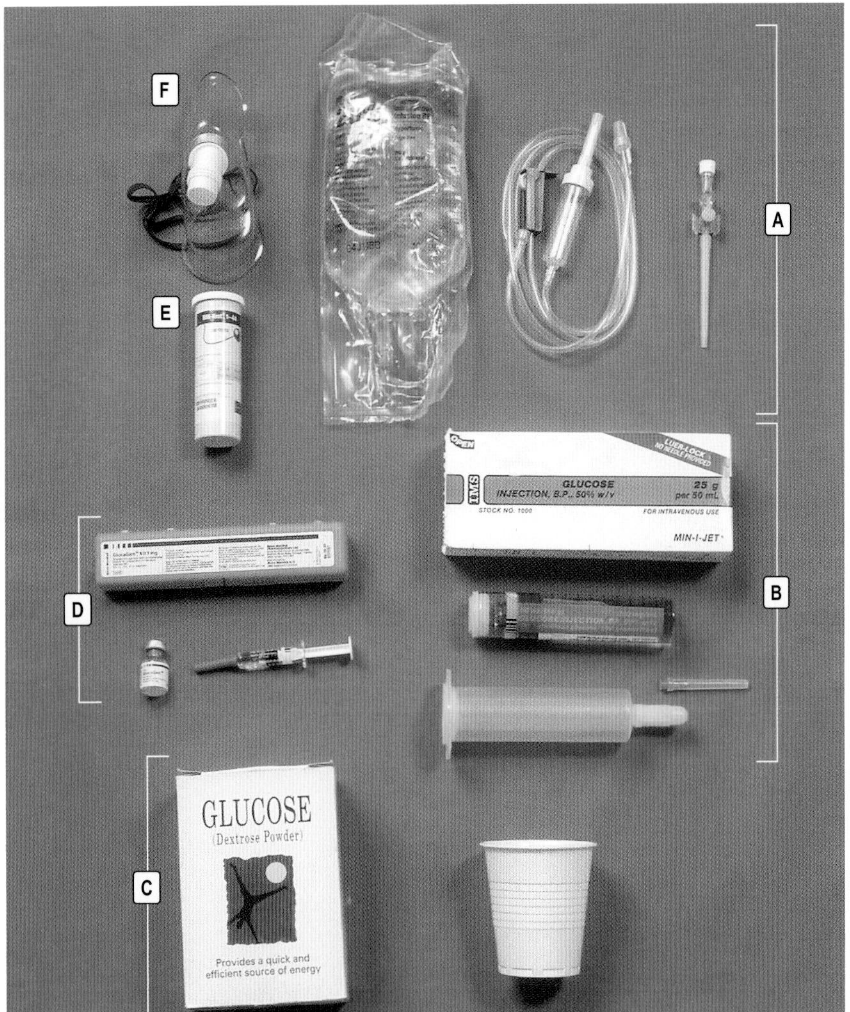

• **Fig. 22.1** Typical presentations of drugs used to treat hypoglycaemia. All these options may be available in a hospital or clinic, whereas only glucose and glucagon are currently the professional requirements for UK primary dental care.

A. Infusion set with 20% glucose.
B. Glucose 50% in Min-I-Jet format. The yellow plastic cover is removed from the back (left-hand end) of the syringe barrel and front of the glass cartridge and the cartridge is screwed into the syringe barrel. Available in two types, with needle fitted and with luer lock fitting for a conventional needle (shown). After removing front cover and fitting needle, if required, use as a conventional syringe.
C. Glucose powder, dissolve 20 g in up to one cup of water.
D. Glucagon emergency set with vial of lyophilised powder. Dissolve by injecting water for injection already in the syringe, and draw up for injection.
E. Blood glucose dipstick test strips.
F. Oxygen mask, give 5 litres/min.

levels are higher at this time. Ensure that the patient has eaten and taken his medication as usual.

A more rapidly accessible glucose formulation might have helped. Glucose powder is useful for nonurgent uses, but a ready-to-use solution is best for emergency use.

Further Points

◆ What are the Oral Complications of Diabetes?

Oral complications of diabetes include:

- Reduced resistance to infection. Infection requires effective treatment early
- Increased severity of periodontal disease and susceptibility to periodontal abscess
- Xerostomia may also be a problem and may further predispose the patient to oral candidosis
- Sialadenosis (asymptomatic salivary gland swelling for hormonal, metabolic or nutritional reasons)
- Oral hypoglycaemics may be associated with the development of lichenoid reactions
- Oral burning and taste disturbances
- Peripheral mononeuropathy in the oropharyngeal area is a very rare effect.

Case 23

A Tooth Lost At Teatime

VINOD PATEL AND ALEXANDER CRIGHTON

Summary

A 78-year-old female patient lost a tooth while eating. What is the cause, and what will you do?

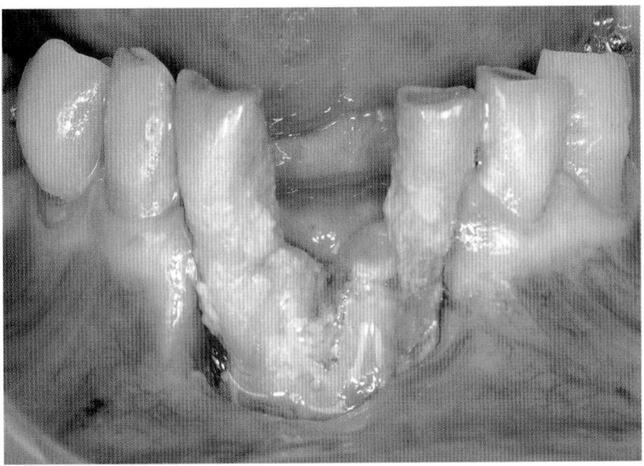

• **Fig. 23.1** The patient on presentation.

History

Complaint

The patient reports that one of her front lower teeth had become loose recently. The tooth simply fell out yesterday when she was eating a biscuit. There was no pain before, during or after losing the tooth.

History of Complaint

This woman has attended your practice for many years and has a well-cared-for mouth, a low caries rate and minimal periodontal disease. She is concerned that a healthy tooth has come out so easily and also that she has had no pain or bleeding from the area since.

Medical History

Five years ago, the patient fractured her arm in a fall, and a diagnosis of osteoporosis was made at that time. She takes calcium supplements daily and alendronate (Fosamax) weekly.

Examination

Extraoral Examination

Oddly, there is no lymphadenopathy, no tenderness to palpation over any area of the facial skeleton and no obvious halitosis.

Intraoral Examination

The patient is partially dentate and wears dentures. Her mucosa is normal, the mouth is not dry, there is no active caries and no pocket depths exceed 3 mm.

There is an area of exposed bone in the anterior mandibular alveolus and a socket from which a lower incisor has been lost, as shown in Fig. 23.1. The adjacent teeth in the exposed bone are mobile in their sockets and are also in danger of spontaneous exfoliation. The attached gingiva in the region is missing and the buccal soft tissue margin of the lesion is lax and can be lifted to allow a dental probe to be inserted down almost to the patient's chin. No pus is present.

◆ How Do You Interpret the Findings So Far?

The lack of bleeding and sensitivity suggest necrotic bone and nonvital teeth. Despite bacterial plaque and debris accumulating on the exposed bone, there seems to be no infection, even though there is a deep soft tissue pocket extending to the chin. The surrounding mucosa is hardly inflamed, suggesting that local trauma and infection are not responsible.

The appearances are very characteristic, and it is possible to make a fairly confident diagnosis without any further investigations.

Diagnosis

◆ What is Your Diagnosis?

Medication-related osteonecrosis of the jaws (MRONJ) is almost certainly the diagnosis on the basis of asymptomatic necrosis of bone without pain. The patient has taken alendronate, a bisphosphonate drug, for several years, and this is a recognized complication.

◆ What Alternative Diagnoses Have You Excluded, and Why?

Chronic osteomyelitis would seem a possibility, but the presentation is not correct for this diagnosis. Relatively mild pain or discomfort would probably be present, as would bad taste, discharge of pus indicating infection and possibly sequestration of nonvital bone. There would also normally be both a cause and a predisposing factor. If dental infection were the cause, it would be evident clinically or radiographically, or there might be a history of trauma such as a fracture or dental extraction. Patients who develop osteomyelitis usually have some systemic predisposing condition such as diabetes mellitus or immunosuppression. It seems that this option is most unlikely, although a radiograph would help exclude or confirm it by the presence of periosteal reaction and new bone formation.

Acute osteomyelitis is even less likely. Acute infection would be accompanied by the cardinal signs of inflammation, including pain, erythema and swelling. There is severe, deep, boring pain in acute osteomyelitis, with systemic signs of infection.

Necrotizing periodontitis could cause necrosis of soft tissue and exposed bone but would be associated with other signs and symptoms. It is almost exclusively found in severe immunosuppression, usually in late or untreated human immunodeficiency virus (HIV) infection. Necrotizing periodontitis is usually painful and limited to the gingiva and alveolar margin. It would not cause extensive soft tissue separation from bone, as here.

Cancrum oris (noma) is a necrotizing mixed bacterial infection that sometimes develops from acute ulcerative gingivitis. It causes tissue necrosis of large parts of the face or other tissues, including bone. The disease is almost confined to malnourished and debilitated children younger than 8 years of age in developing countries.

◆ What is the Difference Among Osteomyelitis, Osteitis and Osteonecrosis?

Osteomyelitis is an infection in the medullary cavity of bone. It is usually bacterial. The resulting increased pressure in the medullary space and the inflammatory reaction devitalize bone marrow by compressing its blood supply and parts of the bone undergo necrosis. After an acute and intensely painful phase, pus drains, and osteoclasts separate the necrotic bone to form sequestra. If the sequestra can be shed, the bone may heal. If not, infection persists in the sequestrum and is difficult to treat, the disease becomes chronic and the surrounding bone becomes sclerotic.

Osteitis is a superficial inflammation of bone, such as is seen in the exposed bone of dry socket (see Case 15). Small sequestra may form but infection does not penetrate into or spread within the medullary cavity.

Osteonecrosis refers to death of bone. The cause is related to bone-modulating medications such as bisphosphonates or denosumab. The necrotic bone is sterile, at least initially, and only becomes colonized by bacteria once exposed to the exterior. Osteonecrosis can follow irradiation of bone because this induces endarteritis, which is narrowing of blood vessels with eventual necrosis. Osteonecrosis is increasingly recognized in patients taking bisphosphonate drugs for the prevention or treatment of osteoporosis, management of bone metastasis in cancer or treatment of metabolic bone diseases.

◆ What are Bisphosphonate Drugs, and Why are They Used?

Bisphosphonate drugs reduce bone turnover. The drugs are adsorbed onto bone surfaces, where they remain bound for a prolonged period. They are taken up by osteoclasts at the sites of bone resorption and interfere with adenosine triphosphate (ATP) metabolism or membrane function. Osteoclasts either die or become unable to resorb bone. Bone formation then exceeds bone resorption, remodelling is slowed and bone density increases or stabilizes.

These drugs have a variety of uses:

- To prevent further bone loss in osteoporosis
- To prevent malignant tumours in bone releasing excess calcium into the bloodstream
- To prevent bony metastases from enlarging by inhibiting bone resorption around them
- To reduce bone turnover in Paget's disease of bone
- To increase bone mass in osteogenesis imperfecta.

◆ Are All Bones Affected Equally?

No, the effects are systemic but the effects are much more pronounced in the mandible and the maxilla. The reasons for this are not clear, but these sites may be subjected to higher drug levels because of their good blood supply. They are also close to the surface such that the bone is readily exposed. Bisphosphonate-induced osteonecrosis affects the mandible twice as often as the maxilla but is almost never seen in other bones.

◆ Are There Other Prescribed Drugs Implicated in Osteonecrosis of the Jaw?

Yes. Bisphosphonates were essentially the first group of drugs in which this complication was regularly seen. Since then, a host of novel drugs (Table 23.3) have been implicated in MRONJ. These medications are divided into two broad categories:

- Bone-modulating drugs
- Antiangiogenic drugs

Bisphosphonates fall under the bone-modulating drug category, as does denosumab, a human monoclonal antibody. This novel drug is given subcutaneously for almost the same indications as those for bisphosphonates. The risk of osteonecrosis is the same as intravenous bisphosphonates when given on a monthly basis for treating malignant disease. For osteoporosis, the medication is prescribed as a 6-monthly dose; by 6 months, the drug effect is eliminated, allowing the bone physiology to return to its previous state, hence the need for repeat injections. This drug characteristically provides an ideal opportunity to provide any dental extractions required, await healing and then recommence the medication with little impact on the patient's osteoporosis and very low risk of osteonecrosis. Such an approach would require communication and planning with the medical prescriber. Dental care remains the same after medication or if osteonecrosis develops, as discussed for bisphosphonates.

A host of novel oncology medications termed 'antiangiogenics' has been introduced. The aim of these drugs is to starve solid tumours of blood supply, on which they are reliant for growth. Restricting the blood supply leads to either lack of further growth or even reduction in tumour size. Medications can be either oral or intravenous, and both types subsequently have a systemic effect, hence it's antiangiogenic effect in the oral cavity can lead to MRONJ. When these drugs are taken solely, the risk of osteonecrosis is less than 1%; however, in metastatic malignant disease, they are often combined with either bisphosphonates or denosumab. This heightens the risk, with some reports showing an osteonecrosis risk as high as 14%. Dose and duration play a key role and need to be considered carefully to determine relevant risk.

TABLE 23.1 Bisphosphonate Drugs and Their Relative Potency

Drug	Relative Potency
Nonnitrogenous	
Etidronate	1
Clodronate	10
Tildronate	10
Nitrogenous	
Pamidronate	100
Neridronate	100
Olpadronate	500
Alendronate	500
Ibandronate	1 000
Risedronate	2 000
Zoledronate	10 000

◆ Why Does the Tissue Undergo Necrosis?

The drugs interfere with inter- and intracellular signalling and inhibit the growth of new blood vessels. The tissue of bone marrow becomes avascular and dies. Bone also becomes depleted of both osteoclasts and osteoblasts because the two cell populations are interdependent. Osteocytes are not replaced by maturing osteoblasts and eventually die. Both bone and soft tissue undergo slow necrosis without symptoms.

As the overlying mucosa partly relies on blood supply from bone and periosteum, it may also undergo necrosis. This is most commonly seen in areas where the mucosa is very thin, typically over the mandibular tori and on the posterior lingual aspect of the mandible where there are few muscle attachments.

◆ What is the Risk of Developing Osteonecrosis?

The risk depends on the total dose of the drug administered, which is a function of it's dose, frequency and duration of administration.

The many different bisphosphonate drugs have varying potencies, as shown in Table 23.1. Non-nitrogenous drugs cause osteoclast death, and nitrogenous drugs inhibit osteoclast function. The more potent drugs are much more likely to cause MRONJ. This is especially so when the drug is given in high doses intravenously, as for metastatic malignancy.

The proportion of patients who are taking bisphosphonates and are affected by osteonecrosis is estimated to be only 0.05%. However, the number of patients being prescribed these medications is increasing with an ageing population and improving survival rates in cancer. Oncology patients are often prescribed the more potent intravenous formulations and hence face a larger risk of osteonecrosis, whereas patients with osteoporosis are routinely prescribed the oral formulation. It is estimated that 4 years of oral administration is required before there is a significant risk of osteonecrosis, whereas the risk becomes significant after 4 months of intravenous administration. In clinical practice, the potency of the drug is not the overriding factor because lower-potency drugs may be administered in larger amounts over longer periods. The total dose administered is the key risk factor.

Investigations

◆ What Investigations Would You Perform?

Investigations are not helpful in diagnosis but may provide useful information for treatment. The vitality of the teeth in and around the exposed area of bone must be determined.

Obtaining radiographs of the area might seem the logical next step. However, you will find that on the radiographs, mandibular bone appears completely normal. This is because osteonecrosis is caused by loss of viable marrow. The disease does not alter the mineralized component that is responsible for the appearance of the radiographic image. This is very different from chronic osteomyelitis, in which there is patchy radiolucency and sclerosis, with separation of sequestra.

There is no completely satisfactory method for showing the areas of bone that are dead in a patient with osteonecrosis. This is unfortunate because it would be useful to know the extent of necrosis in case extraction or surgery is required in other parts of the jaw.

◆ Can More Specialized Investigations Help?

Radioisotope scanning measures bone turnover and should show lack of uptake in osteonecrotic bone, but image resolution is too poor to be useful.

Magnetic resonance imaging (MRI) is probably the most useful modality, but it is expensive and only available in hospitals. Different types of MRI images define vascularity and fat content. MRI shows clearly the loss of bone marrow in affected areas, as shown in Fig. 23.2, where the normal marrow has a high signal (bright) and the affected marrow appears dark. This is currently the best method to identify the extent of osteonecrosis, but it is only useful in the mandible because the maxilla has little medullary space.

It has been suggested that serum levels of C-terminal telopeptide of type 1 collagen (CTX-1), a bone turnover marker, reflect bone suppression by bisphosphonates. This small peptide is released into serum when collagen in bone is resorbed. It provides an indication of bone turnover in the body as a whole, but whether this is a useful reflection of the risk of osteonecrosis in the jaws remains unclear. The currently proposed risk values are shown in Table 23.2, but even a high value cannot guarantee that an extraction is completely without risk.

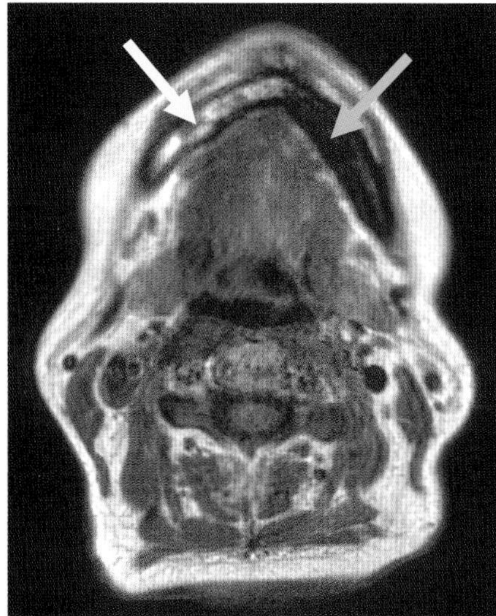

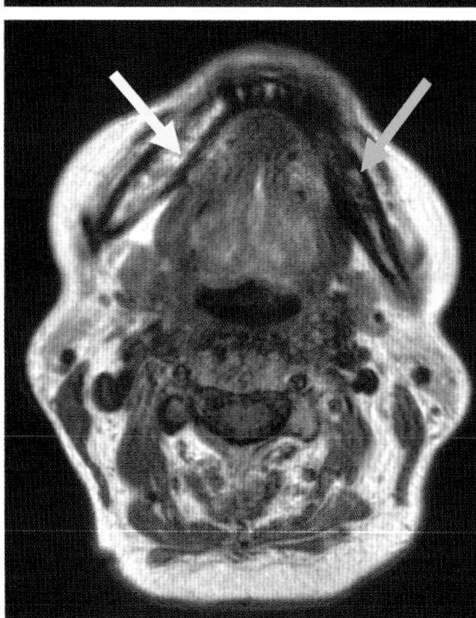

• **Fig. 23.2** Two adjacent axial magnetic resonance imaging scans through the body of the mandible. The normal bright marrow signal is indicated by the yellow arrow, the abnormal avascular marrow in the osteonecrotic bone by the green arrow.

You decide that no investigations are likely to be useful at this stage. You find that the teeth in the exposed bone do not respond to any tests of vitality. The adjacent teeth give an equivocal result.

Treatment

◆ What Will You Do for the Teeth in the Exposed Bone?

The teeth each side of the socket are pain free but mobile. They are best extracted before problems develop and for proper cleaning of the area. If the teeth were firm, they might be left in situ but would probably cause problems in the future. It is not clear whether the teeth in osteonecrotic bone retain their own independent blood supply. If they do not respond to any tests of vitality, the prognosis is likely to be poor.

◆ What Should Be Done for the Exposed Bone?

Once the teeth are removed, the patient should be instructed to keep the mucosa and exposed bone as clean as possible by using simple oral hygiene measures and topical chlorhexidine, as needed. Any prominent bone or sharp edges can be trimmed and removed without local anaesthesia. This should prevent trauma to the oral soft tissues and make the area easier to clean (Fig. 23.3).

The aim of treatment in MRONJ is very different from that in osteomyelitis or osteoradionecrosis. In these latter conditions, necrotic bone is limited in extent, and its

TABLE 23.2 Determining Osteronecrosis Risk Based on Serum CTX Levels

Serum CTX Value	Osteonecrosis Risk
>150 pg/ml	Minimal
150–100 pg/ml	Moderate
<100 pg/ml	High

CTX, C-terminal telopeptide of type 1 collagen.

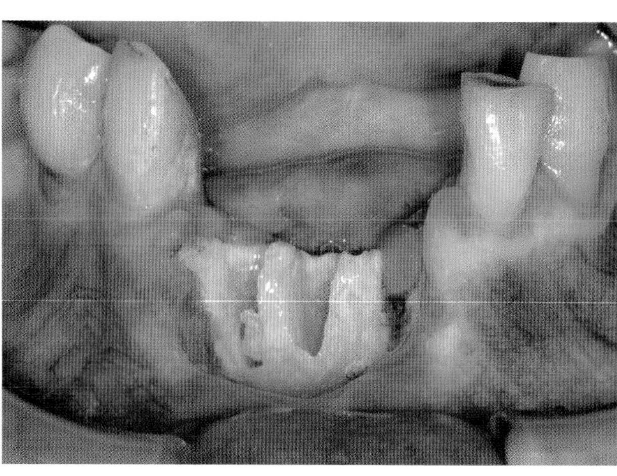

• **Fig. 23.3** The patient after extractions and debridement.

removal exposes healthy, vital bone, which can heal well. In bisphosphonate osteonecrosis, the area of bone involved is very extensive, cannot be removed and is not surrounded by healthy bone. The MRI scan of this patient (see Fig. 23.2) suggests that the entire anterior area and one body of the mandible are involved. Trimming back bone and attempting closure of soft tissue surgically usually result in wound breakdown.

◆ Will the Exposed Bone Get Infected?

Infection can develop but is surprisingly infrequent. The bone will have been colonized by the oral flora as soon as it was exposed, but this is contamination rather than infection. Bone is not invaded by bacteria, and there is no host response in the avascular tissue, no inflammation and no immune response.

Simple cleaning and topical antiseptics are the most effective methods of keeping the flora at bay. Antibiotics are ineffective. Drugs cannot enter bone because it lacks blood supply.

Sometimes, a more aggressive infection will develop in the soft tissues at the margins of the wound, and this must be treated according to conventional principles. A microbiological sample should be taken for culture and sensitivity before commencing empirical antibiotic therapy. In most cases, metronidazole is an appropriate choice, but this can be supplemented by amoxicillin, if needed. In low-grade infection, doxycycline works well and can be used for a longer period compared with metronidazole and amoxicillin.

Very rarely, there is extensive sequestration of bone and aggressive perilesional infection, as shown in Fig. 23.4. Open surgical debridement is then required, and antibiotics may need to be given intravenously. Debridement in such cases may aim to reduce the sharp and loose edges and bony sequestrum rather than achieving complete healing.

◆ What Would You Do if the Site Became Painful?

Sensing pain requires an intact nerve and blood supply. Bone is insensitive, and any pain must arise from the mucosa. Significant infection must be suspected and excluded, but the cause is usually a local problem with tissue hygiene, and it can be managed with simple cleaning and application of topical antiseptics.

◆ Will the Bone Ever Heal? Should the Bisphosphonate Be Stopped?

The continuation of the bisphosphonate drug must be reviewed with the patient's medical practitioner or specialist clinician. When the drug is given for malignant disease, it may not be possible to stop it without risking major adverse effects.

If the bisphosphonate can be withdrawn, the bone will gradually recover with no intervention other than cleaning. This recovery is very slow, and it may take many months to see an improvement. However in 1–2 years, most lesions will show significant improvement. Detached periosteum will reattach, and the mucosa will grow to cover the revascularizing bone. Fig. 23.5 shows regrowth of the mucosa to cover the exposed bone around a defect in the maxilla. An oroantral fistula remains, but the bone is now protected from infection.

Those patients who continue to need medication may be switched to an alternative drug such as raloxifene or teriparatide, which do not seem to cause osteonecrosis. However, these medicines have potentially serious side effects and must only be prescribed by a medical specialist.

◆ Is Dental Treatment Safe in a Patient On a Bisphosphonate Drug?

The risk is best avoided by instituting an effective preventive regimen for caries and periodontitis. An enhanced programme of oral hygiene improvement, dietary instruction and topical fluoride preparations would be appropriate for all patients on bisphosphonates.

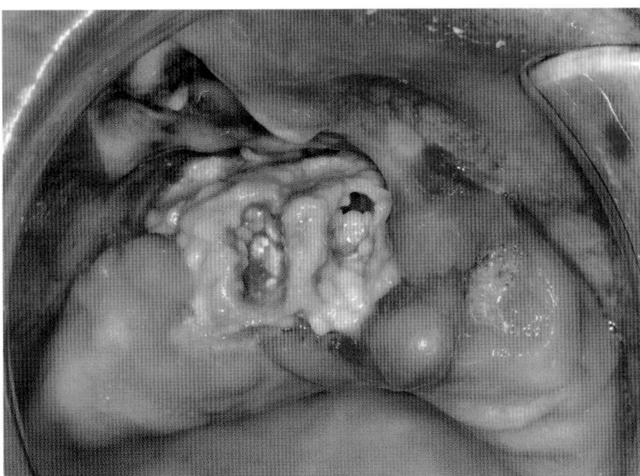

• **Fig. 23.4** A different patient who has developed extensive infection in the soft tissues surrounding a zone of maxillary osteonecrosis.

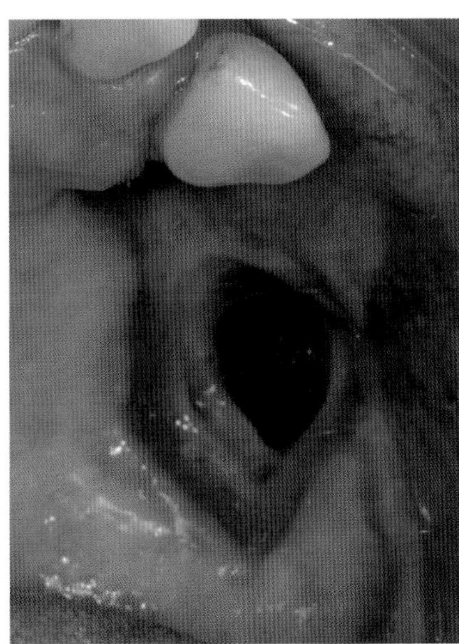

• **Fig. 23.5** A different patient with resolving osteonecrosis.

The safe period of 4 years after starting oral bisphosphonates and 4 months after starting an intravenous regimen gives a window of opportunity to deal with any sepsis or teeth with a dubious prognosis and to initiate prevention.

Routine restorative dentistry can be performed without problems. It may be a sensible precaution to use a local anaesthetic without, or at a reduced amount of, a vasoconstrictor for infiltration anaesthesia, but this is not based on any sound evidence. Oral surgery and dental implants are best avoided if the patient has been taking bisphosphonates for a prolonged period.

◆ What Do You Do if a Tooth Needs Extraction in a Patient At Risk?

Most patients will have no problems after an uncomplicated extraction. Complications are reported to develop in less than 1% of patients. It is important to discuss the risk with patients before starting treatment and give them a risk information leaflet (see further guidance at the end of this chapter). Extractions should be performed as atraumatically as possible and flap surgery avoided. No exposed bone should be seen at 8 weeks after the extraction. If bone is still visible at that time, the patient should be referred for assessment by a local dental specialist in osteonecrosis management.

Every effort should be made to avoid extraction by root filling teeth and retaining decoronated roots in a similar fashion to overdenture abutments. Temporarily withdrawing bisphosphonate drugs for a period before and after the extraction (a 'drug holiday') is not thought to reduce the risk of bone necrosis because of their long activity. In contrast, in patients receiving denosumab, performing an elective extraction in the month prior to the next drug dose will likely reduce the risk of osteonecrosis because the drug's activity will be at its lowest. All patients taking bisphosphonates should be expected to have slowly healing extraction sockets, even when no osteonecrosis develops.

◆ Could I Be Considered Negligent if Osteonecrosis Develops?

No, provided the risk has been identified and managed appropriately and the patient has been informed of the risks and has given consent for the extraction. Good record keeping will provide evidence of this.

Dental extractions or surgery appear to be a precipitating factor in one-third to one-half of cases. However, this is a complication of drug treatment, not of dental surgery. The bone may well have been necrotic without symptoms for some time; dental extraction simply unmasks the process by exposing the bone. Many patients develop spontaneous lesions without any dental interventions.

◆ Should Antibiotic Prophylaxis Be Given for Extractions in Patients Taking Bisphosphonates?

No. The disease is not caused by bacteria, and drugs do not penetrate bone because it has no blood supply. Use of antibiotics risks adverse effects and microbial resistance for no benefit. Similarly, chlorhexidine mouthrinse will not prevent problems with the bone, although it may help keep the soft tissues disease-free during the healing process which may sometimes be slow. However, some patients taking bisphosphonates may also be taking other medications such as immunosuppressants (e.g. methotrexate, mycophenolate mofetil, azathioprine, corticosteroids). These medications place patients at a small increased risk of postsurgical infection. Hence, on the basis of individual clinical judgement, antibiotics may be prescribed, but this should not be done solely because patients are taking bisphosphonates. Furthermore, the addition of immunosuppressants for patients taking bisphosphonates increases the risk of osteonecrosis but for those taking oral bisphosphonates the risk still remains less than 1%. Both immunosuppressants and bisphosphonates will lead to slower healing, and this should be expected.

Table 23.3 provides a number of additional drugs implicated in MRONJ and their indications for use.

TABLE 23.3 Drugs Implicated in Osteonecrosis of the Jaw and Their Indication for Use

Classification	Drug Group	Drug Name	Indication for Use
Bone-modulating	Monoclonal antibody	Denosumab	Osteoporosis, bone metastases, unresectable giant cell lesions
Antiangiogenic	Monoclonal antibody	Bevacizumab	Colorectal cancer, small cell lung cancer, renal cancer, breast cancer, ovarian cancer, glioblastomas
	Tyrosine kinase inhibitor	Sunitinib	Metastatic renal cell carcinoma, gastrointestinal stromal tumours, breast cancer, colorectal cancer, non–small cell lung cancer, neuroendocrine tumours
		Sorafenib	Hepatocellular cancer, locally advanced or metastatic thyroid carcinoma, renal cell carcinoma
		Cabozantinib	Metastatic medullary thyroid cancer, renal cell carcinomas
		Axitinib	Renal cell carcinomas, thyroid cancers

Further Guidance

American Association of Oral and Maxillofacial Surgeons. Position paper: Medication-related osteonecrosis of the jaw – 2014 update. Available at: https://www.aaoms.org/ and search 'MRONJ'.

Scottish Dental Clinical Effectiveness Programme. Oral health management of patients at risk of medication-related osteonecrosis of the jaw – 2017. Available at: http://www.sdcep.org.uk/ and search 'osteonecrosis'.

Case 24
A Problem Overdenture

JONATHAN TURNER AND DAVID R. RADFORD

Summary

A 67-year-old lady is referred to your general dental practice with a complaint that her denture has never 'seemed right' from the day it was fitted.

History

Complaint

The patient complains that a small filling has recently been lost from one of the upper canine roots below her overdenture. However, it quickly becomes clear that this has caused no symptoms (the tooth has been root treated) and that she is dissatisfied primarily with her upper complete overdenture. She can wear the denture in the morning, but by about 3 o'clock in the afternoon, it becomes too uncomfortable, and if she is at home, she likes to take it out.

History of Complaint

The patient successfully wore an acrylic upper partial denture until 6 months ago, but failure of restorations and root treatments led to loss of several upper teeth. She was provided with an upper overdenture on the two retained upper canine roots. The denture was fitted 3 months ago, reviewed on four occasions and minor adjustments made to the base extension. The patient is happy with the retention and fit of the denture. It does not move during eating. She reports no problems with her lower teeth.

Medical History

The patient is taking low-dose aspirin (75 mg/day) following a myocardial infarction and a statin for high serum cholesterol.

Examination

Extraoral Examination

There is no lymphadenopathy. The temporomandibular joint is free of crepitus and clicks, and no muscle tenderness can be elicited in the muscles of mastication. With the denture in place, there is no facial asymmetry. You notice that the patient has a slightly open lip posture when she is seated in the dental chair.

Intraoral Examination

The patient has a well-developed upper alveolar ridge with limited resorption, consistent with the relatively recent loss of several upper teeth. There is slight redness of the palate under the denture-bearing area, but the ridge is not tender on palpation at any site, and there is no bleeding on probing around the canine roots and no detectable sinus. One of the root-treated canine teeth has lost a small restoration from the access cavity. The remainder of the oral mucosa is normal.

There is an almost complete lower arch of natural teeth. These are adequately restored, many with large amalgam restorations, and there is no caries. The occlusal plane is relatively even. There has been slight mesial tipping of the lower second molars as a result of loss of both first molars.

The denture appears clean and without obvious defects, and there is a definite post dam along its posterior margin.

◆ On the Basis of What You Know So Far, What are the Likely Diagnoses, and Why?

The patient has successfully worn a denture and the transition to an overdenture from an upper acrylic partial denture should have been relatively straightforward. It might have been more difficult if the previous denture had been metal based. If the patient has persevered for 3 months without success, she almost certainly has a valid complaint.

There appears to be no problem of displacement of the denture during eating, speaking or other facial movements. This makes it unlikely that the overdenture is poorly adapted or overextended or that the teeth lie outside the neutral zone. Occlusal discrepancies of some kind would appear to be the most likely cause, and the vagueness of the complaint – predominantly inability to tolerate the denture – is consistent with an occlusal problem. A further reason to suspect an occlusal problem is the difficulty arising from a complete upper denture occluding against a lower natural arch.

It must also be borne in mind that some denture patients are particularly conscious of appearance and the construction of dentures that satisfy the expectations of such patients can be very challenging. Sometimes, a mismatch between

TABLE 24.1 Examination of the Denture

Feature	Method
Check base extension. Is the denture correctly extended into the sulcus?	This is done visually where possible, checking the relationship between the denture border, sulcus depth and soft tissue mobility at rest and under tension. In less visible areas such as lateral to the tuberosity palpation may be required.
Does the posterior border extend back to the vibrating area? (Displaceable tissue)	Identify the vibrating area by observing the soft tissue moving when the patient says 'Ahhh', and/or apply pressure with a blunt instrument such as a ball-ended burnisher to define the extent of displaceable tissue.
Is the denture retentive?	Check by pulling down on the upper denture in the premolar region. Check retention of the post dam by trying to displace the denture with forward pressure behind the anterior teeth.
Is there close adaptation of the denture base to the mucosa? NB recent extraction in the last 6 months	Look at the fit surface and check for voids between tissue and denture with a disclosing material such as low-viscosity silicone.
Make an assessment of the occlusal vertical dimension and patient's rest vertical dimension.	Measure the facial height at rest and with the denture in occlusion. Subtract to identify the freeway space. (See below.)
Is the occlusion correct in retruded position?	Check whether the denture meets the natural teeth correctly in retruded position. Are there any premature contacts?
Are the natural teeth affecting the occlusal plane significantly?	Check the occlusal plane to ensure that the natural standing teeth do not place excessive destabilizing forces on the prosthesis. Assess, in particular, whether the denture is stable on lateral excursive movements.
Appearance	Check tooth shade, shape and set-up. Carefully question the patient as to whether they are satisfied with the appearance. Check the soft tissue support provided by the denture, particularly over the canine roots.
*If there were a **lower** complete denture, you should check to ensure that the teeth lie in the neutral zone, and for denture stability. (Not directly relevant in this case.)*	*Look at the denture when the patient's mouth is half open. Is the lower denture displaced by the tongue or lips?*

the denture appearance and desired facial self-image may manifest as dislike of the denture or complaints about relatively minor features. There is always a potential cosmetic problem of an overcontoured labial flange when canine roots support an upper overdenture because the roots preserve the labial aspect of the alveolar bone.

◆ What Specific Features of the Dentures Would You Examine, and How?

All features of the denture should be reviewed (Table 24.1). Denture complaints may have multifactorial causes, and only by examining all features can an accurate diagnosis be made.

Having examined the patient, you find that the denture is correctly extended, stable and retentive. The denture was not displaced on lateral excursion. This leaves the vertical dimension as the most likely cause of an occlusal problem.

◆ What Methods Can Be Used To Assess Vertical Dimension? What are Their Problems?

Initially, it is most straightforward to simply observe the vertical dimension with the denture removed (Fig. 24.1) and in place (Fig. 24.2).

Note the open lip posture (see Fig. 24.2) when the denture is inserted. This is an important indicator that there

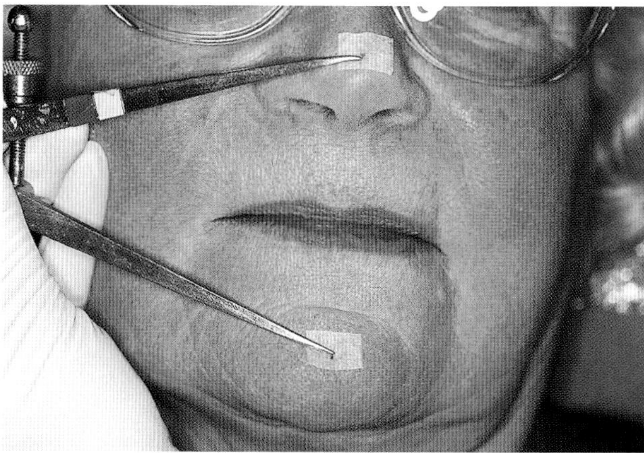

• **Fig. 24.1** Rest vertical dimension with the upper prosthesis removed.

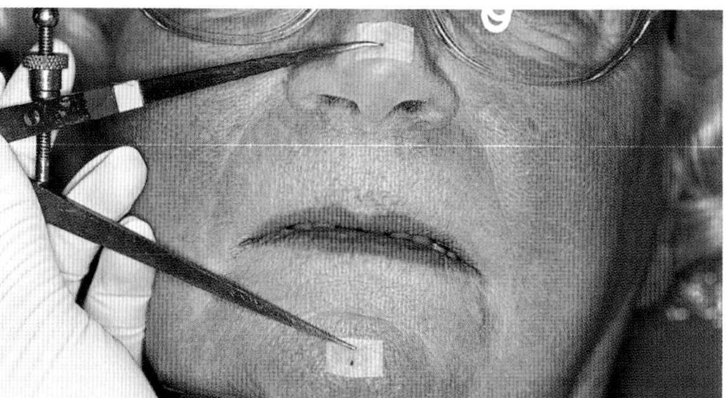

• **Fig. 24.2** Vertical dimension with the upper overdenture in place.

may be an error in vertical height, and a more accurate assessment must be made.

There are three common methods that might be used, the first two of which are essentially similar and have some of the same problems. These both measure the lower facial height at rest and with the dentures in occlusion. The rest value should be greater than the value with dentures in occlusion. The difference between these measurements, with the occlusal vertical dimension subtracted from rest vertical dimension, is the value of the freeway space. The head must be in a natural vertical position supported by the neck muscles. A fixed support such as a head rest can alter the freeway space. In most instances, these methods are satisfactory and readily applied, but sometimes, it may be appropriate to use all three methods to establish the correct vertical dimension.

Dividers/Calipers Method. Marks or adhesive markers are placed on the chin and nose and their distance apart is measured with calipers or dividers. One problem is that the markers are fixed to the skin and may move through muscle activity, particularly pursing of the lips. All suitable sites on the skin may move to some degree, so it is necessary to ensure that the patient remains relaxed during the procedure.

This method is shown in Figs 24.1 and 24.2. The calipers are set to the resting face height (see Fig. 24.1). When the denture is inserted (see Fig. 24.2) the increase in vertical dimension is clearly seen and is about 3–4 mm. The patient, thus, has a negative value for freeway space.

Willis Bite Gauge. This measures lower face height from the lower border of the nose to the lower border of the mandible. It is important to use the same pressure when recording rest and occlusal height, otherwise compression of the tissues will affect the reading. More importantly, the instrument has to be used at a consistent angle at the base of the nose. This is particularly difficult when making complete dentures against lower standing teeth because removing the upper denture to record rest height removes the denture support of the upper lip, which is used as a landmark.

Closest Speaking Space Method. This method provides a rough estimate of the presence of a freeway space but does not involve direct measurement. The patient is asked to say words that include prominent 'ss' sounds, such as 'Mississippi' and 'Tuesday'. These sounds are more difficult to make in the absence of freeway space. Unfortunately, patients adapt their speech to both increased and decreased occlusal heights, and this method can only be considered an adjunct to the more accurate methods above.

◆ How Large Should the Freeway Space Be?

This depends on the patient. The average freeway space is 2–4 mm measured in the premolar region, and dentures may be constructed to this dimension for most patients. However, there are some circumstances in which this clearance needs to be increased. Some patients become habituated to an increased freeway space, either because of wearing of artificial teeth or because of faulty denture construction. In some cases, the freeway space may exceed 1 cm, and it would be unreasonable to expect such patients to accommodate rapidly to the normal freeway space. Provided the increased freeway space is not associated with any problems, a compromise increased freeway space is appropriate.

Diagnosis

◆ What is Your Diagnosis, and Why is This the Most Likely Possibility?

Error in Occlusal Vertical Dimension. There is clearly an increased occlusal vertical dimension, based on the measurements described above, and this is beyond the tolerance level of most patients. This fault is frequently associated with a history of being able to cope with the denture for a few hours and then having to remove the prosthesis. The open lip posture is also often associated with an increased occlusal vertical dimension. Some patients naturally have an open lip posture, so this sign is only an indication of potential problems. Until the fault is corrected, it is not really possible to consider any alternative explanation.

◆ What Possible Diagnoses Have You Excluded? Explain Why for Each Possibility

Error in Retruded Position. Dentures with this fault produce pain on the ridge and pain on eating. If this were suspected, it would be necessary to take a precontact occlusal check record and to remount the dentures on an articulator to make a definitive diagnosis. Adjustment of the occlusion to the correct record should cure the symptoms, and this will confirm the cause. This possible error needs to be kept in mind in all such cases. If the occlusion is ignored and the denture base adjusted, the area of soreness will move to another area with each adjustment, progressively destroying the fit surface of the denture.

Difficulty Becoming Accustomed To Acrylic Palatal Coverage. Patients normally become accustomed to a new denture design in 3 months, even when there is a change to acrylic palatal coverage. In the very elderly or in those who have worn dentures for many years, this period may need to be extended, and a few patients need training bases or simple acrylic partial dentures before definitive complete dentures or overdentures. However, no patient should be expected to become accustomed to a denture with an increased vertical dimension.

Denture-Related Stomatitis. Redness of the denture-bearing area almost certainly indicates denture stomatitis (chronic atrophic candidosis). However, this condition is asymptomatic and not normally noticed by patients.

Patient's Expectation of Appearance Has Not Been Met. Both men and women may be embarrassed to admit that their dentures do not fulfil their cosmetic expectations. This may not just be the fault of the denture but also result from patients seeking to recapture their youthful appearance. Although this may not be unreasonable, it may be physically impossible. Sometimes, hurtful comments from relatives, friends or acquaintances may change the patient's opinion about an otherwise satisfactory denture. This problem may be expressed as repeated minor complaints that do not make sense clinically or, as in this case, a dislike or complete rejection of the denture. This problem can only be diagnosed through careful and considerate questioning.

In the present case, this possible diagnosis is unlikely, given that there is a fault in the vertical dimension and the patient appears happy with the appearance of the denture.

Miscellaneous and Other Unusual Complaints. These include complaints of irritation from a high residual monomer content in an incorrectly processed denture base or, very rarely, hypersensitivity to acrylic. In both cases, the denture-bearing area, and sometimes the whole mouth, would be sore. This patient has inflammation of the denture-bearing area, but this is much more likely to be related to denture plaque or perhaps candidal infection, and these should be excluded before considering the alternative causes. Another complaint, sometimes unfairly ascribed to dentures, is mucosal burning in an otherwise healthy mouth. This is usually psychogenic and associated with depression. Nothing in the history of this patient suggests this diagnosis.

◆ How Would You Manage the Case?

Replace the missing restoration in the canine root to prevent caries.

To solve the denture problem, the denture must be remade with an appropriate freeway space, but the denture stomatitis must first be treated to improve support for the new prosthesis. Treatment will involve improving denture hygiene, ceasing night wear, if appropriate. The possibility of an underlying condition predisposing to candidosis should be considered, especially if the infection involves other parts of the mouth or lips or if treatment fails despite good denture hygiene. In this case, referral to the patient's general practitioner would be indicated for further investigations. Fortunately, denture provision is a less litigious situation; if the patient were unhappy with the denture, a wise practitioner would return the fee because the treatment is reversible, and the patient could find another practitioner or be referred to one who may be more successful.

Case 25

Impacted Lower Third Molars

TARA RENTON AND VINOD PATEL

Summary

A 24-year-old patient is referred to you in your oral surgery-orientated practice for a second opinion on the need to remove his lower third molar teeth. Is this the correct decision, and if it is, how should it be achieved?

History

Complaint

The patient has no complaint at present but has been advised by his general dental practitioner to have his lower third molars extracted. He is very nervous about the extractions and requests a second opinion before deciding on treatment.

History of Complaint

The patient has had two episodes of pericoronitis around the lower left third molar. The first episode was relatively mild, but the second episode, which occurred about 3 months ago, was associated with inability to open the mouth and slight facial swelling, necessitating a course of oral antibiotics.

Medical History

The patient is fit and well. He has had general anaesthesia previously to reduce and fix a compound fracture of his arm, which has been permanently plated. He has had no problems with bleeding after trauma.

Examination

Extraoral Examination

The left submandibular lymph nodes are palpable but not tender. There is no facial asymmetry.

Intraoral Examination

◆ **What Particular Features of the Intraoral Examination are Important and Why?**

See Table 25.1.

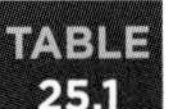

TABLE 25.1 Important Features of Intraoral Examination

Feature	Reason
Interincisal opening	One feature determining access for surgical removal and affecting the difficulty of extraction. Trismus may also reflect infection or inflammation in the muscles of mastication.
Condition of rest of dentition	If the first or second molars have a poor prognosis through caries or are extensively restored, transplanting the third molars in their place might be considered.
Oral hygiene	Poor oral hygiene increases the risk of dry socket, soft tissue infection and delayed healing.
Position of lower third molars	The degree of eruption, angulation and proximity to the second molars are important. Partially erupted vertical or distoangular lower third molars are more at risk of pericoronitis than mesio-angularly impacted ones.
Position of upper third molars	Nonfunctional upper third molars may overerupt and traumatize the operculum over the lower third molar or erupt buccally and traumatize the cheek. Both situations might contribute to symptoms.
Position of external oblique ridge	If this lies close behind or over the impacted tooth, access is poor, and considerable bone removal may be required if the tooth is large or impacted.
Condition of lower second molars	The lower second molar is at risk of iatrogenic damage during surgical removal of the third molar. Crowns or large restorations, especially those involving the distal surface, will be at risk and may increase the difficulty of the extraction.
Presence of pericoronitis	Has the same effect as generalized poor oral hygiene except that the risk of adverse effects is higher. Surgery should not be performed in an infected field.
Miscellaneous features	Factors such as a pronounced gag reflex, poor patient compliance and anxiety may all affect treatment.

In this case, the patient has normal mouth opening and a full unrestored dentition without evidence of caries, periodontal disease or poor oral hygiene. The lower third molars are partially erupted and appear vertically orientated, and there is mild inflammation of the attached gingivae surrounding both crowns. The upper third molars are over-erupted and nonfunctional. The patient demonstrates a pronounced gag reflex when his teeth are examined.

Investigations

◆ Would You Take Radiographs?

Yes, radiographs are required to assess root morphology, degree of bone impaction, proximity to inferior dental nerve and the possibility of associated disease (e.g. cysts, hypercementosis and periodontal bone loss).

◆ Which Views Would You Take, and Why?

The views to be possibly taken are listed, with their advantages and disadvantages, in Table 25.2.

There is little to choose between the two-dimensional radiographic views in terms of radiation dose, provided fast films and appropriate intensifying screens are used. However, cone beam computed tomography (CBCT) does involve a higher dose.

In this case, the patient's gag reflex prevented the taking of paralleling-technique periapicals, and so a panoramic radiograph was taken. It is shown in Fig. 25.1.

◆ What Does the Radiograph Show?

The patient is fully dentate, with no restoration or caries visible on the film. The lower third molars are vertically orientated and impacted against soft tissue rather than against the second molars. The impacted teeth are of normal size, and the surrounding bone appears to be of normal density. The roots of both teeth appear to be closely related to the inferior dental nerve canal; there is darkening, but no narrowing or deflection of the bony wall of the canal, suggesting that it does not contact or pass through the tooth root.

◆ What Additional Value Might Cone Beam Computed Tomography Provide in Mandibular Third Molar Surgery?

It allows clear visualization of the localization and proximity of the inferior dental nerve canal in relation to the tooth as well as the tooth position and anatomy such as number of roots and any dilacerations. In addition, any other findings such as cyst can be seen, including their extension. This information is highly useful in both surgical planning and provision. Its value in a different case is shown in Fig. 25.2.

TABLE 25.2 Radiographic Views

View	Advantages	Disadvantages
Periapicals of upper and lower third molars	Provided the periapicals can be taken with a paralleling technique these are the ideal views. They provide a geometrically accurate projection with true relationships to the adjacent structures. They are also convenient for single extractions. These views are the first choice.	Unfortunately, it may not be possible to obtain radiographs by using the paralleling technique because of patient tolerance. Placement of the film in the ideal position, showing the teeth and inferior dental nerve canal, is uncomfortable. If films are angled then a degree of distortion is inevitable.
Oblique laterals	Readily taken without specialized equipment. Show both upper and lower third molars without superimposition. Give a good view of the surrounding bone when adjacent lesions (e.g. cysts) are present.	Suffer a degree of distortion as the beam is angled upwards, so the relationship to adjacent structures is not accurate.
Panoramic radiograph	Convenient survey film if equipment available. Gives a good view of the surrounding bone when adjacent lesions (e.g. cysts) are present. Panoramic films are often used and in practice usually provide sufficient information to assess extractions.	Poor image quality because the view is a tomograph. In addition, there is superimposition of the opposite angle of mandible over upper and lower third molars. The upward beam angle distorts the relationship between teeth and adjacent structures and the image is magnified. Root morphology can be difficult to assess on panoramic radiographs because of superimposition, shadowing and the two-dimensional nature of the radiograph.
Lower oblique occlusal	Useful when the lower third molar lies horizontally and is seen end-on in a periapical view. Provides information on bucco-lingual orientation. Useful if tooth lies out of the line of arch. Used only rarely.	
Cone beam computed tomography	Low-dose computed tomography available in a dental setting, high definition three-dimensional imaging showing accurate relationships between tooth and inferior dental canal and other structures.	Not available in all centres and requires additional training in assessment and interpretation.

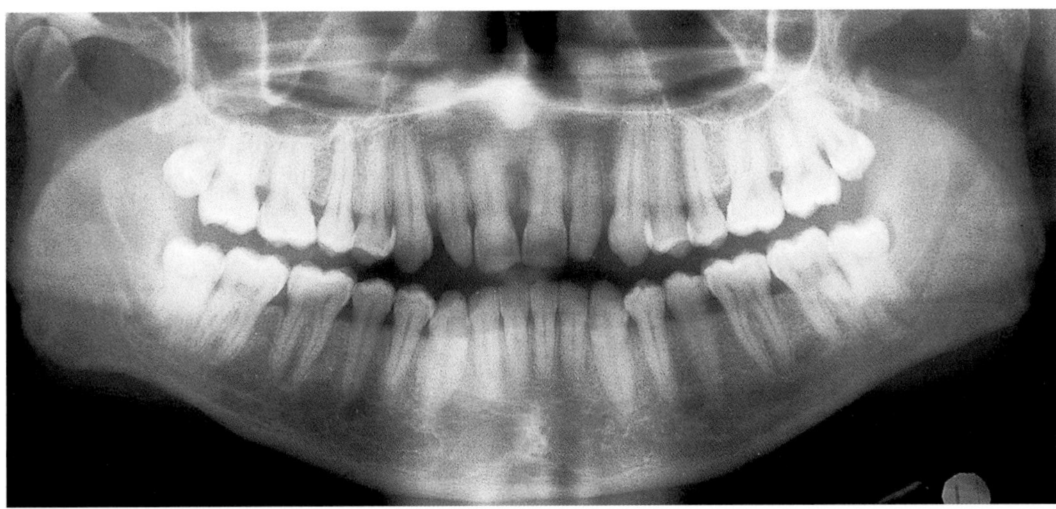

• **Fig. 25.1** Panoramic radiograph.

◆ What Do You See in the Cone Beam Computed Tomography Images in Fig. 25.2?

These images from another case demonstrate the value of this more complex imaging technique. They are selected views from the imaged volume, which is manipulated in three-dimensions on a computer monitor. On the left is an axial slice (almost occlusal view) through a horizontally impacted lower third molar. The image is round because this system images a vertical cylinder of tissue that is being seen end-on. Unlike medical computed tomography (CT), CBCT images are conventionally viewed from the top, so the patient's right is on the left of the figure. On the right is a sagittal slice. The inferior dental canal (C) can be seen clearly, outlined by thin cortical bone as it passes in contact with and between the apices of two roots (A).

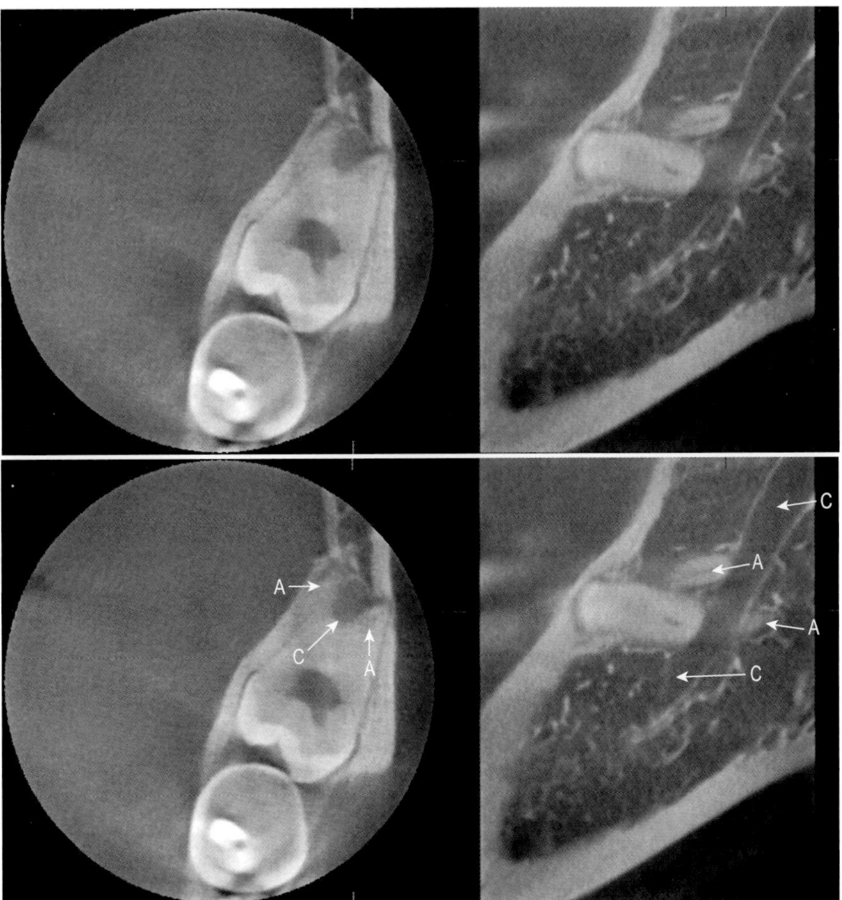

• **Fig 25.2** Cone beam computed tomography (CBCT) images of another patient.

There is no cortex visible where the canal contacts parts of the tooth, so the roots probably penetrate the wall of the canal.

◆ You Now Have Sufficient Information To Decide Whether or Not the Third Molars Should Be Removed. What are the Indications for Removal?

There has been much debate about the indications for the removal of third molars, and those for the removal of asymptomatic third molars are particularly contentious. Mandibular impacted third molars (MITMs) are very common, affecting approximately 75% of 20- to 30-year-old patients. Surgery is unpleasant, carries risks and is expensive to the state and the patient; thus, following current UK guidance (National Institute of Clinical Excellence [NICE] 2000) is essential unless there is high risk of distal caries developing in the second mandibular molars. Current UK guidance is now somewhat dated and is being revised at the time of this writing.

The suggested indications for removal are:

- Recurrent pericoronitis and pericoronitis with acute spreading infection
- Unrestorable caries of MITM or adjacent teeth
- Untreatable periapical inflammation
- Periodontal disease associated with the MITM or adjacent teeth
- Internal or external resorption of MITM or adjacent teeth
- MITM in fracture line
- Associated cysts or neoplasm
- For tooth reimplantation
- For orthognathic surgery or restorative treatment
- Prophylactic removal may be advised in specific medical conditions (before radiotherapy, cardiothoracic surgery or bisphosphonate treatment).

◆ Should This Patient's Teeth Be Removed, and Why?

Yes, he has suffered two episodes of pericoronitis. There is increasing risk of future episodes as the number of episodes rises, and they are likely to become more frequent and more severe.

◆ How Will You Decide Whether Extraction of This Patient's Third Molars is Within Your Ability?

This is a matter of judgement. You must judge your own ability and experience against the likely difficulty and also consider your ability to manage any complications. In general, the following factors should be considered. The most important of these factors may be remembered by using the mnemonic WHARFE:

W Angulation using **W**inter's lines
H **H**eight of mandible
A **A**ngle of second molar
R **R**oot form and development
F Size of **F**ollicular sac
E **E**xit path of tooth to be extracted

Factors to be considered in assessing the difficulty of extraction are listed in Table 25.3.

◆ What are 'Winter's Lines', and How Might They Help Assess Difficulty?

To apply Winter's lines, three imaginary lines are drawn on the radiographic image (Fig. 25.3). For descriptive purposes,

TABLE 25.3 Factors Contributing To the Difficulty of Extraction

Easier Extraction	More Difficult Extraction
Young patient	Patient older than 30 years of age
Female patient	Male patient
European/Asian racial group	African race
Superficial impaction	Deeply buried
Mesio-angular or vertical impaction	Disto-angular or horizontal impaction
Small crown	Wide crown
Conical root	Multirooted, divergent roots
Lying buccally in relation to line of arch	Lying lingually in relation to line of arch
Clear path of delivery, usually forward and upward	Vertical or distal path of removal required, possibly requiring tooth section
External oblique ridge well posterior to tooth	External oblique ridge overlies tooth
Sound second molar	Crowned, root treated or heavily restored adjacent molar
Normal second molar root morphology	Conical root (risks accidental elevation)
Distant from inferior dental nerve	Adjacent to inferior dental nerve
Large dental follicle	Narrow dental follicle or ankylosis
Good access	Poor access (e.g. caused by trismus)
Not impacted or soft tissue impacted	Impacted against bone or root of second molar
	History of complex or difficult extraction

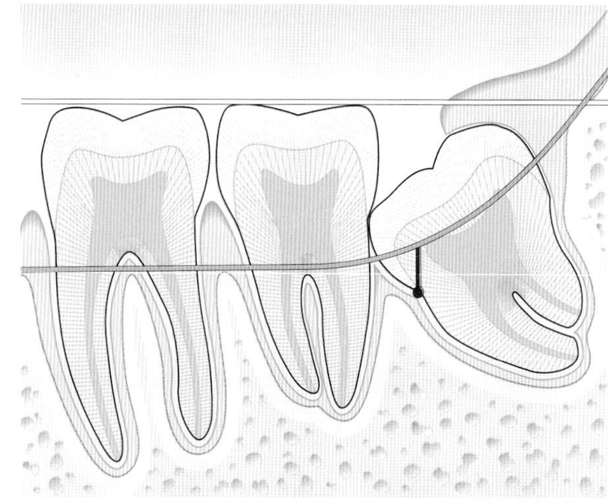

• **Fig. 25.3** Example of the application of Winter's lines.

the lines are assigned colours. The white line runs along the occlusal plane, and the amber line runs along the upper bone surface through the interdental bone crests and along the bone surface behind the third molar (not up the external oblique ridge). The red line passes vertically, at right angles to the white line, to the application point for an elevator. In mesio-angular impactions, the point of elevation lies at the mesial end of the amelo-cemental junction, and for disto-angular impactions, it lies at the distal end of the amelo-cemental junction.

The angle of impaction is judged against the white line. The amber line gives an indication of the amount of tooth that will be visible when the periosteal flap is raised and the amount of bone removal required over the crown. The red line gives an indication of the depth of bone removal required to gain a point of application for an elevator. If the red line is greater than 5 mm in length the extraction is likely to merit the use of general anaesthesia. If it is greater than 9 mm in length, it is likely that extensive bone removal will be required.

◆ What are the Deficiencies of the Winter's Lines Technique?

Winter's lines are useful for mesio-angular impactions, but the length of the red line is almost meaningless in disto-angular impactions, which are always relatively difficult. The technique also ignores the possibility of sectioning the tooth which makes the extraction easier, changing the point of application of elevators and the path of removal. Winter's lines should be applied to a periapical radiograph, preferably a geometrically accurate projection obtained by using a paralleling technique. The method can be used on oblique laterals or panoramic tomographs, but it provides a less accurate estimate of difficulty. In addition, a correction must be made for magnification in the panoral film, which ranges from ×1.2 to ×1.4, depending on the equipment used. Winter's lines would not provide useful information in the present case, but they do provide a way of systematically examining a radiograph to ensure that no information is missed.

◆ How Difficult are This Patient's Extractions Likely To Be?

Both lower third molars are slightly disto-angularly inclined and the external oblique ridge overlies them. Although not very deeply placed, these are moderately difficult to extract. Extraction should not be attempted under local anaesthesia or sedation by anyone other than an experienced or specialized surgeon, regardless of the care setting.

The majority of lower third molars which meet the criteria for extraction will be relatively difficult. This is because the commonest indication is pericoronitis, which affects mostly vertically and disto-angularly impacted teeth.

Prior to surgery, you must warn the patient about the complications of removal. List the possible complications, and give an indication of their frequency.

The complications are listed in Table 25.4. The top four are relatively common and should be discussed with patients as a matter of routine.

◆ What Warnings Would You Give To the Patient About Extraction?

Deciding exactly which complications to warn patients about can be difficult. The decision must be made individually for each case. The patient must be provided with sufficient information to be able to give informed consent, and the clinician must answer all the patient's questions correctly. It is generally considered mandatory to warn the patient about both the sequelae and the significant complications of extraction. Sequelae may be induced by surgery or anaesthesia and should be differentiated. Surgical sequelae include swelling (for 48 hours), pain (for approximately 48 hours), bleeding (for about 2 hours), sore temporomandibular joint and trismus, sensitivity of adjacent teeth, and remodelling of the sockets for approximately 10–12 weeks. Complications which must be described are the risk of dry socket (5%) and the risk of temporary (2%) and permanent (0.5%) damage to the lingual and inferior dental nerves. Warnings concerning damage to adjacent teeth or restorations, or displacement of teeth into the antrum, are usually reserved for patients who are at particular risk.

◆ Does the Patient Require Antibiotic Cover Before Surgery To Prevent Infection of the Bone Plate in His Arm?

No, this is not necessary.

◆ Would You Prescribe Postoperative Antibiotics for These Extractions?

Evidence does not support providing antibiotics perioperatively for dental extractions. Antibiotics do not significantly affect the incidence of dry socket and should not be given without a good reason. They would be indicated if there were an increased risk of infection, as in a patient with diabetes or immunosuppression, after radiotherapy, or if infection were present at the time of operation. However, in normal individuals, antibiotics are probably less important than local measures for preventing infection. A chlorhexidine mouthrinse before the operation and/or debridement of teeth and below the operculum are highly effective in reducing the incidence of postoperative infection and bacteraemia.

In some centres, antibiotics are given routinely whenever bone removal is required, although the value is disputed. If antibiotics are provided, patients having extractions under local anaesthesia usually receive an oral course of amoxicillin or metronidazole. When general anaesthesia is used, a suitable regimen would be a single intravenous bolus dose of either co-amoxiclav or metronidazole.

◆ Is General Anaesthesia Required or Desirable?

The choice of anaesthesia will depend on the indications for treatment, the assessment of difficulty and the anaesthesia risk assessment for the particular patient.

This patient requires extraction of all four third molars. The indications for removal do not, in themselves, require general anaesthesia. However, the surgery is likely to take

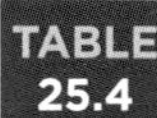

TABLE 25.4 Possible Complications of Removal of Mandibular Impacted Third Molars

Complication	Frequency
Postsurgical pain, haemorrhage, trismus, swelling and ecchymosis	These affect all patients to some degree and in a proportion of cases may be prolonged. Inability to eat and enjoy food is considered a significant complication by patients.
Alveolar osteitis (dry socket)	Affects 1–35% lower third molar extractions, depending on difficulty and technique. An average for surgical extractions is 5%.
Sensory nerve damage, neuropathy which may present with dysaesthesia, paraesthesia or anaesthesia or a combination of all three	Affects 10–20% of cases though almost all recover spontaneously. A degree of permanent damage of inferior dental or lingual nerves affects 0.5% of cases. Temporary lingual nerve effects are seen in 2%.
Acute temporomandibular joint pain/dysfunction (arthromyalgia)	About 4% of cases, higher in patients with pre-existing symptoms and those whose teeth are removed under general anaesthesia. A mild degree of muscle and joint discomfort is probably much commoner.
Iatrogenic fracture	Fracture of the mandible is fortunately rare, occurring in 1 per 10 000 cases. If minor fractures of the alveolar or lingual plates or tuberosity are included, the incidence is 2–4% of cases, but apart from tuberosity fracture these are mostly of little consequence.
Incorrect or incomplete extraction	Less than 1%.
Acute/chronic postoperative infection including osteonecrosis	Rare, affecting 2–3 per 100 000 cases.
Injury to adjacent structures, including teeth and periodontium	Relatively common; occurs in 3 per 1000 cases.
Oroantral fistula	Rare.
Introduction of tooth or fragment into another tissue space (antrum, tissue space, inhaled into lung or swallowed)	Rare.
Systemic medical/surgical complications related to surgery and/or anaesthesia	Sore throat, adverse reaction, etc. Patients must not drive or operate machinery for 48 hours after sedation or general anaesthesia.
Death under outpatient general anaesthesia	1–2 per 400 000. Increased risk in children. May be related to halothane-induced cardiac arrhythmias.

longer than 20 minutes on each side under local anaesthesia. Arguably, this procedure could be performed under local anaesthesia in two visits by an experienced clinician, but many patients find this unacceptable. The patient's gag reflex is one factor suggesting that general anaesthesia or sedation would be appropriate, and the patient appears to have no medical contraindication. The patient must be fully informed of the risks of sedation or anaesthesia before making a decision. The risks of general anaesthesia are such that it is never the anaesthesia of choice for routine or straightforward extractions. The flow chart (Fig. 25.4) illustrates some factors in selecting a suitable type of anaesthesia.

◆ What Surgical Technique Should Be Used To Remove the Lower Third Molars?

There is much debate about the best method for removal of lower third molars. In the UK, the standard of care is usually removal via a buccal approach with a surgical hand piece if required for complete extraction. In this approach, no lingual flap is raised, and no lingual nerve retraction is performed, so this method carries minimal risk of permanent lingual nerve damage. This is the standard method used in Europe and the US and is increasingly used in the UK, replacing the traditional lingual and buccal flap methods.

However, additional approaches are slowly increasing in popularity, often because of concerns regarding risk of inferior dental nerve injury. When CBCT is available to accurately identify a high risk of inferior alveolar nerve injury, coronectomy can be considered.

◆ What is Coronectomy, and When Can It Be Offered?

Coronectomy is the elective removal of the crown of a tooth leaving the roots undisturbed in the socket. This is an alternative surgical approach for mandibular third molars close to the inferior dental nerve canal and is only considered after the risk has been assessed by using appropriate imaging, and there remains a genuine concern regarding nerve injury resulting from the extraction. The technique is not exclusive to third molars and can be used for any impacted mandibular teeth posing the same risk.

Although the procedure of removing the crown appears simple, it can prove to be technically challenging, particularly in deeply impacted mandibular third molars. Amongst many factors, success is imperative on the removal of the

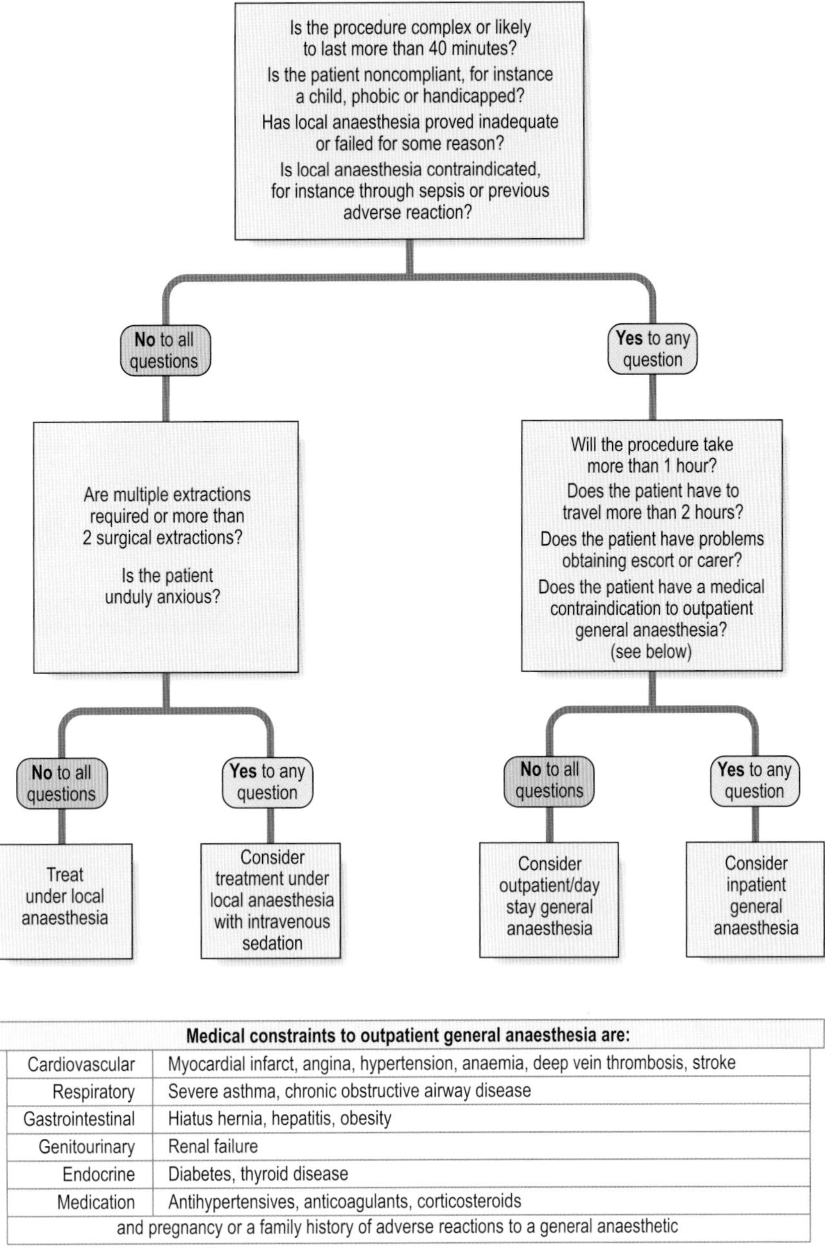

Medical constraints to outpatient general anaesthesia are:	
Cardiovascular	Myocardial infarct, angina, hypertension, anaemia, deep vein thrombosis, stroke
Respiratory	Severe asthma, chronic obstructive airway disease
Gastrointestinal	Hiatus hernia, hepatitis, obesity
Genitourinary	Renal failure
Endocrine	Diabetes, thyroid disease
Medication	Antihypertensives, anticoagulants, corticosteroids
and pregnancy or a family history of adverse reactions to a general anaesthetic	

• **Fig. 25.4** Flow chart for selection of patients for general anaesthesia.

crown at the cemento-enamel junction with no enamel retained on the residual roots.

The principle of retaining the roots in situ requires that the tooth is healthy with no pulpal or periapical disease to allow the retained roots maintain their vitality. In the medium-term healing phase, an osteodentine bridge forms to seal off the pulp, maintaining the root in situ without symptoms. The result of a coronectomy in a different case is shown in Fig. 25.5.

◆ What are the Indications and Contraindications for Coronectomy?

The only indication for coronectomy is to treat a mandibular tooth that merits removal on currently accepted guidelines, but that has roots close to the inferior dental canal risking nerve damage on complete removal. Pericoronitis and even a dentigerous cyst need not contraindicate coronectomy because these processes are associated with the crown. Contraindications for coronectomy are:

- Caries involving the pulp
- Apical periodontitis
- Internal or external resorption
- Mobile tooth
- Periodontal involvement.

◆ Are There Any Further Complications and Risks That Should Be Included When Obtaining Patients' Consent for Coronectomy?

Yes, in addition to the standard warnings for third molar surgery, there are a few specific issues that should be highlighted when discussing coronectomy as a treatment option with the patient. These are detailed in Table 25.5.

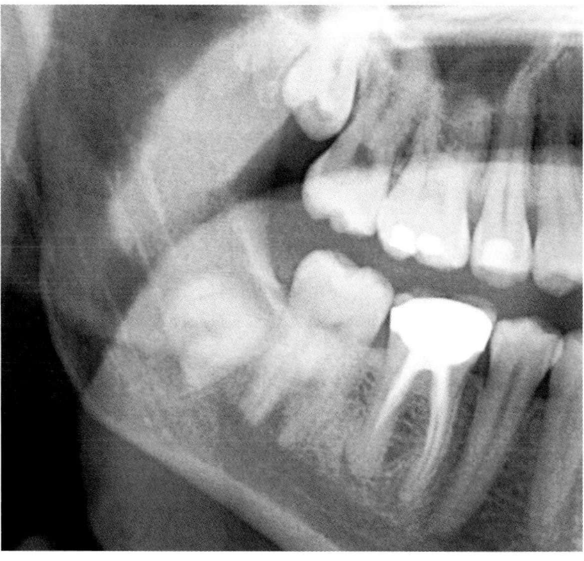

• **Fig 25.5** Shows a lower right third molar tooth before coronectomy with superimposition beyond the inferior dental nerve canal and darkening of the root suggesting a risk for nerve injury if extracted (left) followed by a postcoronectomy radiograph 9 years later, with the roots still buried with overlying bone and no suggestion of apical periodontitis (right). The roots have migrated coronally but still remain superimposed over the inferior dental nerve canal.

TABLE 25.5 **Complications and Risks Associated with Coronectomy**

Complications and Risks	Overall Frequency	Additional Information
Root accidentally mobilized during surgery	3–9%	Mobilized roots are usually caused by incorrect surgical cuts and excessive force used to decoronate or in young females who have a conical root form. Subsequently the mobilized root requires extraction, placing the patient at potential risk of nerve injury.
Inferior dental nerve injury	<1%	All studies have shown coronectomy carries a lower nerve injury risk compared with complete extraction. However, the risk will vary, depending on the complexity and intimacy of the tooth to the nerve. Nerve injury is more likely if the root is accidentally mobilized, or if the nerve canal is close to the crown of the tooth, the latter usually only in deeply impacted teeth.
Damage to adjacent tooth	<1%	This can occur during the smoothing of the retained root where the adjacent tooth roots are in close proximity.
Delayed healing or nonhealing socket	<1%	Usually related to a mobilized root left unnoticed causing infection or because of retained enamel on the root surface.
Migration of roots	14–81%	This is the commonest long-term consequence of coronectomy. Technically, it is not seen as a complication, but this may be noticed on subsequent radiographs. Although the roots remain buried and asymptomatic, regular radiographs are not indicated.
Eruption of roots	0–6%	Continued migration can lead to eruption of the roots into the oral cavity. If symptomatic, this would be an indication for removal.

Case 26

A Patient Presenting with an Avulsed Central Incisor

SERPIL DJEMAL AND RAVI CHAUHAN

Summary

A 26-year-old female presents with an avulsed upper right central incisor and brings with her the tooth wrapped in tissue paper. How will you manage this clinical scenario?

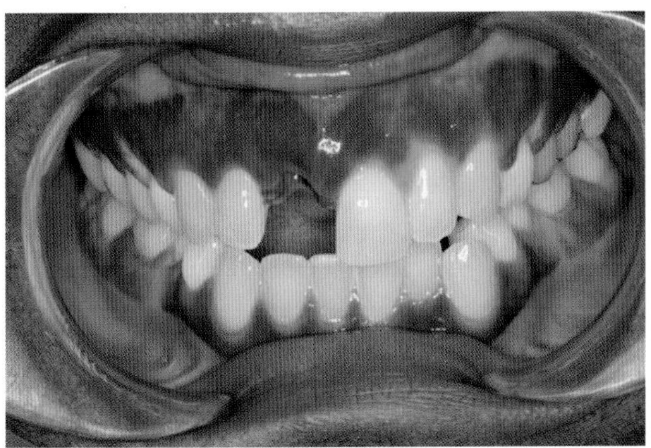

• **Fig. 26.1** An anterior view of the patient's dentition in occlusion, on presentation. © Serpil Djemal.

History

Complaint

A 26-year-old female patient presents to your practice in the morning with her central incisor wrapped in tissue. The patient fell over in a nightclub in the early hours of the morning and knocked her upper central incisor out. She went to a hospital Accident and Emergency (A&E) department, where she was cleared of any other injuries and was asked to see her dentist as soon as possible about her tooth. Fig. 26.1 shows the patient on presentation.

◆ What Further Information Would You Want From the Patient?

Are There Any Other Injuries? It should be established whether there has been any loss of consciousness or signs of concussion. Disorientation and impaired response to simple questions may indicate a brain injury that would require immediate hospital assessment. Dealing with these might be a higher priority than the avulsed tooth. *In this case, the patient did not lose consciousness and was cleared of head injuries at her local A&E department.*

Is There Any Relevant Medical History? Reimplantation of an avulsed tooth is contraindicated in a patient predisposed to infective endocarditis or is immunocompromised in any way. Any known clotting defect could result in problematic bleeding from a tooth socket. *The patient was medically fit and well in this instance.*

Is the Patient Up To Date with Tetanus Immunization? The patient would require a booster if the injury involved soil contamination. Because the injury occurred in a nightclub, her tetanus status was not relevant, but it is good practice to check this for all patients. *The patient was up to date her tetanus immunization.*

What is the Stage of Root Development? The management of a permanent tooth with an immature root is different from a permanent tooth with a fully developed root. An avulsed tooth with a fully developed root will always require root canal treatment within 7 days from the date of injury, regardless of the length of time the tooth was out of the socket. An avulsed tooth with an immature root should always be given an opportunity to revascularize if the extra oral dry time is less than 60 mins. *In this case, the tooth had a fully developed root.* A primary tooth should not be replanted because of the risk of damage to the permanent successor.

When Did the Accident Happen? The length of time the tooth is out of the socket, the extraoral dry time (EODT), will influence the length of time the tooth is splinted and the overall prognosis. An avulsed tooth that has an extended EODT (>60 minutes) will need to be splinted for **4 weeks**. An avulsed tooth that has a shorter EODT (<60 minutes) will need to be splinted for **2 weeks**. The longer the EODT, the poorer the prognosis. *In this case, the tooth had been wrapped in tissue for 5 hours.*

What Has the Tooth Been Stored in? A successful outcome requires a healthy viable periodontal ligament on the surface of the root, and in this case, because of the EODT of 5 hours, a significant inflammatory response is anticipated with resultant replacement resorption and ankylosis. An appropriate transport medium is essential, and the key parameter is its osmotic pressure. Hanks balanced salt solution is the best transport medium but is not readily available at scenes of trauma. It has been shown that the periodontal ligament cells can survive for up to 6 hours if placed in milk. The best outcome is seen if the tooth is reimplanted at the scene of the accident.

Examination

◆ What Will You Look for in the Clinical Examination?

- **Soft tissues.** Check the soft tissues for any lacerations that may require the removal of foreign material and suturing.
- **The dentition.** Check the adjacent teeth and those in the opposing arch for any other injuries such as fractures and other possible laxation/displacement injuries. A disturbance in the bite may indicate a displaced tooth. Also, check for the presence of periodontal disease and/or caries and the level of oral hygiene.
- **The avulsed tooth.** The tooth should be examined and cleaned by rinsing with isotonic saline taking great care not to handle the root surface. Any soft tissues adhering to apex should be left, as they may contain Hertwig's sheath remnants with potential for continued apical maturation.

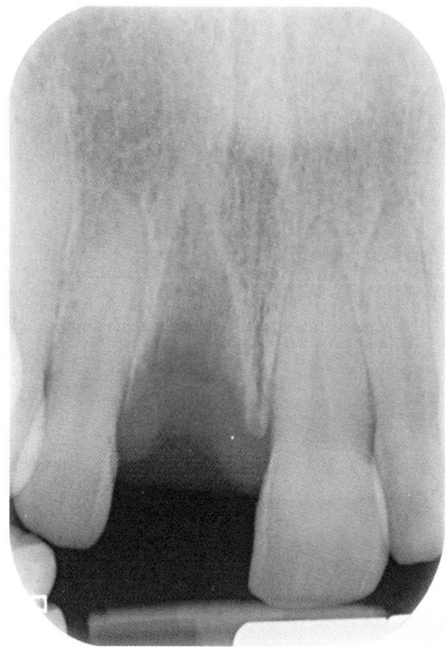

• **Fig. 26.2** A long cone periapical radiograph of the upper anterior teeth and empty socket. © Serpil Djemal.

Special Investigations

◆ What Additional Investigations Will You Undertake?

- **Sensibility testing.** Cold testing or electric pulp testing of the avulsed tooth is not indicated.
- **Radiographs.** A long cone periapical radiograph of the socket and adjacent teeth should be taken to detect any potential remaining root fragments, any associated dento-alveolar fracture and injuries to the adjacent teeth.
- **An upper standard occlusal radiograph** is useful if a root fracture is suspected.

Fig. 26.2 shows the long cone periapical radiograph of the upper incisor teeth, including the upper right central incisor socket.

The periodontal ligament spaces around the upper incisor teeth are even with no obvious changes.

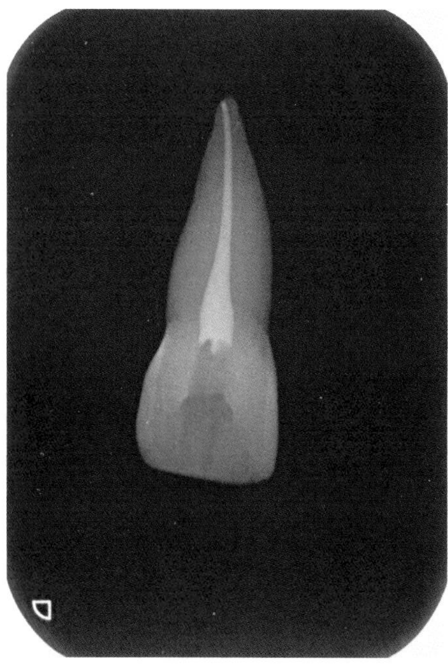

• **Fig. 26.3** A radiograph of the upper right central incisor following extraoral root canal obturation. © Serpil Djemal.

Treatment

◆ How are You Going To Manage the Upper Right Central Incisor?

Avulsed teeth with an EODT of less than 60 minutes should be rinsed and reimplanted under local anaesthesia.

In this case, the EODT was 5 hours (>60 minutes), so root surface preparation is indicated to try to remove all the dead cells and reduce the risk of root resorption. Root surface preparation is as follows:

- Soak the tooth in sodium hypochlorite for 5 minutes
- Rinse the tooth with saline
- Soak the tooth in 0.5% sodium fluoride for 20 minutes
- Root canal treatment within 7–10 days, or if there is time, root canal treatment extra-orally before reimplantation.

The upper right central incisor was root treated extraorally, and a radiograph of the completed root treatment can be seen in Fig. 26.3.

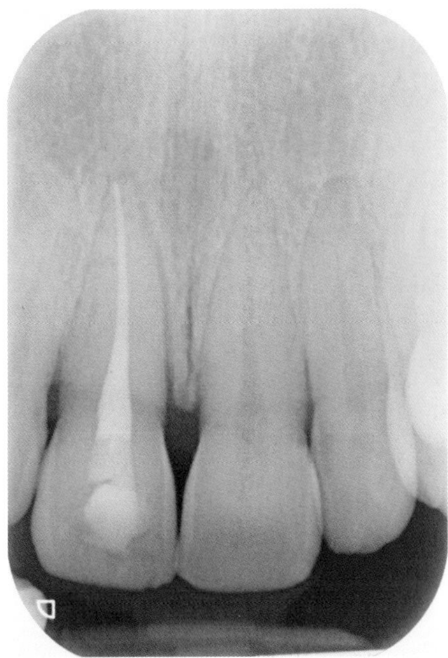

• **Fig. 26.4** Periapical radiograph of the upper right central incisor after reimplantation. © Serpil Djemal.

The reimplantation protocol is as follows:

- Anaesthetize the buccal and palatal tissues
- Remove part of the blood clot in the socket by using a periodontal probe in the central portion rotating it to cause some bleeding
- Digitally reimplant the tooth by holding the crown of the tooth and applying sufficient pressure in an apical direction to position the tooth as near to its original position as possible
- Correct repositioning can be checked by asking the patient to bite together and observing if the patient can bring the teeth together into maximum intercuspation
- Temporarily hold the tooth in position to the adjacent teeth using either a sausage of resin composite or a light cured acrylic material such as TRIAD™
- Take a check periapical radiograph to ensure the tooth has been correctly positioned.

Fig. 26.4 shows the upper right central incisor in the correct position with a relatively even periodontal ligament space.

The splinting protocol is as follows:

- Cut enough 018 stainless steel orthodontic wire to extend from the upper right lateral incisor to the upper left central incisor for flexible splinting
- Prepare resin composite balls of 3 ×4 mm and 3 × 2 mm
- Prepare the teeth by using acid etch and then fully cured unfilled resin on each tooth to be splinted
- Place the 4mm balls onto each tooth, embed the wire into the resin composite and part cure them to secure the wire in position
- Place the smaller 2mm balls on top of each of the 4mm balls encasing the wire and fully light cure each tooth

Fig. 26.5 shows the splinted teeth.

Postoperative instructions include the following:

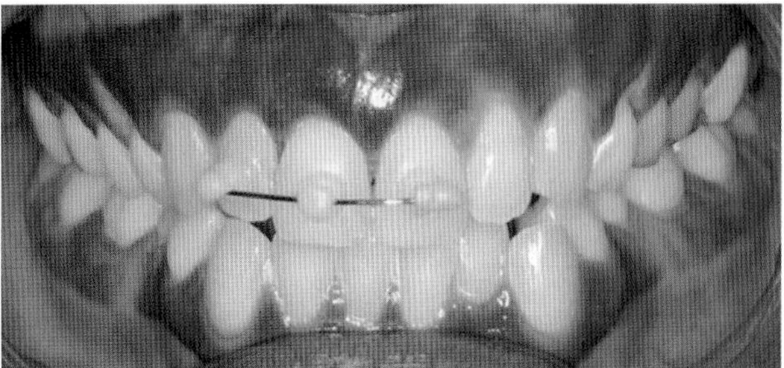

• **Fig. 26.5** Labial view showing the flexible splint on the teeth. © Serpil Djemal.

- Advise the patient not to bite anything with the front teeth and to cut up food and eat using the posterior teeth
- Advise the patient to brush teeth normally.

◆ What Would You Do Next?

Because of the extended EODT, the splint should be removed after **4 weeks**.

The patient will then need to be reviewed at 3 months, 6 months and then annually after the traumatic incident. Each follow-up visit should include the following:

- A clinical examination that should include an assessment of mobility, tenderness to percussion and palpation and the possibility of a draining sinus of the avulsed tooth for any signs of inflammatory or replacement resorption
- The adjacent teeth also need full assessment, as described above, including a note about any possible discoloration indicating loss of vitality
- A periapical radiograph to detect any signs of inflammatory or replacement resorption of the avulsed tooth
- Sensibility testing of the adjacent teeth should be carried out after splint removal.

Throughout this period, the need for good oral hygiene should be reinforced.

◆ How Do I Manage a Tooth That Has an Extraoral Dry Time of Less Than 60 Minutes?

The root does not need to be conditioned with sodium hypochlorite and sodium fluoride. The tooth should be replanted as soon as possible and splinted in the same manner for **2 weeks**. Root canal treatment should be commenced within 7 days from the date of injury.

The follow-up period for an avulsed tooth with an EODT **less than 60 minutes** is at **2 weeks** for **splint removal** and then at 3 months, 6 months and then annually.

In teeth with immature roots (**open apices**), **revascularization** should be attempted with continued root development.

◆ What are the Main Complications of Replantation of an Avulsed Permanent Tooth? How are They Managed?

See Table 26.1

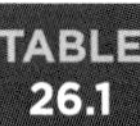

TABLE 26.1 The Main Complications of Replantation of an Avulsed Permanent Tooth and Their Management

Complication	Features	Management
External inflammatory root resorption, thought to be the result of bacteria or their products passing from the pulp chamber through the dentine tubules to induce inflammation in the periodontal ligament and resorption of root and bone.	Recognized radiographically as irregular, crescentic areas of resorption on the external root surface and radiolucent areas in the adjacent alveolar bone. Prompt diagnosis and treatment are essential as the process may be very rapid, especially in immature teeth.	The infected necrotic pulp tissue or existing root filling must be removed as soon as possible and the root canal should be dressed with calcium hydroxide. A definitive root canal filling should not be placed until the inflammatory resorption has been arrested.
External replacement resorption. After ankylosis, the tooth becomes fused to bone and is remodelled and progressively replaced by bone as part of the process of normal bone turnover.	The ankylosed tooth has a high percussion sound, reduced mobility and eventually becomes infraoccluded as a result of reduced alveolar growth. Radiographically, there is loss of definition of periodontal ligament space and dentine. Replacement resorption takes place more rapidly in the growing child.	There is no treatment for external replacement root resorption. In teeth with open apices, as soon as ankylosis is seen, decoronation should be attempted to prevent further disfiguring infraocclusion.

Long-Term Prognosis

◆ What are the Aims of Treatment and Chances of Success?

The aim of reimplantation is to maintain the tooth, thus avoiding the need for prosthetic replacement for as long as possible.

The periodontal ligament heals in 90% of cases if the tooth is replanted immediately but in only 25% of cases if the tooth is incorrectly stored or replantation is delayed. In one large prospective study of 400 replanted teeth followed up for 5 years, 30% were eventually lost. Immature teeth have a worse prognosis compared with mature teeth because the chances of successful revascularization of immature teeth are low (34%).

Treatment Options if Reimplantation is Not Possible

◆ Suppose Re-Implantation is Not Possible for Example, if the Tooth is Not Available, What Treatments are There?

1. Acrylic partial denture
2. Chrome partial denture
3. Resin-bonded bridge
4. Implant
5. 'Mesialization' of the lateral incisor – in the presence of a crowded malocclusion, orthodontic treatment to move the adjacent lateral incisor into the missing central incisor position, as well as to address the malocclusion, can be considered. The size of the lateral incisor will need to be checked carefully to ensure that the emergence profile of the tooth once recontoured to mimic the central incisor will be adequate from an aesthetic point of view. Similarly, the size and shade of the canine tooth must be assessed to ensure that it will be possible to adequately mimic the lateral incisor.
6. Autotransplantation – if a patient is going to undergo orthodontic extraction with one of the premolars being transplanted into the central incisor position.

◆ How Would You Manage an Avulsed Tooth Primary Incisor?

No attempt should be made to reimplant an avulsed primary incisor. Parents should be informed that any attempt to reimplant a primary tooth could result in damage to the permanent successor. A space maintainer with a prosthetic tooth would be advisable to allow for eruption of the permanent successor. If this is not provided, and space is lost, delayed eruption may result.

Case 27
Discoloured Anterior Teeth

MICHAEL THOMAS

Summary

An 18-year-old female presents with concerns regarding the appearance of her teeth. What is the cause, and what treatment would be appropriate?

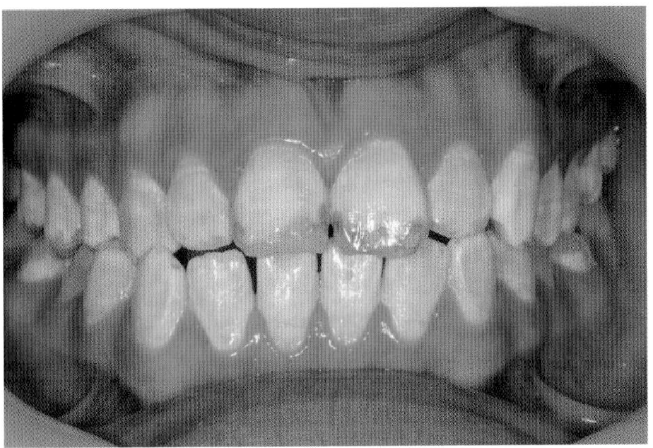

• **Fig. 27.1** Anterior clinical view in occlusion (intercuspal position) showing the dentition on presentation.

History

Complaint

The patient remarked that this appearance has been present since the teeth had erupted into position, but this had caused her no concerns regarding her appearance until now. She has no discomfort from her teeth.

Dental History

The patient has been a regular attendee at the same dental practice all her life. She had received minimal dental treatment and had attended to see a dental hygienist on two occasions in her early teenage years for advice on effective cleaning and diet management.

She brushes her teeth every morning and evening with a rotary electric toothbrush and fluoride-containing toothpaste. She occasionally uses a proprietary mouthwash but uses no further hygiene aids.

Medical History

The patient is fit and well and has no relevant current or historical medical conditions.

Examination

Examination revealed a healthy dentition, with no restorations present. Twenty-eight teeth were present, with early indication of all four third molar teeth being due to erupt shortly. No caries was present, her oral hygiene was excellent and all soft tissues, including the periodontium, were in good health. There was a mottled appearance to the enamel of all teeth, with white striation, brown discolouration and chipping of the enamel on the incisal third aspect of both upper central incisor teeth (Fig. 27.1). There was a small amount of brown discolouration and minor areas of chipping to the remaining maxillary teeth.

◆ What are the Possible Causes of Discolouration of Teeth? What are the Visual Indicators That Assist in Achieving a Diagnosis?

The possible causes of tooth discolouration, which may require aesthetic intervention, are considered in Table 27.1 below. Clinical presentations may include:

- Trauma
- Hypoplastic conditions
- Dental caries
- Crowding
- Missing teeth
- Tooth wear.

Tables 27.1–27.4 show causes of dental discolouration.

◆ What Specific Questions Would You Ask This Patient?

Is She Aware of Any Childhood Illnesses Suffered During the Development of the Teeth (From Birth to Age 7 Years)? Metabolic disorders such as alkaptonuria, congenital hyperbilirubinaemia or congenital erythropoietic porphyria, although rare, will result in discolouration of the dentition during development. Enamel defects may also be observed in cases of vitamin D–dependent rickets, epidermolysis bullosa, Ehlers-Danlos syndrome and pseudo-hypoparathyroidism. Acquired defects, resulting from trauma, systemic infectious disease, localized infection, excessive fluoride intake or administration of tetracycline antibiotics during childhood or to the mother during pregnancy, may affect the dental tissues to a varying degree.

Is There a History Within Her Family of a Similar Appearance To Her Teeth? Hereditary defects such as hypodontia, amelogenesis imperfecta and dentinogenesis imperfecta may affect both the primary and secondary dentition equally.

TABLE 27.1 Developmental Defects Resulting in Dental Discolouration

Cause of Discolouration	Features	Visual Changes
Hereditary Defects		
Hypodontia	Missing teeth, resulting from many possible causes	Spacing of remaining teeth
Amelogenesis imperfecta	Fourteen different subtypes Disturbance of mineralization or matrix of enamel formation	Yellow-brown to dark yellow appearance
Dentinogenesis imperfecta	Type I – disorder of type I collagen	Bluish or brown in appearance, opalescence on transillumination
	Type II – hereditary opalescent dentine	Opalescent primary teeth Enamel chips away to expose EDJ Once dentine exposed, teeth show brown discolouration
	Type III – brandywine isolate hereditary opalescent dentine	Outwardly similar appearance to types I and II Multiple pulpal exposures in primary dentition Dentine production ceases after mantle dentine has formed
Metabolic Disorders		
Alkaptonuria	Incomplete metabolism of tyrosine and phenylalanine Promotes build-up of homogentisic acid	Brown discolouration
Congenital hyperbilirubinaemia	Deposition of bile pigments in the calcifying dental tissues	Purple or brown discolouration
Congenital erythropoietic porphyria	Accumulation of porphyrins in teeth	Red-brown discolouration Red fluorescence under ultraviolet light
Vitamin D dependent rickets	Defects in enamel matrix formation	Pitting and yellow-brown discolouration
Epidermolysis bullosa	Pitting of enamel, possibly caused by vesiculation of the ameloblast layer	Pitting and yellow-brown discolouration
Ehlers-Danlos syndrome	Areas of hypoplastic enamel and irregularities in region of enamel–dentine junction	Pitting and brown or purple-brown discolouration
Pseudo-hypoparathyroidism	Defects in enamel matrix formation	Pitting and yellow-brown discolouration
Molar incisor hypomineralization (MIH)	Unknown aetiology Hypomineralized enamel affecting incisors and permanent first molars	Asymmetrical appearance in arch Enamel defects vary from white to yellow to brown areas

To the Best of Her Knowledge, Has She Received Fluoride Supplements or Lived in an Area with a High Natural Level of Fluoride in the Water Supply? Excessive fluoride ion administration and intake will affect ameloblast function during enamel formation and maturation. The effects are related to age and dose, and both the primary and secondary dentition may be affected by the resulting fluorosis. This may manifest as small areas of flecking to opaque mottling of enamel. Increased porosity of enamel may result in extrinsic staining materials producing an internal effect.

To What Degree is She Concerned About the Appearance of Her Teeth, and Why Has She Sought Advice for Possible Treatment At This Time? Any proposed care plan needs to be patient centred to ensure that fully informed consent is obtained and that the necessary lifelong care of any treatment is appreciated. It is, therefore, important to determine the patient's precise perception of her dental appearance and the outcome that she is seeking to achieve at this time and for the future. Management of patient expectations is critical in such cases.

In response to these questions, the patient commented that her only concern was to improve the appearance of the two upper central incisor teeth. She also did not wish for perfect appearance of these two teeth because she was aware that this would not match with her remaining teeth. She was also aware of the importance of a minimum-intervention approach because a friend of hers had received treatment with

TABLE 27.2 Causes of Intrinsic Dental Discolouration

Cause of Discolouration		Visual Changes
Acquired Defects		
Trauma	Pulpal haemorrhage may lead to accumulation of haemoglobin or other iron-containing haematin molecules within the dentine tubules	Grey-brown to black
Internal resorption	Increased volume of pulpal space and pulpal tissue	Pink
Systemic infectious disease (e.g. rubella)	Generalized hypoplasia due to disturbance of the developing tooth germ	Pitting or grooving leading to yellow-brown discolouration
Localized infection	Localized hypoplasia caused by disturbance of the developing tooth germ	Pitting or grooving leading to yellow-brown discolouration
Excessive fluoride intake	Enamel most often affected Change in mineral matrix from hydroxyapatite to fluorapatite	Flecking to diffuse mottling Colour changes range from chalky white to dark brown appearance
Administration of tetracycline	Chelation to form complexes with calcium ions on the surface of hydroxyapatite crystals, mainly in dentine but also in enamel	Depends on type of tetracycline used, dosage and duration of administration Yellow or brown-grey discolouration.
Amalgam	Migration of tin ions into the dentine tubules	Grey-black discolouration to dentine
Eugenol and phenol containing endodontic materials	Staining of the dentine	Orange-yellow discolouration

TABLE 27.3 Causes of Extrinsic Dental Discolouration

Cause of Discolouration			Visual Changes
Direct stains	Food and drink (e.g. tea, coffee, red wine) Smoking	Usually multifactorial Chromogens incorporated into the plaque or acquired pellicle	Varies from mild yellow to more severe brown – black discolouration
	Chromogenic bacteria.	Incorporated into plaque	Varies from yellow to green – black discolouration
Indirect stains	Chlorhexidine and other metal salts in mouthwashes.	Precipitation of chromogenic polyphenols onto tooth surface	Brown to black discolouration

TABLE 27.4 The Effect of Caries on Dental Discolouration

Cause of Discoloration			Visual Changes
Caries	Cariogenic bacteria, fermentable carbohydrate, susceptible tooth surface, time	Demineralization and eventual proteolytic destruction of organic matrix	White spot lesion to black arrested decay

porcelain laminate veneers and had experienced problems with sensitivity and the veneers debonding on repeated occasions. The patient had chosen to attend at this time because she was planning to leave home to commence university studies shortly.

The patient had not been brought up in an area with a high level of fluoride in the water supply and had not received, to her knowledge, fluoride supplements during her growing years. Her siblings did not have the same characterization to their teeth.

Investigations

◆ What Further Investigations Would You Carry Out?

The teeth should be examined, preferably with magnification, in a dry state and also in a wet state. By examining the teeth when dry, this allows observation of the surface texture and any porous defects. In addition, it becomes easier to observe banding or chronological defects.

Photography is a valuable aid to record the appearance of these teeth to allow discussion with the patient and to record, in much greater detail, the appearance than with text alone. This is an important aspect of dental record keeping, and digital imaging is readily available. It is important to remember, however, that photographs constitute patient personal data and, therefore, must be considered in the same manner as written records as mandated by General Data Protection Regulation. In addition, examining the teeth in fluorescent or polarizing lighting conditions or obtaining fluorescent or polarized images may enhance your ability to observe changes within the tooth structure. This can be achieved by using filters on cameras or commercial devices such as DIAGNOCam (KaVo) (https://www.kavo.com/dental-instruments/diagnocam-small-devices-0#patient-cases) or D-Light Pro (GC) (Fig. 27.2).

When taking intraoral images, it is advisable to use a standard colour scale to act as a visual reference to account for lighting/ambient conditions.

It would be prudent to determine the pulp sensibility of any discoloured teeth.

Radiography is not indicated unless there are concerns regarding the apical status of the teeth, the levels of bone support or to assist in cases of trauma where fracture is suspected. The current history does not indicate the need for radiography.

Your investigations reveal that the incisor teeth give a normal response to both cold and electrical sensibility testing. The levels of fluorescence are even across the teeth. You are able to observe, under magnification, porosity to the surface of the teeth when dry.

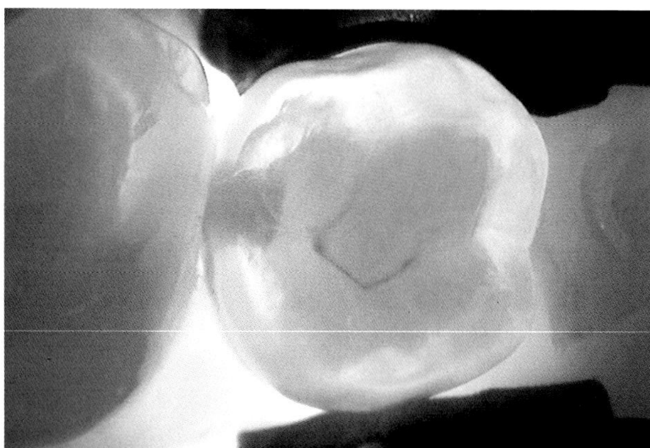

• **Fig. 27.2** DIAGNOCam image that shows a darker shadow on the distal surface of a lower left premolar tooth, indicating the possible presence of a carious lesion.

◆ What is Your Diagnosis?

The diagnosis is enamel hypoplasia of unknown origin. The discolouration is not typical of developmental defects or of metabolic or drug-induced conditions such as tetracycline staining (although this is now so rarely encountered that the use of tetracycline medication during the period of tooth development is discouraged).

Fluorosis would produce a similar appearance, but the lack of history of fluoride supplementation or living in an area with a high natural level of fluoride appears to preclude this.

There is no definitive test for determining the causes of hypoplasia, but with the condition identified, management options can now be considered and discussed with the patient.

◆ What are the Management Options Available? What are Their Advantages and Disadvantages?

See Table 27.5.

◆ How Would You Decide Which Management Approach To Use?

The treatment and overall management of the case should involve the patient at every stage. This is the concept of shared decision making. The Montgomery ruling (Montgomery v Lanarkshire Health Board, 2015, UKSC 11) requires that clinicians translate their professional knowledge into something meaningful for the average patient as well as for the particular patient sitting in front of them. The beneficent aspect of care should be balanced against the nonmaleficent desire to avoid harm, where possible. Consent needs to remain valid through all stages of treatment.

To obtain valid consent, the patient needs to be informed of:

- The options for treatment, the risks and the potential benefits
- Why you think a particular treatment is necessary and appropriate for them
- The consequences, risks and benefits of the treatment you propose
- The likely prognosis
- Your recommended option
- The cost of the proposed treatment
- What might happen if the proposed treatment is not carried out
- Whether the treatment is guaranteed, how long it is guaranteed for and any exclusions that apply.

Leaflets, online material, discussion using visual aids such as photographs of the patients' teeth and other resources may assist in obtaining informed consent. The discussions need to be documented, and it is good practice to allow a period of reflection so that the patient can consider the options before committing to treatment.

(See D'Cruz, L. (2017). Dento-legal considerations about an MI approach. *British Dental Journal, 223*(3), 199–201.)

TABLE 27.5 Management Options

Option	Advantages	Disadvantages
Bleaching, using hydrogen or carbamide peroxide	Works best with extrinsic stains and quite well for many intrinsic stains Easily applied using customized trays Noninvasive treatment. Can be repeated if required Endpoint determined by patient May be used in combination with other treatment options	Limited effect on tooth translucency Unpredictable outcome, length of treatment and durability (rebound effect) Does not affect the appearance of existing restorations Possible sensitivity experienced during treatment Varying licensing regulations for supply between countries May encourage further treatment with products not suitable for dental use
Resin infiltration	No tooth preparation required Good aesthetics possible	Unpredictable outcome Only effective for small areas of mild discolouration/hypoplasia Surface repolishing will be required over time
Direct resin composite application	Good appearance possible No tooth preparation required Predictable outcome Can be used in combination with techniques such as microabrasion	Some tooth preparation is required unless a greater thickness of the labial surface is acceptable The emergence profile must be maintained to allow effective cleaning Repolishing and/or repair of the material will be required over time
Indirect restorations – ceramic veneers or crowns	Good aesthetics possible Durable surface finish reducing need for re-polishing or repair Can be effective for masking dark and extensive areas of discolouration	Preparation of tooth structure required – high biological cost in weakening tooth Possible indirect pulp damage resulting from preparation Outcome for veneer restorations relies on successful cementation procedure Margins may compromise gingival and/or periodontal health Not readily amenable to repair if chipping or fracture occurs

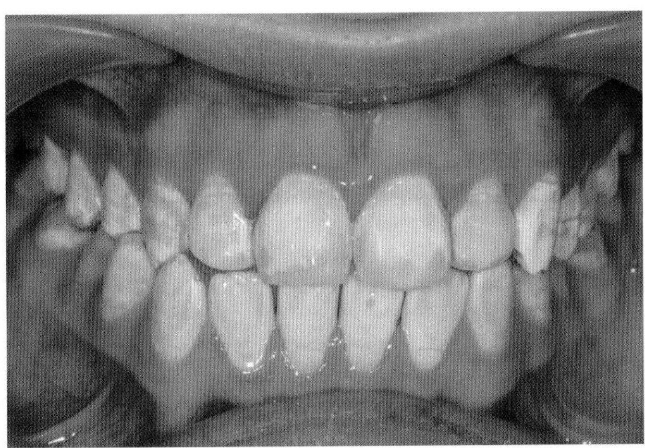

• **Fig. 27.3** Anterior view showing the appearance following a course of vital bleaching and microabrasion of the areas of greatest discolouration and application of resin composite.

◆ What Would Be the Most Appropriate Treatment in This Case?

The patient has advised that she is only concerned with the appearance of the two upper central incisor teeth and was not seeking a 'perfect' appearance because she was aware that this would make these teeth look different compared with her remaining dentition. On the basis of her friend's experience, she was also aware of the effects of tooth preparation and the unpredictable results of using porcelain veneers.

A minimally invasive conservative approach such as using a hydrogen or carbamide peroxide bleaching agent may result in an appearance that is satisfactory to the patient. This technique has the advantage that no tooth structure removal is required and the treatment may be repeated again in the future, if required. However, if this technique does not produce an outcome that is satisfactory for the patient, alternative techniques such as microabrasion to remove the areas of greatest discolouration, followed by surface application of flowable resin composite material, may be used. *This was the completed treatment for the patient* (*Fig. 27.3*).

Prognosis

The appearance of the teeth after this treatment was not perfect, but there was a marked improvement from that at presentation, which allowed the patient to move to her new academic environment with increased confidence in her dental appearance. Importantly, the patient was satisfied with the outcome, and this was documented, along with the whole management process, contemporaneously in the dental notes.

The prognosis for the teeth remains good. The resin composite will require repolishing to maintain the surface lustre and, in due course, will require repair and possible replacement. However, this can be carried out with a careful technique, preferably with magnification, to minimize the risk of tooth structure damage or removal of teeth. *The patient has been informed of this.*

Case 28
A Very Painful Mouth

PEPE SHIRLAW AND SANDEEP JOSHI

Summary

A 20-year-old man presents at your general dental practice, feeling ill and with a very sore mouth.

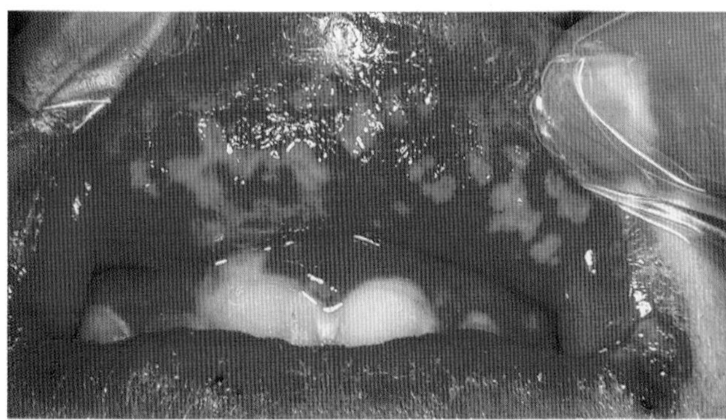

• **Fig. 28.1** Appearance of the patient's mouth.

History

Complaint

The patient complains of pain which is preventing eating and hampering drinking. He also feels unwell.

History of Complaint

He first noticed feeling unwell 4 days ago and thought he had the flu. He was slightly feverish and had a headache. His mouth was sore, but it was not until about 1 day later that it became very painful. Because he felt unable to take time off work, he took the remains of a course of an unknown oral antibiotic that had been prescribed for his brother who had an infected cut on his arm. This did not appear to have led to any improvement. He has had no similar attacks before.

Medical History

The patient is otherwise fit and well.

Examination

Extraoral Examination

The patient has enlarged cervical lymph nodes that are slightly tender, mobile, soft and firm rather than hard. Apart from this finding, no abnormalities are found in a routine examination of the head, neck and hands.

Intraoral Examination

◆ What Do You See in Fig. 28.1?

On the labial mucosa, there are numerous ulcers with the following characteristics:

Site	Labial mucosa and attached gingiva
Size	A few millimetres in diameter
Shape	Well defined, rounded, sometimes coalescing to form larger irregular ulcers
Colour	Covered by a yellow-grey fibrin ulcer slough, no well-defined rim of periulcer erythema
Background	The surrounding mucosa appears uniformly inflamed

In addition, one large ulcer lies at the commissure, and there are small bloodstained crusts around the lips.

If you were able to examine the patient, you would discover that more ulcers affect much of the oral mucosa, including the gingivae, palate and tongue, and that they extend back into the oropharynx.

◆ Give a Differential Diagnosis On the Basis of the Information You Have So Far.

- Primary herpetic gingivostomatitis
- Erythema multiforme.

◆ Justify This Differential Diagnosis.

Primary herpetic gingivostomatitis and other oral viral infections typically cause multiple round, small ulcers of acute onset, sometimes coalescing, on a background of inflamed mucosa. The patient feels unwell and has enlarged tender lymph nodes, suggesting infection. Primary herpes simplex virus (HSV) infection usually affects much of the mucosa and has a predilection for the keratinized masticatory mucosa of the gingiva. The patient is older than is normally expected for a primary infection. However, the average age of patients with this infection has increased over the last few decades because improved living conditions have resulted in fewer individuals coming into contact with the virus during their childhood.

Erythema multiforme (Stevens-Johnson syndrome) is possible. The acute onset and bloody crusts on the lips suggest this diagnosis, and the age of the patient is compatible. However, the distribution of ulcers is not particularly suggestive of this condition. Erythema multiforme affects primarily the lips and nonkeratinized lining mucosa of the anterior mouth, and the ulcers have ragged margins, whereas the irregular ulcers in the picture seem to be formed by coalescence of small, round ulcers. A trigger for erythema multiforme is sometimes identified, and antibiotics, particularly sulphonamides, are sometimes the cause. This patient has recently taken antibiotics, but only after the symptoms appeared. Erythema multiforme is typically recurrent, and a history of previous attacks and their periodicity is important in making the diagnosis. However, in a first attack, the features may be milder, and, as in this case, there is no history of similar attacks.

◆ What Diagnoses Have You Discounted, and Why?

Other oral viral infections do not produce a clinical picture of this severity. Herpangina and hand, foot and mouth disease are milder and usually affect the soft palate of children. Varicella zoster would be expected to cause chicken pox in this age group, although children are more typically affected; oral zoster usually affects older patients and is unilateral.

Herpetiform aphthous stomatitis should be considered but is readily excluded. The ulcers may be numerous, small and coalescing and may have an erythematous background. However, they are usually limited to the anterior or posterior area of the mouth, do not affect keratinized mucosa and are not accompanied by systemic illness. Attacks are recurrent.

In a mild primary attack of HSV infection in an adult, the ulcers may be limited to the gingiva, raising the possibility of acute necrotizing ulcerative gingivitis. However, in this case, the ulceration is too extensive for necrotizing gingivitis to be considered, and in any case, it is usually clinically characteristic.

◆ What Further Questions Would You Ask, and What Further Examinations Would You Perform, and Why?

Do You Suffer From 'Cold Sores'? If the patient has had recurrent HSV infection, usually in the form of herpes labialis, then the present ulcers could not have been caused by a primary herpetic infection. Recurrent herpetic infection is sometimes a trigger for attacks of erythema multiforme and a cold sore 1–2 weeks before onset would raise this possibility. *In answer to this question, the patient indicates that he does not suffer from cold sores.*

Have You Been in Contact with Anyone with Cold Sores? Identification of a possible source of HSV infection 1–2 weeks before the ulcers would give further credibility to this diagnosis. Contact with *Herpes zoster* is not significant in this case, but in less clear-cut cases, it would be prudent to ask about any exposure to chicken pox and shingles. The patient has no known exposure to any viral disease.

Did You Notice Small Blisters in Your Mouth Before the Ulcers Appeared? This would suggest herpes virus infection, each ulcer being preceded by a small, round vesicle. Larger vesicles and blisters are also found in erythema multiforme, but these are irregular and usually limited to the vermilion border of the lips and the floor of mouth.

Have You Taken Any Drugs or Medicines in the Last 3 Weeks? This will clarify the possibility that medication has triggered an attack of erythema multiforme. *The patient has taken no medication apart from the antibiotic noted in the history.*

Have You Any Rash Anywhere On Your Body? Erythema multiforme is associated with a variety of rashes (hence its name), and the patient should have a skin examination. The presence of typical target lesions indicates erythema multiforme but other less characteristic rashes should also be noted, along with their time of onset. *No rash is present.*

Take the Patient's Temperature. This simple investigation is easily forgotten, but often valuable. A raised temperature in the early stages indicates infection. The temperature is not raised in erythema multiforme even when severe (unless there is infection of skin lesions). *The patient's temperature is 38°C.*

Diagnosis

Differential diagnosis in such cases sometimes poses problems. If the patient has erythema multiforme, he should be treated with a moderately high dose of systemic steroids, but this should be avoided if he has a viral infection. A certain amount of time must elapse before the results of investigations will be available.

◆ Can You Make a Diagnosis and Commence Treatment?

Yes. In this case, there is sufficient evidence to make a working diagnosis of primary HSV infection. Investigations should be performed to confirm the diagnosis but need not delay treatment. Investigations are probably only available to those in hospital practice. Practitioners confident in their diagnosis may well initiate treatment without confirmatory results from laboratory tests.

Investigations

◆ What Investigations Might You Consider, and What are Their Advantages and Disadvantages?

See Table 28.1.

In the current case, a viral swab was taken for PCR confirmation of HSV infection.

Treatment

◆ What Treatment Would You Provide?

The patient should be reassured that he has a common viral infection, which, although unpleasant, has no significant

TABLE 28.1 Investigations To Be Considered

Test	Advantages and Disadvantages
Smear for light microscopy	Simple and rapid. Characteristic viral changes may indicate herpes virus infection, provided the epithelial cells from the ulcer margin are present in the smear. Most hospitals should be able to give the result the same day. However, a smear will only be positive for the first few days of ulceration. As a result, a positive result on smear analysis indicates infection but a negative result cannot exclude it in all cases.
Viral culture	Simple but takes several days. In general terms, this test has the advantage of being able to detect a wide range of viruses, but in this differential diagnosis, the broad specificity is not particularly helpful.
Viral antigen screen	Simple and moderately fast. A small number of viruses may be identified from their antigens in a swab with ELISA (enzyme-linked immunosorbent assay). Results may be available in 24 hours, but this test is only available in some centres.
Polymerase chain reaction (PCR)–based viral detection	Obtaining the smear is simple, but the laboratory procedure is complex. Highly specific and moderately fast. Results should be available in 24–48 hours. The test is only available via a virology lab. The swab is taken and placed in a culture medium. The PCR test is now the 'norm' for for identifying HSV infected ulcers.
Electron microscopy	Very specific and relatively simple, but, again, only available in specialized centres. The result is usually available the same day.
Viral antibody level	Serum for antibody to herpes and other viruses is simple to obtain and provides the result in about 48 hours. A high titre of antiviral immunoglobulin M (IgM) indicates acute infection (though it may take a day or two to rise to a detectable level), and a low stable titre of IgG denotes a previous infection. In the absence of raised IgM, taking two samples several days apart to demonstrate an increasing IgG level is required for a confident diagnosis of primary infection. This test is widely available and frequently used.
Biopsy of ulcer	Relatively readily performed but almost never necessary in herpes simplex virus (HSV) infection (except for the unusual chronic infections found in the immunosuppressed). Will give the diagnosis of herpetic infection in almost all cases. Also diagnostic in most cases of erythema multiforme.

implications. It will run its course for up to the next 10 days or so, but it is unlikely to worsen significantly now that it is in its fifth day. Some adult patients may confuse this condition with genital herpes and require some additional explanation.

While he feels unwell, the patient should rest and maintain a good fluid intake. This is especially important in children who refuse fluids and become dehydrated rapidly. A sedative antihistamine such as promethazine is sometimes suggested for very small and fractious children who have difficulty sleeping during the acute phase. It also has the advantage of drying the reflex salivation.

The patient should be warned about infectivity. The virus is transmitted only through close contact, but while there are vesicles or ulcers in the mouth, the saliva is infectious. Care should be taken to avoid close contact with other individuals, especially children. In the nonimmune patient (by definition, anyone with a primary infection), other sites may also become infected, and particular care should be taken to avoid saliva coming in contact with the eyes.

Antiviral treatment with aciclovir should be considered. Aciclovir is only effective in the earliest stage of the infection when the virus is replicating. It must be taken in the first 48 hours for best effect while vesicles, rather than ulcers, are present. Aciclovir is not indicated in this case because of the delay in presentation (although it might be considered in an immunosuppressed patient). A dose of 200 mg five times daily is recommended for immunocompetent patients. Related drugs giving higher levels in blood such as valaciclovir, are usually reserved for varicella-zoster virus (VSV) infection.

Preparations for symptomatic relief of the oral ulceration are indicated. Tetracycline mouthwash (250 mg capsule of a soluble preparation dissolved in water, used four times daily) or 100 mg doxycycline, also used topically, is very useful in reducing discomfort and would be an appropriate choice in this patient, who has presented too late to benefit from aciclovir. Antiseptic mouthwashes such as chlorhexidine are also effective. These presumably reduce oral discomfort by preventing bacterial infection of the ulcers. Chlorhexidine would also compensate for inability to carry out oral hygiene procedures. Analgesic mouthwashes such as benzydamine are an alternative.

Prognosis

◆ What is the Risk That This Patient Will Suffer From Cold Sores in the Future?

Between 15 and 30% of individuals who come into contact with the virus develop recurrent infection. It is not clear whether those who suffer a symptomatic primary infection such as gingivostomatitis have an increased risk. Although this percentage seems high, many patients with recurrent herpes infection suffer only very occasional lesions.

What are the Mechanisms and Significance of Recurrent Infection?

During infection, HSV is transported back along axons of sensory nerves to their nuclei. There, the neurones are infected but do not die, and the virus becomes latent – that is, virus persists but no infectious virions are produced.

A viral latency gene and the cell-mediated immune response contribute to the balance between latency and reactivation. If infection is reactivated, the virus travels down the nerve to cause a localized recurrent infection of the mucosa or skin – a cold sore. Because the virus is intracellular for most of this life cycle, antibodies of the humoral immune response are not effective in preventing recurrences. Environmental triggers for cold sores include ultraviolet light, illness and stress.

Latent infection has important consequences. Subclinical reactivation may result in the virus being shed from the mucosa without the individual realizing that he or she has an active infection. This may be one of the mechanisms of spread in the population. Latent infection in the geniculate ganglion is one cause of Bell's palsy, and very occasionally, the virus may spread along the nerves to the brain, causing herpetic encephalitis.

Labial recurrences are painful and unpleasant but relatively readily treated because there is often a characteristic prodromal sensation of burning or itching and the vesicles are easily seen. Early treatment is, therefore, possible, and antiviral drugs can be very effective. Topical preparations of 5% aciclovir are available without prescription.

When Would You Ask the Patient To Return?

The patient should return in about 1 week to check that healing is progressing, but earlier if symptoms worsen or new signs develop.

At some stage during treatment or follow-up, the patient should be warned about not taking medications that are prescribed for others. The antibiotic prescribed for the patient's brother was apparently a harmless drug, but inappropriate for this patient. Those who take drugs prescribed for others run the risk of hypersensitivity, drug interaction or other unwanted reaction. The importance of completing the prescribed dose should be emphasized to all patients receiving antibiotics, to ensure effective treatment and because this is critically important in preventing the emergence of resistant strains in the community.

Final Outcome

The next day, the polymerase chain reaction report shows positivity for HSV type 1 DNA. The diagnosis of herpetic gingivostomatitis is confirmed.

Case 29

Caution! – X-Rays

NICHOLAS DRAGE AND ERIC WHAITES

Summary

A 25-year-old female patient attending your practice for the first time is worried about having radiographs taken. How should her concerns be addressed?

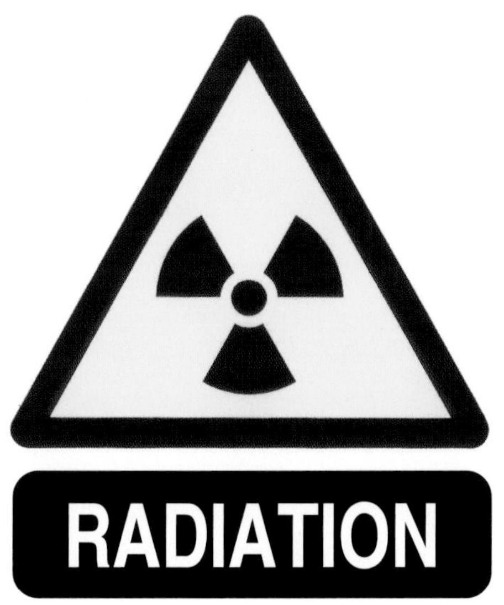

• **Fig. 29.1** The international warning sign for radiation, known as the trefoil.

History

Complaint

After a full clinical oral examination, you decide that taking radiographs is justified. The radiographs you decide to take and the reason for each are shown in Table 29.1.

TABLE 29.1 Radiographic Views Required for the Patient and the Clinical Justification

View	Reason
Right and left bitewings	*To assess existing restorations and periodontal status.*
Periapical radiograph of the lower left first molar	*This tooth is tender to percussion and may need extraction or root canal treatment.*
Panoramic radiograph	*To assess partially erupted lower third molars as there is a history of recurrent pericoronitis.*

The patient is concerned about radiation. Current regulations require you to have a meaningful discussion with the patient regarding the risks and benefits of the radiographic investigation, so you start to provide dose and risk information.

◆ What Three General Guiding Principles Must You Follow in Deciding Whether or Not To Undertake Any Radiographic Examination?

Justification. Each radiation exposure must have a net positive benefit.

Optimization. The exposures must be at a dose that is As Low As Reasonably Practicable (ALARP), taking social and economic factors into account.

Limitation. The dose to individuals must not exceed the recommended limits.

The principles are set out by the International Commission on Radiological Protection (ICRP), which also sets the recommended dose limits for staff.

◆ What is the Patient Dose Associated with Exposure of These Radiographs?

Radiation dose measuring is complex. The effective dose (absorbed dose corrected to compensate for the type of radiation and susceptibility of different tissues) is usually quoted. The effective dose for an intraoral radiograph (periapical or bitewing) is in the range of 0.0003–0.022 millisieverts (mSv) and for a panoramic radiograph 0.0027–0.075 mSv, depending on the equipment used.

◆ Because These Technical Terms Do Not Mean Much To Most People, How Can You Reassure the Patient?

The patient can be reassured that the doses are very small and equivalent to a tiny fraction of the natural background radiation (ubiquitous radiation) to which we are all exposed every day. If the patient wants to know actual figures, then she should be told that the annual dose from background radiation varies around the world, but, for example, the average is 2.3 mSv in the UK and is 3.1 mSv in the US. The dose for the radiographs required equates to approximately 8 hours of additional background radiation for an intraoral radiograph and 3 days for a panoramic radiograph.

◆ The Patient Accepts This But Points At the Hazard Warning Sticker On Your X-Ray Cubicle. What Exactly are the Risks?

At these low absorbed doses, there is only one significant risk, that of cancer induction. This is a very low frequency and completely random (stochastic) effect induced by damage to DNA either directly or indirectly.

The risk of developing a fatal malignancy as a result of taking a periapical radiograph varies, depending on the equipment used and dose delivered, but in 'best practice' radiography using modern equipment and techniques, it is estimated to be about 1 in 10 000 000.

In panoramic radiography, the risk, again, varies, depending on the equipment used and the type and speed of the image receptor (film/screen combination or digital) but is estimated to be around 1 in 1 000 000.

◆ The Patient Wants To Know How You Ensure That She Will Receive the Minimum Dose of Radiation Necessary. What Methods are Used To Optimize Dose To Patients, and How Do They Work?

After the radiographic image has been justified, the radiation doses can be optimised by using modern x-ray equipment and techniques, as shown in Table 29.2.

◆ The Patient Has Decided To Go Ahead with the Radiographic Examination and Asks Whether She Should Wear a Lead Apron During the Procedure. Is a Lead Apron Advised for Dental Radiography?

Lead aprons are no longer considered necessary for intraoral radiography in some countries, including the UK. Instead, emphasis is now placed on reducing the dose from the main beam by the factors outlined below in Table 29.2.

TABLE 29.2 Methods of Dose Optimization

	Precaution	Reason
Clinical judgement (justification)	Patients should only be x-rayed if the investigations are clinically necessary (i.e. they can be justified after a thorough clinical examination).	Unnecessary radiographs give an unnecessary x-ray dose.
	Published evidence-based 'selection criteria' should be used during the justification process.	Weighing the benefits of radiography with the potential adverse effects is complex and best performed by experts. Follow their guidance.
Equipment	The x-ray sets for intraoral radiography should operate at 60–70 kV and ideally should be constant potential units.	This produces the optimal-energy x-rays for dental radiography, the best balance between tissue penetration and image contrast.
	The x-ray set should contain aluminium filtration in the beam path.	To absorb most of the low energy x-rays that would otherwise be absorbed by the skin. These would increase patient dose and would not contribute to the radiographic image.
	X-ray sets for intraoral radiography should have a rectangular collimated beam.	To reduce the width of the beam to the minimum required to cover the image receptor. This makes it more difficult to aim the beam accurately, and so an image receptor holder and a beam aligning device will be required.
	The x-ray set should be checked for safety on installation and regularly thereafter.	This must include, in particular, checks on the tube kilovoltage, as this determines dose, and to ensure no x-rays leak from the back and sides of the unit.
	Image receptors should be as sensitive as possible (i.e. digital receptors or F-speed film) to ensure the shortest exposure times.	Faster detectors reduce the dose required. Digital receptors are the most sensitive.
	Extraoral radiographs should be taken by using digital receptors or cassettes containing rare earth intensifying screens.	Intensifying screens amplify the x-ray signal within the cassette and thus reduce the dose required.
Radiographic technique	Radiographs should be taken as geometrically accurately as possible by using image receptor holders and beam-aiming devices for intraoral radiography. The minimum number of images should be taken. Retakes should be avoided. Processing (conventional or digital) should be carried out correctly by following manufacturers' instructions	This will reduce the number of inadequate images caused by malpositioning of the beam or image receptor.

You are planning to take the radiographs by using a photostimulable phosphor plate digital imaging system (PSP system). The benefit to the patient depends on the diagnostic information, or yield, provided, and this, in turn, is dependent on the quality of the radiographic images produced. To achieve this, a quality assurance (QA) programme in dental radiography is highly desirable and in some countries, including the UK, is a mandatory legal requirement. The World Health Organization (WHO) has defined QA in radiography as 'an organized effort by the staff operating a facility to ensure that the diagnostic images produced by the facility are of sufficiently high quality so that they consistently provide adequate diagnostic information'.

◆ What are the Aims of a Quality Assurance Programme?

The aims should include the following:

- To produce diagnostic radiographs of a consistently high standard
- To reduce the number of repeat radiographs
- To determine all sources of error and allow for their correction
- To increase efficiency
- To reduce costs
- To reduce the radiation dose to patients and staff.

◆ What Areas or Topics Should a Digitally Based Quality Assurance Programme Address?

There are five main areas or topics of concern that should form the basis of the QA programme. These include:

- Personnel and training
- Image quality
- Working procedures
- Patient dose and equipment, including the
    - X-ray set
    - Digital imaging receptor type (solid state detector/PSP) and digital processing
    - Viewing screen (monitor)
- Clinical audit.

The essential procedures for each should be laid down in writing and should be the responsibility of a named person.

◆ How Can the Quality of Digitally Captured Images Be Assessed in General Dental Practice?

One way to assess image quality is to visually compare every radiograph with a good quality standard reference image and to subjectively rate the quality using the 2-point scale as recommended by Public Health England/Faculty of General Dental Practitioners, shown in Table 29.3.

TABLE 29.3 Quality Ratings for Radiographs

	Quality	Basis
A	Diagnostically acceptable	No errors or minimal errors in either patient preparation, exposure, positioning, image (receptor) processing or image reconstruction and of sufficient image quality to answer the clinical question
N	Diagnostically not acceptable	Errors in either patient preparation, exposure, positioning, image (receptor) processing or image reconstruction which render the image diagnostically unacceptable

◆ What Should Be Done with the 'Not Diagnostically Acceptable' Category 'N' Images?

They should be analyzed over a suitable period (e.g. a week or a month). This analysis is often referred to as *image reject analysis*. The category 'N' images are assessed as to why they have been rejected and to identify the causative error. Changes to practice can then be instituted to avoid the error being repeated. This process should be documented for best practice and for future reference.

◆ The Following Five Intraoral Digitally Captured Radiographs All Have Errors. What is Wrong with Each, and What are the Possible Explanations?

◆ What is Wrong with the Image in Fig. 29.2?

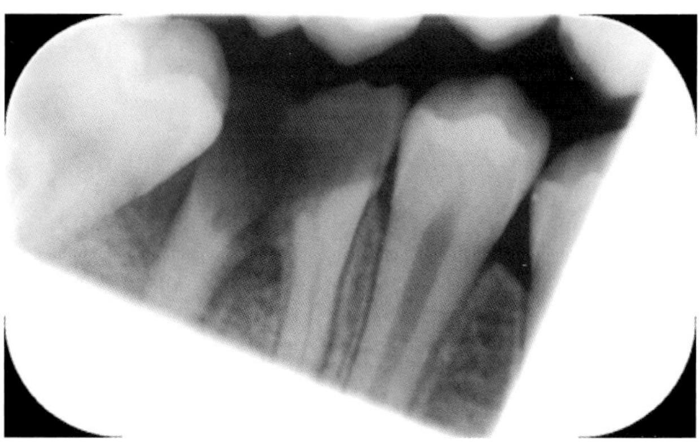

• **Fig. 29.2** Periapical radiograph of the lower right first molar.

This is a periapical radiograph of the lower right first molar (grade 'N' quality rating). The image is 'coned off' – part of the image receptor has not been exposed. Typically, this happens when the spacer cone is not aligned correctly to the image receptor. In this case, the main reason for the 'coning off' is incorrect orientation of the rectangular collimator within the open-ended spacer cone. Note also that even if the rectangular collimator had been aligned properly, it is unlikely the apices of the teeth would be fully visualized because the incorrect photostimulable phosphor plate (PSP) size has also been selected.

What is Wrong with the Image in Fig. 29.3a?

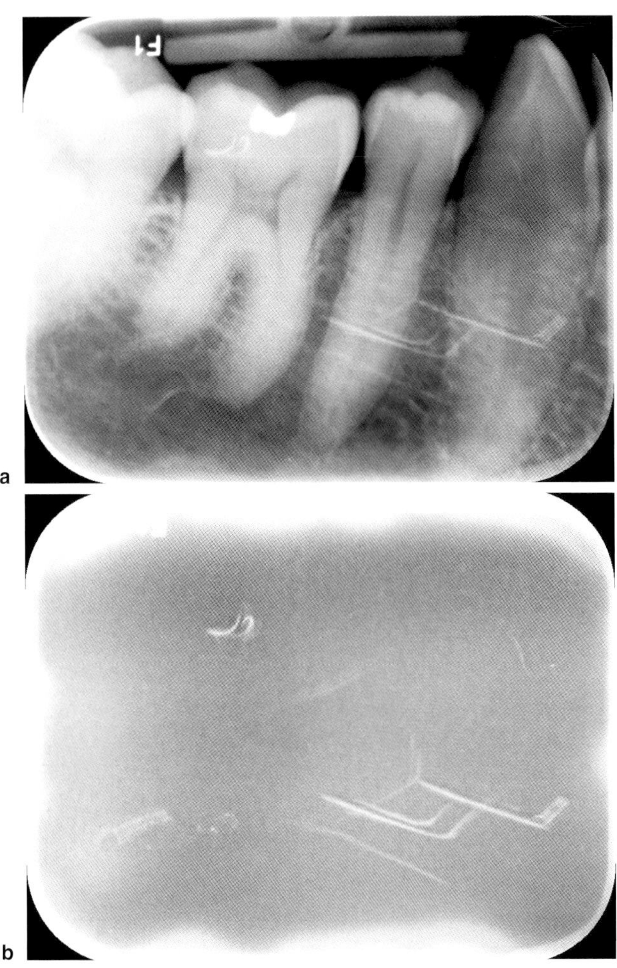

• **Fig. 29.3 a,** Periapical radiograph of the lower right first molar. **b,** radiograph of the same PSP.

This is a periapical radiograph of the lower right first molar (grade 'A' quality rating). The image shows several white lines/marks on the image. These are artefactual due to scratching of the phosphor layer. A well-organized quality assurance (QA) programme should include visually inspecting the photostimulable phosphor plate (PSP) for scratches and checking for image uniformity by exposing the image receptor to radiation. Fig. 29.3b is a radiograph of the same PSP, which has been exposed to radiation as part of QA testing. This demonstrates the scratches and also shows areas of image nonuniformity along the long edges of the image receptor. Although in this case the radiographic image of the lower teeth is diagnostically acceptable, this PSP needs to be removed from clinical use.

What is Wrong with the Image in Fig. 29.4?

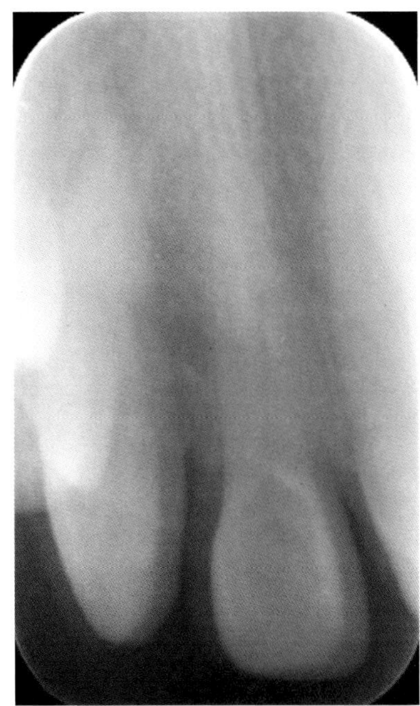

• **Fig. 29.4** Periapical radiograph of the upper right lateral incisor.

This is a periapical radiograph of the upper right lateral incisor (grade 'N' quality rating). The image is blurred. This is caused by movement of the patient or of the image receptor during the exposure.

What is Wrong with the Image in Fig. 29.5?

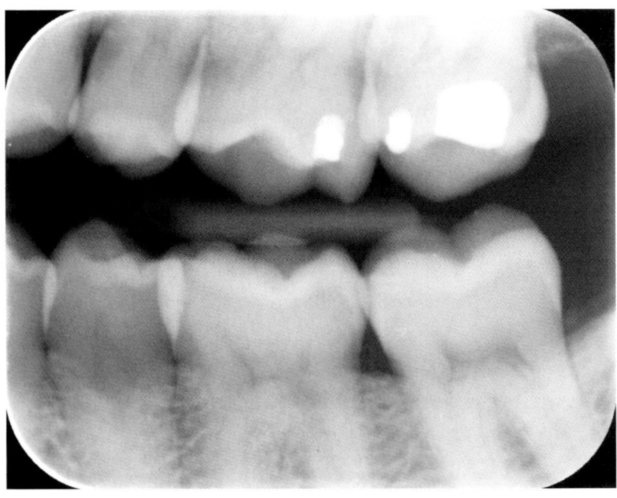

• **Fig. 29.5** Left bitewing radiograph.

This is a left bitewing radiograph (grade 'N' quality rating). The image is distorted, and there is severe overlap of the contact points, making caries assessment impossible. Although an image receptor holder and beam aiming device have been used, the image receptor has not been placed parallel to the dental arch. Consequently, the x-ray beam does not pass through the contact areas leading to overlap.

◆ What is Wrong with the Image in Fig. 29.6?

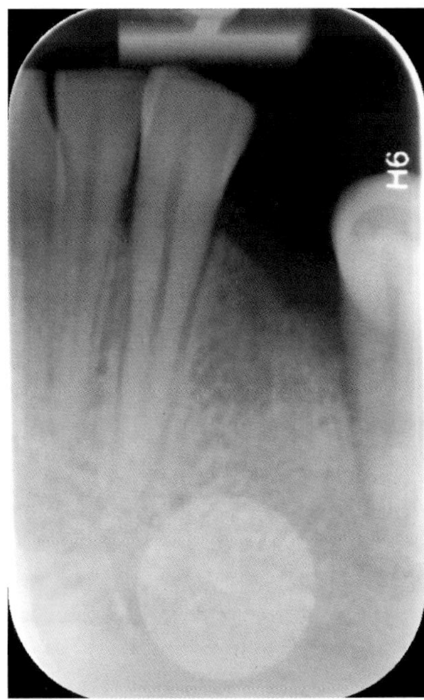

• **Fig. 29.6** Periapical radiograph of the lower right lateral incisor.

This is a periapical radiograph taken to show the lower right lateral incisor (grade 'A' quality rating). There is a round radiopacity on the lower part of the image. This is caused by the image receptor being placed in the mouth back to front. This particular brand of PSP has a round metal magnet on the back to allow introduction of the PSP into the scanner. It is the magnet that has caused the radiopaque shadow. Although this image is still of diagnostic value, it must be flipped in the horizontal plane before the image is saved because it is currently displayed as if the image is of the left side.

◆ What are the Advantages of Digital Radiography Over Film-Based Systems?

The use of digital radiography has a number of advantages. One of the most important is that the image receptors are more sensitive than film, allowing a lower patient dose. In addition, image production is quicker allowing an almost immediate assessment of image quality. The images can be enhanced digitally to extract useful diagnostic information from underexposed or overexposed images and may be optimized to assess specific dental conditions such as dental caries or periodontal bone levels. Finally, electronic storage of data means that images can be accessed quickly. Digital radiography is, therefore, in the patient's interests, with around 75% of dental practices in the UK now using digital systems.

◆ What Regulations Must UK Dentists Comply with in Regard To Ionising Radiation?

The regulations governing the use of ionising radiation in the UK are called the *Ionising Radiations Regulations 2017 (IRR 2017)* and the *Ionising Radiation (Medical Exposure) Regulations 2017 (IRMER 2017)*. Because the European Directive applies to all European Union (EU) countries, the regulations in the EU countries will have similar content to those of the UK. The United States Environmental Protection Agency (EPA), the US Food and Drug Administration (FDA) and the American Dental Association (ADA) provide guidance on dental radiography in the US.

The UK regulations encompass the general principles of the International Commission on Radiological Protection (ICRP) – of **Justification**, **Optimization** and **Limitation**. After the introduction of IRMER 2017, there is now a requirement to provide the patient with risk and benefit information as part of the consent process prior to the radiographic exposure. This information should be provided in a qualitative rather than a quantitative manner.

Both sets of UK legislation are criminal law; therefore, failure to comply with it could result in serious consequences, including, in extreme cases, a possible custodial sentence. As IRMER 2017 is designed to protect patients, failure to comply with it, potentially putting patients at risk, could also result in a practitioner's 'fitness to practise' being investigated by professional regulatory bodies whose primary function is to protect patients.

Further Guidance

For the UK

Ionising Radiation (Medical Exposure) Regulations 2017 (IRMER 2017): http://www.legislation.gov.uk/uksi/2017/1322/pdfs/uksi_20171322_en.pdf

Ionising Radiations Regulations 2017 (IRR 2017): http://www.legislation.gov.uk/uksi/2017/1075/pdfs/uksi_20171075_en.pdf

PHE and FGDP 2020 *Guidance notes for dental practitioners on the safe use of x-ray equipment.* 2nd Edition. Public Health England, London and Faculty of General Dental Practice (UK) of the Royal College of Surgeons of England. Available from: https://www.fgdp.org.uk/

For Europe

European Council Directive: https://eur-lex.europa.eu/legal-content/EN/TXT/?uri=CELEX%3A32013L0059

For the US

American Dental Association recommendations for patient selection and limiting radiation exposure: https://www.ada.org/~/media/ADA/Publications/ADA%20News/Files/Dental_Radiographic_Examinations_2012.pdf?la=en

Case 30

Whose Fault is It This Time?

JONATHAN TURNER AND DAVID R. RADFORD

Summary

You seem to be having trouble communicating with the dental laboratory. How will you tackle the problems that have arisen?

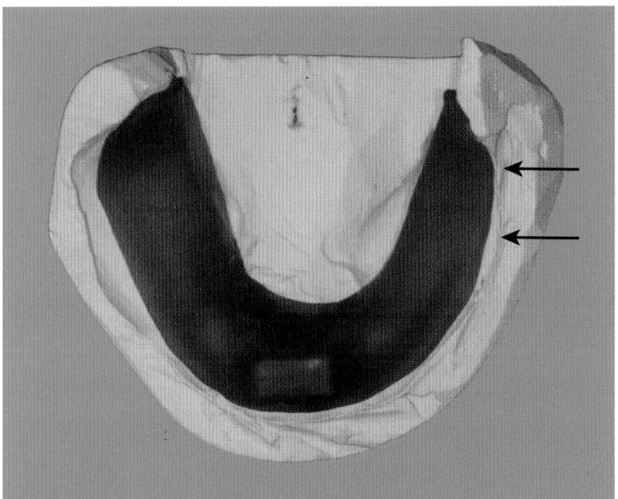

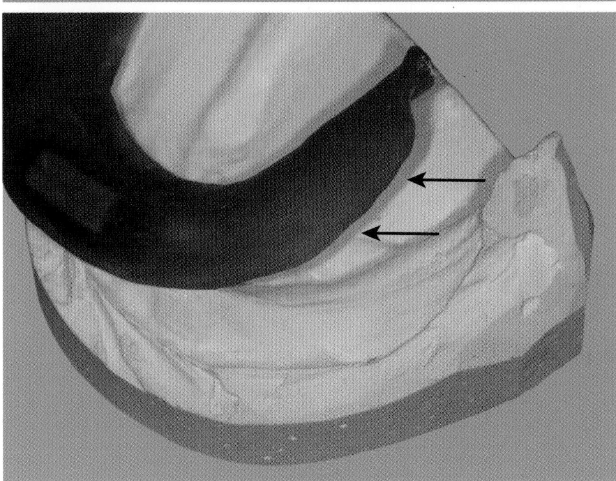

• **Fig. 30.1** The lower tray.

FIRST PATIENT

Complaint

Your nurse takes the special trays out of the laboratory package for you to record secondary impressions of an edentulous patient. They are not as 'special' as you had intended.

History of Complaint

You are constructing new complete dentures for a patient who has been a poor complete denture wearer. She has lost her lower denture and does not like the upper, so you have decided to make a new set from first principles rather than use a copy denture technique.

The upper primary impression was taken in alginate, and the lower was recorded in a stock tray adapted with silicone putty and covered with an alginate wash to record detail. This was because the upper edentulous stock tray conformed well the patient's edentulous anatomy; however, the lower tray did not fit well. You were going to take both upper and lower secondary impressions in close-fitting trays by using a light-bodied silicone elastomeric material. Traditionally, close fitting impressions have been recorded in zinc oxide and eugenol (ZoE); however, although more expensive, elastomeric materials are increasingly being used because they are easier to handle. They have the disadvantage of tending to be hydrophobic, as opposed to ZoE, which is hydrophilic, so good moisture control is important.

Diagnosis

◆ The Lower Special Trays are Shown in Figs 30.1 and 30.2. What is Wrong?

The lower tray is asymmetrical: The extension on the patient's left is considerably shorter than that on the right. However, when you look at the cast, you see that your impression was short in that area and that the laboratory has extended the tray as much as possible. The laboratory was correct not to have extended the tray over the land area on the stone cast (the 'land area' is that peripheral part of the model not recorded in the impression that the technician creates to preserve the rolled borders of an

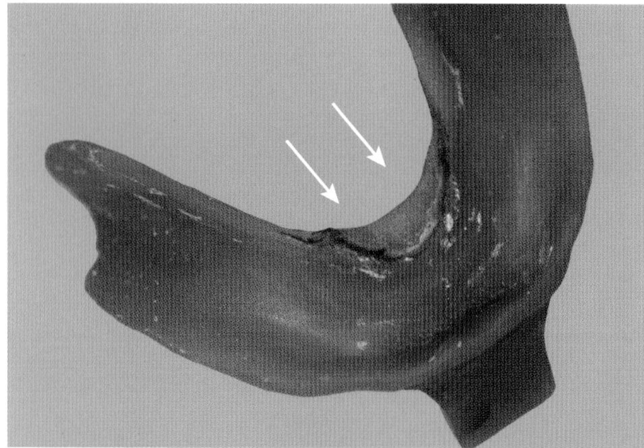

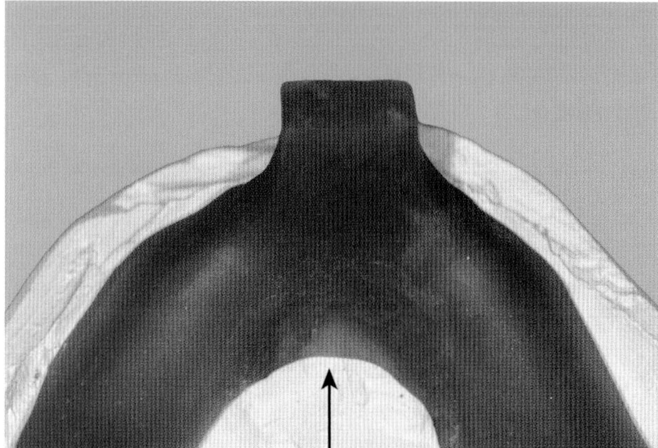

• **Fig. 30.2** The lower tray.

impression). The result is that the tray is underextended on the left buccal shelf. This is important because the lower denture will need to be extended here to gain good support.

Conversely, the tray has been overextended onto the land area in the floor of the mouth, and this will need to be altered prior to recording a secondary impression.

◆ The Upper Special Tray is Shown in Fig. 30.3. What is Wrong?

This shows a well-constructed upper special tray, but it has been perforated and spaced for an alginate secondary impression. The tray is properly extended, but spaced trays always look slightly overextended on a primary model because it sits lower after the spacer has been removed. Your heart sinks.

You look at the laboratory request sheet to see what you prescribed and read: 'Please cast upper and lower primary impressions. Construct upper and lower special trays. N.B.: Lower close fitting for silicone.'

Your error is lack of suitable detail in your communication. Many dentists and clinical dental technicians (CDTs) use alginate in a spaced tray for upper impressions. You had expected that the laboratory would assume that if one tray was close fitting, then the other one would be, too. You make a note to be more careful in the future.

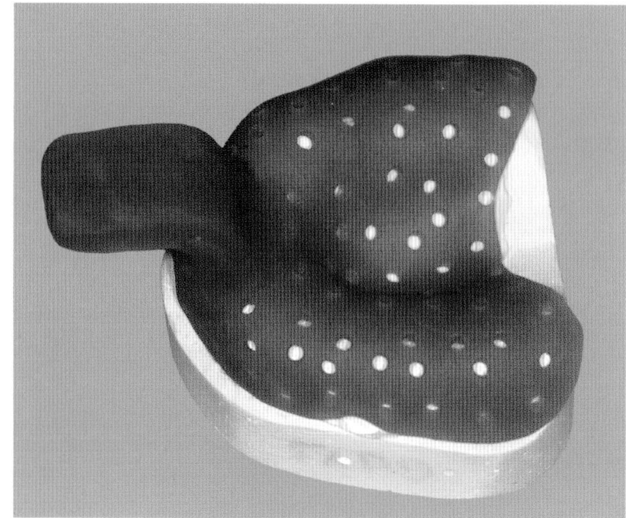

• **Fig. 30.3** The upper tray.

TABLE 30.1 Upper Tray Solutions

Possible Solution	Disadvantages
Record the impression as planned with either a medium-bodied addition-cured silicone, because it will flow less, or, as intended, a light bodied material.	Will certainly be very messy, even with a heavier bodied material.
Record the impression with alginate.	It is difficult to control the thickness of the rolled border with alginate. Unless you are using a modern 5-day-stable alginate, impressions need to be cast as soon as possible. Unless making a new tray, this would be the best solution.
Block the perforations with composition or cold curing acrylic.	Time-consuming, but the tray would still have the wrong spacing for a light-bodied silicone.
Have a new tray made.	Technically the best solution, but there are time and cost implications for the patient and you.

Solutions

There are several things you can do to save the patient a further appointment and yourself the additional cost of extra trays.

◆ What You Can Do About the Upper Tray?

There are a number of options, but all have problems (Table 30.1). The only alternative would be to request a new tray.

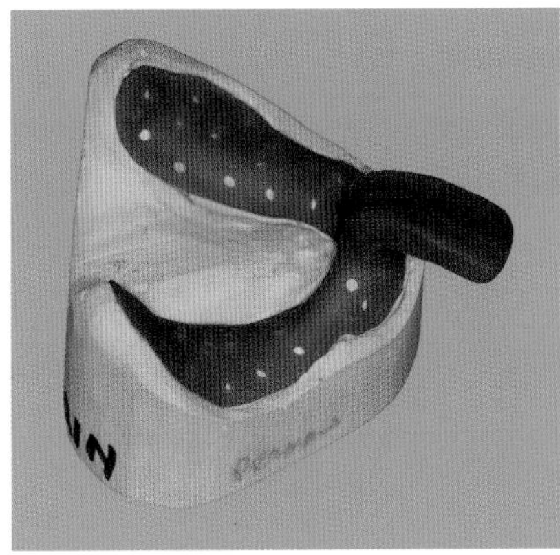
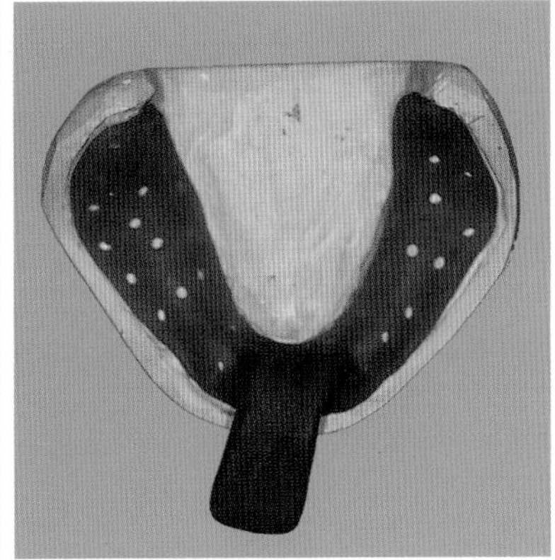
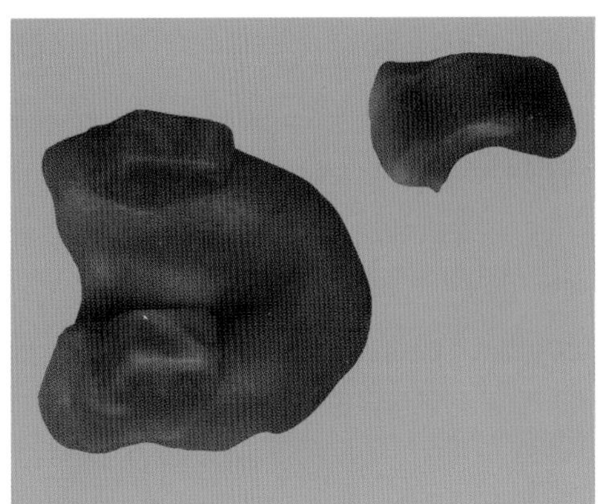

• **Fig. 30.4** Potential handle faults.

◆ What You Can Do About the Lower Tray?

This has one laboratory fault (overextension) and one fault resulting from your original impression (underextension). Again, you could take a new primary impression and request new special trays, but the lower tray is more easily dealt with. The best solution is to extend your tray over the buccal shelf by using a material such as green or pink stick composition (pink is much easier to use because it flows at mouth temperature). The lingual overextension can be trimmed back with a bur to the correct extension, which is marked as a black line on the undersurface in the upper panel of Fig. 30.2.

◆ What Else Should You Check Before Trying To Adapt the Trays?

The extension should be checked in the patient's mouth to ensure that the other areas are correct. Other common errors in tray construction relate to handle design. You need to check the handles to ensure that they are properly constructed. Prosthodontists can become excited about tray handles, but there are no absolute rules regarding what can and cannot be used. However, some tray handle designs could cause you and your patient problems.

◆ Are These Handles Suitable?

As indicated by the appearances in Figs 30.1–30.3, the laboratory has provided well-made and well-designed handles. Faults to look for are shown in Fig. 30.4. Can you identify them and the reasons for the deficiencies?

The left and central images in Fig. 30.4 show the same tray that has been poorly constructed. The handle will almost certainly get in the way of the lower lip, risking displacement during use and distortion of the sulcus. As you are aware, complete dentures develop retention from a correct border seal, and this might be more difficult to achieve in the master impression if the tray handle distorts the lips. This fault usually arises because the tray is left sitting on the bench before light curing, during which time the handle sags under the influence of gravity. A stub handle would be better, as seen in Fig. 30.1.

The handle also deviates from the midline, so it will be very difficult for the user to centre and seat the tray without the handle as a guide. This would certainly be the case with a spaced perforated upper special tray for use with alginate.

The image on the right shows that the handle has fallen off. This is because the light-cured materials were not processed in the light box at the same time. With use of this type of material, a handle cannot be added at a later stage without using a special adhesive because the material has a high filler content. It is unlikely that you would have this adhesive in your surgery. This problem may only come to light when removing the impression. A well-recorded impression is normally very retentive and can be difficult to remove. The clinician has to first release the border seal in the buccal aspect of the premolar region and then remove the impression using the handle. It is a bit embarrassing if the handle falls off!

Also, the technician has placed posterior stub handles. These are not normally used on maxillary trays and have no advantage there. Their sole advantage is to help prevent the clinician's fingers from distorting the buccal sulcus when taking impressions of an edentulous lower ridge.

SECOND PATIENT

Summary

You are constructing a new upper complete denture over a lower metal-based partial denture for a 52-year-old male when things start to go wrong. How will you rectify the mistakes?

History

Complaint

The patient dislikes the worn appearance of the upper anterior teeth on his complete denture and complains that it is becoming loose.

History of Complaint

The patient lost all his upper teeth because of decay in his late 20s and early 30s despite extensive dental care. He has had five dentures over a 20-year period and managed with them fairly well. The current lower metal-based partial denture was his first partial denture. He dislikes the back of the denture lifting up during function but copes with this reluctantly.

Examination

The upper complete denture lacks retention, and no peripheral seal is evident when seated. There is some wear of the anterior teeth.

The lower partial denture has wear on the prosthetic teeth, and they are no longer in occlusal contact. The patient has an inadequate posterior occlusion (posterior support).

Solution

◆ What Will You Prescribe?

Both dentures must be replaced. Relining the upper denture is pointless if the teeth are worn. The lower partial denture needs replacing because it is not retentive and is worn out. The posterior occlusion will have to be reconstructed with two new dentures because neither is currently correct.

Replacing the upper denture alone might cure the aesthetic problem. However, lower natural teeth occluding against a complete denture with no lower partial teeth or with worn teeth will accelerate alveolar bone loss and risk formation of a fibrous ridge ('flabby ridge').

You decide to construct a new metal-based partial denture for the lower arch and a new complete upper denture by using a copy denture technique.

◆ In What Order Do You Plan To Provide This Dental Care? Why?

It would be best to start with the metal-based partial denture first. If the copy technique for the upper denture goes to plan, four visits will be required without reviews. If the metal-based partial denture goes to plan, even ignoring the altered cast technique, it will require six visits without reviews. Some laboratories prefer 3 weeks to make a metal framework, and you do not want to be recording the definitive upper impression too early in the treatment schedule.

The most efficient plan is shown in Table 30.2.

TABLE 30.2 Dental Care Plan

Visit	Complete Upper Copy Denture	Metal-Based Lower Partial Denture
1		Primary impressions (then denture designed)
2		Tooth preparations and secondary impressions
3	Copy upper denture in silicone putty and send to the laboratory	Metal try-in and optional altered cast technique impression
4	Secondary impressions and jaw registration	Definitive jaw registration
5	Wax try-in	Wax try-in
6	Fit	Fit
7	Review	Review

The metal framework is shown in Fig. 30.5. It looks beautiful and fits the model well. Everything seems to be going to plan until you notice that the laboratory seems to have omitted the cingulum rest and minor connector for the lower left canine.

Before reaching for the phone to call the laboratory and complain, you look at the design that you sketched on the prescription card, shown in Fig. 30.5.

◆ Is Anything Wrong with Your Prescription? If So, What?

There are several errors:

- You have mixed up left and right, producing a mirror-image prescription – easily done if you look at an impression to help with the design.
- You have failed to consider the need for indirect retention.
- In your drawing, the minor connector on the lower right second premolar passes over the distal aspect of the lingual cusp.

In your diagram, no reciprocation has been indicated for the clasp on the lower right second premolar, next to the bounded saddle. Luckily the laboratory has realized this and has put a reciprocal on the framework.

◆ Will These Design Faults Cause Problems? Why?

Yes, probably. The patient is not keen on wearing a lower partial denture and complains of lifting of the free end (distal extension) saddle. A cingulum rest on the lower left canine would provide indirect retention (see Case 54) against this movement. As well as causing problems in function, the saddle lifting posteriorly would cause the lingual bar, which lacks support from the anterior teeth, to impinge on the soft tissues. This would cause soreness under the major connector.

◆ What Can You Do To Rectify These Errors?

There are four options:

1. **Ignore the indirect retention** on the basis that there is good direct retention with three clasps. If the framework fits, it might be possible to take a chance and go ahead. If this works, you will owe the laboratory thanks for remembering to add the reciprocal arm to the premolar because this contributes significantly to the overall retention by ensuring that the clasp is guided, reciprocated and engaged.
2. **Have a separate rest and connector cast**, and ask the laboratory to try to laser weld that on. This is difficult, carries a cost implication and the fit might not be very satisfactory. It carries a risk of failure.

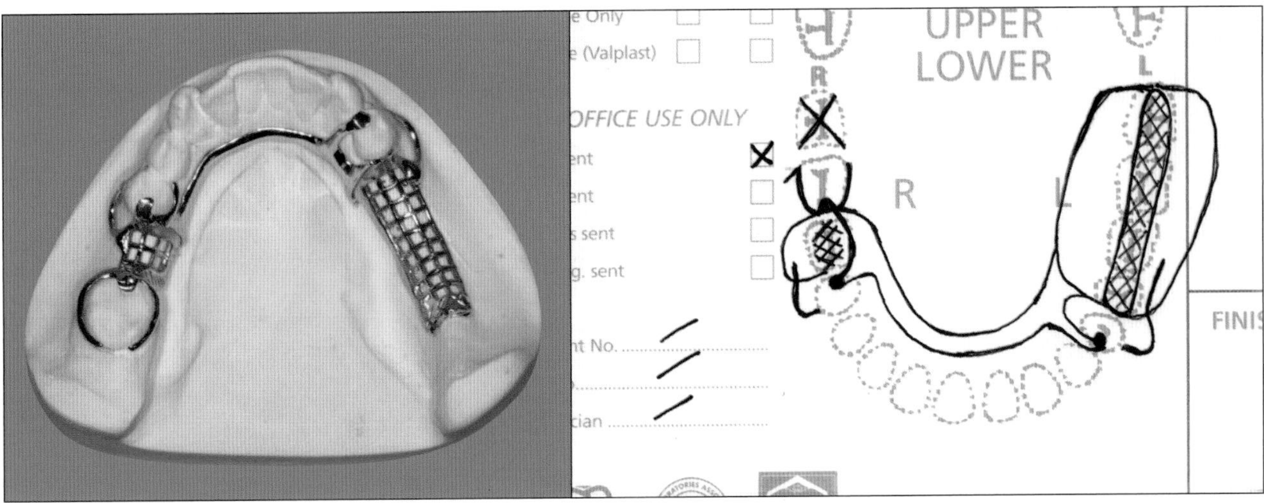

• **Fig. 30.5** The framework back from the laboratory (**a**) and your original instructions (**b**) (vertically mirrored).

3. **Make a new framework** either on the existing master cast, if it has not yet been disposed of or damaged in any way, or record a new secondary impression and make a new framework – the optimal clinical solution, but with cost and time implications.

As the patient is already waiting, you decide at least to try-in the framework. If it does not fit, the option of adding an indirect retainer is not practical.

◆ How Do You Decide Whether the Framework Fits?

Check systematically that:

1. the rest seats are fully seated
2. there are no gaps between the soft tissues and the major connector
3. there is not an anterior–posterior or lateral rock
4. clasps and reciprocals are in close contact with the teeth
5. guide planes provide a clear single path of insertion
6. clasp tips engage in undercuts.

Bear in mind that the saddle is not supported with acrylic resin under the mesh and that if you place vertical force on the saddle at this stage the framework will lift anteriorly, even if it fits well.

When you seat the framework, it seems to fit well, and it appears that you may be able to adapt it. Confidently, you ask the patient how the framework feels. Unfortunately, he says it is lifting at the back and on both sides, not just the side with the distal extension saddle. Closer inspection reveals that the clasp on the lower left second molar is not providing any retention.

◆ A Close-Up of the Clasp is Shown in Fig. 30.6. What is Wrong?

Lack of retention indicates that the clasp tip is not in an undercut relative to the path of insertion. The fault could lie with the construction of the clasp or the lack of undercut relative to the path of insertion.

There is a design fault in the molar clasp. The clasp arm starts below the survey line and is, therefore, in the undercut relative to the path of insertion. The clasp tip is in contact with the tooth but above the survey line, which lies at the level of the gingival margin. In such situations, the clasp is usually so inflexible in the first third that it is impossible to seat the framework in that area.

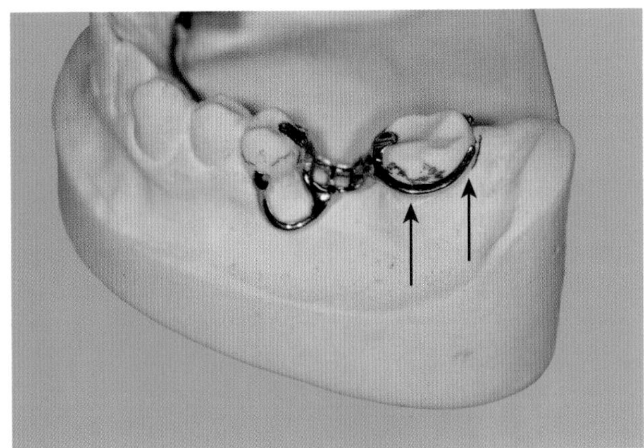

• **Fig. 30.6** The molar clasp.

This cannot be sorted out in the surgery. You warn the patient that a new impression and framework will probably be required.

◆ How Will You Take This Up with the Laboratory?

If you have a good dental laboratory, you cannot afford to lose its confidence or support. You will be aware that metal-based dentures have to be designed using a team approach, especially if you are not an expert (see Case 54).

You are responsible for the several prescription errors, which significantly contribute to the failure of the framework. Conversely, if the laboratory had phoned to query the design faults, they might have been rectified.

You should already have a service level agreement with the laboratory, specifying what each party expects and provides. The laboratory will expect you to provide:

- patient identification
- an accurate legible prescription

- identification of teeth with poor short- and long-term prognosis
- dates that stages are required back in the surgery
- accurate and correctly extended impressions
- adherence to accepted infection control procedures.

In return, you will expect the laboratory to contact you if it has any advice about your design or consider that it could be improved. You would expect it to contact you before changing your design, and you must be willing to take calls as often as necessary for minor queries.

The agreement should include what should be done in the event of errors and provides a basis for negotiating a fair solution. Errors will arise, but often, both parties will need to take some responsibility for them.

Unless you have a surveyor in your practice, you would not have been able to identify that there is no undercut on the distal aspect of the tooth. The dental technician should have pointed out that a better solution would be a circumferential ring clasp, engaging the mesio-lingual undercut from the distal aspect. This is exactly the sort of potential problem that is easily solved through good communication.

◆ What is the Optimal Design for This Framework?

After discussion with the laboratory and a resolution to improve communication on both sides, the laboratory manager offers to make the framework again free of charge. This is a welcome and significant gesture of good will.

The final framework is shown in Fig. 30.7.

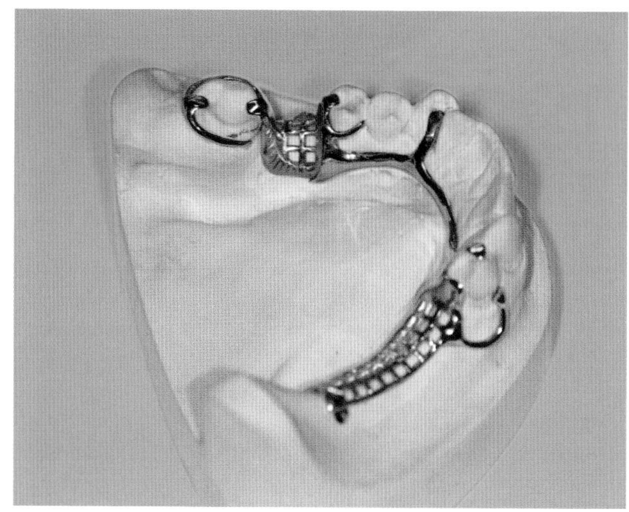

• **Fig. 30.7** The new framework.

The rest on the lower left canine provides indirect retention, and the circumferential clasp of the lower left second molar now engages an undercut from above the survey line. This design is likely to be successful, although it is not necessarily the single best solution. All designs involve some compromise with regard to mechanical properties, patient acceptability, reducing the damaging potential of the prosthesis, and the cost.

Acknowledgement

We are grateful to PWS Direct Ltd, Bolton, for the examples of correct and incorrect laboratory work specially prepared for this problem.

Case 31

Ouch!

CHRIS DICKINSON

Summary

You sustain a substantial percutaneous injury to your foot. What should you do?

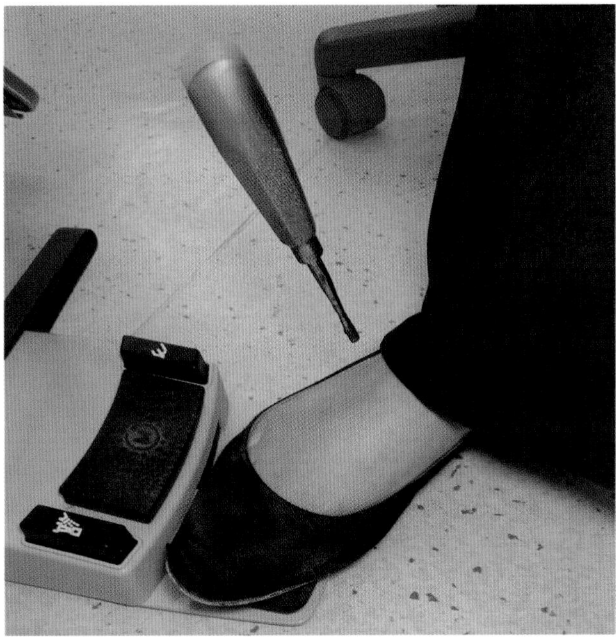

• **Fig. 31.1** Murphy's law in action. (Nice shoes – fine for a sunny summers day out, but not appropriate for clinical wear!)

History

You are extracting a difficult tooth and have used a luxator to loosen the tooth prior to elevation. While transferring the luxator to the bracket table, you drop it (Fig. 31.1). The luxator impales itself in your foot.

◆ What Diseases of Significance May Be Transferred By the Injury?

Most infectious diseases can be transmitted by a percutaneous (sharps) injury, but the main concerns are hepatitis B, hepatitis C and human immunodeficiency virus (HIV) infection.

◆ What Would You Do Immediately?

Encourage bleeding at the injury site, and wash it with soap and water, but without scrubbing the wound. Antiseptics should not be used because their effects on the local defence mechanisms are unknown. Free bleeding should be initially encouraged.

◆ What is the Most Urgent Priority and Why?

The most urgent priority is to assess whether there is a significant risk of transmission of blood-borne virus (BBV) infection. Postexposure prophylaxis (PEP) with antiretroviral drugs can significantly reduce the chance of transmission of HIV, but for maximum effectiveness, it is recommended that it be administered within 1–2 hours. The reduction in risk of HIV transmission may be as high as 81%. There is some evidence that some protection of transmission is still possible, even if the administration of the PEP is delayed, even by as much as 48–72 hours.

◆ How Could You Obtain Postexposure Prophylaxis, if Required?

The Health Act 2006 requires every National Health Service (NHS) employer to have a policy on the management of exposure to high-risk body fluids such as blood. 'Saliva associated with dental treatment' is also classified as high risk because of its likelihood of being contaminated with blood during treatment. Saliva alone is classified as low risk. The policy must ensure that advice is available 24 hours a day and where to obtain that advice and any recommended treatment.

PEP is only available following a formal risk assessment for each individual injury. This involves determining the severity of the injury and the risk that the patient is carrying HIV infection.

The procedure for obtaining a formal risk assessment varies with local circumstances. In hospitals, the infection control consultant(s), hospital casualty or occupational health department will perform the risk assessment and provide the appropriate medication. Those in general practice must contact their local hospital casualty department, which will follow its local guidelines. Each dental practitioner should know the contact number and name/position of the appropriate local department or the nominated person.

When you telephone, you will be asked for details of the injury and of the patient. You will then be told whether or not the injury carries a risk of transmission. To provide this information, you or a member of your team will need to carry out a risk assessment on the patient.

◆ What is the Risk of Developing HIV Infection After a Sharps Injury?

The average risk for transmission of HIV is estimated at 3 infections per 1000 injuries. Comparatively, the risk of contracting hepatitis C is 10 times greater, and for hepatitis B, it is 10 times greater (if the recipient is not protected by vaccination).

◆ What Factors Affect the Risk of Transmission?

An increased risk of occupationally acquired HIV infection is associated with:

- a deep injury
- visible blood on the device that caused the injury
- injury with a needle that has been in a blood vessel
- a high viral load in the source patient.

The viral load is a measure of the concentration of the virus in blood. It is higher during the primary infection (the so-called window period), reduces with early infection but then rises with symptomatic and late-stage infection (acquired immunodeficiency syndrome [AIDS]). It is reduced with effective treatment.

The risk from a needlestick injury, where the needle has been used to administer a local analgesic, is therefore lower because the needle would not be expected to have been placed in a blood vessel (if an aspirating technique) was used. PEP is therefore often unnecessary for a needlestick injury from a dental anaesthetic needle.

Splashes of infected blood carry a low risk. Splashes on to broken skin or mucous membranes, including the eye, carry a risk of transmission estimated as being less than 0.1%. It is considered that there is no risk of transmission from a splash of blood on to intact skin.

Your injury is a deep injury caused by a sharp instrument covered with blood, and therefore there is a risk of transmission of HIV.

◆ The Patient Has Returned To the Waiting Room with Your Nurse. What Will You Say and Do?

In a private area, you should explain to the patient exactly what has happened and that there has been an accident involving a surgical instrument. Inform the patient that there is a practice policy, which is derived from national policy that should be carried out when this happens. Introducing the HIV assessment of the patient in this way depersonalizes the incident and avoids making difficult judgements and discriminating against perceived 'high-risk' groups for HIV infection.

The patient should be asked to give informed consent for blood to be taken and tested for HIV, hepatitis B and hepatitis C and for storage of serum. If infection has been transmitted, it will be necessary to compare the patient's sample and the sample of your blood for industrial injury benefit or insurance purposes.

Lengthy pretest counselling is now no longer a requirement prior to testing for HIV. It is only necessary to provide it if the patient requests it or needs it. The benefits of testing to both the dentist and the patient should be stressed. If the patient has an undiagnosed HIV infection or hepatitis, then an earlier diagnosis is more likely to lead to effective treatment, and the dentist can have the most effective prophylaxis to prevent infection. Most patients will be happy to give a sample of their blood under these circumstances. If not, then the reason for the refusal should be explored as sensitively as possible. It may be that patients have an impression that they have, in some way, done something illegal or hold a false belief about the virus itself.

The general population has little knowledge of hepatitis, but many understand that it is a serious disease and may be aware that it can be transmitted sexually. At a minimum, blood should be obtained to store serum in case testing is required at a later date.

The dentist will most likely not have the facilities to take blood, and the patient can be asked to go to his or her general medical practitioner with a request or to attend the local Accident and Emergency (A&E) department. If the dentist does carry out the test, then the patient should collect the results from his or her general medical practitioner.

The possibility that the patient might be HIV positive will have to be addressed to assess the risk of transmission. This must be done in a sensitive manner, preferably in a private room and with reassurance about the confidentiality of any answers given. These questions should not be asked by the recipient of the needlestick injury because it is difficult to be objective if you are feeling anxious or distressed. However, in dental practice, there may be no other person suitable to handle this issue, and you may have to ask the questions yourself. As an alternative, you could consider asking the patient to speak on the phone to the local casualty officer responsible for the PEP, sexual health clinic medical staff, a sexual health counsellor or other suitably experienced person.

You should remember that it is not the risk factor that denotes the risk of transmission but how the activity that dictates the relative risk takes place (Table 31.1).

◆ What Questions Would You Ask?

- Are you a regular blood donor in the UK? (Blood donations are screened for hepatitis B and C, and HIV).
- Have you ever had a blood donation refused?
- Have you ever been diagnosed with hepatitis B or C, or HIV?
- Have you ever lived in HIV high-prevalence areas such as Africa or Asia?
- Have you ever had a blood transfusion or surgery abroad?
- Have you ever had an injury when you have been exposed to someone else's blood?
- Have you ever injected drugs into a vein?
- Have you ever been imprisoned?
- Do you have sex without using a condom?

A positive answer to any of these questions requires further questioning to understand the degree of risk of

TABLE 31.1 Risk Factors for Human Immunodeficiency Virus (HIV) Infection

Type of Risk	Risk Factor	Relative Risk
Parental infection	Transfusion	There is a small risk of infection to recipients of blood transfusion given between the mid-1970s and 1987. Most of those exposed will already have developed the infection, and there is a very small risk for those who are not positive. Donor screening since 1987 has reduced this risk to a minimal level.
	Haemophilia	Recipients of factor VIII–containing blood products before 1985 had a high risk of infection – almost 80%. Most of those exposed will already have developed the infection, and there is a very small risk for those who are not positive. All UK factor VIII sources are now screened.
	Injecting drug users (IDUs)	The risk depends on whether the needle is shared and how much contamination occurs. Needle exchange programmes have reduced the incidence of HIV in IDUs. IDUs without access to needle exchange programmes represent a high-risk group for acquiring HIV.
	Needlestick injury	The risk is 0.3%, but depends on the type of injury, volume of blood transmitted and the infectivity of the blood.
Sexually transmitted infection	Vaginal intercourse	A risk to both partners but greater for the female. Properly lubricated condoms offer good protection.
	Prostitution	Unprotected intercourse with a prostitute is a high-risk practice, but the risk varies greatly in different parts of the world.
	Oral sex	Transmission has been documented, but the risk is considered lower than with vaginal sex.
	Anal intercourse	The highest-risk sexual activity. Condoms reduce risk but failure is common. Prisoners may have consensual or coerced sex, and lack of access to condoms means they represent a high-risk group for acquiring HIV.

acquiring hepatitis B or C or HIV through the activity. In practice, asking these questions does not usually constitute a problem because, in almost all cases, there will be either no risk or a very low risk. Similarly, most HIV-positive individuals will readily disclose the information in this situation.

◆ What are the Risk Factors for Contracting HIV infection?

In the UK, in 2016, an estimated 54% of new diagnosis of HIV infection acquired it through men who have sex with men (MSM). In contrast, the numbers of new infections acquired through heterosexual sex were 19% for men and 22% for women.

◆ If the Patient Discloses That He or She is HIV Positive, What Information Would You Like To Know? What is the Significance of the Answers (Fig. 31.2)?

Answers and significance are shown in Table 31.2. The answers to these questions would be invaluable to the person making the risk assessment.

◆ If the Patient Indicates That He or She is Not HIV Positive But Agrees To an HIV Test, Can You Carry It Out?

Yes, UK National Guidelines for HIV Testing say that it should be within the competence of any trained healthcare worker to obtain consent and conduct an HIV test.

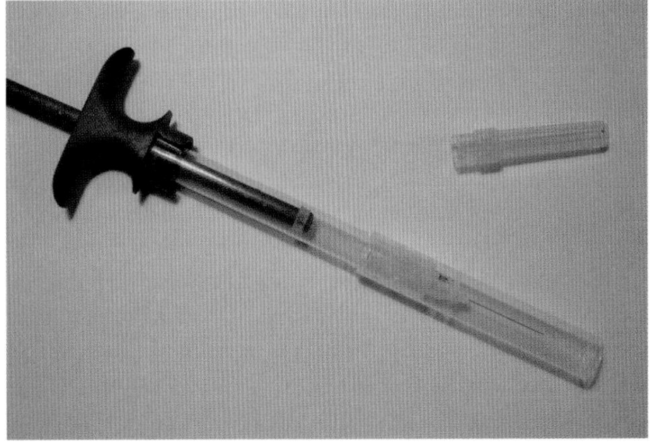

• **Fig. 31.2** A 'safety' local anaesthetic needle system. Note the retractable sheath over the needle tip.

If you do not have the facilities to perform the test, then you can ask the patient's general medical practitioner to carry out risk assessments, advise, test and provide PEP, if indicated. Your local A&E centre may also have facilities for the urgent, out of hours, assessment and treatment of body fluid exposures in healthcare workers. The result of the test should be given back to the patient by a person qualified to answer any initial questions that the patient may have and who has knowledge of the local specialist services for a prompt referral. This is often the patient's general medical practitioner.

TABLE 31.2 Information From Human Immunodeficiency Virus (HIV)–Positive Patients and Its Significance

Information	Significance
Whether patients are generally well	Patients with asymptomatic HIV infection have low viral load and lower infectivity.
Their CD4 (T-helper cell) count	An indicator of immunosuppression, the stage of disease and effectiveness of treatment.
Their viral load and when it was last checked	A direct measure of infectivity.
The names of any medications they are taking	The same drugs would be avoided for postexposure prophylaxis (PEP) if they are not being effective in the patient.
Whether patient's medication has changed recently and why	Recent changes in medication may indicate their strain of HIV becoming drug resistant, and this must be taken into account in choosing the drugs for PEP.
The address of the patient's HIV clinic	To contact for further information. Obtain consent to do this, and respect the patient's confidentiality.

◆ What is PEP? Why Not Simply Take the Drugs Regardless of the Relative Risk?

PEP is preventive treatment started immediately after exposure to an agent that causes infection. The regimes for PEP after exposure to HIV are complex. New drugs are being developed, and knowledge is continually acquired about HIV and the emergence of drug-resistant strains. This, along with the desire to reduce the side effects of PEP to increase compliance, means that the regime for PEP is constantly under review. At the time of writing (2008), the regimen includes a combination of tenofovir, emtricitabine, lopinavir and ritonavir. This is continued for 4 weeks.

The side effects of these drugs include nausea, diarrhoea, dizziness, headache, muscle weakness and skin rash. These effects can be debilitating, and automatic prophylaxis for every sharps injury cannot be advocated. Pregnancy is not a contraindication for PEP, but the evidence for its safe use in pregnancy is limited.

◆ What if the Patient Indicates a Risk of HIV Infection To You But You Cannot Obtain a Formal Risk Assessment Within 1 Hour?

You should not delay starting PEP while awaiting either a formal risk assessment or the testing of the patient's sample of blood. PEP is at its most effective within the first few hours, and preferably the first hour.

◆ Do I Have To Give a Blood Sample for Testing?

You will be asked to give a blood sample for storage of serum. This is because you may need to prove that infection was not present at the time of the injury. If the patient is subsequently shown to have an infection, you will be asked to provide a sample for testing 12 weeks (at a minimum) after the injury, or cessation of PEP if it was prescribed.

◆ What is the Risk of Transmission of Hepatitis B Through This Injury?

This should be minimal. All members of the dental team should be vaccinated against hepatitis B. Once they have achieved a satisfactory antibody response of 100 mIU/ml to the vaccine, a single booster may be given after an inoculation injury. Nonresponders will receive anti–hepatitis B immunoglobulin on an occupational exposure. If recent evidence of the effectiveness of the recipient's vaccination is not available, the recipient should have his or her antibody titre checked.

If the recipient is not immune, the risk of transmission has been estimated as high as 30%, especially if the patient is e-antigen positive. Infection can follow transmission of as little as 0.1 ml of blood. Hepatitis B is so infectious that the degree of injury is almost immaterial. In the unlikely event that a nonimmunized individual receives a sharps injury, specific hepatitis B immunoglobulin provides passive immunity and can give immediate but temporary protection after accidental inoculation or contamination with hepatitis B–infected blood.

◆ Does This Mean I Have To Give Blood Even if I Know That My Hepatitis B Vaccination is Successful?

You must also ensure that your serum is stored because you may need to show that hepatitis infection was not present at the time of injury.

◆ How Can You Determine Whether the Patient is Infectious for Hepatitis B?

Blood must be screened for hepatitis B antigens and antibodies (Table 31.3).

◆ What is the Risk of Contracting Hepatitis C?

The risk of contracting hepatitis C through a needlestick injury is 3% if the donor is infected. This risk is therefore higher than for HIV infection but, as for HIV infection, is dependent on the amount of virus present in blood. The consequences can be severe. As many as 75% of individuals who become infected will become chronic carriers. Of these, 20% will go on to develop serious sequelae, for example, cirrhosis, liver cancer or liver failure.

It is estimated that 4 in 1000 individuals in England in the 15–59-years age group is infected with hepatitis C. The majority remains undiagnosed. The prevalence of hepatitis C in intravenous drug users has been estimated to be between 3% and 42%.

◆ Is Prophylaxis Against Hepatitis C Available?

No PEP is available. However, early treatment of acute hepatitis C infection may prevent chronic hepatitis C infection.

TABLE 31.3 **Hepatitis B Antigens and Antibodies and Their Significance**

Antigen or Antibody	When Found	Significance for Infectivity
HBs (surface) antigen or 'Australia' antigen	Becomes detectable in late incubation and is present during acute hepatitis. Declines over 3–6 months but persists in carriers, whether asymptomatic or with chronic active hepatitis	Indicates past infection and potential current infectivity, although not necessarily high infectivity
Antibody to HBs (surface) antigen	Seen in recovery, reflecting immunity against the virus. Also found in those immunized against hepatitis B	Probably indicates no risk of infection. Denotes past exposure and immunity (including by active vaccination) to the virus and a possible need for further investigation to determine infectivity
HBc (core) antigen	Only present in the liver; not used for determining infectivity	
Antibody to HBc antigen	Found in acute disease, recovery and in carriers, whether asymptomatic or with chronic active hepatitis	Indicates past infection but a high level indicates an infection risk
HBe (envelope) antigen	Becomes detectable in late incubation and is present during acute hepatitis. Persists in carriers with chronic active hepatitis but not usually in asymptomatic carriers	Indicates acute infection or a carrier state of high infectivity
Antibody to HBe antigen	Develops as HBe disappears. Sometimes persists in chronic asymptomatic carriers	Indicates either recovery from acute infection or a carrier state of low infectivity

◆ How Can the Risk of Needlestick or Sharps Injury in the Dental Setting Be Minimized?

Sharps injuries do not always result from needles. Burs, hand instruments (as you have just found out) and other contaminated sharps all constitute a risk. You should:

- utilize 'sharps-safe' devices such as safety needle and scalpel systems, that have in-built covers that protect the needle point or blade after use. This is now law under the European Safer Sharps legislation of 2013. This legislation requires clinicians to risk assess the nonsafety sharps used in their practice and replace with safer sharps alternatives, if available, as long as procedural outcome quality can be maintained
- ensure that the entire dental team is trained in the disposal of sharps
- Identify and dispose of needles and other sharps immediately after use in the appropriate sharps container
- *always* pass instruments with the sharp end pointing away from any person
- remove burs and ultrasonic tips from handpieces immediately after use
- pick up instruments individually
- retract the patient's cheek with a mirror while administering local analgesia
- never resheath a needle holding the sheath in a hand: If a sharps-safe device is not available, then use a one-handed technique (Fig. 31.3), or dispose of the needle immediately
- never place your finger or your assistant's finger in front of a sharp instrument such as a scalpel or luxator
- always use a firm finger rest while scaling

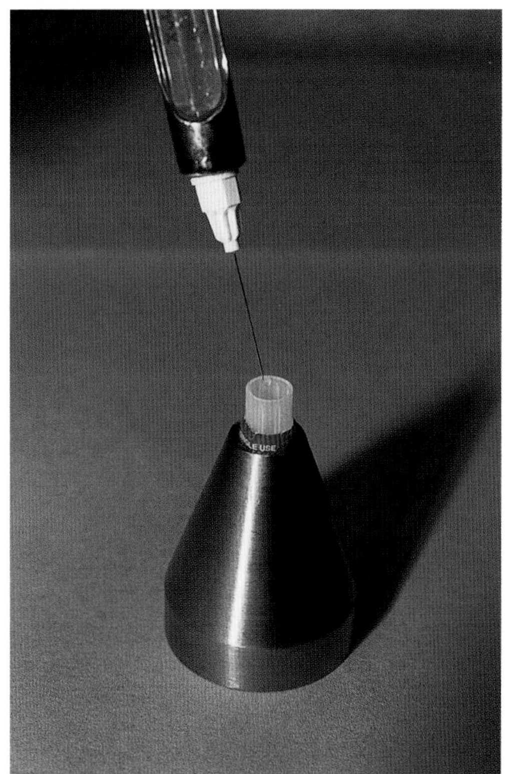

• **Fig. 31.3** A simple needle sheath holder. The holder is not intended to hold the syringe upright, only to hold the sheath during resheathing.

- dispose of sharps into a solid container (approved to BS 7320)
- ensure that sharps are disposed of by incineration and by an authorized person registered to collect such waste

- use heavy-duty gloves when cleaning instruments prior to autoclaving
- keep your working area well organized and uncluttered with sharps in a separate area. Do not place waste material such as swabs or tissues, over instruments
- always wear appropriate masks, visors or protective eye protection. Modern minimalist designer glasses offer little protection
- footwear should cover the top of the foot. You would not have a problem today if you had worn footwear appropriate for the dental surgery.

◆ What is Your Last Duty Before You Can Turn Your Back On This Unfortunate Episode?

You must remember to fill in an incident report as required by law (the Reporting of Injuries, Disease and Dangerous Occurrences Regulations 1995) and submit it to your employer. If seroconversion occurs, you will need to inform the Health and Safety Executive and the General Dental Council. This will be important evidence for industrial injury benefit or insurance purposes, together with the records in your notes.

◆ This Injury Has Ruined Your Day. This Has All Proved So Complex That Next Time You Might Just Wash the Injury and Ignore It. Why Not?

The main reason is the worry that you might contract a blood-borne virus infection from an unsuspected carrier. The effectiveness of PEP – reducing the risk of transmission by greater than 80% – cannot be ignored. Also, it would be unethical for a dentist not to follow up the possibility of developing an infection that could jeopardize the wellbeing of his or her patients. There would also be a risk of transmission to the dentist's sexual partner(s).

Acknowledgement

The editors would like to acknowledge the previous contributions of Guy Palmer.

Further Reading

AVERT: Global Information and Education on HIV and AIDS.

Health and Safety (Sharp Instruments in Healthcare) Regulations 2013. Guidance for employers and employees. Health and Safety Executive. Health Services Information Sheet 7.

Case 32

A Swollen Face and Pericoronitis

TARA RENTON

Summary

A 23-year-old woman presents in your hospital Accident & Emergency department with a painful swelling of the right side of the face and neck. What is the cause, and what treatment would you provide?

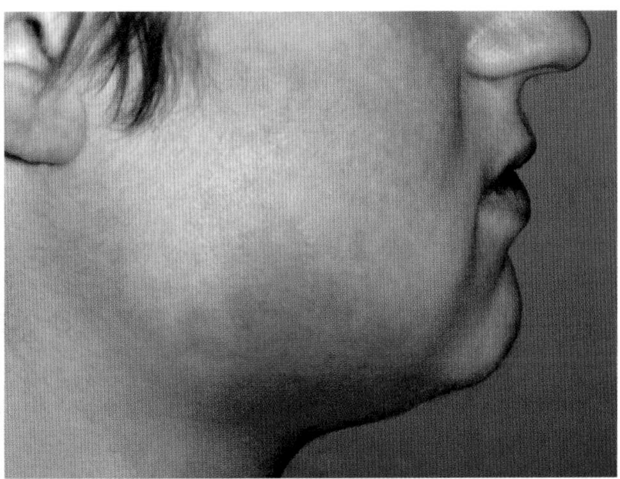

• **Fig. 32.1** The patient on presentation.

Further information on the diagnosis of soft tissue infection will be found in Case 49.

History

History of Complaint

The patient has suffered worsening pain 'from her wisdom tooth' on the lower right side for 5 days. There has been some swelling of the gingiva around the tooth, and she has been unable to bite her teeth together for a few days. Yesterday, she noticed pain in the floor of her mouth and found that moving her tongue was painful. Today, she awoke to find the facial swelling; she feels unwell and has difficulty eating, swallowing and opening her mouth. (see Fig. 32.1)

She had an episode of pericoronitis a few months ago and is on her local hospital waiting list to have all third molars extracted. Until the swelling developed, she thought this was just another attack of pain from her wisdom teeth. She has not had facial swelling before and has come straight to hospital.

Medical History

The patient is otherwise fit and well.

Examination

Extraoral Examination

There are palpable tender lymph nodes in the upper deep cervical chain and submandibular triangle. Opening is limited to 15 mm interincisal distance.

There is swelling below and around the lower border and angle of the mandible and extending back towards the neck. The swelling is hot, tender, very firm and a dusky red colour centrally. The swelling is not pointing to the skin. There is a marked halitosis.

Intraoral Examination

Trismus hampers examination. The lower right third molar can be seen to be partially erupted, the operculum is swollen and pus exudes from below it on gentle probing. The second and third molars appear caries free.

The floor of the mouth is very tender and firm on the right side.

◆ What Additional Examinations or Investigations Would You Perform? Explain Why.

It is extremely important to take the patient's temperature to determine whether the infection is exerting systemic effects.

She has a temperature of 37.8°C (normal temperature 36.8°C) and is therefore pyrexic.

There is a need to confirm that pericoronitis is the cause. It would be prudent to exclude the possibility that this is infection from a nonvital molar, and tests of vitality should be performed. If there were a suggestion from the examination that a lower molar was nonvital, a radiograph might be indicated; otherwise, radiographs would provide little useful information for diagnosis unless another lesion were present.

Diagnosis

◆ What Do These Findings Tell You?

The combination of inflammation (swelling, pain, redness and heat), together with local lymphadenitis and pus seen intraorally, indicates an infection. Pericoronitis is present, and this appears to be the primary source of the infection. Trismus is an important sign, indicating that the infection or inflammation has spread to involve the muscles of mastication.

The patient is pyrexic and feels unwell. These features indicate that the infection is exerting a systemic effect. Infection appears to be spreading relatively fast because the swelling has appeared overnight, and there are already systemic signs.

◆ Which Type of Infection is This?

It is difficult to tell because the tissues involved are deeply sited. Pus is draining from under the operculum, indicating abscess formation, but this might extend into a soft tissue space or be limited to the tissues around the unerupted tooth. The rapid spread, firmness and tenderness of the tissues ('brawny' swelling) indicate cellulitis. This might continue to spread or develop into an abscess. There is probably a mixed infection with a local pericoronal abscess and a spreading cellulitis.

◆ To Which Tissue Spaces May Infection Spread From a Lower Third Molar? What are the Boundaries of These Spaces?

Pus from lower third molars may track to many spaces, and spread is unpredictable, depending on many factors including the angulation of the tooth, the size of the follicle, relationship to the second molar, degree of bone loss around both teeth and the anatomical relationships between teeth, bone and muscle attachments in the region. Pus may drain into the mouth from under an operculum, into the buccal or lingual sulcus or into one or more tissue spaces. The routes of spread to tissue spaces are shown in Fig. 32.2 and are described in Table 32.1.

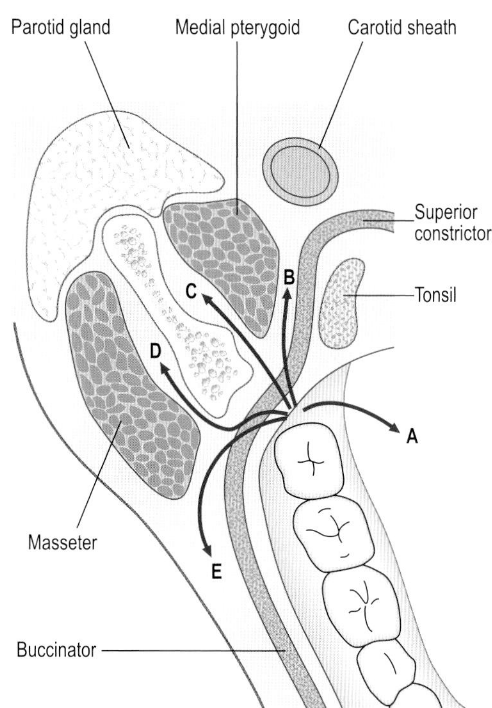

• **Fig. 32.2** Paths of spread of infection into tissue spaces from third molars: A, into the sublingual and submandibular space; B, into the parapharyngeal space; C, into the pterygo-mandibular space leading to the infratemporal fossa; D, into the submasseteric space; E, into the buccal space.

Pus from lower third molars tends to perforate the lingual plate, which is closer and thinner than the buccal plate. Infection is deflected to either the sublingual or submandibular space by the attachment of the mylohyoid muscle.

◆ In What Tissue Spaces is the Present Infection Tracking, and Why?

This swelling appears to be in the submandibular space. The main infected tissue is not visible and lies around the submandibular gland deep to the body of the mandible. The swelling just spreads round the lower border of the mandible onto the face. Moderate trismus is typical. It is relatively common for this tissue space to be involved in pericoronitis.

There may well be early sublingual space involvement. Infection readily tracks between the submandibular and sublingual spaces around the submandibular gland and the posterior edge of the mylohyoid muscle. In addition, infection may spread through the mylohyoid muscle, which is thin, perforated by blood vessels, and a poor barrier to spread of infection. There is not yet an established sublingual space infection because this would cause extensive swelling of the floor of the mouth and deflect and limit any movement of the tongue. Swelling from sublingual space infection would be readily visible in the lingual sulcus and causes considerable oedema in the loose tissues rather than the firmness and tenderness seen in this patient.

◆ Is This a Potentially Life-Threatening Infection?

No, but it is serious. The patient's airway will be at risk if the infection continues to spread posteriorly. This would be potentially fatal, and dyspnoea may develop unexpectedly and with great rapidity. Vigorous treatment of the infection must be commenced immediately.

◆ What is Ludwig's Angina? Is This a Risk?

Ludwig's angina is a bilateral infection involving the submandibular and sublingual spaces. It is frequently caused by cellulitis when the classic 'brawny' (board-like) induration of the neck is seen. Spread of infection involves the epiglottis or parapharyngeal spaces rapidly and causes airway obstruction. Death may also result from septicaemia, disseminated intravascular coagulation, or spread in the fascial planes of the neck to the mediastinum. Early diagnosis and prompt surgical intervention combined with definitive airway management are necessary to prevent serious morbidity or mortality.

◆ Is There a Risk That the Patient Might Develop This Condition?

It would be possible for this patient's condition to progress to Ludwig's angina, but this is not likely to be imminent

TABLE 32.1 Paths of Spread of Infection From Lower Third Molars

Direction of Spread	Tissue Space	Boundaries
Medially above the attachment of the mylohyoid muscle	Sublingual space, A	Lies between the floor mouth and the mylohyoid muscle with the body of the mandible laterally.
Medially below attachment of the mylohyoid muscle	Submandibular space, A	Lies between the mylohyoid muscle and platysma, with the hyoid bone medially and the lower border of the mandible laterally. Contains the submandibular gland.
Posterior and medial to the mandibular ramus, medial to the lateral pterygoid muscle	Parapharyngeal space, B	Lies between the superior constrictor muscle and the pterygoid muscles with the pterygoid plates.
Posterior and superior, between the mandibular ramus and the lateral pterygoid muscle	Infratemporal space via C, which communicates with the cavernous sinus	Base of skull superiorly, laterally sigmoid notch of mandible and temporalis muscle, medially lateral and posterior wall of maxilla.
Posterior and medial to mandibular ramus, lateral to the lateral pterygoid muscle	Pterygomandibular space, C (and potentially on into the infratemporal space)	Lies between the lateral and medial pterygoid muscles and the ascending ramus of the mandible. Extends up to base of skull.
Posterior and lateral to mandible ramus	Submasseteric space, D	Lies between the masseter muscle and the ascending ramus of the mandible.
Posterior and superiorly, lateral to buccinator	Buccal space, E	Between the buccinator muscle and skin.

and treatment will prevent this complication. However, she could also develop airway problems from spread via other routes.

Treatment

The principles of treatment of odontogenic soft tissue infection are described in Case 49. It is necessary to drain pus, remove the cause of the infection, if possible, and provide antibiotics in selected cases.

◆ Where Should This Patient Be Treated?

Admission to hospital will be necessary for this patient because she has systemic effects of infection and there is a risk that infection might impinge on the airway.

◆ Is Pus Present? If So, How Will You Drain It?

It is unclear at this early stage of infection whether an accumulation of pus, as well as cellulitis, is present in the submandibular space. Incision may not be helpful. Infection at less important sites might be treated with vigorous antibiotic therapy and removal of the cause, followed by drainage, if required, 1–2 days later. However, because of the proximity of the airway, incision must be performed if there is suspicion of abscess formation. Even within cellulitis, there will be small collections of pus or necrotic tissue. Drainage is the safer option in this case.

The submandibular space must be drained through an extraoral incision, ideally 2 cm below the lower border of the mandible (to avoid damage to the mandibular branch of the facial nerve). In practice, this may not be the appropriate site and a soft spot centrally in the hard swelling is the best place to incise. Distortion of soft tissues makes the position of the mandibular branch difficult to predict. Forceps use or an incision must extend up medially to the mandible to drain the submandibular space. A drain will be required.

Drainage of the sublingual space is not indicated in this case and is rarely necessary. It could be achieved via an incision in the floor of the mouth (taking care to avoid damage to the lingual nerve).

Pus should be released from the pericoronal tissue through either an intraoral incision or extraction of the tooth.

◆ How Will You Remove the Cause?

General anaesthesia will be required to drain the swelling. Fibreoptic-guided intubation may be necessary because of trismus and infection around the airway. In a more advanced case with airway oedema or infection, intubation of a conscious patient may be required because paralysis for intubation prevents the patient from keeping the airway open voluntarily. Perforation of the pharynx during intubation is possible if it is oedematous or displaced, and this might drain pus into the upper airway. Forcing the mouth open under anaesthetic may have the same effect.

It may well be possible to remove the third molar at the same time despite the poor access. This breaches the general surgical principle that surgery is best avoided in an infected field, but with effective antibiotic treatment, postoperative complications are rare. Obviously, the decision will depend on the difficulty of the extraction. Removal of the opposing third molar could also speed recovery and reduce the chances of another episode of pericoronitis. Removal of the lower third molar may have to await resolution of the infection.

◆ Would You Provide Antibiotics? If So, Which?

Yes, prescription of antibiotics is required in such a case. An initial bolus of intravenous metronidazole would be appropriate, with an oral regimen for a few days afterwards. There is further discussion of antibiotics for odontogenic infections in Case 49.

Further Guidance

http://www.sdcep.org.uk/ and search 'bacterial infection'.

https://www.fgdp.org.uk/ and search 'antimicrobial prescribing'.

Case 33

First Permanent Molars

MIKE HARRISON

Summary

A 7-year-old girl has pain from a first permanent molar. What is the cause, and how might it affect her dental development?

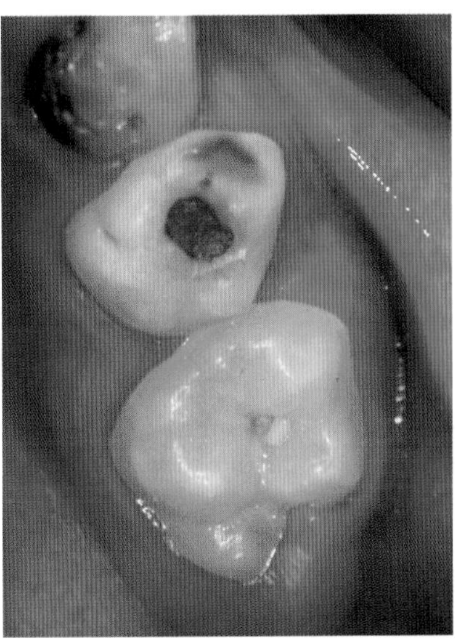

• **Fig. 33.1** The occlusal view on presentation of the upper left quadrant.

History

Complaint

The patient's mother reports that the child suffers intermittent spontaneous discomfort from the upper left teeth.

History of Complaint

The symptoms have been vague, no sleep has been lost and there has been no facial swelling. The patient has complained of the pain three or four times over the last month.

Medical History

The child is fit and well.

Dental History

The child has been a regular patient since the age of 3 years. She has required restorations in four primary molars, with one requiring local analgesia. You have identified a high caries risk in her. Despite intensive preventive advice and diet analysis, new carious lesions have been present at each recall visit.

Examination

You ask the child to point to the painful tooth, and she points to an apparently sound upper left primary canine.

◆ The Appearance of the Upper Left Quadrant is Shown in Fig. 33.1. What Do You See?

- An amalgam restoration with ditched or raised, defective margins on the palatal aspect of the first primary molar
- An apparently sound amalgam restoration in the second primary molar
- Possible caries in an occlusal pit on the second primary molar
- An erupting first permanent molar with the occlusal surface not fully through the mucosa
- An occlusal cavity in the confluence of the mesial fissures of the permanent molar
- Plaque or food debris in the fissures.

◆ How Do You Interpret the Information So Far, and What are the Likely Diagnoses?

The child is probably pointing at the wrong tooth; the canine appears intact. Children are often poor historians, and they often have difficulty localizing the source of pain if the pain is not present at the time of examination.

Pulpitis appears likely because the pain appears poorly localized and is relatively intermittent. A history of hot or cold or sweet exacerbating factors would point to this diagnosis. The likely causes are caries beneath a restoration or carious or traumatic pulpal exposure in one of the primary molars. Any primary molar with an unrestored carious cavity or even a clinically sound restoration should be examined closely for signs of pulp necrosis.

◆ What Features Might Suggest a Necrotic Pulp?

- Extension of caries or fracture into the pulp
- Discoloration of the crown
- Swelling or tenderness in the buccal sulcus adjacent to the tooth

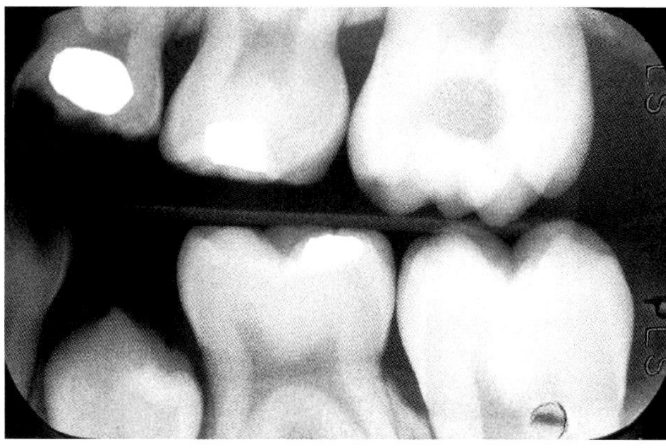

• **Fig. 33.2** The left bitewing radiograph.

- Pus draining from a sinus in the mucosa, usually buccally, but occasionally lingually or palatally
- Pus draining from the gingival margin
- Facial swelling
- Well-localized pain.

None of these symptoms and signs is present. Therefore pulpitis seems likely.

Investigations

◆ What Investigations are Indicated? Why?

- Bitewing radiographs to check the proximity of restorations to the pulp, the extent of the occlusal caries in the permanent molar and to detect small proximal surface carious lesions
- Clinical examination of the other permanent molars for caries
- Tests of sensibility of primary and permanent molars are unlikely to help because the results of such tests are often unreliably reported in children.

◆ The Left Bitewing Radiograph is Shown in Fig. 33.2. What Do You See?

See Table 33.1.

TABLE 33.1 Features Seen in Fig. 33.2

Tooth	Features
First primary molar	The restoration appears to be in the pulp chamber but reinspection of the tooth clinically will remind you that the restoration is on the palatal aspect of the tooth and is only superimposed on the pulp chamber. No proximal surface caries is present.
Second primary molar	The restoration appears sound, with no radiolucency between the base of the restoration and the pulp to suggest caries. There is sufficient sound dentine (approximately 1–2 mm) between the restoration and the pulp to make pulp exposure unlikely. No proximal surface caries is present.
First permanent molar	There is an extensive dentine radiolucency under the small occlusal cavity, indicating caries. The deep aspect of the lesion is ill-defined, indicating rapid progression. The lesion extends close to the disto-buccal pulp horn, and there may be involvement of the pulp.

Diagnosis

◆ What is Your Final Diagnosis?

Pulpitis in the upper left first permanent molar in response to a deep occlusal carious lesion. On the basis of the report that pain has been intermittent, the pulpitis is probably reversible, but the rapid progression of the caries and proximity to the pulp may herald involvement of the pulp. Caries must be excavated to discover the true extent of the caries.

◆ How Can Caries Be So Extensive Beneath Such a Small Enamel Cavity?

This pattern of caries is sometimes referred to as *occult* or *hidden occlusal caries*. This presentation was much less common prior to the 1970s, when caries was more prevalent, lesions larger and fluoride products less available. It has been speculated that the widespread use of fluoride toothpaste has resulted in enamel that is more resistant to smooth-surface caries. Fluoride in toothpaste has little effect on the progression of dentine caries and is less effective against fissure caries. Carious lesions in fissures that progress to dentine might well be able to enlarge greatly before the occlusal enamel cavitates significantly. In a partly erupted tooth such as this, there is no significant occlusal force to fracture away any unsupported enamel. This 'traditional' hypothesis seems feasible, but there is currently no evidence that the prevalence of such occult lesions is actually affected by exposure to fluoride. An alternative hypothesis is that there was a developmental defect of dentine mineralization in this tooth. After tooth eruption, cariogenic bacteria at the depths of the fissures could penetrate a more porous enamel–dentine junction and spread rapidly through the defective dentine. This is considered unusual, but it is difficult to prove that it was not present after caries supervenes without pre-eruption radiographs. Radiographs are required to diagnose occult lesions.

◆ Does This Discovery Have Significance for Other Teeth?

Yes, it will be necessary to examine all the other permanent molars clinically again. Carious lesions may have been missed. The discovery of this large lesion should make you more suspicious, and you should consider exploration of any other suspicious fissures as well as obtaining a right-side bitewing radiograph.

Further Investigation

The child has been cooperative for restorative care under local analgesia in the past, so you make an appointment to investigate and, hopefully, restore this tooth. *When you open the small occlusal cavity, you discover that the underlying coronal dentine has been almost completely destroyed by caries. Caries extends into the pulp.*

◆ Why Did the Child Not Experience the Severe Symptoms of Irreversible Pulpitis?

There is no clear correlation between symptoms and pulp vitality or histological evidence of inflammation in mature or immature teeth. The concept of irreversible pulpitis is a useful one for making treatment decisions, but it is only an average reflection of symptoms. It is not unusual for teeth to become nonvital through caries without any significant symptoms. This is even more likely in multirooted teeth or teeth with open apices in which the pulp has a better blood supply.

◆ Can the Tooth Be Saved with Root Canal Treatment?

Root canal treatment in immature permanent molars is difficult and the outcome is unpredictable. The canals are wider and generally more accessible than in older patients, but it is virtually impossible to create an effective apical seal with gutta percha in the open apices. If endodontic treatment were necessary and the child could cooperate for the several long sessions of treatment required, nonsetting calcium hydroxide dressings could be placed to induce calcific barrier formation apically. This would require changing every 4–6 months until an apical barrier is felt on gentle instrumentation and a longer-term filling of calcium hydroxide powder or mineral trioxide aggregate could be placed. However, the chances of success are reduced because of the multiple canals. The tooth would remain compromised for future use, for instance, as orthodontic anchorage. The tooth is almost certainly better extracted.

◆ If the Pulp Reacted Positively To Sensibility Testing Under a Similar Deep Carious Lesion, What Would You Do?

The guiding principles for the minimally invasive, selective removal of carious tissue are as follows:

- Preserve nondemineralized and remineralizable tissues
- Achieve an adequate seal by placing the peripheral restoration onto sound dentine and/or enamel, thus controlling the lesion and inactivating remaining retained bacteria
- Avoid discomfort/pain and dental anxiety, as both significantly influence treatment/care planning and outcomes (operative methods that are less likely to lead to dental anxiety are preferable)
- Maintain pulp health by preserving residual dentine (avoiding unnecessary pulpal irritation/insult) and preventing pulp exposure (i.e. leave softer, contaminated dentine in close proximity to the pulp, if required).

To adopt a 'minimally invasive' approach to carious tissue removal, selective removal to soft dentine should be performed and pulp exposure avoided, where possible.

Care Planning

◆ What are the Effects of Extraction of a First Permanent Molar On the Developing Permanent Dentition?

- The spaces created close more by mesial movement of posterior teeth than by distal movement of anterior teeth.
- There would be only a small effect on any anterior crowding and minimal effect on the position of the midline.
- Spaces close more rapidly in the upper arch than in the lower. Space closure in the lower arch is frequently incomplete, unless much of the space can be occupied by distal movement of a crowded second premolar.
- Lower second molars tend to tip mesially and roll lingually, producing poor proximal contacts that are prone to food packing and periodontitis in the long term. Upper second molars rotate mesio-palatally as they drift mesially but produce much better proximal contacts than in the lower arch.
- More satisfactory space closure and proximal contacts are produced in the lower arch if the first molar is extracted before eruption of the second molar (see below).

◆ Do You Require an Orthodontic Opinion?

Yes. If at all possible, an orthodontic opinion should be sought prior to the extraction of any permanent tooth in a child. In this particular case, the patient may well benefit from compensating or balancing extractions. This is a complex area and will require an orthodontic examination to assess crowding, the occlusion of the buccal segments, overbite and overjet.

◆ What are Compensating and Balancing Extractions, and What are Their Benefits?

Compensating extractions are those of the opposing molar; balancing extractions are extractions of the contralateral tooth.

Compensating extractions prevent overeruption of the opposing molar to maintain the correct occlusal level. Balancing extractions maintain the symmetry of the arch.

◆ How Will the Orthodontist Decide Whether To Perform Compensating or Balancing Extractions?

The decision depends on weighing several factors:

- The presence of the other permanent teeth, including third molars
- The condition of the other permanent molars – whether they are already compromised by caries or large restorations
- The presence of crowding in the buccal and labial segments
- The acceptability of overbite and overjet
- The stage of dental development
- The patient's likely future need and wish for orthodontic treatment and their likely compliance.

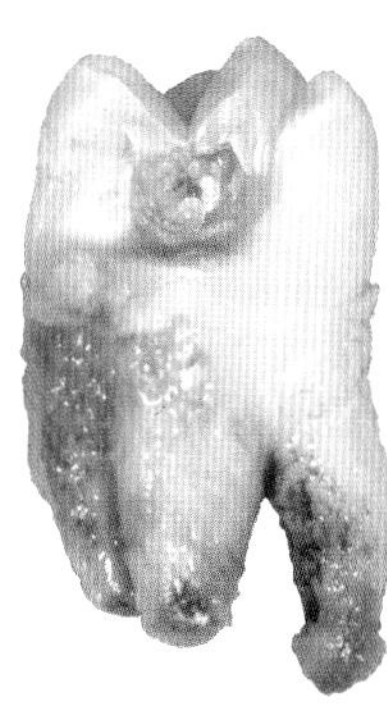
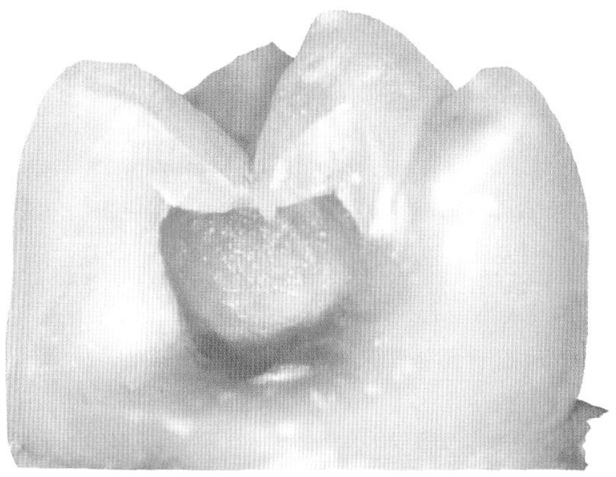

• **Fig. 33.3** The extracted tooth.

◆ What is the Ideal Age To Extract First Permanent Molars?

Extraction must be performed at the ideal time to minimize the adverse effects of extraction listed above. The stage of dental development, rather than the chronological age, is important. The crucial factor is the stage of development of the lower second molar because this determines how satisfactorily the space in the lower arch will close. The range of acceptable development is from crown completion to mineralization of one-third of the root, but primarily before it has erupted into the mouth. A frequently held opinion is that the appearance of an interradicular crescent of bone in the second molar indicates the optimal stage for first molar extraction (at approximately 9.5 years of age). More recent evidence suggests that other factors may be involved in favourable eruption of the second molar and that early extraction is not problematic. Radiography is required to confirm the stage of development and to ensure that the third molars and the second premolars are present and normal.

Late extraction of poor-quality first molars is to be avoided, wherever possible, specifically when the unerupted second molar is no longer completely encased within bone, as seen radiographically.

◆ Does Extraction of First Permanent Molars Complicate Orthodontic Treatment?

It used to be said that extraction of all four first permanent molars doubled orthodontic treatment time and worsened the prognosis. This held good only for removable appliance treatment and does not apply to fixed appliance treatment. However, closure of residual lower first molar spaces does pose complex anchorage problems, and it will sometimes be preferable to delay the extraction of compromised but symptom-free first molars until the second permanent molars have erupted. This is a further reason why a full orthodontic assessment is required.

◆ How Can You Change the High Caries Risk?

Providing dietary advice to prevent dental caries, use of age-appropriate fluoride toothpastes and topical application of high-concentration fluoride varnishes are important tools to address an identified high caries risk. Bonded resin sealants on vulnerable pits and fissures must be carried out carefully to ensure a good seal, and if moisture control is difficult when molars are partially erupted, blocking out fissures with provisional glass-ionomer cement sealants is to be encouraged.

Children can be members of a family with a high caries risk, possibly with low expectations of dental health, and changing family behaviours can be challenging. You should aim to work with the family to identify achievable goals. Contemporaneous notes of all discussions with the patient and the carer must be recorded.

Further Information

◆ The Extracted Tooth is Shown in Fig. 33.3. What Do You See?

Part of the crown has been removed to expose the carious cavity. On the left, you can see a small periapical granuloma at the apex of the palatal root. The pulp was therefore nonvital despite the lack of symptoms. On the right, you can see a large defect extending from the enamel to the pulp. The central occlusal enamel is completely unsupported but has not fractured. The carious dentine is hardly discoloured because it is progressing rapidly.

Case 34
A Sore Mouth

DAVINDER BAINS AND HELEN MCPARLAND

Summary

A 55-year-old Afro-Caribbean woman presents to you with a complaint of a sore mouth. You must make a diagnosis and institute treatment.

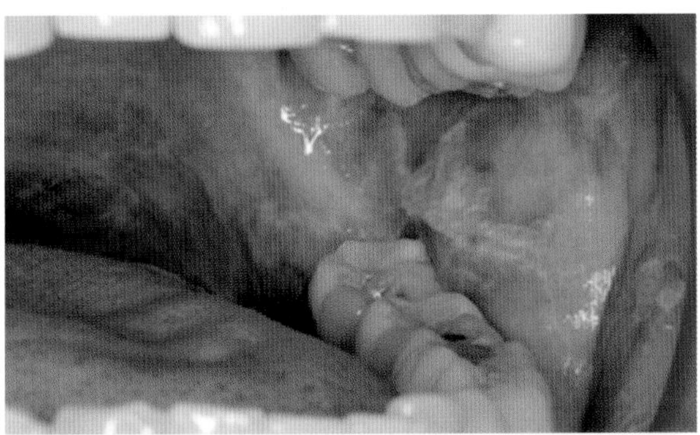

a

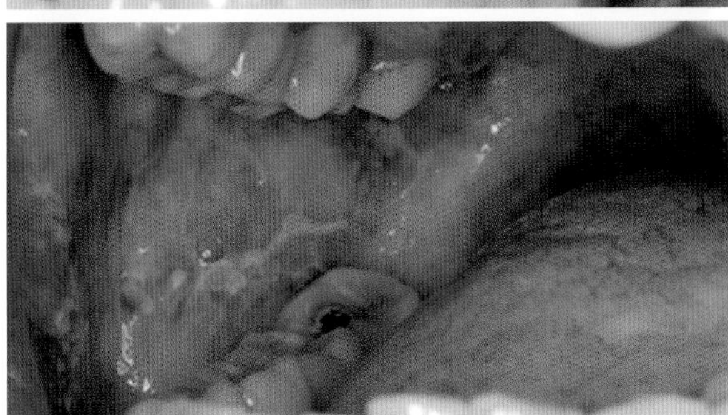

b

• **Fig. 34.1** The patient's left **(a)** and right **(b)** buccal mucosa.

History

Complaint

The patient complains of occasional soreness on the inside of her cheeks and white patches on the inside of her lips.

History of Complaint

The patient first noticed a burning sensation 3 months ago. She notes that the soreness is brought on particularly when she eats sour and mildly spicy foods. She had noticed that the white patches on her lips started around the same time, and she thinks these patches are spreading.

Medical History

The patient is generally fit and well. She is not on any current or recent medication. She has never smoked and consumes less than 5 units of alcohol a week.

Examination

Extraoral Examination

The patient appears fit and well. There are no rashes on her face, and no cervical lymph nodes are palpable. White patches were visible on the upper lip.

Intraoral Examination

The mouth is well lubricated with saliva, and the patient has good oral hygiene. There is discolouration of the occlusal surface of the lower posterior molars and only minimal occlusal amalgam restorations. The appearance of the left and right buccal mucosa are shown in Fig. 34.1 and of the palate in Fig. 34.2.

◆ Describe What You See On the Buccal and Palatal Mucosa.

The buccal mucosa is affected bilaterally by reticular white striae and associated poorly defined diffuse brown pigmentation found mostly at the periphery of the striae. The white striae extend from the posterior buccal mucosa

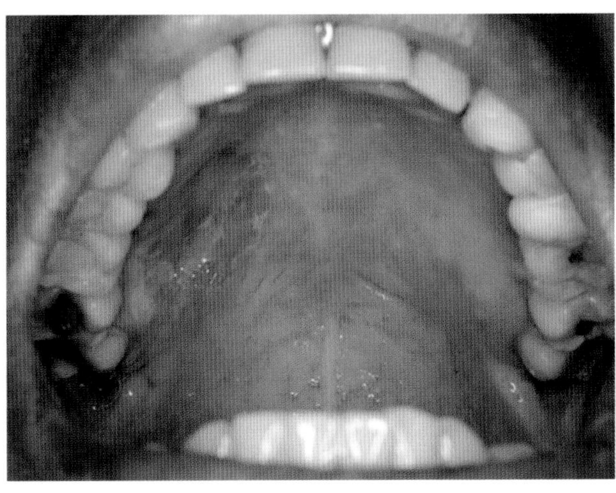

• **Fig. 34.2** The appearance of the palate.

to the commissural region. In the left buccal mucosa (see Fig. 34.1a), there is a central solid patch of white mucosa. Poorly defined striae are seen in the right soft palate. In the right buccal mucosa, the white appearance of the buccal mucosa is most prominent in the occlusal plane (see Fig. 34.1b). There are no obvious red patches and no ulceration.

◆ What is Your Differential Diagnosis?

1. Lichen planus
2. Lupus erythematosus (systemic [SLE] or discoid [DLE])
3. Lichenoid drug reaction.

◆ Justify This Differential Diagnosis.

The combination of reticular and diffuse white areas on a background of slight redness almost certainly indicates one of these three conditions. The lesions cannot always be diagnosed by their clinical appearance alone, although there can be some differentiating features to each condition.

Lichen Planus. This condition is the commonest of the three possible diagnoses and most prevalent in women in their 5th and 6th decades of life. The striae and lacy patterns on the buccal mucosa are distinctive of lichen planus and are typically bilateral. Lichen planus can also cause white patches on the lip and palate as in this patient, although this is less common.

Lupus Erythematosus (LE). The mouth may be involved in lupus erythematosus, either as part of SLE or in DLE. In both conditions, clinical features of oral mucosa resemble those of lichen planus and lichenoid reactions, but some findings may help in the diagnosis. LE is more frequent in females, and there is a higher prevalence in patients of Afro-Caribbean ethnicity. Lesions in LE often have a central ulcer or erythematous area around which the striae tend to radiate, rather than follow the random pattern of lichen planus. Lesions are also typically asymmetrical and affect the hard and soft palates, which are less frequently involved by lichen planus or lichenoid reactions. LE is much rarer than either of the other two possibilities but unilateral involvement of the palate and lip involvement, as well as the patient's ethnic background, indicates that LE should remain a consideration in this case.

Lichenoid Reaction. Oral lichenoid reactions may be localized (in response to topical triggers such as restorations) or more widespread, in which case they are usually caused by medication. Some features that point to a lichenoid drug reaction rather than lichen planus include acute onset, extensive ulceration, asymmetrical distribution and severe involvement of the dorsum of the tongue. Lesions may also affect sites that are less commonly affected by lichen planus such as the floor of the mouth. Lichenoid reactions may be clinically indistinguishable from lichen planus. In this case, a lichenoid drug reaction can probably be ruled out because the patient is not on any medication, although double-checking recently discontinued prescriptions and over-the-counter drugs is necessary to be certain. The location and distribution of the lesion do not correspond to any dental restorations so a topical lichenoid reaction can be ruled out.

◆ How Do You Explain the Darker Pigmented Areas?

The combination of white patches and striae with pigmentation is potentially confusing, but the pigmentation is almost certainly a secondary effect called *inflammatory* or *postinflammatory pigmentation*. In diseases where the epithelium is damaged or becomes inflamed, melanin pigment formed by melanocytes in the epithelium fails to transfer into the epithelial cells and 'drops out' into the underlying connective tissue. Here, it is recognized as a foreign material and phagocytosed by macrophages and only slowly degraded, producing patchy brown discolouration. Inflammatory pigmentation is usually seen in dark-skinned individuals.

◆ What Further Questions and Examinations are Appropriate? Explain Why.

See Table 34.1.

On further questioning, the patient reports an itchy rash on the flexor surface of her forearms (Fig. 34.3) and shins which developed around the same time as her oral white patches.

Her rash is consistent with cutaneous lichen planus, which typically presents as raised itchy red/purple lesions. She has never had a facial rash, and she reports no other symptoms. Rashes in lupus typically affect the head and neck and sun-exposed skin.

Investigations

◆ Is a Biopsy Indicated? Why?

Yes. Ideally, biopsy should be performed in the majority of white lesions in the mouth, especially if the patient reports high alcohol or any tobacco consumption. When there is extensive mucosal involvement, ulceration or atrophy, or when the clinical presentation is not typical, other conditions need to be excluded through biopsy for example in this case, lichenoid reactions and LE. It is not always possible to distinguish between these three diseases histologically but microscopic characteristics may help favour one of these three entities. Histological features always need to be interpreted within the context of the clinical presentation and the results of other tests. A biopsy is also useful to exclude unexpected diseases, particularly dysplasia. Proliferative verrucous leucoplakia and other potentially malignant disorders can be misdiagnosed as lichen planus, particularly when the lichen planus forms plaques rather than striae. A further reason for biopsy is that lichen planus itself is considered to have a very low risk of malignant transformation.

For this patient, incisional biopsy is indicated.

TABLE 34.1 Further Questions

Subject	Questions and Reasons
Rash	Is a rash present? The patient should be questioned about any skin, nail or scalp problems and about any genital symptoms. Ask about and examine the flexor surface of the wrist and the extensor surface of the shins. These are common sites for skin lesions of lichen planus and lichenoid reactions. The typical skin lesions of lichen planus are purplish polygonal papules with faint striae (Wickham's striae). They are usually very itchy. Severe lichenoid reactions may be accompanied by an extensive erythematous rash. Only a minority of cases with oral lichen planus or lichenoid reaction will have skin lesions on presentation. This is because the skin lesions often resolve spontaneously after a few years or with topical steroid treatment. In contrast, oral lesions may persist for many years and are often resistant to treatment. Therefore, ask about previous rashes. The skin lesions of SLE are different from those of lichen planus and may be of several different types, including 'discoid' rashes, erythema nodosum and other more nonspecific papular, erythematous and blistering rashes. Rashes in DLE are often confined to the face, neck and scalp and present as well-demarcated, round or oval, red, scaly patches (discoid rash). The dorsum of the hands may also be affected, with sparing of the knuckles. Typically the face is affected by a butterfly rash on the malar region of the face. Rashes elsewhere on the body tend to be photosensitive so are worse on sun-exposed areas.
Signs and symptoms of SLE	Although it is a less likely diagnosis, the patient should be asked some questions to exclude systemic involvement. Questioning and examination should be more thorough if the oral lesions suggest lupus erythematosus by virtue of their appearance, distribution or the young age of the patient. SLE has numerous signs and symptoms, including rashes (above), photosensitivity and hair loss. Vasculitis can affect most organs. There may be glomerulonephritis, arthritis, anaemia and central nervous system involvement, causing infarction and/or psychiatric manifestations. The patient should also be questioned about symptoms of fatigue or arthralgia.

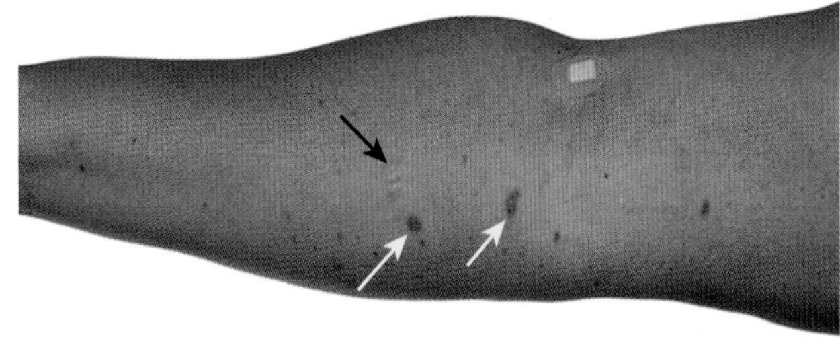

• **Fig. 34.3** Clinical appearance of the rash on the arm. There are white papules centrally (black arrow), measuring several millimetres. The papules usually become flattened after several months and leave pigmentation (yellow arrows) that may become hypertrophic.

◆ Which Part of the Lesion Would You Remove for Biopsy?

The biopsy specimen should be taken from the most clinically representative area, including both red and white areas, if present. If there is ulceration, it should be avoided because the epithelium is required for diagnosis, and there will be florid inflammation masking the histological features. The specimen should be elliptical, about 8–10 mm long, 5–6 mm wide and an even 3–4 mm deep. *In this case, a biopsy specimen was removed from the left buccal mucosa, as shown later in Fig. 34.4.*

◆ What Other Investigations Would You Perform?

Autoantibody Screen. If SLE is a possibility, an autoantibody screen may provide evidence to support the diagnosis. A serum sample should be sent for antinuclear antibody (ANA) extractable nuclear antigen (ENA) and double-standed DNA (dsDNA) assessment. Four-fifths of patients with systemic disease are ANA positive, often having high titres. A high titre of anti-dsDNA antibody is almost exclusive to SLE but is positive in only 50% of cases. Autoantibodies against Smith (Sm) antigen (part of the ENA screen) is also highly specific for SLE. In DLE blood tests are less helpful for diagnosis because few patients have a positive ENA or ANA. Individuals with lichen planus or lichenoid reaction are likely to have a negative autoantibody screen.

Microbiological Tests. When lichen planus or a lichenoid reaction is widespread or becomes symptomatic, the possibility of superimposed candidal infection should be considered. The thick keratotic epithelium is more prone to infection compared with normal epithelium. A smear from the surface of the lesions on each side is an ideal investigation. Saliva sampling for candidal counts may also be helpful. This has the advantage that the organism is cultured for complete identification and sensitivity testing to antifungal agents. The disadvantage is that it cannot distinguish candidal infection from candidal carriage. *In this case, saliva sampling was done.*

Other Tests. Because the patient has oral mucosal and cutaneous involvement, she may be a candidate for systemic medical management. Therefore baseline renal and liver function screens may be useful for monitoring any adverse drug effects. Furthermore, renal function tests may be useful in eliminating possible kidney involvement in LE.

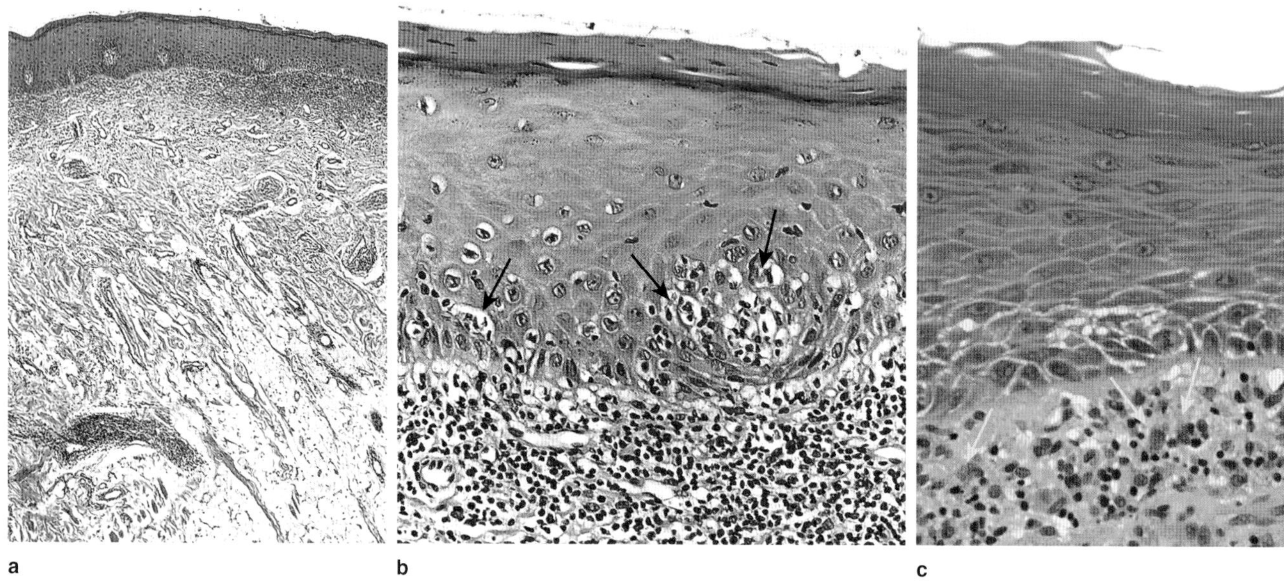

• **Fig. 34.4** Buccal biopsy: **a**, low-power view; **b**, higher-power view; **c**, higher-power view of adjacent area.

◆ In the Biopsy Specimen Shown in Fig. 34.4, What Do You See?

The left image (a) at low power shows mucosa with underlying fat. The surface epithelium is slightly thinner than normal buccal epithelium and has a red layer of keratin just visible at the surface. There is a well-demarcated inflammatory cell infiltrate in a band immediately below the epithelium within the superficial connective tissue. The band is denser towards each side of the picture. At this magnification, the cells cannot be definitely identified as inflammatory cells, but this is the most likely explanation for the very cellular zone. There are also several foci of inflammatory cells in the deeper tissues, one particularly large one associated with a vessel near the bottom of the picture. The basement membrane is prominent.

The middle image (b) is a higher-power view and shows the interface between the epithelium and connective tissue. The very cellular layer seen in (a) is composed of lymphocytes. Lymphocytes have infiltrated into the basal and suprabasal layers of the epithelium and caused the basal epithelial cells to undergo apoptosis. Apoptotic cells are visible as shrunken, very pink cells with nuclear remnants (black arrows). There is no remaining clearly defined basal layer of epithelial cells, and the cells lying at the basement membrane have the appearance of prickle cells. The surface is parakeratinized. Buccal epithelium is normally nonkeratinized, except along the occlusal line as a result of friction.

The image on the right (c) is from an area adjacent to (b) at similar magnification. The surface here is orthokeratinized, a feature that is abnormal for the buccal mucosa. As in (b), cells in the basal layer have the appearance of prickle cells. The basement membrane is thickened. Within the lamina propria, there are macrophages containing melanin pigment (yellow arrows), which has 'dropped out' of the overlying epithelium. This explains the pigmentation seen clinically.

◆ How Do You Interpret the Histological Findings?

The dense band-like infiltrate of lymphocytes and lymphocytic infiltration of the basal cells with focal basal cell degeneration, apoptosis, loss of basal cells and a thickened basement membrane are typical of lichen planus. There are no histological features to allow definitive diagnosis of LE over lichen planus, although the perivascular infiltrate seen in Fig. 34.4a may be suggestive of the fomer. For this reason, the biopsy diagnosis is 'consistent with lichen planus or a lichenoid reaction or LE'. The histological findings should be correlated with clinical features before finalising a diagnosis.

Other Results

In this case, the autoantibody screen result was negative, and no Candida was found in the saliva or biopsy sample. The full blood count, as well as the haematinic, renal and liver function screen results were normal.

Diagnosis

◆ What is Your Final Diagnosis? Explain Why.

The final diagnosis in this case is lichen planus with oral and cutaneous involvement. Lichenoid reaction has been excluded because the patient is not on any medication, and the distribution of the lesions do not correspond to any dental restorations. The cutaneous findings are not typical of LE and the autoantibody screen was negative. With

TABLE 34.2 Treatment Options

Treatment Option	Indications and Use
Analgesic relief	Topical benzydamine (a nonsteroidal anti-inflammatory agent) provides temporary analgesia to the oral mucosa. It can also be useful prior to toothbrushing to help maintain good oral hygiene.
Topical medium-potency corticosteroids	These can be prescribed in the form of mouthwashes, sprays, ointments or in the form of aerosol inhalers used for asthma. This option would be the mainstay treatment for most patients with mild to moderate symptoms. Options include beclomethasone inhaler and betamethasone mouthwash.
Topical high-potency corticosteroids	Topical high-potency drugs such as clobetasol ointment should be considered for more severe or generalized conditions. In general, this option should be provided in a secondary or tertiary care setting.
Systemic corticosteroids and disease-modifying agents	Systemic corticosteroids (e.g. prednisolone) and disease-modifying agents (e.g. hydroxychloroquine, azathioprine and mycophenolate mofetil) are used for severe cases that do not respond to topical treatments and should only be used in a secondary or tertiary care setting. Regular monitoring for the adverse effects of these drugs is required.

these other options excluded, the diagnosis of lichen planus is made despite the unusual distribution of disease in the mouth.

Treatment

◆ How Would You Manage This Patient's Oral Symptoms?

The aim of management of lichen planus is to relieve symptoms because the underlying disease process is not easily influenced without the use of drugs that have significant adverse effects. Many patients with lichen planus have no symptoms and therefore do not require any active treatment. Several options are listed in Table 34.2, and choice of treatment largely depends on severity of symptoms. Gingival lichen planus is aggravated by plaque, and in some patients, maintaining optimal oral hygiene can be difficult because of pain. Patients should be helped to maintain a high standard of oral hygiene. Some patients also find the detergent sodium lauryl sulphate (SLS) in certain toothpastes an irritant, and they should switch to an SLS-free toothpaste. Highly flavoured toothpastes should also be avoided.

In this case, the oral symptoms were managed with 0.5 mg betamethasone dissolved in 5–10 ml water as a mouthwash for 2–3 minutes up to three times daily. *The patient was referred to her general medical practitioner for the management of her skin lesions. At the review appointment, the patient reported that she was much more comfortable and that her oral symptoms were under control.*

◆ What Considerations Would You Take Into Account When Determining the Frequency of Follow-Up Appointments?

The frequency of review appointments depends on whether or not systemic medication has been prescribed, because this may require monitoring for adverse effects and the clinical appearance. There is also a very low risk of malignant transformation in oral lichen planus. There is controversy surrounding the exact rate of malignant transformation, but it is likely to be less than 0.1%. Some authorities suggest that malignant change is more common in nonreticular forms of oral lichen planus. Lesions in high-risk sites such as the floor of the mouth, should be monitored. Patients should be instructed to look out for changes in the clinical appearance of the lesions.

Further Advice

An example of a patient information leaflet from the British Society of Oral Medicine can be found at http://www.bsom.org.uk/, under patient information.

Case 35
A Failed Bridge

SOPHIE WATKINS

Summary

A 40-year-old man has had a missing upper incisor replaced by a spring cantilever bridge. This has become decemented, and you must assess the options for replacement.

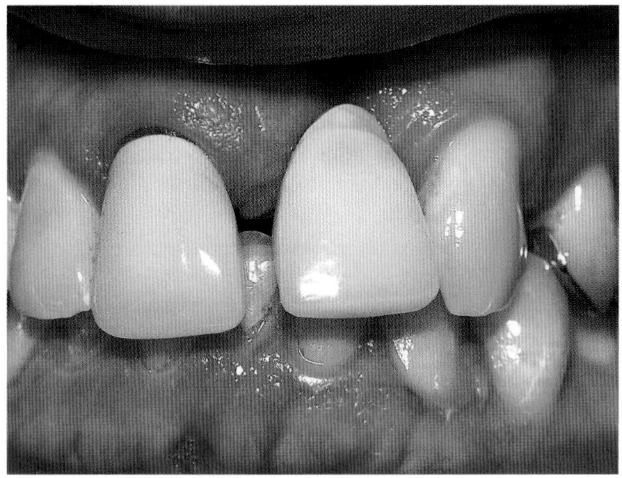

• **Fig. 35.1** Anterior view of the patient at presentation with the bridge which replaced the upper left central incisor reinserted.

History

Complaint

The patient complains that his anterior bridge has become detached. He would like it recemented or replaced.

History of Complaint

The bridge had been satisfactory for many years but became detached about 2 years ago. It was recemented and had been firm until yesterday when it fell off the teeth without warning.

Dental History

The upper left central incisor was lost as a result of a bicycle accident when the patient was 16 years of age. The tooth was completely avulsed, and the adjacent upper right central incisor was fractured. The missing central incisor was initially replaced by a simple spoon denture and a few years later by a spring cantilever bridge attached to full-coverage crowns on the left first and second premolars. The other upper central incisor was root treated and a post crown fitted. The present bridge is a replacement made about 8 years ago after the cantilever spring fractured. The patient has never had an upper left lateral incisor.

Examination

Intraoral Examination

The patient's dentition is in good condition, with a few carious lesions and a small number of restorations. The upper left premolars are the abutment teeth and have conservative crown preparations. There is superficial caries over much of the surface of the first premolar crown preparation and a larger cavity at the distal gingival margin. The mesial surface of the second premolar is also carious. Both abutment teeth are vital. The gingival condition is good except for bleeding on probing between the abutment premolars. Here, the probing depth is 4 mm. The bridge can be replaced, and the appearance with it fully seated is shown in Fig. 35.1. The caries in the first premolar is exposed below the crown margin.

◆ What is the Prognosis for This Bridge? Why?

Hopeless. Fig. 35.1 shows that the aesthetic result is not good. The bridge pontic has moved buccally and upwards, probably a combined result of alveolar ridge resorption and distortion of the spring cantilever. It also appears to have moved distally, increasing the median diastema. The abutment teeth will both require re-restoration, and the first premolar appears to be very carious. In the long term, both abutment teeth are likely to be compromised because of the risk of further caries and periodontitis.

◆ Why Was This Method of Replacing the Central Incisor Chosen Originally?

Although a well-designed partial denture should not compromise the health of the remaining dentition, most patients prefer a fixed prosthesis without palatal coverage for a single tooth replacement.

The spring cantilever design was considered suitable in this case for the following reasons:

- It allows spacing (diastemas) between adjacent crowns. The spaces would have been present because the lateral incisor on that side was developmentally absent. A fixed-fixed bridge restoring the space, utilizing adjacent teeth as abutments, would not allow spacing to be maintained, resulting in a pontic that was either too wide, or with uneven, asymmetrical spacing between the anterior teeth on the other side.

- The upper right central incisor was not a suitable abutment tooth for conventional fixed bridgework, having been traumatized, root filled and crowned with the use of a prefabricated post.

◆ What Replacement Restorations Would You Consider? Explain Your Choices.

A new spring cantilever bridge. For the reasons noted above, the spring cantilever design remains a good choice, and it has served this patient fairly well. However, the abutment teeth will require restoration and may no longer be suitable abutments. The initial design in this case utilized linked abutment teeth (a 'double-abutted' design), which is no longer considered appropriate because forces placed on the bridge tend to result in the loss of cementation of one of the retainers; this is difficult to identify on clinical examination and results in caries in the associated abutment tooth, as occurred here. In addition, double abutting also hampers oral hygiene measures, and this may predispose the patient to periodontal involvement and marginal caries, as may also have occurred in this case. Therefore if a new spring cantilever were to be constructed, it would be advisable to modify the design to incorporate a single abutment tooth. This, as with all abutments, would need to be sufficiently robust to support a spring cantilever design with sufficient coronal tooth structure, clinical crown height for retention and resistance form and periodontally sound.

An adhesive bridge could be supported on the upper left canine, with the central incisor replaced by a cantilevered pontic. This would be possible because the lateral incisor is missing but would not normally be practical in this situation. This alternative has the advantage of minimal/no tooth preparation and allows maintenance of the median diastema. Success is dependent on the area of enamel available for adhesive bonding on the palatal aspect of the canine, and the occlusal relationship. This is a realistic option because canines typically make good abutment teeth for adhesive bridgework because of their large crown offering a larger surface area of enamel for adhesion and a robust supportive root form. This also has the advantage that the existing abutment teeth could be restored independently, reinstating their embrasures to help prevent further caries and periodontitis.

A single tooth implant would allow a restoration independent of the adjacent and abutment teeth. It would permit both mesial and distal spacing and would therefore provide an aesthetically acceptable restoration, comparable with the appearance achieved by the spring cantilever bridge. However, an implant would entail surgery, more protracted treatment and higher patient costs. A provisional restoration would be required until the definitive coronal restoration is placed. An implant should provide a successful long-term restoration, provided the patient is motivated and does not have any active periodontal disease. As with the adhesive bridge, the original abutment teeth would no longer be involved in the restoration of the anterior segment and can be restored independently, which may enhance their long-term prognosis.

The above options should be presented to patients in a way that allows them to make an informed decision with regard to which one they prefer. It is essential that the advantages and disadvantages are explained in a way patients can understand and that discussions relating to this are carefully and clearly documented in the contemporaneous clinical record, with written information given to patients in the form of a letter outlining the options to allow them time to make their decision away from the clinical environment. In this case, discussion regarding the upper right central incisor will also be relevant because this tooth is somewhat aesthetically compromised and may also have a guarded long-term prognosis. It is not suitable as a bridge abutment for the reasons described above and may be a candidate for replacement at some stage. This may influence the patient's decision-making process.

After discussing the options, the patient opted to have the bridge replaced by a single tooth implant, thus maintaining the upper right central incisor for the time being because it is still functioning well.

◆ What are the Components of a Typical Single Tooth Implant?

1. The implant or fixture that is osseointegrated to the surrounding bone. Anterior single tooth implants are normally between 10 and 13 mm in length and approximately 4–5 mm in diameter.
2. An abutment that is attached to the implant by an abutment screw. Abutments are provided in various designs (according to use) and lengths. For single tooth restorations, it is important to have an antirotational lock which prevents rotation between implant and abutment and crown.
3. The crown, which can be made of porcelain or porcelain bonded to metal. This is made on a prefabricated component that fits the abutment precisely. Single tooth implant crowns can either be screw retained as an integral part of the abutment or cemented onto the abutment, depending on the orientation of the implant and whether the screw access hole, which will be in the long axis of the implant, emerges on the palatal or labial aspect of the crown. If labially/palatally placed, a cemented crown would be required to conceal it. From a maintenance perspective, a screw-retained crown may be considered preferable because this is more easily removed to allow access to the implant. This option may not always be possible because of factors affecting the positioning of the implant itself, including the available bone quantity, quality, position, or how this affects the emergence profile of the final restoration.

Investigations

◆ What Further Features Require Examination or Investigation To Assess Suitability for an Implant? How Would You Assess Them, and Why Need They Be Considered?

See Table 35.1.

Treatment

◆ What Precautions Must Be Taken When Inserting an Implant?

The implant is inserted into a hole which must be made with a drill matched to the implant. A surgical stent (see Table 35.1) is

TABLE 35.1 Features Requiring Investigation

Feature	Method	Reason
Edentulous ridge height and width, labial contour of ridge keratinsed gingiva and fraenal attachments	Visual inspection and palpation	To ensure that sufficient alveolar ridge remains for the final restoration to have an acceptable appearance. There must be keratinised gingival tissue where the gingival margin of the new restoration will lie.
Bone height and width Absence of bone abnormality at site	Plain radiography – ideally, a periapical view taken using a paralleling technique and sectional or cone beam tomographs to show bone width	To assess whether sufficient bone is present to accommodate the implant. A minimum height of 10mm and a width of 6mm are required to place a standard 4 mm-diameter implant. Tomography and palpation help detect concavities in the labial plate of bone resulting from resorptive remodelling of the ridge. These would dictate implant angulation because the implant must lie inside the cortical plates.
Desired result from functional and aesthetic points of view	Ideally, mock up the final result as a provisional restoration, or construct a diagnostic wax-up. Check the occlusion. Remember to check the old restoration and copy any desirable features	To assess the appearance of the final result and assess the relationship of the crown position to the implant position. Models are used to construct a surgical stent to facilitate ideal positioning of the implant.

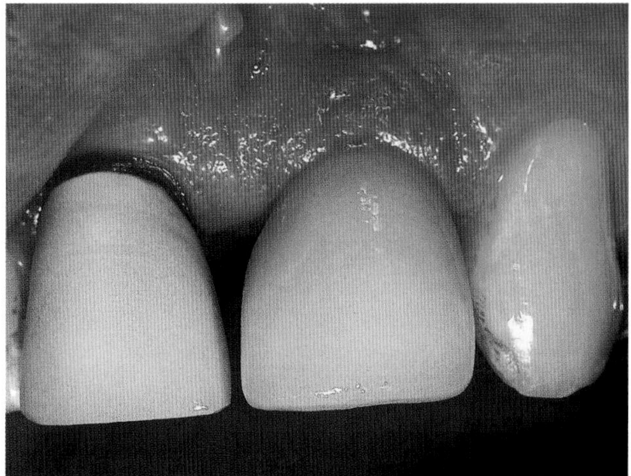

• **Fig. 35.2** Anterior view of the final result 3 years after completion.

used to ensure that the implant is placed at the correct angulation and depth so that the implant does not perforate the cortical bone and allows the final restoration to be constructed with a suitable emergence profile. Careful sterile technique is essential, and particular care must be taken to ensure that the bone is not damaged by overheating. Copious irrigation and slow drill speeds are required. The exact method of insertion and subsequent restoration depends on the type of implant and the manufacturer. The implant is normally left in place for 3–6 months to allow osseointegration before loading. A partial denture would provide a satisfactory temporary replacement during this period.

◆Fig. 35.2 Shows the Result 3 Years After Completion and Fig. 35.3 the Corresponding Radiograph. Is the Implant Osseointegrated and Successful? How Can You Tell?

Osseointegration is the direct structural and functional connection between living bone and the surface of a load-bearing implant. This implant was firm and symptomless and appears successful radiographically. There is bone in close apposition to the implant surface along its whole length. The head of the implant is level with, or only just above, the surrounding bone. Failure would be indicated by mobility, signs of infection, peri-implant radiolucency or progressive marginal bone loss.

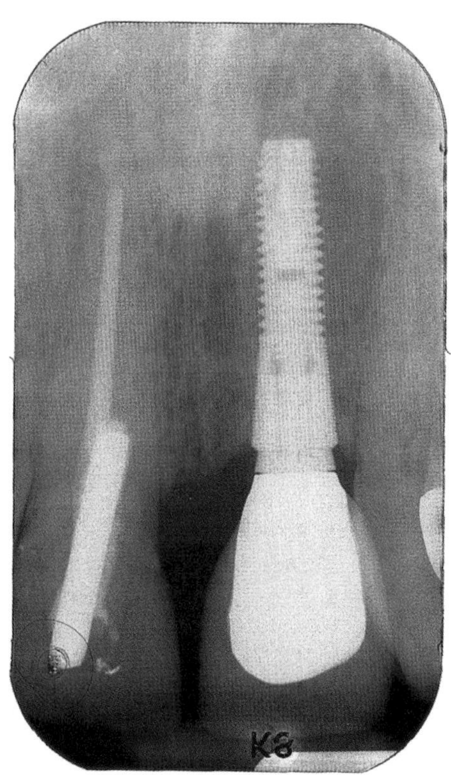

• **Fig. 35.3** Periapical radiograph of the maxillary anterior teeth taken 3 years after completion.

◆ What Factors are Important in Achieving and Maintaining Osseointegration, and Why?

See Table 35.2.

◆ At Each Review, How Would You Determine Whether the Implant is Successful?

- The implant is immobile when tested clinically.

- A periapical radiograph does not reveal any peri-implant radiolucency.
- Radiographs taken at annual visits should reveal stable crestal bone levels after the first year of loading. This can be assessed with periapical radiography using the paralleling technique, to allow reliable comparison between successive radiographs. Ideally, the threads of the implant should be clearly defined to allow accurate assessment of crestal bone levels.
- Vertical bone loss, assessed radiographically, should be less than 0.2 mm per year in subsequent years.
- There is absence of signs and symptoms such as pain, infections, elevated probing, or, for mandibular implants, neuropathies, paraesthesia or a violation of the mandibular canal.
- The aesthetic result remains acceptable.

Acknowledgement

With acknowledgement to Prof. Richard Palmer for the images in this chapter.

TABLE 35.2 Factors Important in Achieving and Maintaining Osseointegration

Factor	Reason
Implant biocompatibility and design	Implants of commercially pure titanium osseointegrate successfully. Titanium alloys and hydroxyapatite are also used but may be less effective.
Implant surface characteristics	A degree of surface roughness is desirable for osseointegration, and much research is currently directed at enhancing optimal surface characteristics. Currently used implant surfaces include machined, blasted, etched, plasma-sprayed or hydroxyapatite-coated types. It is unclear whether any of these offer a significant advantage.
Surgical technique	It is vital that the bone is not overheated during the preparation process. Elevation of the temperature to 47°C for a short period will cause bone cell death, subsequent bone resorption and failure of integration. A careful surgical protocol ensuring drill speeds are not too fast, excess pressure is not applied, and appropriate irrigation for cooling during placement are all important. As with all surgical procedures, careful handling of hard and soft tissues is important.
Bone quality	It is important that the implant is stable immediately after placement for predictable osseointegration. Mobility induces fibrous tissue encapsulation rather than osseointegration. If bone quality is poor, delayed loading may be advisable (see below).
Bone volume	There must be sufficient bone height and width to accommodate the physical size of the implant. In certain circumstances, bone grafting can be used to augment bone volume, but this can affect success rates.
Loading of the implant	It was initially recommended that an implant not be loaded for several months after placement. Most protocols advise a period of healing of 3–6 months. More recently, protocols have changed because evidence has suggested that this is not always necessary, depending on the initial stability of the implant at the time of placement, bone quality and whether grafting was required, and in some cases, immediate restoration and loading are performed. The exact period of healing required depends on bone quality, the type of loading and the implant type and dimensions.
Occlusion	Overloading may result in loss of osseointegration or component failure.
Maintenance care	The patient must achieve and maintain a good level of oral hygiene to avoid peri-implant disease. Regular recall visits are recommended, including assessment of oral hygiene, probing depths around the implant and regular radiographs to monitor bone around the implant.

Case 36

Skateboarding Accident?

JENNIFER C.HARRIS

Summary

A 6-year-old boy with a facial injury attends late one afternoon without an appointment. Assess the child, and decide what treatment he needs.

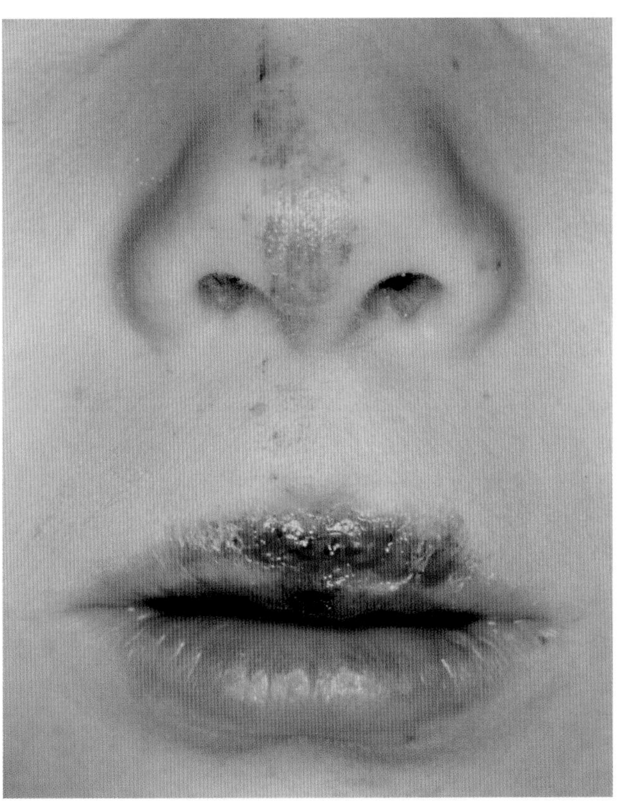

• **Fig. 36.1** The patient's face on presentation.

History

Complaint

The child complains of loose front teeth and that his mouth is sore and it hurts to eat.

History of Complaint

The child's mother says that he fell off his skateboard and banged his teeth. The injury occurred the previous evening when he was playing at a friend's house.

Dental History

The family attend your practice occasionally. The patient had some primary molars extracted under general anaesthesia 6 months ago and has since missed two appointments for review.

Medical History

The patient is otherwise fit and well.

◆ What Do You Need To Know About the Accident?

Further details, including the exact time, whether it was witnessed by others and who was responsible for looking after him at the time, must be sought: Was he knocked out when he fell? What type of surface did he fall on? Were the abrasions or mouth contaminated with soil or other dirty material? Is the patient's tetanus immunization up to date?

Examination

Extraoral Examination

The child looks anxious and withdrawn. Abrasions are present on the tip of the nose and the upper lip, as shown in Fig. 36.1. These have a parallel vertical pattern consistent with scraping on a pavement but are not visibly contaminated by debris. When asked if he has injuries elsewhere, he does not respond at first and then shows abrasions on his knees and elbows.

On examining his face, you notice faint parallel lines of petechial bruising running horizontally across the left side of his neck (Fig. 36.2) and bruising on both the outer and inner surfaces of the right ear (Fig. 36.3). No other injuries are visible on those parts of his arms and legs that are not covered by clothing.

Intraoral Examination

The patient's upper anterior teeth and lip are shown in Fig. 36.4.

◆ What Do You See?

He is in the early mixed dentition, has poor oral hygiene and no obvious caries. There are abrasions on the vermilion border and inner surface of the upper lip. The upper labial frenum is torn and bruised. The upper left primary central incisor has bleeding around the gingival margin and is displaced palatally.

On examination of the patient, you find that both upper primary central incisors are slightly mobile and tender to pressure. The displaced incisor is not causing occlusal interference.

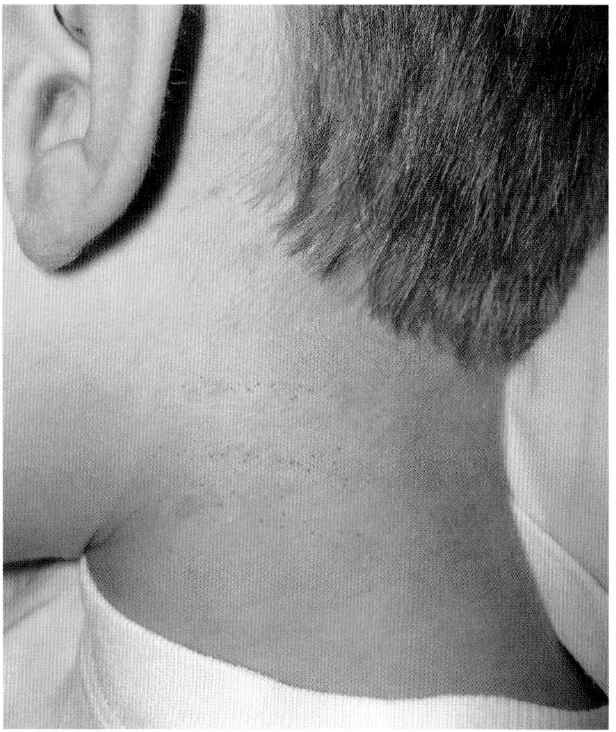

• **Fig. 36.2** The left side of the patient's neck.

◆ You Should Already Be Suspicious About Some Aspects of This History. What Further Information Would You Ask?

Whether he has already received any medical attention and why dental care was not sought sooner. Who was looking after the child when he was injured?

You should also ask the child himself about the cause of the injury, particularly allowing him to talk and volunteer information without asking leading questions.

When you ask the patient what happened to him, he looks away and says nothing. When you note the marks on the neck and ear, his mother looks uncomfortable and says, 'He fell off a wall last week. He's very accident prone.'

Investigations

◆ What Radiographs Would You Take and Why?

A periapical view of the primary upper incisors should be taken to show the extent of physiological root resorption, any displacement or root fractures and the proximity of the developing permanent incisors. As well as aiding diagnosis, the radiograph will act as a baseline for future monitoring.

If a periapical film is too uncomfortable to hold, an occlusal view or occlusal taken with a periapical film or detector may prove more acceptable.

◆ The Radiograph is Shown in Fig. 36.5. What Do You See?

All permanent incisors are present and appear to be relatively distant from the primary tooth roots. There is resorption of the upper primary central incisor roots, consistent with the patient's age.

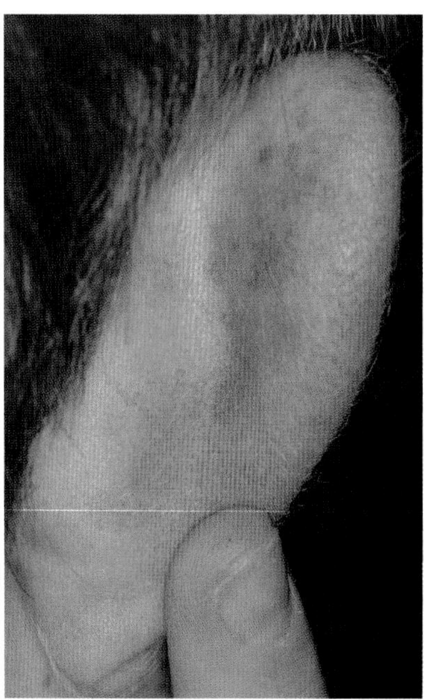

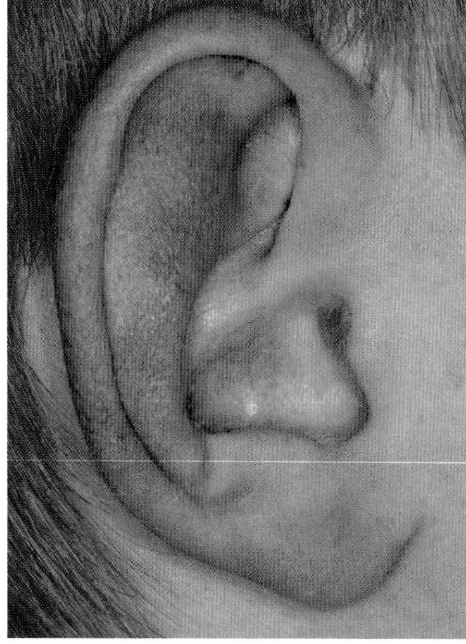

• **Fig. 36.3** The patient's right ear.

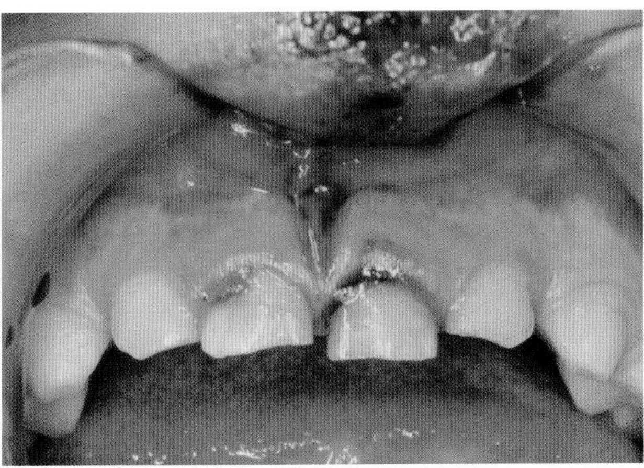

• **Fig. 36.4** The mouth at presentation.

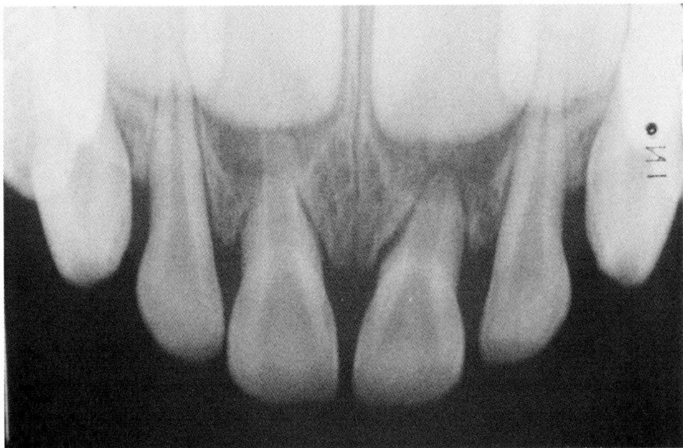

• **Fig. 36.5** Radiographic image.

There is increased periodontal ligament space and displacement of the upper left primary central incisor, but no other abnormalities.

Diagnosis

◆ What is Your Diagnosis?

Facial abrasions, intraoral soft tissue injuries, subluxation of the upper right primary central incisor and lateral luxation of the upper left primary central incisor.

The findings are consistent with the history of an accidental fall from a skateboard but are accompanied by bruises on the neck and ear, which give cause for concerns about possible physical abuse.

◆ What Factors in the History Make You Concerned That This May Be Child Abuse or Neglect?

- The history is vague and does not fully explain the injuries observed.
- There was some delay in seeking dental care, without satisfactory explanation.
- There was possibly a lack of adult supervision to ensure his safety.

◆ Why Does the History Not Explain the Injuries?

- There are injuries to soft tissues not overlying bony prominences: in this case, the neck and ear.
- There are injuries to both sides of the body: the left side of the neck and right ear.
- The pattern of bruising on his neck is suggestive of a slap mark. There are parallel lines of petechial haemorrhages between the fingers, where blood was forced out of capillaries by the force of the slap.
- Bruising on both inner and outer aspects of the pinna of the ear suggests injury from pinching or pulling.
- The neck and ear are rarely injured in accidental falls because they lie in a 'triangle of safety', protected by the shoulder and the parietal area of the skull.

You might also have a sense of unease about the boy's behaviour and interaction with his mother. The patient seems unwilling to talk about the cause of the injury.

◆ How Certain Can You Be That Injuries are Not Accidental?

Care must always be exercised when interpreting injuries. It is important to realize that there are no specific injuries that are diagnostic of abuse, even though some patterns of injury are highly suggestive of it. There will almost always be a degree of uncertainty, especially with the type of injuries seen in a dental setting. In all such cases, you are likely to be weighing evidence from a variety of sources and must come to a judgement yourself. There are no easy answers.

A torn labial frenum used to be considered diagnostic of abuse, but it is now recognized that it may also result from an accident. In this case, accompanied by other intraoral injuries, it would not, in itself, cause you to suspect abuse. However, if seen in a young child who is not yet walking and is, therefore, unlikely to have fallen, it is a sign that should always be taken seriously and discussed with an experienced colleague.

◆ What General Risk Factors for Child Abuse are Recognized?

Recognized risk factors are shown in Table 36.1. Such features may be noted during the appointment, be identified from previous knowledge of the family or be present in your dental records. They may be helpful when deciding how to interpret your findings and in deciding what to do.

Treatment

◆ What Dental Treatment is Necessary?

Advise analgesia, as required; the drug of choice in this age group is paracetamol suspension. Recommend a soft diet. Give instruction in oral hygiene, including use of chlorhexidine gel applied twice daily for a week. Advise the mother and patient to return if there is increasing pain or swelling.

Inform the parent of the possibility of damage to developing permanent teeth and the need for follow-up. Make the first follow-up appointment after 1 week.

TABLE 36.1 Risk Factors for Child Abuse and Neglect

Parental	Social	Child
Parents needing additional support to meet child's needs	**Families living in adverse social environments**	**Children in need of additional help to safeguard their welfare**
Young parents	Poverty	Babies and toddlers are most vulnerable
Single parents	Social isolation	Children with disabilities
Parents with learning difficulties	Poor housing	Older children, particularly girls, are more vulnerable to sexual abuse
Mental health problems	Family violence	Children with behavioural problems
Drug and alcohol abuse		Children looked after in foster care or residential care

Splinting the teeth is unnecessary and would hinder the recommended oral hygiene procedures.

◆ What Else Should You Do?

The injuries to the mouth were probably caused in a skateboard accident. They are consistent with this explanation and accompanied by injury on the elbows and knees. However, there are unexplained injuries on the neck and ear. You need to decide what must be done about these additional injuries.

It is often helpful to discuss the case with a suitably experienced colleague or advisor such as a nurse or social worker from the local safeguarding children advisory service. Telephone numbers for advice and referral should be available in the practice. A flowchart to guide your actions is shown in Fig. 36.6.

In this case, it is likely that you would be advised to make an immediate referral to children's services (alternatively known as 'social services'). A full assessment of the child is needed to determine whether the unexplained injuries have occurred as part of a pattern of sustained and deliberate child abuse or may be the result of momentary loss of control by a frustrated parent (or other individual inside or outside the family). This child may urgently need protection, or the family may need advice and support.

◆ What Do You Say To the Child and the Parent?

Explain that you are concerned about the marks on his neck and ear and that you need to arrange for someone else to look at him. Ask for consent to phone children's services to share this information. If the parent questions whether this is really necessary, you will need to stand your ground and give further explanation. You should explain that your responsibility is not simply the health of the boy's teeth but also his general welfare and safety and that you recognize that his mother will want that too. Research shows that being open and honest from the start results in better outcomes for children.

◆ Are There Any Circumstances in Which You Would Not Discuss Child Protection Concerns with the Parents?

Although it is generally considered good practice to explain your concerns to the child and his or her parents, there are certain exceptions:

- Where discussion might put the child at greater risk
- Where discussion would impede a police investigation or social work inquiry
- Where sexual abuse by a family member or organized/multiple abuse is suspected
- Where fabricated or induced illness (formerly known as *Munchausen syndrome by proxy*) is suspected
- Where parents or carers are being violent or abusive, and discussion would place you or your staff at risk
- When parents or carers are not present and it is not possible to contact them without causing undue delay in making the referral.

In these circumstances, first seek advice from your dental defence organization or from senior child protection professionals. Reasonable judgement must be made in each case.

◆ What Do You Do Next?

Phone children's services to make a child protection referral. You will be asked to give the full name of the child, date of birth, address, gender, school and the name of the person(s) with parental responsibility. Discuss your concerns, and agree on what will happen next. Agree with the social worker what you will tell the parent and child and what will happen next.

◆ Anything Else To Remember?

You need to keep comprehensive contemporaneous clinical records, including any explanation given by the parent and the child in their own words. You should include both a written description and a diagram of the injuries. Differences between fact and your opinion should be clearly stated. You should include a summary of the discussions with the child and the parent.

If other members of the dental team have been involved, they also should record their observations.

◆ What Action is Required Later?

The telephone referral must be followed up in writing within 48 hours. Children's services should confirm receipt of the referral, decide on the next course of action and give feedback to you.

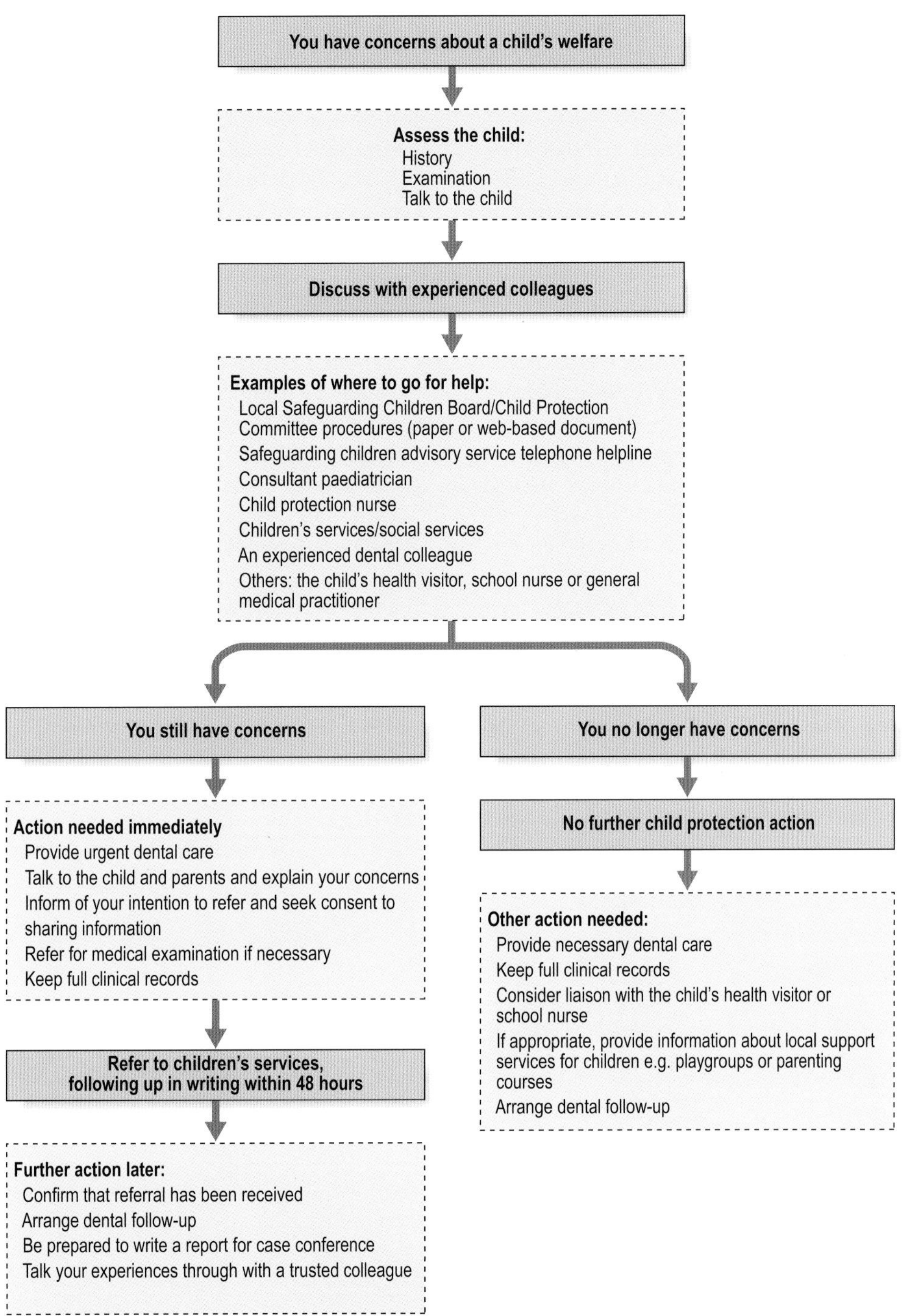

• **Fig. 36.6** Flowchart for child protection action. (Adapted with kind permission of Committee of Postgraduate Dental Deans and Directors (COPDEND), from Harris, J., Sidebotham, P., Welbury, R., et al. (2006). *Child protection and the dental team: An introduction to safeguarding children in dental practice.* Sheffield: COPDEND. Available at: www.cpdt.org.uk, www.bda.org/childprotection, updated 2013.)

If you hear nothing, you should telephone again to confirm that your referral has been received and acted on. You should be prepared to write a report for a child protection case conference, if requested to do so. You will also need to ensure that the child receives a follow-up dental appointment.

It is important to acknowledge that involvement in child protection cases can be distressing. If necessary, take time to talk through your experiences with a trusted colleague, or seek further advice from the safeguarding advisory service.

Research shows that dentists do not always respond effectively when they recognize signs of child abuse and neglect. This is a serious matter: It may be some years before another opportunity arises for someone to take action to protect the child from the misery of ongoing maltreatment. Furthermore, to ignore suspicions about abuse could result in a complaint against you and may put your registration at risk or lead to a professional negligence claim. The General Dental Council's ethical standards guidance makes it clear that all members of the dental team must 'follow local child protection procedures if you suspect that a child might be at risk because of abuse or neglect'.

When dentists are asked why they do not follow child protection procedures correctly, they often say that they want to be really certain before taking action. You can be reassured that the responsibility for making a diagnosis of abuse is not something you have to shoulder alone but is always shared by a multiagency team. Discuss your concerns with the experts and refer early.

Do not fear that the family will suffer drastic action. Children are only removed from their families when there is no safe alternative. Emphasis is usually given to supporting the family to protect their own children.

You may be concerned about possible litigation if you get it wrong, yet the law places the child's welfare as paramount and protects healthcare professionals who make child protection referrals in good faith. This is a challenging area of practice, but expert help is available.

◆ Is Dental Neglect Abuse?

Child abuse is defined in four categories: physical abuse, emotional abuse, sexual abuse and neglect. Abuse or neglect may be by inflicting harm or by failing to prevent harm. Recently, there has been increased agreement that severe untreated dental disease can indicate neglect and should prompt a child protection referral.

Under the United Nations Convention on the Rights of the Child 1989, children have a right to 'the enjoyment of the highest attainable standard of health and to facilities for the treatment of illness and rehabilitation of health'. To enjoy optimal oral health, children need their parents to provide a suitable diet, facilities for and help with oral hygiene and access to dental treatment when needed. There is no doubt that oral disease can have a significant impact on a child's general health and can cause pain, loss of sleep and even poor growth and quality of life. Once dental problems have been explained to parents or carers, and appropriate and acceptable dental treatment has been offered to restore oral health, the following would be of concern:

- Repeated missed appointments
- Failure to complete planned treatment
- Repeatedly returning in pain
- Requiring repeated general anaesthesia for dental extractions.

Preschool children are particularly vulnerable, and in such cases, it is recommended that you contact the child's health visitor to discuss how you might work together to support the family to ensure that the child's needs are met. This contributes to 'safeguarding' children, namely, not only protecting children from abuse and neglect but also taking a wider range of measures to promote their health and development and to minimize risks of harm. In many cases, lack of knowledge and difficulty accessing care account for the apparent neglect. However, if a child is suffering significant harm from untreated dental disease, it will be necessary to make a child protection referral without delay.

Case 37

An Adverse Reaction

CHRIS DICKINSON

Summary

A 38-year-old woman becomes unwell during routine dental treatment at your general dental practice. What would you do? What is the cause?

History

Complaint

The patient is to have a crown preparation performed on her lower second molar and a very small amalgam placed in an upper premolar on the same side. You have given an infiltration of 1.0 ml lidocaine (lignocaine) 2% with adrenaline (epinephrine) 1:80 000 (12.5 µg/ml) and used a further 2-ml cartridge to give an inferior dental and lingual nerve block. Having finished injecting, you turn away to prepare some instruments. Almost immediately the patient says she feels ill. She is clearly apprehensive and is holding her chest complaining of palpitations.

Dental Treatment History

The patient is in the middle of her first course of treatment in many years. She has been scared about visiting a dentist for some years. You have started a course of treatment and carried out several simple restorative procedures. You had seen her only 2 days ago to place several direct restorations, using three cartridges of a local anaesthetic. These restorations and one extraction have all been carried out under local anaesthesia using lidocaine (lignocaine) 2% with adrenaline (epinephrine) 1:80 000.

Medical History

The patient is apparently fit and well. The medical history indicates no allergies.

◆ What Would You Do?

- Reassure the patient; encourage regular breathing.
- Have her lie down supine or with her head slightly down.
- Feel the skin and take her pulse.
- Prepare oxygen in case it is needed.

This approach applies unless the patient were pregnant or obese, in which case having her lie flat on her side would be more appropriate.

◆ One Minute Later, the Patient Feels No Improvement. What Would You Do?

- Take the blood pressure, and monitor her pulse.
- Check for pallor.
- Check for rash or urticaria.
- Wait and observe for dyspnoea while considering possible causes.

◆ What Causes Would You Consider?

Intravascular injection of the local anaesthetic appears to be the most likely cause of her symptoms because they started immediately after the inferior dental block. However, vasovagal attacks are common, and an acute medical or mental health problem unrelated to dentistry should not be excluded. Thus, possible causes include:

- vasovagal attack
- adverse reaction to the local anaesthetic
- hypersensitivity reaction
- myocardial infarction or angina attack
- acute anxiety (panic) attack.

◆ Is This a Vasovagal Attack? Explain Why.

The features of a vasovagal attack are pallor, apprehension, restlessness, nausea, bradycardia, weak slow pulse and loss of consciousness (fainting). The loss of consciousness may be immediate. In more severe attacks, there may be clonic muscle contractions or rigidity as a result of cerebral hypoxia. None of these symptoms is seen in this patient. In addition, vasovagal attacks are usually caused by fear or anxiety and so may precede the injection. Patients will usually be able to explain that they feel faint either before or after the attack.

◆ Is This is Myocardial Infarction?

No. The symptoms and signs of myocardial infarction are crushing central chest pain, sometimes radiating to the arm or the neck, dyspnoea and possibly vomiting, which may be followed by cardiac arrest. There is usually, although not always, an individual or family history of angina, coronary artery disease or hypertension.

TABLE 37.1 **Unwanted Effects of Local Anaesthesia**

Type of Reaction	Unwanted Effect	Signs and Symptoms
Immediate	Neuralgic pain from needle penetrating nerve	Electric shock pain on injection, sometimes followed by prolonged anaesthesia
	Vasomotor effect of intravascular injection of vasoconstrictor	Tachycardia without hypertension, in overdose arrhythmias. Occasionally, skin blanching on face or neck in the event of arterial injection
	Facial paralysis from intraparotid injection	Paralysis of one or more branches of facial nerve; may mimic Bell's palsy
	Anaphylaxis caused by hypersensitivity to one or more of the components of the anaesthetic solution	Anaphylactic shock, local or systemic oedema, urticaria, asthma, hypotension, pulmonary oedema, tachycardia, breathlessness and circulatory collapse
	Drug interaction	Although theoretically many are possible, none is a practical possibility at normal dosage
	Central nervous system stimulation or depression caused by overdose of lidocaine (lignocaine)	Only seen in large overdose. Sometimes initial apprehension, excitability or confusion or muscle spasm followed by respiratory and cardiac depression
	Rare complications such as needle breakage or infection	
Delayed	Trismus or local trauma from injection, haematoma formation or damage to analgesic tissue caused by the patient	Vary with effect
	Transmission of infection	Vary with infection

◆ What are the Unwanted Effects of Local Anaesthesia with Lidocaine (Lignocaine) and Adrenaline (Epinephrine)? What are Their Causes and Signs and Symptoms?

See Table 37.1.

While these possibilities run through your mind, the patient remains conscious but nervous and agitated. She gradually calms down and says that the palpitations are reducing. She takes a few breaths of oxygen but refuses more after a few minutes and says that she feels better. Her pulse is 105 beats/min and her blood pressure is 140/90 mmHg.

Differential Diagnosis

◆ What is Your Differential Diagnosis, and Why?

Intravascular injection is the most likely diagnosis, the patient's symptoms being caused by the vasoconstrictor component of the local anaesthetic. The solution contains 1:80 000 adrenaline (epinephrine), which causes tachycardia felt by the patient as palpitations. Intravascular injection is most common after inferior dental blocks and posterior superior dental blocks because of the high vascularity of the injection site.

Anxiety can itself produce a significant level of adrenaline, but levels rise more slowly; and the patient would have to be very nervous, positively phobic, to generate endogenous adrenaline to the levels found in intravascular injection of the local anaesthetic. This patient is nervous but has recently accepted routine dental treatment without problems. A vasovagal attack would be a much more likely effect of marked anxiety, but a panic attack brought on by the emotional response to the tachycardia will need to be managed.

◆ Could the Local Anaesthetic Given 2 Days Ago Contribute To This Reaction?

No, the adrenaline (epinephrine) will have been rapidly moved into the circulation from the site of injection in spite of its intrinsic vasoconstrictor effect. Its action is then terminated quickly by reuptake into the noradrenergic fibres and other cells and tissues. Metabolism takes place within these at various sites throughout the body by the action of the enzyme catechol-*O*-methyl transferase and to a much lesser degree by monoamine oxidase in the liver before undergoing renal excretion.

As far as the local anaesthetic component is concerned, the symptoms experienced by this patient are not typical of an overdose, and in any event, the half-life of lidocaine (lignocaine) is only of the order of 90 minutes. Therefore, this event being related to either the local anaesthetic or the vasoconstrictor given at the previous appointment can be safely ruled out.

TABLE 37.2 Maximum Recommended Doses

Drug	Maximum Dose	Equivalent Cartridges for a 70 kg Male
Lidocaine (lignocaine) and mepivacaine	4.4 mg/kg	For 2% solutions, about eight 1.8-ml or six-and-a-half 2.2-ml cartridges For 3% mepivacaine, five-and-a-half 1.8-ml or four-and-a-half 2.2-ml cartridges
Prilocaine	6 mg/kg	For 3% prilocaine, about seven 1.8-ml or six 2.2-ml cartridges For 4% prilocaine, about five-and-a-half 1.8-ml and four-and-a-half 2.2-ml cartridges
Articaine	7 mg/kg	For 4% articaine, about six-and-a-half 1.7-ml and five-and-a-half 2.2-ml cartridges

◆ Is an Overdose Possible? What are the Maximum Recommended Doses of Local Anaesthetic Solutions Used in Dentistry?

Although theoretically possible, it is actually quite difficult to administer an overdose of a local anaesthetic in dentistry. Because of the nature of the cartridge syringe and needle system used, doses are accurately counted and monitored, and the need to change a cartridge affords 'thinking time' for the operator. This is in contrast to the use of a local anaesthetic in the other areas of the body where large volumes of drug can be administered into body spaces more easily.

However, one cannot be complacent. In recent years, the recommendations for maximum safe doses of local anaesthetics in the head and neck area have been reviewed. Because of the vascularity of the region and the recognition that vasoconstrictors do not hold the drug in place for as long as was previously thought, the recommendations have been rationalized and the maximum recommended doses reduced.

It is important to realize that advice based on a recommended number of cartridges or fixed dose does not take into account different formulations. Some cartridges contain only 1.8 ml of solution, whereas others contain 2.2 ml and, therefore, 22% more drug. Thus, four cartridges of the larger volume will contain almost the same dose of the local anaesthetic and vasoconstrictor as five of the 1.8-ml cartridges. The concentration of drug also varies from preparation to preparation. Importantly, patients come in different shapes and sizes, and fixed dose recommendations are based on the safety limit for the elusive 'fit 70-kg man'!

Another way to consider the safe total dose is to relate it to body weight and the amount in a dental local anaesthetic cartridge (which varies among drugs).

Thus, 2% lidocaine in a 2.2-ml cartridge is equivalent to 44 mg of drug. With a maximum safe dose of 4.4 mg/kg, a single cartridge could be administered for every 10 kg of body weight. For a 70-kg male, the maximum safe dose would be seven cartridges, and for a 20-kg child, the maximum safe dose would be two cartridges.

Current recommendations are expressed in the form of the maximum safe dose per kilogram of body weight given over a period of treatment of 1 hour. The maximum recommended doses are shown in Table 37.2.

These limits apply to all preparations of local anaesthetics irrespective of the presence of or type of vasoconstrictor. It is no longer considered that larger doses are safe to be given in one treatment session if the preparation contains vasoconstrictor.

◆ Immediately After Calming Down, the Patient Claims That She Must Be Allergic To the Local Anaesthetic. Is This Possible?

It is possible but is extremely rare. Only a handful of cases of genuine lidocaine (lignocaine) hypersensitivity have been recorded. Very few older patients have given a convincing history of allergy to local anaesthetics, in some cases backed up by hospital investigations. This is because older preparations contained preservatives such as benzoates to which hypersensitivity was possible. The worst offending preservatives are no longer used, although a reaction to sodium metabisulphite preservative has been reported on rare occasions. Patients can be tested for hypersensitivity to anaesthetic agents, but this is only worthwhile when a typical allergic reaction is suspected.

Hypersensitivity is unlikely to follow repeat administration of lidocaine (lignocaine) for dental anaesthesia. A much more potent cause is repeat application of lidocaine (lignocaine) creams to the skin. Local anaesthetic pastes and solutions should be handled with care; the dentist is more at risk compared with the patient.

◆ Would a Switch To Prilocaine with Felypressin in the Future Be Prudent?

No, lidocaine (lignocaine) with adrenaline (epinephrine) has been used successfully in the past for this patient, and there is no evidence of an idiosyncratic or allergic response to the preparation itself. Prilocaine produces a shorter period of analgesia, and the patient should not be subjected to suboptimal pain relief because of the remote possibility of another intravascular injection. There is no evidence that prilocaine, with or without felypressin, is safer.

Such a switch would reinforce the patient's perception that she is allergic to local anaesthetics. A spurious history of allergy might compromise the patient's general health. Lidocaine (lignocaine) is used in the emergency treatment of myocardial infarction and in many other medical situations.

◆ How Can the Risk of Intravascular Injection Be Minimized?

Good injection technique is the key to reducing the risks associated with intravascular injection because it ensures that the minimum amount of anaesthetic solution is used. The solution should be injected slowly, thus reducing the risk of injecting a bolus into a vessel. An aspirating technique should always be used, even though it does not always guarantee success; because of the narrow needle diameters used in dentistry, aspiration is relatively poor.

It is impossible to completely avoid the tip of the needle entering a vessel. Indeed, in some very vascular areas, penetration of a vessel is not the cause because the solution can be absorbed into blood almost as rapidly as it can be injected. Nothing can guarantee the prevention of complications of intravascular injection.

Another Possibility

◆ If the Patient Had Genuine Anaphylaxis, What Causative Agents Would You Consider?

Anaphylaxis to other agents is considerably commoner than hypersensitivity to local anaesthetics. A number of other agents used in dental surgery should be considered before the local anaesthetic is suspected.

Latex hypersensitivity is increasing in prevalence and is commoner in patients with atopia and those who have come into contact with latex repeatedly such as healthcare workers, those with spina bifida or those who are subjected to multiple surgical procedures. Rubber dam, gloves and even traces of rubber from local anaesthetic cartridges or drug vials can trigger reactions. Other less obvious items that may contain latex are face masks with elastic components, amalgam carriers, plastic syringes, aspirator tubes, orthodontic elastics and emergency equipment such as ventilating bags and sphygmomanometer cuffs.

Although some items containing natural rubber latex may still exist, most are being phased out now and are being replaced by silicone or the synthetic 'nitrile' rubber (acrylonitrile butadiene rubber, Buna-N, NBR), which is a copolymer. However, allergies to nitrile products have been reported, albeit extremely rarely.

These usually cause type 1 reactions such as urticaria, asthma or anaphylactic shock. Glove powder is a particularly potent vehicle for dissemination of the latex allergen into the atmosphere; therefore, to reduce the risk of allergy developing among the dental team, use of powdered gloves should be avoided. In addition to allergy to latex, staff and, more rarely, patients may develop hypersensitivity to acrylics, composite resins, dentine bonding agents, eugenol, cleaning and disinfection solutions and metal alloys. Almost all materials may be allergenic to some individuals. The formulations of the worst offending agents have been changed, and the most notorious ones, particularly some synthetic impression materials and self-curing acrylics, are no longer available in their original forms. It is worth remembering that many of these agents are irritant as well as allergenic and that rashes may not be true hypersensitivity reactions.

Case 38

Advanced Periodontitis

MANDEEP GHUMAN

Summary

A 49-year-old woman has periodontitis. Diagnose and plan management of her condition.

History

Complaint

The patient complains of two loose upper back teeth, and the teeth feel fleetingly sensitive to hot and cold.

History of Complaint

She is an irregular dental attender at your practice and had last seen your colleague 3 years ago prior to his retirement. The clinical notes show that he had diagnosed generalized severe chronic periodontitis and carried out a course of nonsurgical periodontal treatment, but the patient did not attend for review because of her busy work schedule. Despite the past treatment, on presentation, several teeth are loose, and the patient reports dental sensitivity as well as occasional soreness when gums are inflamed. She also recalls having gum abscesses on at least two occasions in the past and being prescribed antibiotics.

Besides having all her third molars extracted 20 years ago, she cannot recall having any other extractions.

Medical History

The patient reports being fit and well, takes no medications, and has no allergies, as revealed by her medical history questionnaire.

◆ What Additional Specific Questions Will You Ask the Patient? Explain Why

Oral Hygiene Regimen. The patient tells you that she cleans her teeth twice daily with an electric toothbrush. She uses floss on her anterior teeth every day and only occasionally on her molars and premolars, where access is more difficult.

Current or Past Smoking. Smoking increases the risk of periodontitis five-fold. This patient has never smoked.

Presence of Diabetes or Any Other Condition Causing Susceptibility To Infection. Poorly controlled diabetes has a strong association with periodontitis. This is relatively severe periodontitis, and there is a history of multiple abscesses. These features do not necessarily indicate an underlying condition, but it would be worthwhile to exclude diabetes and ask the patient to see her doctor to be tested. Another feature that might suggest diabetes is rapid attachment loss within a short period in middle age, suggesting type 2 diabetes.

Family History of Premature Tooth Loss. A positive family history can be associated with development of periodontitis at a younger age.

Stressful Life. Patients who cope poorly with stress are more likely to develop periodontitis.

Examination

Extraoral Examination

No cervical lymphadenopathy is present. The temporomandibular joint and mandibular movements appear normal.

Intraoral Examination

The other mucosa and soft tissues of the mouth are normal except for a buccal sinus just anterior to the upper right first premolar. All teeth, with the exception of the third molars, are present. All remaining molars and two premolars contain small- to medium-sized amalgam restorations. No caries is detected.

◆ How Will You Assess the Patient's Periodontal Health and Oral Hygiene?

On examination of the mouth, the inflammatory status of the gingival tissues should be assessed visually, noting any redness, swelling and increased inflammatory exudate. The presence, location and extent of any visible plaque or calculus should also be noted, and can be recorded by using various indices. A common index used is the Plaque Control Record (Fig. 38.1), where a disclosing solution is painted on all exposed tooth surfaces. After the patient has rinsed her mouth, using a probe, the operator examines each stained surface for plaque at the gingival margin. If plaque is found, the information is recorded on the form in the appropriate spaces. After all the teeth are examined and scored, the index is calculated by dividing the number of plaque-containing surfaces by the total number of available surfaces.

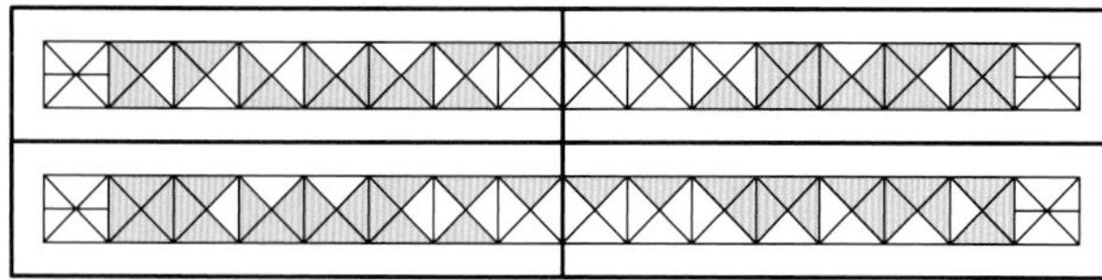

• **Fig. 38.1** An example of a plaque control record. Plaque was detected on 67 of the 112 surfaces, giving a score of 60%.

In this case, previous clinical records have documented pre-existing periodontitis, and this should trigger a full periodontal assessment immediately. In the case of a patient who has not previously been encountered and does not present with historical periodontitis ascertained through history and examination (interproximal recession), the health of the periodontal tissues should be screened by performing the Basic Periodontal Examination (BPE) with a World Health Organization (WHO) probe.

The measurements that form a full periodontal assessment are:

- probing depths with bleeding on probing
- recession
- mobility
- furcation involvement

Probing depth and recession and measurements are made at six points around the circumference of a tooth: mesially, at the midpoint and distally on the buccal and palatal surfaces. Probing depths are measured from the gingival margin to the base of the periodontal pocket. Presence or absence of bleeding on probing should always be recorded in conjunction with a six-point pocket chart. The presence and extent of palpable subgingival calculus should also be briefly noted. The distance from the cemento-enamel junction to the gingival margin indicates the amount of recession. The sum of recession and probing depth gives the extent of clinical attachment loss (CAL).

Measurements are described in Table 38.1.

Clinical photographs and results of these examinations are shown in Figs 38.2 and 38.3, respectively. The patient's clinical appearance is not immediately suggestive of severe periodontal problems, and the relatively minor amount of clearly visible plaque and gingival inflammation appear disproportionate to the extensive CAL. This highlights the patient's susceptibility to periodontitis and the importance of periodontal screening and subsequent comprehensive clinical assessment.

On closer inspection, gingival inflammation is more noticeable palatally, and suppuration can be seen to be associated with the upper left lateral incisor distally, upper right first molar and upper left first premolar teeth. Furthermore, loss of the papilla between the upper central incisors could be indicative of previously treated periodontitis.

Investigations

◆ What Radiographs Would You Take, and Why?

See Table 38.2.

◆ Selected Periapical Radiographs Were Taken, As Shown in Fig. 38.4. What Do You See?

The radiographs show widespread bone loss extending to or beyond the middle or apical third of the roots of most teeth, correlating with the probing depths. Angular intrabony defects are associated with the upper second molar, upper right first premolar, upper right canine, upper left lateral incisor and all lower molar teeth. These are interspersed with areas of moderate (<33%) horizontal bone loss. Furcation bone loss is associated with all upper molar and lower right molar teeth. Periapical radiolucencies are associated with the upper right first molar and the upper left first premolar.

◆ Full Mouth Periapical Radiographs Were Also Taken 4 Years Previously, As Shown in Fig. 38.5. What Differences Can You See Between the Two Sets of Views?

The bone loss is less severe, and there has been rapid progression in multiple areas within a relatively short period (5 years).

◆ What Further Examinations or Investigations Would You Perform?

Sensibility tests are indicated for all teeth with severe attachment loss for possible pulp involvement. This would include all molars, the upper right canine and the first premolar, and the upper left lateral incisor and the first premolar.

◆ Are Any Other Investigations Necessary?

Yes, the patient should be advised to see her general medical practitioner to exclude diabetes. At a later appointment, she reported that the diabetes test result was negative.

Diagnosis

◆ What is Your Diagnosis?

Under the previous periodontal disease classification system (1999), this case would have been diagnosed as generalized severe chronic periodontitis. Additional diagnoses include endodontic–periodontal lesions of the upper right first molar, upper left first premolar and lower left second molar.

The periodontal disease classification system has since been revised (2017), and staging and grading of periodontitis is now similar to staging and grading in oncology. The system has been simplified by the British Society of Periodontology to make it workable for clinicians (see References). Staging of periodontitis reflects the severity and extent of the disease and is based on radiographic bone loss (Table 38.3). Periodontitis should also now be graded to estimate future risk of disease progression and responsiveness to standard management. If previous radiographs are not available to assess the rapidity of bony destruction, grading is calculated using the ratio of percentage bone loss adjusting for age (see Tables 38.3 and 38.4). In this case, because previous radiographs were available (see Fig. 38.5) clearly showing evidence of rapid destruction, calculating the ratio was not necessary. When known risk factors are

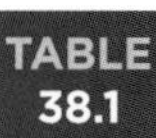

TABLE 38.1 Measurements for Full Periodontal Assessment

	Meaning of Score	Significance of Score
Pocket Depths		
0–3 mm	Normal range	
4–5 mm	Mostly likely reflects mild to moderate periodontitis (stage I or II in 2017 classification)	Nonsurgical periodontal therapy likely to be indicated
6 mm+	More likely to have severe or very severe periodontitis (stage III or IV 2017 classification)	Additional therapy may be needed
Recession		
	Indicative of attachment loss caused by past disease	Important to record, in addition to probing depth, to assess true extent of periodontal tissue loss
Bleeding on Probing		
Absent	None	Inactive site – periodontitis progression unlikely
Present	Bleeding	Active inflammation, but not necessarily indicative of disease progression N.B. In smokers, bleeding may be less than expected for the disease activity.
Tooth Mobility		
Degree 1	Movement of the crown of the tooth between 0.2 and 1 mm in a horizontal direction	Minor movement, possibly physiological If periodontal disease present, treat conservatively
Degree 2	Movement of the crown of the tooth exceeding 1 mm in a horizontal direction	Caused by loss of attachment The degree of mobility depends on remaining periodontal support and the shape of the roots Conical roots on molars are more likely to develop mobility than divergent roots on teeth with a similar degree of attachment loss
Degree 3	Movement of the crown of the tooth in a vertical and horizontal direction	Indicates bone loss below the apex and little or no bony support Usually indicates a need for extraction
Furcation Involvement		
Degree 1	Horizontal loss of supporting tissues not exceeding one-third of the width of the tooth	Early furcation involvement Can be treated effectively in the long term with conservative nonsurgical periodontal treatment; predisposes to further and more rapid attachment loss if untreated
Degree 2	Horizontal loss of supporting tissue exceeding one-third but not a 'through and through' lesion	Much more difficult to keep clean Unlikely to respond to conservative treatment alone
Degree 3	A 'through and through' lesion	May be easier to clean depending on soft tissue contour The prognosis for the tooth would depend on the location of the involvement, the remaining amount of periodontal attachment and the length and shape of the roots Indicates susceptibility to furcation caries and risk of loss of vitality

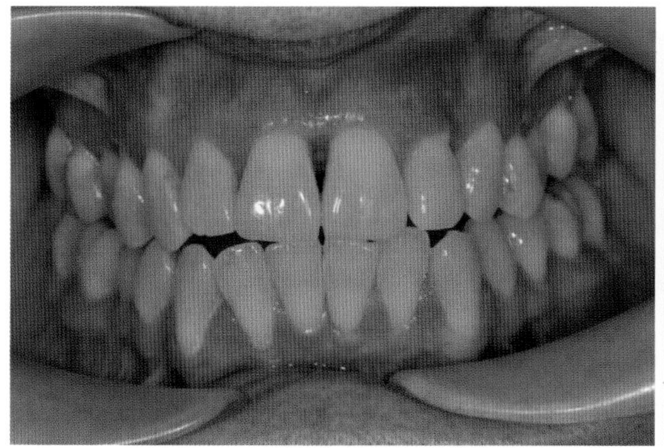
a

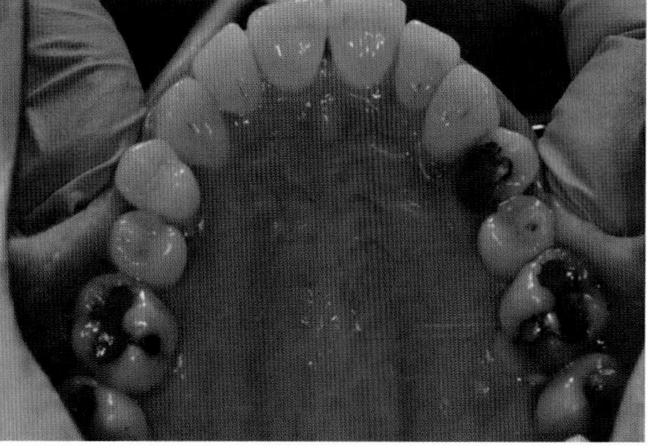
b

• **Fig. 38.2 a,** Anterior, **b,** upper occlusal views at presentation (see text for details).

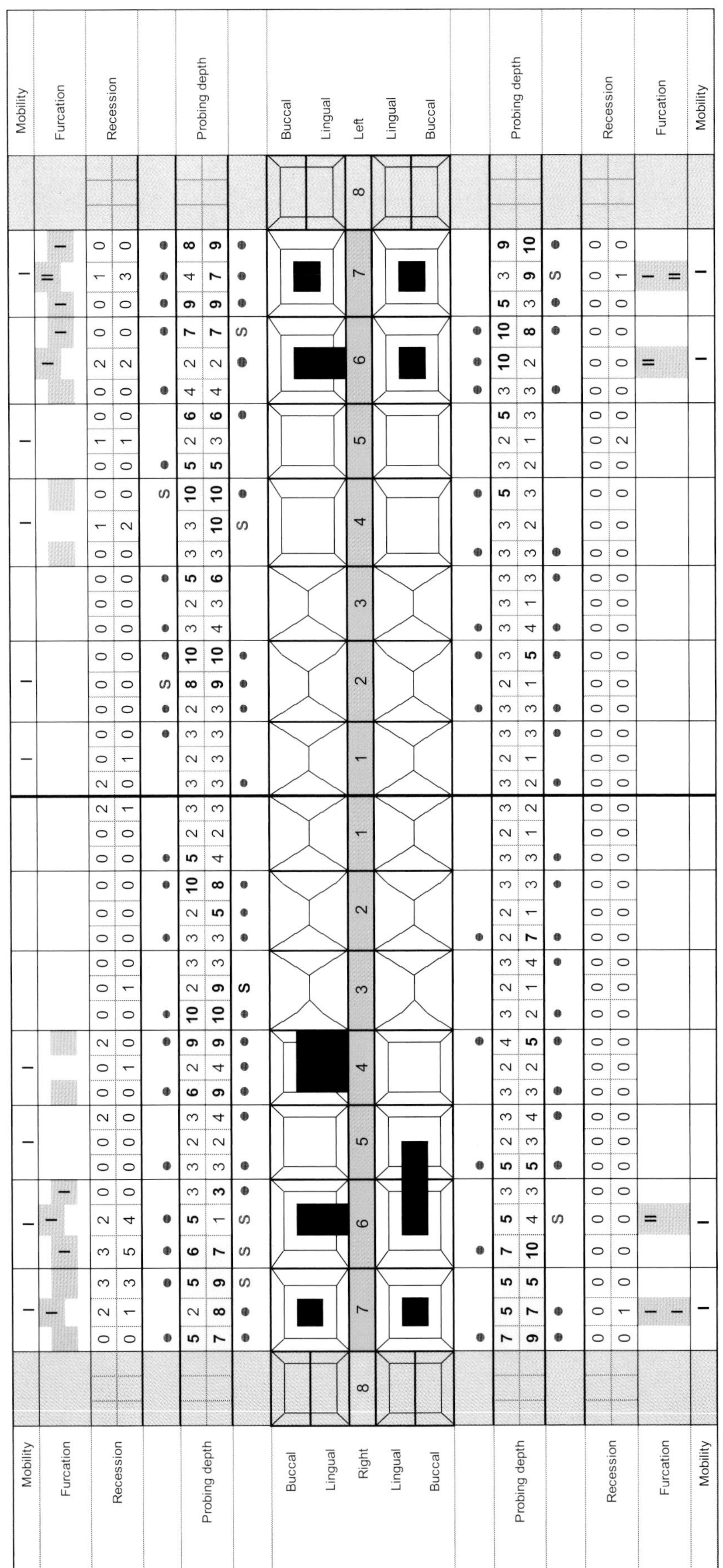

• **Fig. 38.3** Probing depths and recession (in millimetres) at six points, bleeding sites (red dots) and mobility and furcation involvement (grade), recorded for each tooth. S indicates suppuration from probed site.

TABLE 38.2 Options for Radiographic Views to Assess Periodontitis

View	Advantages	Disadvantages
Periapical radiographs	Ideal as excellent detail for assessing bone loss, root anatomy and periapical regions if taken with a paralleling technique. Selected views based on presence of clinical attachment loss are justifiable. Necessary for this case to provide appropriate care planning.	Patients with limited mouth opening or gag reflex may find them difficult to tolerate.
Dental panoramic tomogram (DPT)	Can be used as a general survey for a new patient. May also involve lower dose than a large number of periapical films especially if dose minimized (50% reduction) by excluding parotid and temporomandibular joint regions.	Distortion and low resolution (10 times less than periapicals) make detailed assessment of periodontal bone support, root anatomy, caries and restorative status difficult, especially around incisors.
Vertical bitewings	An option for molars and premolars when there is no more than moderate bone loss.	Cannot record proportion of bone loss because apical regions not visible. Less useful for diagnosis and monitoring compared with periapical views.

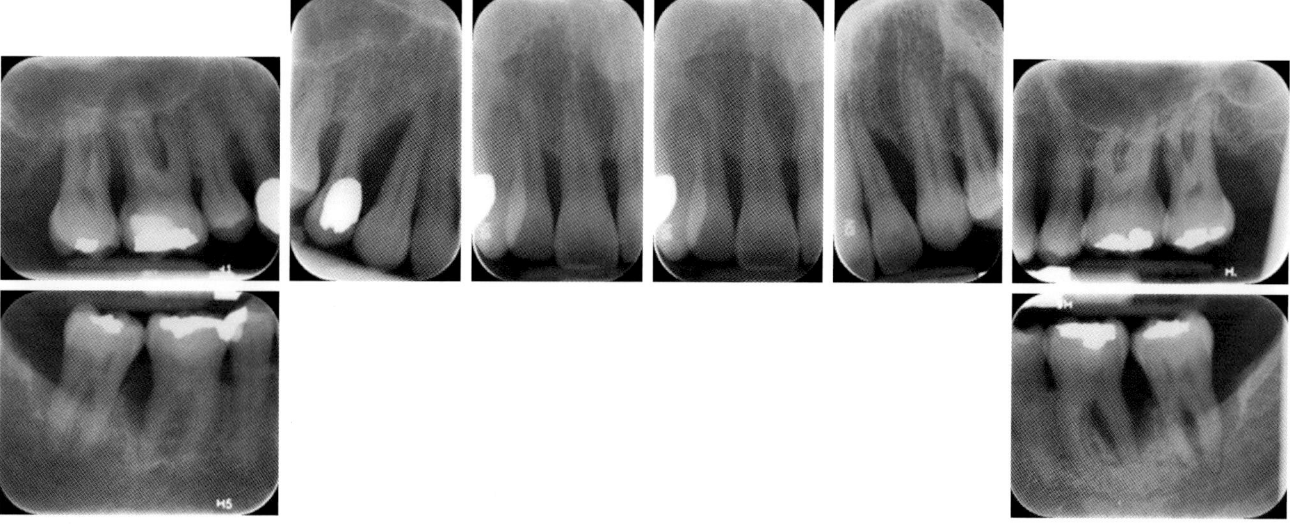

• **Fig. 38.4** Periapical radiographs of the patient at presentation.

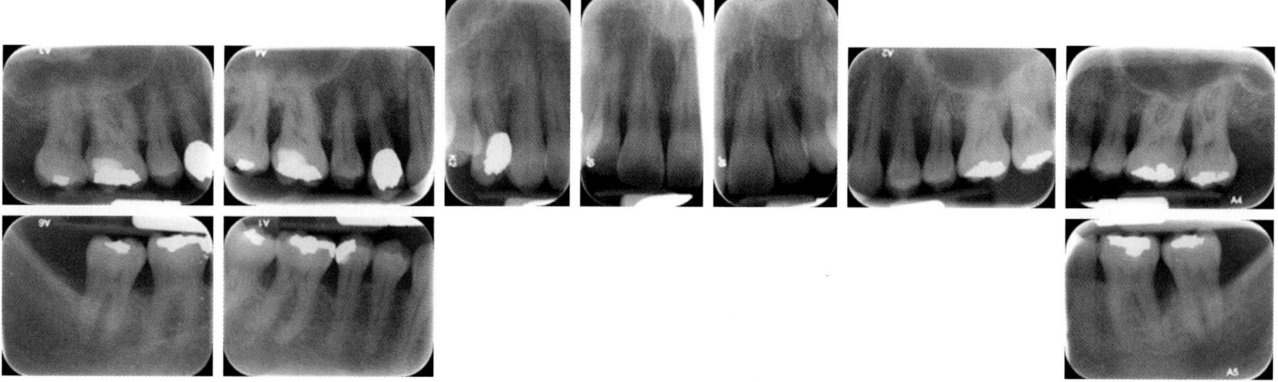

• **Fig. 38.5** Selected periapical radiographs taken 4 years prior to current presentation.

TABLE 38.3 Staging of Periodontitis

	Stage I (Early/Mild)	Stage II (Moderate)	Stage III (Severe)	Stage IV (Very Severe)
Interproximal bone loss*	<15% or <2 mm†	Coronal third of root	Mid-third of root	Apical third of root
Extent	Described as: localized (up to 30% of teeth) generalized (more than 30% of teeth) molar/incisor pattern.			

*Maximum bone loss in percent of root length.
†Measurement in millimetres from cemento–enamel junction (CEJ) if only bitewing radiograph available or no radiographs clinically justified.
Notes:
1. If a patient has interproximal attachment loss but Basic Periodontal Examination codes of only 0, 1 and 2 (e.g. a patient with previously treated, stable periodontitis), and radiographs are not available/justifiable, staging and grading should be performed on the basis of measuring attachment loss in millimetres from the CEJ and estimation of concomitant bone loss.
2. If a patient is known to have lost teeth caused by bone loss likely to have been within the apical third of the root, stage IV may be assigned.

TABLE 38.4 Grading of Periodontitis

	Grade A (Slow)	Grade B (Moderate)	Grade C (Rapid)
% Bone loss/age	<0.5	0.5–1.0	>1.0

TABLE 38.5 Assessment of Stability of Treated Periodontitis

Successfully Treated Periodontitis	Health (Stable)	Gingival Inflammation in a Patient with a History of Periodontitis (Remission)
Probing attachment loss	Yes	Yes
Probing pocket depths (all sites and assuming no pseudo-pockets)	<4 mm (no site >4 mm with bleeding on probing (BoP))*	<4 mm (no site >4 mm with BoP)*
Bleeding on probing	<10%	≥10%
Radiological bone loss	Yes	Yes

*A patient with successfully treated periodontitis, with sites of gingival bleeding, remains at high risk of disease recurrence at those sites and of progressive attachment loss. Therefore, gingival inflammation is defined as bleeding at a shallow site of 3 mm or less rather than 4 mm or less, as is the case in gingival health. Where the probing depth is 4 mm with bleeding, or higher, this is no longer a 'closed pocket' and is assumed to be unstable periodontitis.
It is important to note that a higher probing depth of 5 mm or 6 mm in the absence of bleeding may not necessarily represent active disease, in particular soon after periodontal treatment.

also present (e.g. smoking and diabetes), they are now highlighted to support the diagnosis.

This case would, therefore, be classified as 'generalized periodontitis; stage IV; grade C; currently unstable (pockets >4 mm with bleeding on probing)'. Parameters to assess stability after treatment are shown in Table 38.5.

◆ This Patient Has Many Teeth with Furcation Involvement. What are the Possible Sequelae?

- Further and more rapid periodontal destruction
- Devitalization of the tooth
- Periodontal abscess
- Root caries.

◆ This Patient Has Already Had Nonsurgical Periodontal Treatment. Why Has the Disease Progressed?

Although her oral hygiene was fair, because of her susceptibility to periodontitis, further improvement is necessary to achieve an excellent standard (ideally, a full-mouth plaque score <10%) and to ensure that this is maintained meticulously. Interdental spaces are more effectively cleaned with interdental brushes, and floss should only be used in spaces where they do not fit. Resolution of pocketing where an angular pattern of bone loss with nonsurgical treatment is also more challenging, and multirooted teeth also may present inaccessible furcations. With improvement of oral hygiene, surgical intervention is a management option to reduce probing depths.

The patient is also an irregular attender, and the importance of her role in controlling the condition must be clearly communicated. Because there is no cure for periodontitis (other than extraction!), the patient should be advised that at the outset, she will need to commit to maintaining excellent oral hygiene and attending the clinic regularly for necessary active and supportive periodontal therapy for an indefinite period. The patient's responsibility in the long-term management of this condition should be clearly discussed prior to undertaking any treatment, and should be documented carefully in the patient's records.

Management

Extraction of the teeth with a hopeless prognosis should be advised.

◆ Which Teeth Would You Advise To Be Extracted?

The teeth with endodontic–periodontal lesions require extraction. Because devitalization has occurred as a result of progression of periodontitis rather than endodontic failure, further restorative treatment is highly unpredictable and likely to fail.

The upper second molars have minimal bone support, and unfavourable root morphology will make treatment difficult; therefore, extraction must be considered.

Extensive bone loss around the distal root involving the interradicular region is compromising the lower left first molar. The lower right first and second molars also have severe angular bone loss distally, a poor prognosis and may require extraction in the long term.

However, all molars are in occlusion and functional. With the exception of the upper right first molar, the molars could be preserved in the short or medium term. A definitive decision on extraction could be delayed until an attempt has been made to improve the periodontal condition of these teeth. If these extractions are carried out, the patient may have to accept a premolar-to-premolar occlusion or a prosthesis.

The patient did not wish to have any teeth extracted and accepted a plan to help retain a completely natural dentition for as long as possible. All molars will be retained for the time being. The risk of further bone loss potentially affecting adjacent teeth and of development of pain and abscesses should be clearly communicated to the patient and documented.

◆ At This Stage, What are the Treatment Goals?

1. Improvement of the periodontal condition of the teeth that do not have a hopeless prognosis
   a. Elimination of suppuration and reduction of bleeding on probing
   b. Reduction of pockets depths to below 5 mm
   c. Establishing and facilitating maintenance of periodontal health with the aim of preserving as many teeth as possible in the long term, especially premolar-to-premolar
2. Removal of the teeth with a hopeless prognosis and any necessary replacement if the patient agrees.

A premolar-to-premolar occlusion provides acceptable function, although the appearance may be unacceptable, depending on the visibility of the molar spaces. The upper second molars provide useful occlusion, and, although compromised, may last for many years with conservative treatment.

◆ What Treatment Should Be Provided Initially?

Because of the presence of plaque, palpable subgingival calculus and inflammation, further nonsurgical periodontal treatment was provided, as described below. Prior to provision of the treatment, the benefits and potential side effects were clearly communicated to the patient and documented in the notes – in particular, the possibility of dentine sensitivity, recession affecting appearance and increased food trapping.

1. Oral hygiene advice: The patient was disclosed, and a suboptimal plaque score was revealed – 35%. Toothbrushing technique was checked and modified to ensure that the gingivae adjacent to palatal aspects of the upper teeth and the lingual aspects of the molar were covered. Interdental brushing technique was also checked and modified so that larger sizes were used in the upper interproximal areas, and the importance of daily use was reinforced.
2. Oral hygiene was reviewed and was found to have improved, with the full mouth plaque score dropping to 15%. Supragingival instrumentation and root surface debridement of all quadrants were carried out using ultrasonic and hand instruments under local anaesthesia over two visits. Oral hygiene instructions were reinforced at every visit.
3. Reassessment was performed, with full 6 point pocket charting 2–3 months after completion of root surface debridement.

The patient maintained a more effective cleaning regimen, and over a period of 3 months, the suppuration was eliminated. However, residual pocketing with bleeding was still present, especially in the regions with angular defects. Conservative management was successful in limited areas; because the patient's oral hygiene was good, more complex treatment options and specialist referral were considered. There can be a cost implication to specialist treatment, with potential discomfort from surgery and subsequent follow-up treatment. It is advisable to forewarn the patient of this prior to referral.

The patient opted for specialist referral and had successful regenerative periodontal surgery carried out in the upper anterior and lower right molar regions. She also returned for extraction of the upper right first molar and the upper left first premolar, and an immediate partial denture was fitted (Fig. 38.6).

◆ What are the Long-Term Treatment Options To Restore These Spaces?

See Table 38.6.

◆ What is the Appropriate Solution for This Patient?

Patient-centred decision making requires the patient's views to be carefully taken into account and is crucial for effective

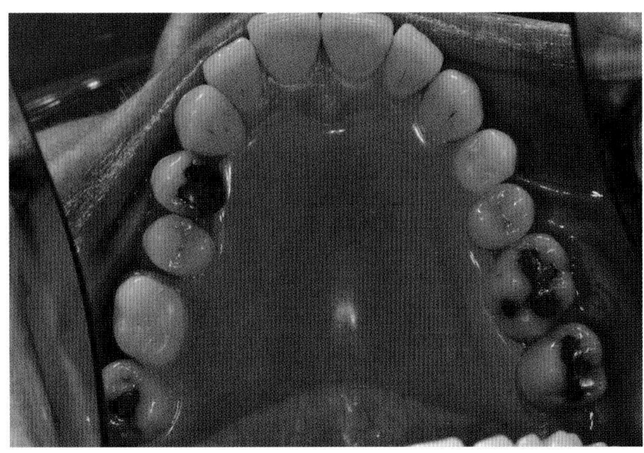

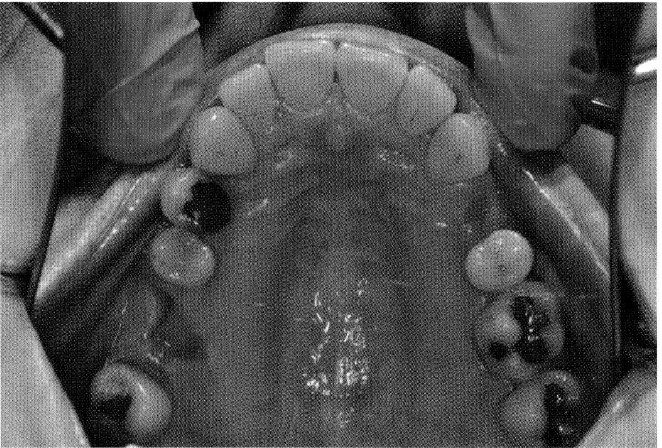

• **Fig. 38.6** Extraction of **(a)** the upper right first molar and **(b)** the upper left first premolar and replacement with an immediate partial denture.

TABLE 38.6 Treatment Options for Upper Right First Molar and Upper Left First Premolar Spaces

Care Plan	Advantages	Disadvantages
Definitive acrylic partial denture	Should other teeth with a poor prognosis need extraction, they can be added onto the denture Good appearance because acrylic can mask soft tissue deficits well	Acrylic dentures predispose to increased plaque retention leading to further deterioration of the periodontal tissues Removable
Definitive cobalt–chrome based partial denture	Less plaque retention than acrylic option and better tolerated with greater tooth borne support	Cost Likely to need remaking with further loss of teeth Still prone to plaque retention Removable
Conventional bridge	Fixed Good long-term survival	Risk of devitalization of abutment teeth Compromise oral hygiene if pontic is poorly designed Difficult to manage if complications/failure arise Need abutment teeth with good support UR6 requires a fixed-fixed design, so minimal support and persistent pocketing on UR7 excludes this option
Cantilevered adhesive bridge	Fixed No/minimal preparation of abutment teeth Minimal/shallow guidance on abutment teeth favour this option for UL4 Easier to manage with failure	Compromise of oral hygiene if pontic poorly designed Need sufficient enamel for good bond strength – ideally sound abutment teeth with good support Cantilever design not ideal for wide spaces Do not survive as long as fixed-design
Implant-retained crowns	Fixed No biological cost to adjacent teeth	Increased risk of peri-implantitis in patients with periodontitis Bone grafting/sinus lifting likely to be required further increasing risk of failure Expensive and require careful monitoring and maintenance
Spaces left as are	Low cost Maintain access for oral hygiene of adjacent teeth	Poor appearance, especially UL4 space Patient may experience impairment of function Potential for overeruption of opposing teeth

clinical management. *The patient disliked wearing a removable prosthesis and did not want another one. Because of the low biological cost, she elected to have a cantilevered, resin-retained bridge to replace the upper left first premolar, but after considering the advantages and disadvantages of the options above, she did not wish to have the upper right first molar space restored (Fig. 38.7). This discussion was carefully documented in the patient's clinical record.*

The specialist also reported that because of the extensive bone loss around the distal root, the lower left first molar was beyond saving with conventional or regenerative periodontal surgical treatment.

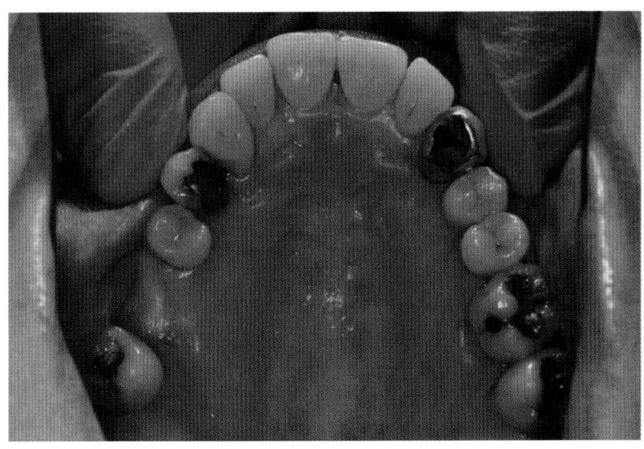

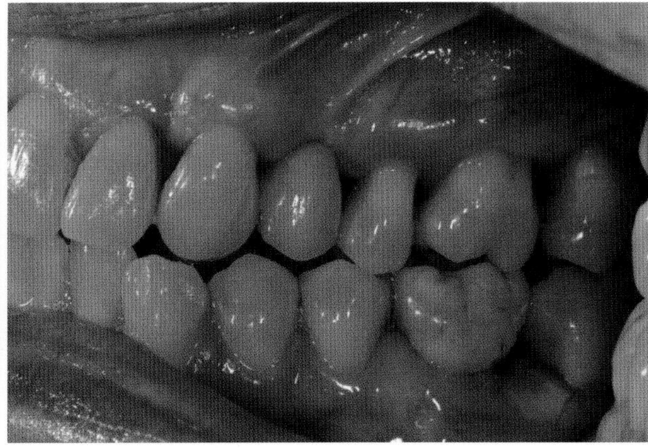

a b

• **Fig. 38.7** Restoration of the upper left first premolar with a cantilevered resin-retained bridge.

TABLE 38.7 Treatment Options for the Lower Left First Molar

	Treatment	Indications and Contraindications
Eliminating tooth	Extraction and replacement options, as highlighted in Table 38.6	Very mobile; poor oral hygiene or compliance; patient wishes; caries in furcation or elsewhere rendering tooth unrestorable; insufficient bone support on either root to conserve. This option has already been discussed and rejected.
Non-surgical	Continue regular supportive periodontal therapy – root surface debridement	Effective only for grade 1 involvement. Inappropriate in this case where furcation cannot be debrided without raising a flap.
Surgical	Tunnel preparation/apically repositioned flaps	Need sufficient residual bone around all roots, not present in this case. Opens furcation for cleaning but also risks caries.
	Root canal treatment (RCT) and hemisection	Difficult procedure; expensive; hemisected tooth loses contact on one side; full coverage restoration required to enclose RCT. Only suitable for teeth with bone far enough below the furcation to allow surgical access.
	RCT and root resection	Simpler than hemisection; expensive; full coverage restoration may be required because of fracture risk with RCT. Only suitable for teeth with bone far enough below the furcation to allow surgical access. More likely to fail because of caries, fracture and endodontic infection. Rarely fail for periodontal reasons.

◆ What are the Treatment Options for the Lower Left First Molar? Under What Circumstances are These Possible and Practical?

See Table 38.7.

Table 38.7 *Root canal treatment and a distal root resection were performed on the lower left first molar. This eliminated the furcation and enabled the patient to use a large interdental brush in the area. The inflammation associated with the mesial root resolved. See Fig. 38.8.*

◆ Do Hemisected or Root-Resected Teeth Require Restoration?

Ideally, yes. The large area of exposed dentine and risk of fracture of the overhanging crown after root resection do demand full coverage restorations. However, complex and expensive treatment is often avoided because hemisected and root-resected teeth are compromised.

Hemisected or root-resected teeth that have proved themselves stable over a period of months or years are best restored. The tooth remains in function and is an excellent semipermanent solution to this patient's problem.

Root treatment, surgery, restoration and maintenance add up to a huge investment in time and money spent on just one very compromised tooth root, and the option of extraction and potential prosthodontic replacement needs to be carefully discussed with the patient and documented.

After completion of the periodontal and restorative periodontal treatment, the patient is receiving ongoing 3-monthly supportive periodontal therapy to maintain the improvements made to her periodontal condition and reduce the risk of relapse.

Medico-legally, it is important to keep detailed records of all discussions regarding diagnosis, management options

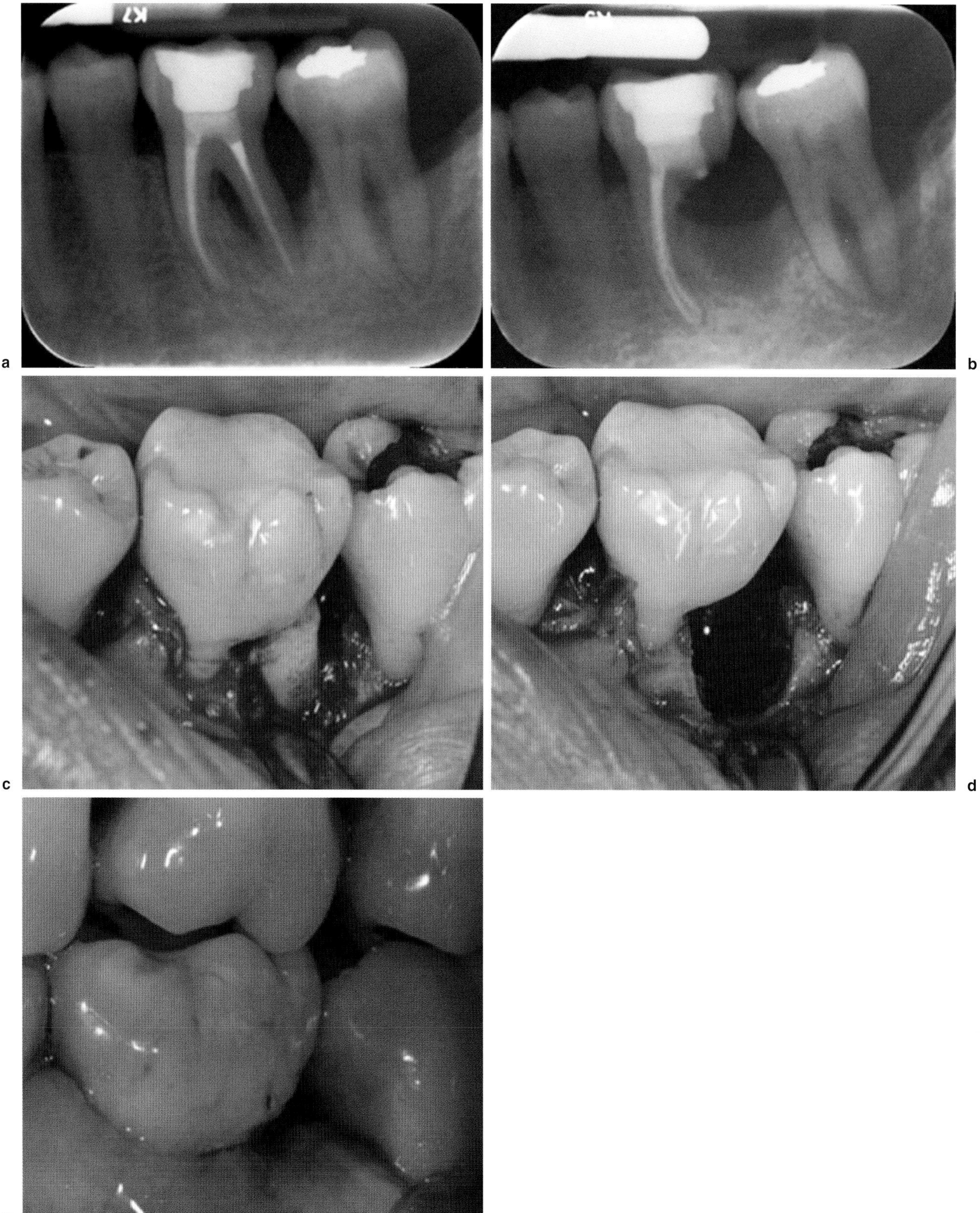

• **Fig. 38.8** Top panel – periapical radiographs of LL6 before **(a)** and after **(b)** distal root resection. Bottom panel – perioperative photos showing separation **(c)** and removal **(d)** of the distal root, followed by healing 6 months after surgery **(e)**. The patient elected to keep the hopeless but functional LL7 until symptomatic.

and treatments carried out. It should be ensured that patients clearly understand the significance of periodontitis and the critical role they play in managing it on a regular basis, especially in relation to plaque control, smoking cessation and diabetes control. Adequate notes detailing advice given at each appointment should be kept. Patients should also be advised of likely consequences if treatment advice is ignored.

Further Reading

Dietrich, T., Ower, P., Tank, M., et al. (2019). Periodontal diagnosis in the context of the 2017 classification system of periodontal diseases and conditions – implementation in clinical practice. *British Dental Journal, 226,* 16–22.

http://www.bsperio.org.uk/publications/downloads/111_153050_bsp-flowchart-implementing-the-2017-classification.pdf

Case 39
Fractured Incisors

SERPIL DJEMAL AND RAVI CHAUHAN

Summary

A 25-year-old man presents to you at your practice after visiting your local hospital dental department. He has fractured his upper central incisors. You must manage the injury and outline a care plan for final restoration.

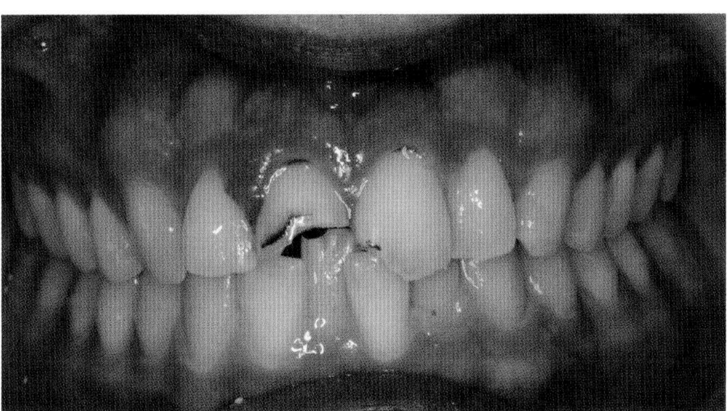

• **Fig. 39.1** The clinical appearance of the anterior teeth on presentation, in maximum stable intercuspation. © Serpil Djemal.

History

Complaint

The patient's upper central incisors have been fractured. They are currently very sensitive to cold air and cold drinks.

History of Complaint

An accident occurred whilst playing hockey the previous evening. The patient was hit in the face with a hockey stick at the start of the match. He was not wearing a mouthguard. He did not lose consciousness and was taken to a local hospital accident and emergency (A&E) department, where head injuries were ruled out. At that time, his teeth and jaws were not examined and intraoral radiographs were not obtained.

He saw his dentist as an emergency and the dentist referred him to a specialist trauma clinic.

You ask the patient whether he has the broken tooth fragments, but he does not have them.

Medical History

The patient is medically fit and healthy and has no known allergies.

Dental History

The patient is a regular dental attender.

Examination

Extraoral Examination

◆ How Would One Assess the Possibility of a Mandibular Fracture?

Fracture is suggested by:

- Pain, swelling and tenderness at the fracture site
- Bleeding, bruising or haematoma at the fracture site
- Displacement or step deformity
- Change in the occlusion
- Mobility of fragments or of teeth
- Difficulty opening the mouth or movement in lateral excursion
- Paraesthesia or anaesthesia in the distribution of nerves involved near the fracture.

◆ How Would One Assess the Possibility of a Fracture of the Zygoma or the Facial Skeleton?

In addition to the features noted above, a fractured zygoma may present with:

- Facial asymmetry and flattening of facial contour (may be masked by overlying soft tissue swelling for a few days)
- Step deformity along the relevant infraorbital margin
- Altered sensation (anaesthesia or paraesthesia) of the cheek, nose, upper lip and teeth
- Circumorbital ecchymosis (bruising around the eye)
- Restricted eye movements and diplopia (double vision).

Extraoral examination did not indicate the presence of a fractured mandible, zygoma or maxilla. There was no restricted mouth opening, no pain on opening and no obvious swelling associated with the temporomandibular joint.

The lips were slightly swollen but not lacerated.

Intraoral Examination

◆ The Anterior Teeth are Shown in Fig. 39.1. What Do You See?

- Good oral hygiene
- Lingually positioned lower right central incisor
- Upper right central incisor – loss of 50% coronal tooth tissue involving enamel and dentine with exposure of the pulp
- Upper left central incisor – loss of 10% coronal tooth tissue affecting mainly enamel
- Lower right central incisor – loss of less than 10% enamel.

◆ What Investigations Would You Ensure Had Been Carried Out At the Patient's First Attendance At the A&E Department? Explain Why.

A posterior–anterior radiograph of the chest should have been taken if the patient had difficulty breathing, to determine whether the lost tooth fragments were inhaled.

Facial radiographs should have been taken to assess the possibility of fracture of the maxilla, zygoma or mandible. A suitable selection of films for this purpose would be a 10-degree and 30-degree occipito-mental view, a posterior–anterior view of the jaws and a panoramic view.

A soft tissue radiograph of the lips should have been taken if a laceration had been present and tooth fragments were unaccounted for. This would exclude the possibility that small tooth fragments have been embedded in the lip. Larger fragments of tooth in the lip are usually obvious on examination, palpation and debridement of the wound. Such fragments may cause infection or exaggerate the amount of scar tissue, affecting the appearance of the lip.

These films may have been overlooked at first examination in the A&E department if the fractured teeth were not recognized or if the hospital's medically trained staff concentrated on excluding more serious head and neck injuries.

◆ What Features of the Anterior Teeth are Important At Examination? How Would You Examine Them?

Mobility of the Teeth. The teeth should be tested gently for mobility in a bucco-palatal direction, using a mirror handle or, if very tender, using the operator's fingers. A further examination of any mobility can be carried out under local anaesthesia when a more accurate assessment can be made. The degree of movement and the position of the fulcrum of movement (to help distinguish between root and coronal fractures, although this is not always easy) should be noted after assessing the upper and lower anterior teeth. *In this case, the upper and lower central incisors were firm and not mobile.*

Occlusion. The occlusion should be assessed to determine whether all teeth make contact in a stable intercuspal position and that no pain is elicited on bringing the teeth together or in excursive movements. *The patient was able to bring his teeth into maximum interdigitation and noted no interferences when doing this.*

Fractured Teeth. The degree of fracture of the teeth should be inspected. Although it is not visible in Fig. 39.1, the pulp of the upper right central incisor was exposed. *Because of tenderness elicited when the crown was palpated, the true extent of the injury could only be assessed under local anaesthesia. The pulps of the adjacent fractured teeth were not involved.*

Percussion Sounds of Teeth. Traumatized teeth should not be tapped to check the percussion sound because it is too distressing for patients and has very little value at the acute stage of management.

Sensibility Testing. These may be thermal tests (e.g. cold test using Endo-Frost at −50°C) or electric pulp testing and are useful to assess pulpal sensibility.

These tests have been shown to give false-negative results for up to 3 months after acute trauma, and so they will not provide any useful information and can make patients more anxious.

◆ How Do You Interpret These Findings?

Because there were no lacerations of the lip, it must be assumed that the tooth fragments have been lost. There was no mobility of the upper incisors, and the patient was able to bring his teeth into maximum intercuspation without any interferences. The extent of the upper right central incisor fracture can only be investigated further under local anaesthesia. The patient must consent to this after it is explained that the tooth may be unrestorable after this and may need to be extracted. The upper left central incisor and lower right central incisor did not have any pulpal involvement.

Investigations

◆ What Investigations Would You Perform?

Intraoral radiographs are required and should include a periapical radiograph of the injured teeth (Fig. 39.2).

An upper standard occlusal radiograph is useful if a root fracture is suspected after clinical examination.

◆ What Do the Radiographs Show?

The periapical radiograph shows:

- Good alveolar bone levels
- Upper right central incisor has loss of 50% coronal tooth tissue extending to the crestal bone level – note the radiographic appearance of an oblique, shear fracture
- Upper left central incisor loss of mesial corner with no pulpal involvement
- No radiolucent lines across the roots or changes in the periodontal ligament space around any of the upper incisor teeth to suggest root fracture.

Diagnoses

◆ What are the Diagnoses in This Case?

1. Upper right central incisor enamel–dentine–pulp fracture
2. Upper left central incisor enamel–dentine fracture
3. Lower right central incisor enamel fracture.

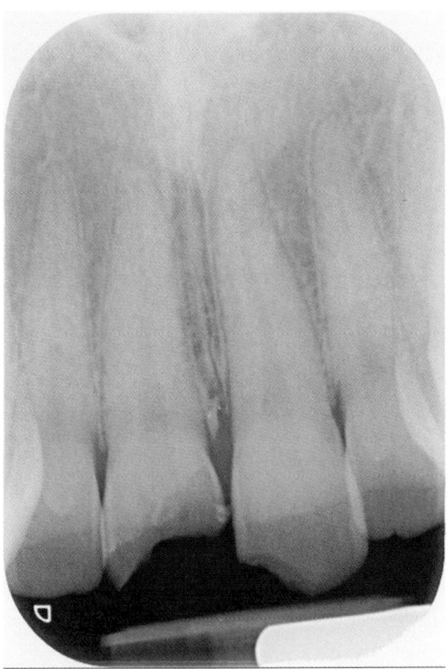

• **Fig. 39.2** Periapical radiograph of the upper incisors. © Serpil Djemal.

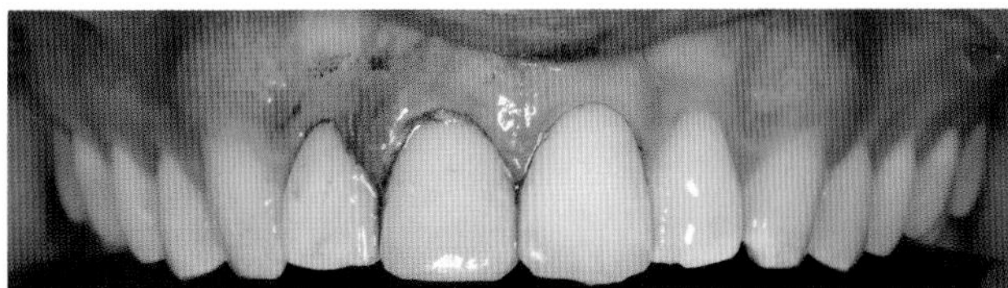

• **Fig. 39.3** Restoration of the upper right central incisor (UR1 or 11) after a pulpotomy and the upper left central incisor (UL1 or 21), both with resin composite. © Serpil Djemal.

◆ What Emergency Treatment Would You Provide?

The patient must consent to an examination under local anaesthesia to investigate the extent of the fractured upper right central incisor.

Once the tooth has been anaesthetized, any loose fragments should be removed. The extent of the fracture can then be visualized and the restorability assessed. If the tooth is unrestorable, upper and lower alginate impressions should be taken to fabricate an immediate partial denture.

If the tooth is restorable, moisture control and access to further tooth tissue for bonding can be gained through the placement of retraction cord or by removing palatal gingival tissue with electrosurgery. The original fragment can be rebonded with flowable resin composite (if available), or the tooth can be built up with resin composite, shade matched to the remaining anterior, hydrated teeth. Crown lengthening surgery can also be considered if there is insufficient tooth tissue remaining.

The aim of management is to preserve pulp sensibility irrespective of the time elapsed since the pulp was exposed, and this is achieved by carrying out a pulpotomy.

◆ How Would You Perform a Pulpotomy?

1. Under local anaesthesia and using a small, round diamond bur and copious water, remove the coronal 2–3 mm of the exposed pulp.
2. Pressure should then be applied by using a cotton wool pledget soaked in sodium hypochlorite. If bleeding does not stop, another 1–2 mm of pulp tissue should be removed and the process repeated. In an **adult** with **closed apices**, bleeding up to the level of the canal orifice indicates the need to abandon the pulpotomy and to **extirpate the pulp.** In children with open apices, pulpotomy should always be carried out, regardless of the level, to support continued root development and, thus, strengthening of the root.
3. The resultant healthy pulp should be dressed with non-setting calcium hydroxide and sealed with glass-ionomer cement. The tooth can then be built back up to full contour with resin composite.

Resin Composite Build-Up. The upper central incisors and the lower right central incisor should be built back up to full contour with resin composite (Fig. 39.3).

Moisture control can be achieved by using a rubber dam or cotton wool roll and gauze. The crevicular fluid can be managed with retraction cord impregnated with astringent or by electrosurgery, as needed.

There is no indication to prescribe antibiotics, and oral hygiene measures should be resumed as soon as possible.

◆ When Should the Patient Be Reviewed?

The patient should be seen again at **3 months** after injury, at **6 months** and then **annually**. Each follow-up visit should include:

- A pain history from the patient
- A clinical examination of the teeth to look for possible discolouration, mobility, tenderness to percussion and the presence of a sinus
- A periapical radiograph to look for changes in the periodontal ligament space or apical radiolucency
- Sensibility testing using cold test (e.g. Endo-Frost at −50°C and electric pulp testing.

The aims of the follow-up visits are to monitor the traumatized teeth for pulp health and, in particular, for signs or symptoms of pulp necrosis.

Root canal treatment should only be initiated if there are **two** of the signs or symptoms of pulp necrosis, as described above.

Throughout this period, the need for good oral hygiene should be reinforced.

◆ What Complications of the Injury Require Follow-Up?

The other anterior teeth should also be monitored for signs and symptoms of pulp necrosis, as detailed above. The composite resin restorations may require repair or replacement because of wear or discolouration in the future.

TABLE 39.1 Types of Definitive Replacement To Be Considered

Type of Prosthesis	Advantages	Disadvantages
Acrylic partial denture	Quick, easy and relatively inexpensive Pink acrylic can mask defective ridges well Can be added to	Removable nature not well tolerated by patients Plaque-retention increases Can cause stripping of the palatal tissues
Cobalt chromium denture	More patient-friendly Can be made stable with use of guide planes, rest seats and clasps Covers less palatal tissues	Multiple appointments and relatively expensive Removable nature not well tolerated by patients Plaque-retention increases
Resin bonded bridge with an adhesive cement (e.g. opaque Panavia 21)	Fixed replacement with no gingival coverage Simple cantilever design possible Well tolerated and survival good Reversible with little or no tooth preparation	Metal showing on incisal edge not desired by patients Less metal coverage reduces lifespan Technique sensitive
Implant	Fixed crown Good function resumed Not reliant on adjacent teeth for retention >20 year survival	Cost Susceptible to peri-implantitis if not maintained Surgical procedure not always welcomed by patients Technical failure with bruxism

◆ What Types of Definitive Replacement Would You Consider if the Upper Right Central Incisor Was Unrestorable? What are Their Advantages and Disadvantages?

See Table 39.1.

◆ Are There Any Medico-Legal Implications?

It is important to fully document when, how and where the injury occurred. Remember that the account from the patient is their version and not a matter of fact. Recording the exact details given by the patient is important. You may be asked for a report at a later date, and so the more details recorded, the better.

All radiographs should be justified, graded and fully reported on in written form and are an important part of clinical documentation.

Consent for taking photographic images as well as informed consent for the treatment proposed should be sought. In addition, warn the patient that once the teeth are anaesthetized, further injuries may come to light that may render the tooth or teeth unrestorable.

Website for Further Information

www.iadt-dentaltrauma.org/www.dentaltrauma.co.uk

Further Reading

Diangelis, A. J., Andreasen, J. O., Ebeleseder, K. A., Kenny, D. J., Trope, M., & Sigurdsson, A. et al. (2012). International Association of Dental Traumatology. *Guidelines: Fractures and Luxations of Permanent Teeth. 29*(1), 2–12.

Djemal, S., Singh, P., Polycarpou, N., Tomson, R., & Kelleher, M. (2016). Dental trauma. Part 1: Acute management of luxation/displacement injuries. *Dental Update, 43*(9), 812–814, 817–818, 820–823.

Djemal, S., Singh, P., Polycarpou, N., Tomson, R., Kelleher, M. (2016). Dental trauma. Part 2: Acute management of fracture injuries. *Dental Update, 43*(10), 916–918, 920–922, 924–926.

Case 40

An Anxious Patient

EMILY SHERWIN

Summary

A 23-year-old student is referred to you for removal of her wisdom teeth. She is very anxious at the prospect of minor oral surgery and has been told that you specialize in treatment under general anaesthesia. Assess the treatment options and their suitability for this case.

History

Complaint

The patient has no presenting complaint.

History of Complaint

The patient has had several episodes of pain, swelling and bad taste related to both lower impacted wisdom teeth during the last year. Her general dental practitioner has diagnosed pericoronitis and prescribed local treatments, but the episodes are increasing in frequency and severity, and the last required systemic antibiotics.

Medical History

The patient has moderately well-controlled epilepsy and suffered her last seizure approximately 4 months ago. She is treated with phenytoin 300 mg daily. She also reports allergy to penicillin and co-trimoxazole (Septrin), both of which have caused rashes.

Dental History

The patient has had a few dental restorations placed since the age of 10 years. Her general dental practitioner has provided intensive preventive treatment because she is very nervous. She can tolerate regular recall consultations but has required no invasive operative treatment for many years. Her last restorative procedure had to be abandoned on two occasions because of acute anxiety and fainting.

Investigation and Diagnosis

The patient has had episodes of pericoronitis and requires extraction of at least her mandibular third molars. Further details of the indications for removal of lower third molars and their radiographic and clinical assessment are provided in Case 25.

The patient has mesio-angularly impacted, but relatively superficial, third molars and you assess them as being relatively straightforward surgical extractions that will require minor bone removal but not tooth sectioning.

Anxiety Management

◆ What Options are Available for Controlling Patients' Anxiety? What are Their Advantages and Disadvantages?

See Table 40.1.

After discussing the options, risks and benefits, the patient elects to have her extractions performed under intravenous sedation.

◆ What Constraints are Placed On the Use of General Anaesthesia for Dentistry?

General Dental Council guidance on the use of general anaesthesia is contained in the Council's document Standards for Dental Professionals (June 2013). This document was active from 2005 to 2013; however, the standards that supersede it make no reference to the provision of general anaesthesia for dentistry, and so the previous document is used as guidance. Failure to comply would render a dentist liable to a charge of serious misconduct.

The guidance states that:

> Dental treatment under general anaesthesia should:
> - only be carried out when it is judged to be the most clinically appropriate method of anaesthesia; and
> - only take place in a hospital setting (see the note below) that has critical-care facilities.
>
> - General anaesthesia may only be given by someone who is:
> - on the specialist register of the General Medical Council as an anaesthetist;
> - a trainee working under supervision as part of a Royal College of Anaesthetists' approved training programme; or
> - a nonconsultant career-grade anaesthetist with a National Health Service (NHS) appointment under the supervision of a named consultant anaesthetist, who must be a member of the same NHS anaesthetic department where the nonconsultant career-grade anaesthetist is employed.

- The anaesthetist should be supported by someone who is specifically trained and experienced in the necessary skills to help monitor the patient's condition and to help in any emergency.
- The publication *A Conscious Decision* defines 'hospital setting' as 'any institution for the reception and treatment of persons suffering illness or any injury or disability requiring medical or dental treatment, which has critical care facilities on the same site and includes clinics and outpatient departments maintained in connection with any such institution'.

◆ What Guidelines are Available Regarding Conscious Sedation and Dental Treatment?

Recent guidelines include:

Intercollegiate Advisory Committee for Sedation in Dentistry. (2015). *conscious sedation in the provision of dental care.* London: RCS. https://www.rcseng.ac.uk/dental-faculties/fds/publications-guidelines/standards-for-conscious-sedation-in-the-provision-of-dental-care-and-accreditation/

Scottish Dental Clinical Effectiveness Programme. (2017). *Conscious sedation in dentistry* (3rd ed.). Edinburgh: NHS Education for Scotland. http://www.sdcep.org.uk/wp-content/uploads/2018/07/SDCEP-Conscious-Sedation-Guidance.pdf

◆ Is Epilepsy a Contraindication To the Use of Intravenous Sedation?

No. Benzodiazepines (e.g. midazolam) are the drugs of choice and have anticonvulsant properties. In any case, this patient's epilepsy is well controlled. An epileptic seizure under sedation is most unlikely.

◆ How Would You Assess the Patient's Fitness for Intravenous Sedation?

The American Society of Anesthesiologists (ASA) classification is useful when assessing fitness for sedation or general anaesthesia (Table 40.2).

TABLE 40.1 Methods of Controlling Anxiety

Method	Advantages and Disadvantages
Behaviour management	Simple to perform but time consuming. Methods include identifying causes of anxiety (which may be visual, auditory or olfactory), modifying anxiety by using desensitization techniques and a 'tell-show-do' approach. Works well in mild or moderate anxiety and for routine dental treatment but is unlikely to be appropriate for surgical extractions.
Cognitive behaviour therapy (CBT)	An evidence-based therapy that can help manage anxiety and phobia, including dental anxiety and needle phobia, by changing the way the person thinks and behaves. It focuses on present and future behaviour rather than past experiences and breaks down the problems into smaller parts, along with providing the person with strategies to manage negative feelings, thoughts and behaviours. It is carried out by a trained practitioner over a number of sessions and uses collaborative work between the individual and the CBT practitioner to work towards specific goals.
Hypnosis	Requires a trained clinician and several relatively time-consuming sessions of training prior to surgery. Can produce pain relief as well as anxiety suppression. If patient has already received hypnotherapy, suggestibility will be known and the preliminary episodes may not be necessary. No after-effects occur, and no drugs are required.
Preoperative oral anxiolytic medication (e.g. diazepam, temazepam)	Suitable for mild anxiety and restorative procedures but unlikely to be sufficient for surgical extraction. May be used in addition to other techniques if the patient is so anxious that he or she may not even attend for the appointment. Unpredictable effect in children.
Inhalational sedation	Requires trained operator and team. Suitable for routine dental treatment for adults and children with mild or moderate anxiety and especially useful in anxiety-related gagging reflex. Ineffective in nasal obstruction or if patient fears mask.
Intravenous sedation	Requires trained operator and team but relatively simple in comparison with general anaesthesia and easily administered in a general practice setting. Fast onset and with few medical contraindications or adverse effects. Patient remains conscious throughout procedure.
General anaesthesia	Seldom the method of choice for minor procedures because of the risk of serious complications. Although very low, this risk is sufficient to contraindicate general anaesthesia for most dental treatment in normal individuals. General Dental Council regulations require general anaesthesia to be administered in a hospital. May be required for patients with severe disabilities or for more complex surgical procedures.

◆ Which Groups Would Normally Be Considered Suitable for Treatment with Sedation in a Primary Care Setting?

ASA groups I and II.

◆ Does This Mean That Patients in ASA Groups III and V Should Never Be Treated Under Sedation?

No. Many patients in ASA groups III and IV may benefit from sedation because it reduces the patient's anxiety and, as a result, their endogenous catecholamine secretion. However, such patients require careful assessment and planning and should be treated in a hospital setting with input from medical teams as necessary.

◆ What Medical Investigation Would You Perform?

The systemic arterial blood pressure must be checked. Normal blood pressure is considered to be 120/80 mm Hg; however, small variations are common, and the systolic blood pressure is often raised in anxious subjects. Hypertension that is well controlled is not a contraindication to sedation. However, patients with a diastolic blood pressure that is consistently above 110 mm Hg should be investigated before sedation is given.

When you take the patient's blood pressure it is 140/90 mm Hg, consistent with her anxious demeanour.

◆ Is This Patient a Suitable Candidate for Treatment Under Local Anaesthesia with Intravenous Sedation?

Intravenous sedation would appear to be an ideal adjunct to local anaesthesia. The patient has practically no experience of dental procedures, has a history of failed treatment under local anaesthesia alone and is anxious about the extractions.

Treatment

◆ What is the Drug of Choice for Intravenous Sedation?

Midazolam is a benzodiazepine, which is well suited to dental sedation. It is soluble in water and presented in a 5-ml ampoule in a concentration of 1 mg/1 ml. This presentation is ideal to titrate for conscious sedation in dentistry.

TABLE 40.2 The American Society of Anesthesiologists (ASA) Classification for Assessing Fitness for Sedation or General Anaesthesia

ASA Group	Definition
ASA I	Normal healthy patient
ASA II	Patient with mild systemic disease
ASA III	Patient with severe systemic disease
ASA IV	Patient with severe systemic disease that is a constant threat to life
ASA V	A moribund patient who is not expected to survive without the operation

◆ Are There Any Contraindications To the Use of Midazolam?

Allergy to benzodiazepines is an absolute contraindication but is extremely rare. Some drugs interact with midazolam, but careful administration of the sedative drug will minimize any difficulties.

◆ What is Meant By 'Titration of the Dose'? Suggest a Suitable Titration Regimen for a Healthy (ASA group I) Adult Patient Being Sedated with Midazolam.

Titration is administration of a drug in small quantities whilst observing the patient's response. Sedation is judged to be adequate when the patient looks relaxed and displays a slight delay in response to questioning of commands (e.g. 'raise your arm'). There is often a degree of slurring of speech.

A suitable regimen would be 2 mg of midazolam injected intravenously over a period of 30 seconds, followed by a pause of 90 seconds, during which the patient's response is observed. If sedation is inadequate, further increments of 1 mg should be administered every 30 seconds until sedation is sufficient. A local anaesthetic can then be administered and treatment carried out in the normal way.

◆ What are the Undesirable Side Effects of Intravenous Midazolam?

Intravenous sedation with midazolam is an extremely safe procedure when the drug is administered according to the above guidelines. However, all drugs have side effects, and the major side effect with midazolam sedation is respiratory depression. There is a dose-related decrease in both respiratory rate and tidal volume, which is most pronounced in the first 10 minutes of sedation.

◆ How Should a Patient Be Protected From This Potentially Dangerous Side Effect?

Clinical monitoring by observing the patient must be carried out by both the dentist and a suitably trained and experienced dental nurse. The use of a pulse oximeter to monitor arterial oxygen saturation and heart rate is mandatory for intravenous sedation.

All suitable pulse oximeters have 'alarm limits'. The minimum acceptable arterial oxygen saturation is 90%. If the alarm sounds, the patient should be encouraged to take deep breaths. If this is not successful, the airway must be opened by using airway manoeuvres such as head tilt, chin lift or a jaw thrust. If breathing is still inadequate as indicated by arterial oxygen saturation and clinical monitoring, supportive ventilation should be provided along with the administration of the reversal agent flumazenil, a benzodiazepine antagonist.

◆ Why Must a 'Second Appropriate Person' Such As a Dental Nurse Always Be Present During Sedation and Recovery?

To help monitor the patient's condition, assist with any emergency and act as a chaperone in case the patient experiences a benzodiazepine-induced sexual fantasy, which might result in accusations being brought against the dentist or another member of the oral healthcare team.

◆ What Postoperative Care is Required?

At the end of the procedure, the patient is slowly returned to the upright position over a period of 3–5 minutes and helped to a supervised rest area. The patient must not be discharged until she has sufficiently recovered so as to be able to stand and walk without assistance.

The patient should be discharged into the care of a responsible adult escort, who must also be given written and verbal postoperative instructions.

◆ What Instructions Would You Give This Patient and Her Escort Following Treatment?

- Do not travel alone: travel home with your escort, by car if possible.
- For the next 8 hours:
  - Do not drive or ride a bicycle
  - Do not operate machinery
  - Do not drink alcohol
  - Do not return to work or sign legal documents
  - Do not use the Internet

◆ Are Benzodiazepine Antagonists Used Routinely To Hasten Recovery After Dental Sedation?

At present, antagonists such as flumazenil are recommended for emergency procedures such as benzodiazepine overdose and should not be used to hasten recovery. However, elective reversal of benzodiazepines may be helpful in some patients such as those who must travel some distance home on public transport. In such cases, it is **important** that the usual postoperative instructions for intravenous sedation are given and adhered to.

Prognosis

◆ Is the Patient Likely To Require Intravenous Sedation for All Future Dental Treatments?

Not necessarily. Sedation will have ensured that the extractions were performed as pleasantly as possible and any existing dental phobia should not have been reinforced. The amnesic effect of benzodiazepines is likely to reduce the patient's memory of the whole procedure. During future visits for dental care, anxiety-reducing methods should be used so that eventually dental care can be provided routinely.

◆ What Documentation Should Be Completed for Intravenous Sedation?

Along with completing the usual contemporaneous clinical notes, sedation-specific information should also be recorded. This should include the names of the dentist and the dental nurse; presedation checks; the dose, site, time, batch number and expiry date of the sedation drug given; monitoring carried out during sedation; and recovery and discharge information.

Case 41

Blisters in the Mouth

BARBARA CAREY, ESTHER HULLAH AND JANE SETTERFIELD

Summary

A 63-year-old female patient of your general dental practice reports severe oral discomfort with blistering. Identify the cause, and outline the appropriate management.

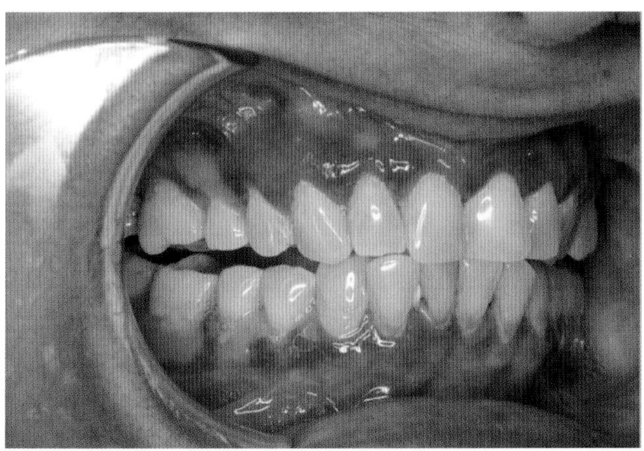

• **Fig. 41.1** The appearance of the gingiva.

History

Complaint

The patient complains of soreness involving the cheeks, gums and palate, which started 12 months ago and has increased in severity since. She reports blisters that burst to release a clear fluid. She is able to tolerate soft foods in her diet but avoids anything hard or sharp as even minor trauma can cause a blister to bursts. When a blister bursts, it leaves a painful ulcer that is slow to heal. Brushing of teeth is painful and associated with bleeding.

She denies any cutaneous or genital blisters. The history is negative for dysphagia and odynophagia. However, she describes recurrent nose bleeds and nasal crusting. There are no ocular symptoms.

Medical History

The only relevant past medical history is hypertension, for which she takes ramipril.

Examination

Extraoral Examination

Extraoral examination is unremarkable, with no cervical lymphadenopathy. The eyes appear normal.

Intraoral Examination

The appearance of the gingivae, shown in Fig. 41.1, demonstrates extensive gingival erythema of the buccal and labial gingiva in all quadrants. There are ulcers on the posterior gingiva on the right side. Inflammation is generally limited to the attached gingiva but extends onto the alveolar mucosa and into the sulci in several places.

Differential Diagnosis

◆ Which Diseases Cause Oral Blisters? How Do the Blisters Form?

Causes or oral blisters are listed in Table 41.1.

◆ What Name is Given To the Gingival Appearance?

This appearance is called *desquamative gingivitis* and is characterized by inflamed, peeling gingiva and separation or loss of the epithelium. The gingiva appears erythematous and oedematous. Unlike plaque-induced gingivitis, the gingival erythema can extend the full width of the attached gingiva and beyond it to the alveolar mucosa. Patients often report gingival discomfort and, sometimes, bleeding.

◆ What are the Main Causes of Desquamative Gingivitis in Order of Prevalence?

- Lichen planus
- Mucous membrane pemphigoid
- Pemphigus vulgaris

◆ Which of These Conditions Would You Include in Your Initial Differential Diagnosis? Explain Why.

On the basis of the answers above, only three conditions commonly cause both oral blisters and desquamative gingivitis:

1. **Mucous membrane pemphigoid (MMP).** A good history of blister formation with subsequent rupture makes

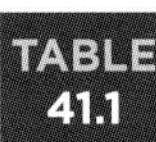

TABLE 41.1 **Causes of Oral Blistering**

Mucous membrane pemphigoid (MMP)	An autoimmune disease with autoantibodies targeting various components of the basement membrane such as the bullous pemphigoid antigens BP180 and BP230. Autoantibody binding activates complement and attracts neutrophils and eosinophils, resulting in degradation of the basement membrane and separation of the epithelium from connective tissue. Oedema fluid collects in the space to form a blister.
Pemphigus vulgaris (PV)	An autoimmune disease with immunoglobulin G (IgG) autoantibodies directed against desmoglein 1 and 3 which are adhesion molecules in the desmosomes that hold the epithelial cells together. Autoantibody binding activates complement, the cells detach from each other (acantholysis) and spaces in the epithelium fill with fluid to form blisters. Mucosal lesions are associated with a predominance of autoantibodies against desmoglein 3 and cutaneous lesions with a predominance of autoantibodies against desmoglein 1.
The bullous subtype of lichen planus (LP)	A T cell–mediated reaction, possibly autoimmune or possibly directed against haptens or extrinsic antigens in the basal cells of the epithelium. Basal cells are killed, and because they maintain the basement membrane, the attachment of the epithelium to the connective tissue is weakened. Usually, the epithelium becomes thin and ulcerates because the dividing cells have been lost, but in the bullous subtype, the weak basement membrane separates, fluid accumulates and a blister forms.
Erythema multiforme (EM) and Stevens-Johnson syndrome	These hypersensitivity reactions, usually triggered by infections such as herpes simplex or mycoplasma (in EM) or drug hypersensitivity (in Stevens-Johnson syndrome/toxic epidermal necrolysis) cause oedema and fluid accumulation below and within the epithelium, raising blisters.
Angina bullosa haemorrhagica (ABH)	The mechanism of blister formation in ABH is unknown, but assumed to be a weakened basement membrane.
Viral infections	Oral viral infections such as herpes simplex and herpangina are 'lytic' infections – that is, the infected epithelial cells lyse to release the virus particles. Clusters of epithelial cells burst beneath the intact surface layers to produce vesicles or small blisters, which later rupture to form ulcers.
Epidermolysis bullosa	A heterogeneous group of inherited defects in the components of the epithelial cytoskeleton or of the basement membrane. Mechanical weakness in the tissue allows fluid filled spaces to open up under mild trauma or spontaneously.
Dermatitis herpetiformis	Autoantibodies against dietary gluten are thought to cross-react with epithelial cell enzymes, bind near the basement membrane, activate complement and cause small foci of separation of the epithelium. The blisters are only small vesicles, not usually clinically evident as blisters.

either pemphigoid or pemphigus the most likely diagnosis. In MMP, 90% of patients with oral lesions have desquamative gingivitis with or without additional involvement of buccal mucosa and palate. The lips and tongue are not frequently affected. MMP is slightly more common in women than in men and often presents after 55 years of age. All these features fit the current presentation, and the nasal crusting and bleeding may signify nasal involvement because nasal, oesophageal, laryngeal and genital mucosae and the eyes may be affected.

2. **Pemphigus vulgaris (PV).** Approximately 70% of patients with PV have oral lesions on presentation, and it eventually involves the oral mucosa in greater than 90% of patients. The oral lesions are usually more extensive than in the current patient, with ragged irregular areas of ulceration derived from ruptured vesicles and blisters in all parts of the mouth. Compared with MMP, PV is less likely to present with gingival lesions alone. It is rare to find intact intraoral blisters in pemphigus, and patients often do not notice them because the epithelium of the blister roof disintegrates quickly. The long history and the absence of skin lesions in the present case also count against PV and make MMP more likely. However, investigations are necessary to completely exclude the possibility of PV.
3. **Lichen planus (LP).** LP is the commonest cause of desquamative gingivitis and gingival ulceration, but it rarely produces blisters. Most patients with LP have buccal mucosal and lateral tongue involvement and only 10% present with gingival lesions alone. Erythema and ulceration are consistent with LP, but other features such as reticular white striae or white plaques are not present in the gingiva of this patient. Occasionally, desquamative gingivitis caused by LP may be associated with genital involvement, and it is important to ask patients whether they have any genital itch or soreness. In females, the presentation of vulvovaginal–gingival LP is associated with significant morbidity and scarring of the affected sites. Although blister formation in LP is rare, when it does occur, the gingiva is a common site.

◆ What Diagnoses Have You Excluded? Explain Why.

Erythema multiforme (EM) is unlikely in this case and only merits consideration because of the presence of blisters. It most frequently occurs in young adults between the ages of 20 and 40 years and exhibits a slight male predilection. Diffuse areas of mucosal erythema, painful erosions, and bullae (large blisters) affect primarily the vermilion of the lip, buccal mucosa, labial mucosa, alveolar mucosa, and tongue. Skin lesions may also be present with a characteristic target-like appearance. EM lesions usually appear over the course of 3–5 days and resolve within approximately 2–3 weeks. EM does not cause desquamative gingivitis.

TABLE 41.2 Investigations

Test	Significance
Biopsy	Definitive diagnosis depends on histopathological examination of the affected tissue and direct immunofluorescence. An elliptical biopsy specimen should be taken across the edge of a lesion and sent in formalin fixative for histological examination. A separate biopsy sample is taken for direct immunofluorescence (DIF) from a perilesional site and placed in special transport medium such as Michel's medium. This specimen should not be placed in formalin because fixation destroys the protein structure and antigenicity of the tissues, making the sample useless for DIF. Taking a biopsy specimen requires careful handling of tissues because the desquamated areas are friable. If the epithelium falls off the mucosa during the biopsy procedure, diagnosis will not be possible.
Serum	A sample of clotted blood should be sent for indirect immunofluorescence to detect circulating autoantibodies. Immunoglobulin G (IgG) antibodies that bind to desmosomes indicate pemphigus, and IgG or IgA antibodies that bind to the basement membrane indicate pemphigoid. In mucous membrane pemphigoid (MMP) and pemphigus vulgaris (PV), the titre of circulating antibody can be a useful tool for monitoring or predicting a change in disease activity. ELISA (enzyme-linked immunosorbent assay) is a more specific alternative to indirect immunofluorescence and can help identify the target autoantigen.

Angina Bullosa Haemorrhagica (ABH). This term is used to describe acute recurrent subepithelial oral mucosal blisters filled with blood that are not attributable to a systemic disorder or haemostatic defect. They typically arise on the palate or oropharynx and heal rapidly. The distribution, slow healing and clear fluid–filled blisters in this patient make the diagnosis extremely unlikely. ABH does not cause desquamative gingivitis.

Drug Reactions. Some may cause lichenoid reactions and, very rarely, produce pemphigus and pemphigoid-like presentations. This patient is taking the angiotensin-converting enzyme inhibitor ramipril, which has been implicated in oral lichenoid reactions. If the presentation were more typical of LP, it would be necessary to investigate the possibility of a drug reaction.

Rare Vesiculobullous Conditions. Those that may affect the mouth can be excluded at this stage. Dermatitis herpetiformis is associated with coeliac disease and usually causes skin lesions. Oral mucosal involvement is rare and may manifest as vesicles, erosions, or erythematous macules on the palate or tongue. Epidermolysis bullosa (EB) encompasses a clinically and genetically heterogeneous group of rare inherited disorders characterized by marked blistering and erosions occurring after minor trauma. There is often scarring of the affected sites.

Other Causes of Oral Blisters. These include viral infections, which present as acute single episodes of vesicles (small blisters), often accompanied by systemic signs and symptoms of viral infection. They may include, for example, herpes simplex (acute primary gingivostomatitis, chicken pox) or coxsackievirus infections (hand foot and mouth or herpangina). Gingival ulcers and erythema are common, but not typical desquamative gingivitis.

◆ What Additional Questions Would You Ask During History Taking? Why?

Do You Have Any Blisters On Your Skin? Cutaneous blistering confirms the presence of a systemic, probably autoimmune, disease; aids in the diagnosis; and provides further lesions for investigation. Cutaneous pemphigus lesions manifest as flaccid blisters that rupture quickly, resulting in painful erosions that bleed easily. In MMP, patients may present with localized blisters or erosions, which often occur on the face, scalp, arms or legs and heal with atrophic white scars. Cutaneous LP manifests as pruritic, purple, polygonal papules or plaques on the skin. Target-like lesions are a hallmark of EM, are often on the hands or feet and may be painful. A history of herpes simplex virus infection (e.g. cold sore) would also suggest a likely trigger for EM.

Do You Have Any Problems Anywhere Else? The oral cavity is the most common site of involvement in MMP. Other sites of involvement include the conjunctiva, skin, pharynx, external genitalia, nasal mucosa, larynx, anus and oesophagus. Pemphigus may affect the oesophagus, upper respiratory tract, eyes and genital or perianal sites.

In this case, the history was negative for cutaneous lesions. The history of recurrent epistaxis and nasal crusting is suggestive of involvement of the nasal mucosa.

Investigations

◆ What Tests Would You Perform, and What is Their Significance?

Tests and their significance are listed in Table 41.2.

In view of your clinical differential diagnosis, you decide to undertake an incisional biopsy for routine histology and a separate biopsy for direct immunofluorescence.

◆ The Routine Histology Specimen is Shown in Fig. 41.2. What Do You See?

The epithelium has separated cleanly from the underlying connective tissue in the plane of the basement membrane. A few erythrocytes lie in the cleft between the two. No cause for the separation is evident. The epithelium appears almost normal, and there are only a few inflammatory cells in the lamina propria.

◆ The Immunofluorescence Stain for Complement C3 is Shown in Fig. 41.3. What Do You See?

The immunofluorescence staining has been carried out on a separate biopsy specimen from the perilesional mucosa, in which there is no epithelial separation. A bright line of

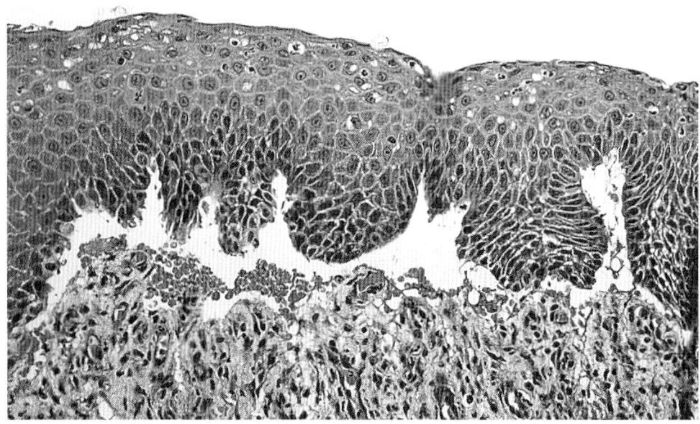

• **Fig. 41.2** Histological appearances of the biopsy specimen stained with haematoxylin and eosin.

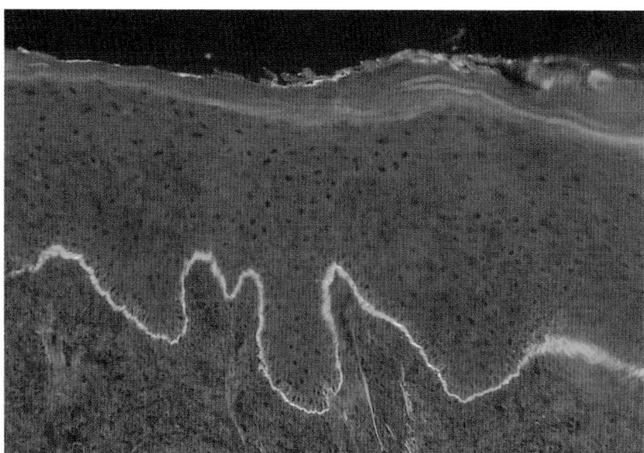

• **Fig. 41.3** Direct immunofluorescence appearance of the separate biopsy specimen.

fluorescence runs along the basement membrane, outlining the rete processes of the epithelium. Immunofluorescence for immunoglobulin G (IgG) gave an identical result.

◆ How Do You Interpret These Histological Features?

Separation of the full thickness of the epithelium at the level of the basement membrane, without epithelial damage, is consistent with a diagnosis of MMP. PV is excluded because of the lack of acantholysis and the level of separation.

For immunobullous disorders, direct immunofluorescence (DIF) is the 'gold standard' diagnostic test, revealing the presence and binding site of autoantibody in tissues. Linear binding of C3, immunoglobulin G (IgG) or IgA at the basement membrane is diagnostic of pemphigoid. There is no intercellular binding of IgG or C3 around the cells in the epithelium to suggest PV. LP is excluded because of the lack of basal cell degeneration and lymphocytic infiltration of the epithelium and positive immunofluorescence findings.

Diagnosis

The patient has pemphigoid, of which there are several types. There is no skin involvement, excluding bullous pemphigoid (a pemphigoid variant predominantly affecting the skin), and so the final diagnosis is mucous membrane pemphigoid.

Treatment

◆ How Should This Patient's Condition Be Managed?

The primary goals of treatment of MMP are to halt the progression of disease, alleviate symptoms, and prevent complications (chronic tissue inflammation and scarring). The treatment options are:

- Symptomatic treatment with agents such as benzydamine hydrochloride mouthwash for pain relief.
- Topical corticosteroids may be effective alone, but only if the disease is very mild. They are more effective when combined with systemic agents in more severely affected cases. Betamethasone 500 microgram soluble tablets used as a mouthwash up to four times daily as a 3-minute rinse (taking care to spit out all remaining mouthwash after use) or clobetasol propionate 0.05% mixed with benzocaine (Orabase) applied directly to the affected areas are frequently used in secondary care.
- Dapsone is frequently used in patients with oral MMP who fail to respond to local therapy or in those who present with widespread oral or multisite disease.
- More potent immunosuppressants such as topical tacrolimus are effective in some patients, and systemic glucocorticoids may be required in refractory disease. Azathioprine or mycophenolate mofetil can be used as 'glucocorticoid-sparing' agents to reduce the required doses of prednisolone and maintain remission after discontinuation of glucocorticoid therapy.

This patient requires multidisciplinary treatment and should be referred to an ophthalmologist to identify and manage any ocular lesions that may be present but not yet identified. The patient may also require referral to an ear, nose and throat (ENT) specialist for management of nasal and laryngeal involvement.

◆ Can This Patient Be Managed in Primary Care?

The investigation and treatment options require that the patient be treated in a secondary care setting, at least until a definite diagnosis is made and the condition is stabilized. After that, the general dental practitioner has an important role in maintaining adequate plaque and calculus control because poor oral hygiene worsens desquamative gingivitis. Patients using systemic or topical glucocorticoids are predisposed to oral candidosis, and this should be monitored at subsequent visits.

◆ Are There Significant Complications?

Yes. The chronic ulceration may lead to varying degrees of scarring. In some patients, the disease may predominantly or exclusively affect the eyes, and scarring causes adhesions between the lid conjunctiva and the surface of the eye (symblepharon formation), restricting movement, infolding the lashes, inflaming the surface of the eye and ultimately causing blindness. The oral mucosa is relatively resistant to scarring, but scarring in the eye, larynx or oesophagus may be severe.

Patients are also at risk of the adverse effects of steroids and other immunosuppressive agents, including bone marrow suppression and increased risk for infection or malignancy.

Case 42

Will *You* See My Son?

WENDY BELLIS

Summary

The mother of a 6-year-old child brings him to your practice to ask for an appointment. She has been to other practices but felt that the dentists were unfamiliar with autism and that her son was not welcome.

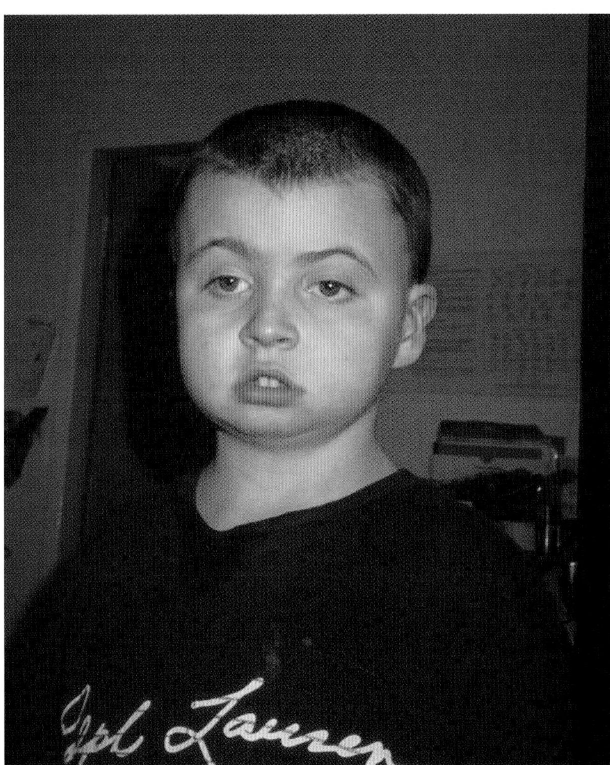

• **Fig. 42.1** The patient on presentation.

History

Complaint

The mother reports that she had asked several dentists to treat her son who has autism, but they all found reasons not to.

History of Complaint

No one has ever been able to perform a proper examination on her son. A recent attempt by another dentist ended in failure, and her son became very distressed. Recently, he has been putting objects into his mouth and biting his clothes. His mother is worried that he may be in pain but is unable to tell her.

Medical History

The patient was diagnosed with autism at 3 years of age. He has no other medical conditions and takes melatonin to aid sleep. His mother thinks that he may be allergic to wheat and dairy produce and consequently tries to exclude these from his diet. He has had no formal allergy diagnosis and no advice from a dietician.

Examination

Extraoral Examination

◆ The Patient is Shown in Fig. 42.1. What Do You See?

Many children with autism look like any other child. However, you notice that this patient fails to make eye contact with you and seems to have a relatively large head, a feature seen in some young children with autism.

While you speak to the mother in the waiting room, the child is flapping his hands and rocking backwards and forwards. He does not seem to be aware of his surroundings.

It appears that you will not be able to perform an examination easily. The mother appears stressed and anxious.

◆ What is Autism Spectrum Disorder?

Autism is a lifelong developmental disability that affects how people perceive the world and interact with others. Individuals with autism can have difficulties with everyday social communication, social interaction, repetitive behaviours and sensory issues.

Autism has a wide range of presentations and so is described as a 'spectrum'.

Approximately 50% of people with autism have learning disabilities; however, some have normal or above normal intelligence.

Asperger's syndrome is a form of autism, in which there may be average or above average intelligence. Specific learning difficulties such as dyslexia or difficulty understanding or processing language may also be present.

Dyspraxia is also common.

There is no cure for autism. However, a range of strategies and approaches to enable learning and development may help some people.

◆ What is the Cause of Autism?

Early suggestions that autism might result from abnormal parenting or having been abandoned. Although the exact cause of autism is still under investigation, there is overwhelming evidence that a combination of both strong genetic factors and weaker environmental factors alter the brain structure and neuron function.

◆ Who is Affected?

Autism affects at least 1% of the UK population and affects all races and socioeconomic groups.

Males are four times more frequently affected compared with than females. However, girls are underdiagnosed because of their better language and social skills and ability to mask their difficulties to fit in with their peers. Because girls are not diagnosed early, they may display secondary difficulties – depression, severe anxiety and eating disorders, especially anorexia.

It is not unusual for siblings to be affected, although this may not be recognized if signs are limited to subtle lack of social skills or failure of language development.

◆ What Features of Autism Will Affect Your Management?

Sensory processing problems are extremely common in children with autism, and sensory issues often trigger anxiety during a dental appointment. A child may be hyposensitive or hypersensitive to sights, sounds, smell, taste and touch – all of which are challenges encountered in a dental surgery.

Oral care may be compromised because the texture of the toothbrush and the strong taste of the toothpaste may not be tolerated. Dietary control and prevention may be made more difficult by rituals around eating or strong preferences for foods with particular packaging, colour or texture. There may be idiosyncratic behaviours such as food having to be arranged on the plate in a certain way.

Aversion to physical contact can make examination, treatment, and the usual means of physical reassurance ineffective.

Self-stimulatory behaviours are common. These repetitive habits ('stimming') can take many forms, including visual or tactile stimulation or movements such as rocking and hand flapping. Stimming is thought to provide reassurance in stressful situations and helps block out other unwanted sensory input. If the child receives too much sensory information, 'meltdown' can occur. This is an uncontrolled emotional or behavioural reaction to overwhelming stress or sensory overload that can trigger a flight-or-flight reaction.

Difficulty in expressing pain is a further sensory issue because these individuals' response to pain may be different. The mother is worried and thinks that her son may be in pain and that because his communication is impaired, he would be unable to tell her. Dental professionals need to look out for alternative indicators of pain such as sleep disruption, random emotional outbursts unusual for the child or problems eating.

Verbal communication is a major problem. Many children with autism never develop functional speech and are reliant on communication aids, often visual aids. These children may have very limited understanding of colloquial speech, jokes and sarcasm.

Nonverbal communication is poorly understood by many children with autism, particularly the facial expressions and tone of voice that indicate emotions. This may mean that you have to adapt things you normally take for granted in managing other paediatric patients. For example, there is often absence of eye contact, which makes it difficult to gain and maintain attention. Also, physical reinforcements such as patting or stroking may not be acceptable to the child.

The child's behaviour might appear disruptive, challenging, frightening or bizarre and may include self-harming. Children with autism lack the 'theory of mind' (the ability to understand other peoples' thoughts and emotions) and are, therefore, not aware of how their behaviour is seen by those around them. The child may dislike or be extremely frightened of new situations and people.

Autism is associated with a strong need for routine. These individuals would like events to be predictable and new experiences may unbalance the whole day. They dislike things that are unfamiliar to them and definitely do not like surprises.

In many cases, diets are unusual because many parents exclude wheat, dairy products or yeast in an attempt to improve the child's condition and behaviour. This and the patient's own dietary demands, mean that you may have to think imaginatively when offering preventive dietary advice.

Children with autism have significantly more eating and feeding problems compared with other children. This is often linked to their sensory issues and is not necessarily associated with the severity of autism.

Other things to consider include the strong genetic element in autism. You may need to take into account the possibility that the parents themselves may suffer from a mild form of the disorder and that their communication and social interaction may appear unusual.

Sleep disruption is very common in children with autism, and this affects the whole family. As a result, parents' resilience may be compromised, and they may resort to anything to influence the child's behaviour.

◆ Are Significant Medical Conditions Associated with Autism?

Yes, 10% of individuals may have other conditions such as fragile X syndrome, tuberous sclerosis or syndromes, including Down's syndrome. These may compound the learning disability or behavioural problems.

Many children with autism have mental health problems such as anxiety, obsessive compulsive disorder and depression. Attention deficit hyperactivity disorder is frequently present, and patients may be prescribed methylphenidate (Ritalin) to address this. Epilepsy is a common association and, if not present in childhood, often manifests in adolescence.

◆ Should This Patient Be Referred for Hospital or Specialist Care?

Given time, you would probably be able to examine and may even be able to carry out simple treatments for the patient by adapting your approach. If you consider that there is pain, infection or other acute condition, then it would be appropriate to make immediate referral to a specialist care centre where general anaesthesia is available.

However, you still need to examine him to establish whether there is disease present.

There is no reason why patients at the more able end of the spectrum cannot be treated in general practice for routine preventive and even simple restorative care.

◆ What Will You Do Next?

It appears that the patient may be in pain. You may want to examine the mouth to determine the cause quickly, but without a careful plan of action, you will probably fail. Before you can proceed, you will need some information from the mother.

◆ What Information Will Help You Plan Treatment?

- Patient's likes and dislikes – useful in establishing a rapport with the child and avoiding any actions which might distress the child
  - Any communication aids that are used (see below)
  - Possible associated behavioural conditions such as attention deficit hyperactivity disorder
  - Possible associated medical conditions such as epilepsy, and medication for them
  - Whether tooth brushing is managed and whether toothpaste is tolerated
  - Whether the child is able to give a degree of cooperation and accept physical contact (experiences such as having a haircut are often good indicators of this)
  - Any therapies being used to help the condition.

In a planned situation, this information would be best collected through a previsit questionnaire.

◆ Might Treatment and Therapies for Autism Affect or Aid Dental Care?

Drug treatments only address symptoms and behaviours. Those commonly used include selective serotonin reuptake inhibitors, antiepileptics, methylphenidate (Ritalin), and melatonin. Although these have some oral adverse effects such as dry mouth, they should not compromise treatment. Of course, any liquid medication must be sugar free.

Early intensive behavioural therapies. A range of communication-based, behavioural and educational approaches are used to support people with autism. These include approaches such as PECS (Picture Exchange Communication System), TEACCH (Treatment of Autistic and Communication Handicapped Children), ABA (Applied Behavioural Analysis), sensory integration and speech and language therapy. ABA can be effective therapy but is very labour intensive, costly and of limited availability. It breaks down learning into tiny chunks, using imitation and reinforcement to encourage children with autism to communicate. Positive responses are rewarded by reinforcers such as food, social interactions, games or toys. Given more time, visits to the dentist could be rehearsed with the patient's ABA teacher and parent. If, as here, this cannot be undertaken, at least knowing the rewards used may be very helpful in reinforcing good behaviour at this and future visits.

Complementary treatments are often sought by parents. Some parents consider that fluorides and some dental materials worsen or even cause autism. Some negotiation and compromise may be required on both sides to allow successful treatment.

◆ What is Your Plan To Examine the Child?

Conventional behaviour management techniques rely on building a positive relationship with the child. However, because of problems with social communication, your approach will have to be adapted substantially, taking into consideration the child's understanding, ability to communicate and sensory issues.

You need to ensure that the visit does not become a negative experience. You will need to reinforce all positive behaviour and regard this as the first of, perhaps several, short visits. These may achieve little more than 'saying hello' and allowing the child to see you, your staff and the surgery and experience its sights and smells. Autistic children are highly anxious in new situations, but repeated exposure helps.

Invite the mother and the child into the surgery. Reassure the mother that her child's behaviour does not worry you or your staff, and try to appear confident. Make sure there is a quiet, calm atmosphere, without distractions such as music playing or telephones ringing. Observe the child's behaviour, and keep in mind that the most likely cause of noncompliance is anxiety.

Do not expect the child to sit in a dental chair. Try engaging him at a sink, playing with running water. Try having him use a toothbrush, if acceptable. This may allow you to view the child's mouth.

Some children develop the habit of repeating what is said to them (echolalia), seemingly understanding, but usually not. One positive aspect of this behaviour is that copying the sound 'ah' may facilitate toothbrushing and also allow you to see inside the mouth.

◆ How Can You Communicate with the Patient?

Try to engage the child. Knowing what he likes and dislikes is most important. Try to identify an activity involving something in the surgery, perhaps moving the dental chair or playing with the light or a toy, that can be used to reinforce good behaviour.

There are some basic rules that will keep you in good stead. Keep the language very simple, and do the following:

- Use the child's name at the beginning of every sentence to get his attention.
  - Always look at the child when you are talking to him.
  - Speak slowly.
  - Avoid idiomatic expressions such as 'take a seat' because they may be taken literally.
  - Humour has no effect and will not be understood.

- Omit unnecessary words, especially social language – 'please' and 'thank you' will only be understood by individuals with mild autism.
- Be patient.

Pictorial communication aids such as Makaton or PECS may be used by some individuals. Makaton uses iconic symbols and line drawings to convey the meanings of words. The more user-friendly PECS system teaches non-speaking children to exchange pictures of things that they want for the item, using their visual skills rather than verbal skills, as shown in Fig. 42.2.

◆ If the Patient is in Pain, What Would Be the Likely Causes?

Without having set up the visit in the way described above, you may only achieve a glimpse of the teeth, and so you will need to know the likely causes in advance. For this patient, these are potentially:

- **Caries** – especially if the diet or behavioural reinforcers are cariogenic
  - **Trauma** from a nonvital deciduous incisor – children with autism can be more clumsy and may have epilepsy, commonly resulting in trauma
  - **Self-mutilation** – some individuals with autism may pick at the gingiva, causing ulceration or inflammation
  - **Mobile lower incisors** – resulting from physiological loss in a child 6 years of age

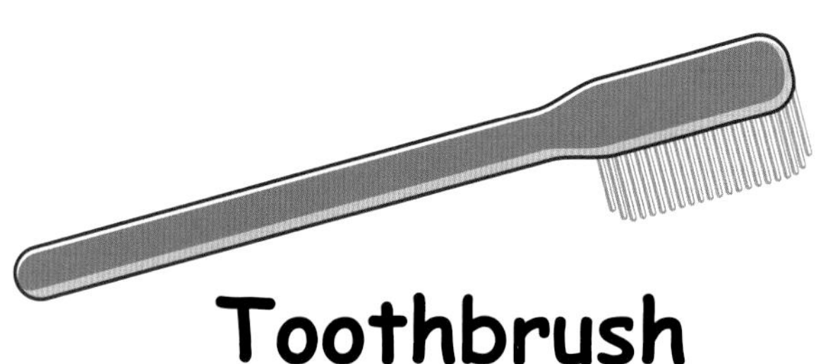

• **Fig. 42.2** A pictorial exchange picture.

- **Discomfort from pericoronitis** associated with erupting first permanent molars.

Using the strategies described earlier, you manage to get the child to let you look at his teeth while his mother brushes them. No caries is obvious, but both lower central deciduous incisors are very mobile. These appear to be the cause of the discomfort, and the mother can be reassured. No intervention is likely to be helpful or possible. This is a self-limiting problem. The parent should be instructed to show the mobile teeth to the child in a mirror to help him understand.

If caries had been noted, there would probably have been no option but to refer the patient for treatment under general anaesthesia. This would have the benefit of allowing a complete examination and radiography, which might otherwise take months to perform successfully. If the first permanent molars had erupted, fissure sealing could also be performed under general anaesthesia.

You ask the mother to bring the child back for a subsequent visit. There will be time for the child to be properly prepared with the use of pictures, as described above, and possibly one or more trips to your surgery waiting room.

◆ What is Your Strategy for Further Visits?

Plan frequent short visits to make progress in small increments until the child accepts dental examination while seated in the dental chair. The aims are to provide an intensive preventive regimen so that treatment is unnecessary and to be able to undertake examinations to ensure the regimen is effective.

A 'social storyline' may help prepare the child for the next dental visit and reduce anxiety. This is a series of pictures or photographs that tell the child what will happen and what can be expected. Different children will respond to different styles and formats of social stories.

Offer to have your photograph taken, together with any images of the practice and staff involved. An example is shown in Fig. 42.3. You will need to investigate the child's own communication strengths.

Dietary analysis is critical, given the unusual diets in many cases, as noted above. Safe reinforcers and snacks

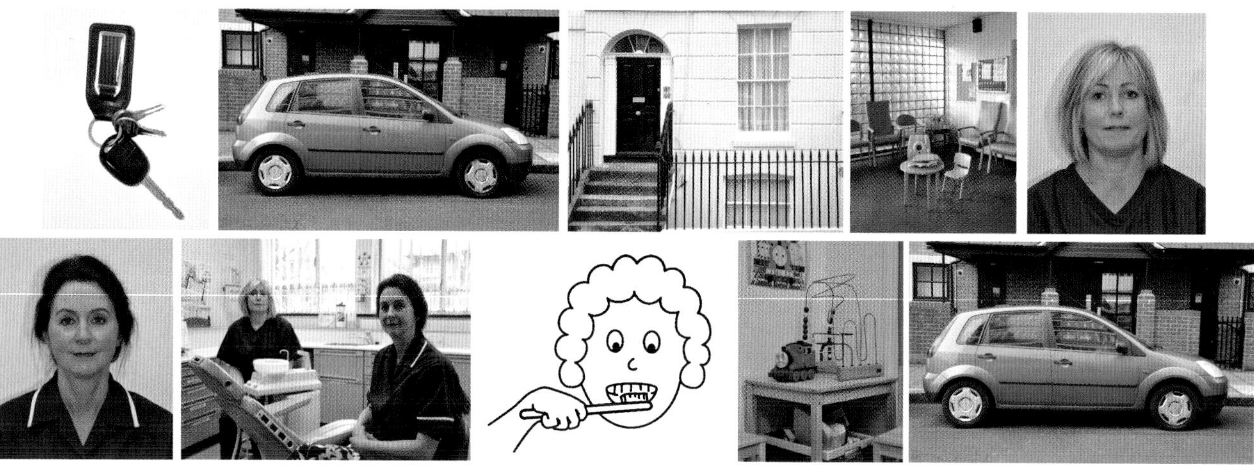

• **Fig. 42.3** Example of social storyline preparing for a visit to the dentist.

may need some imaginative thought because wheat and dairy products may be unacceptable, chronic diarrhoea may have ruled out fruit, and the child may only eat food of one colour. Sugar-free confectionery may have to be considered.

Establishing the habit of toothbrushing is essential for children with autism. Not only does it maintain gingival health but it will also deliver fluoride through the toothpaste. As for other children with disabilities, adults' toothpaste with a high fluoride content is appropriate, given the importance of preventing caries. If the toothbrushing habit has been established, a toothbrush is usually the best way to entice children with learning difficulty to open the mouth.

The mother should bring the patient's own toothbrush and paste. These form a conceptual link for the patient between visiting the dentist and his teeth and also allow you to capitalize on behaviour that is normally part of the patient's home routine.

The dental treatment of children with autism in a general practice can be a challenge, but if the practitioner is willing and able to adapt his or her approach, more able children with autism can be treated. Parents are often disappointed by dental staff who know too little about the condition and who feel they are ill equipped to manage a child with autism. More severely affected children usually require referral to a specialist.

Further Guidance

Further information for dental professionals can be found at the British Society of Paediatric Dentistry website (www.bspd.co.uk), including a questionnaire for parents and information leaflets on autism and dental care for children with autism.

Case 43

Bridge Design

SOPHIE WATKINS

Summary

A 21-year-old woman presents to your general dental practice with a premolar space in the lower left quadrant and missing her lower central incisors. She would like these spaces filled. What options will you discuss with the patient?

History

Complaint

Her complaint is the perceived poor appearance of the gap, which is visible when speaking and smiling.

History of Complaint

The patient suffers from hypodontia and has multiple teeth missing. She has had orthodontic treatment in the past to align her teeth in the upper and lower jaws and now requests a replacement for the tooth missing in the lower left quadrant and those anteriorly. The patient is happy with the maxillary result but would prefer the mandibular edentulous spaces to be filled.

Dental History

The patient first came to your practice 18 months ago and is well motivated and attends regularly for review. The patient consumes a low-sugar diet and has good oral hygiene.

Medical History

The patient is fit and well, with no medical problems.

Examination

Extraoral Examination

No abnormalities are present on extraoral examination. The lower anterior and premolar spaces are visible during normal speech.

Intraoral Examination

The patient has an unrestored dentition with an intact upper arch and the following teeth missing in the lower arch: mandibular second molars, mandibular central incisors and the mandibular left second premolar.

Basic periodontal examination (BPE) revealed scores of 0 or 1 in all sextants.

The buccal segments are well interdigitated, and the teeth are well aligned.

The patient completed orthodontic treatment a few years ago and has been wearing a Hawley retainer, with replacement teeth incorporated into the retainer. The appearance of this is satisfactory, but the patient now requests a fixed replacement for the missing teeth.

◆ What Alternatives are There for Replacing the Missing Teeth, and What are Their Relative Advantages and Disadvantages?

The options are shown in Table 43.1.

◆ What Specific Features of Importance Would You Examine? Explain Why

The vertical height available for the pontic. Where a tooth is missing, there is potential for overeruption of teeth in the opposing arch. It is, therefore, important to assess the dimensions of the edentulous space when the teeth are in occlusion. If there has been vertical movement of opposing teeth, this can be addressed as part of an orthodontic care plan or restoration at increased vertical dimension if no conventional orthodontics is planned. In this case, the opposing premolar had been aligned as part of the orthodontic treatment.

The degree of bone loss of the edentulous alveolar ridge is important. If this is extensively resorbed, an elongated pontic would be necessary to mask the bone loss. This might well be unacceptable if the pontic is easily seen during talking or smiling. Pink porcelain is possible at the gingival aspect of the pontic to mask lost soft tissue height, or this issue could be overcome with surgical ridge augmentation prior to placement of a bridge. This would prolong the treatment and make it considerably more complex as well as expensive. A diagnostic wax-up or computer-aided design may help the patient visualize the potential result if resorption is a problem or if the appearance is critical.

Size and state of existing restorations in potential abutment teeth adjacent to the space. This is the most important consideration for minimal preparation bridges; that abutment teeth require no restorations, or only small restorations, so that there is sufficient enamel for bonding. A small

TABLE 43.1 Replacement Options

Replacement	Advantages	Disadvantages
Removable partial denture	Removable for cleaning; lower cost than a fixed replacement; flange useful to improve appearance if significant bone loss has developed buccally; appearance can be acceptable.	Patients rarely prefer a removable prosthesis and often dislike palatal coverage. If poorly designed and inadequately cleaned, it may compromise the gingival margin around several teeth, leading to periodontal issues as well as caries. Retention can deteriorate with time.
Adhesive (resin-retained) bridge	Appearance can be excellent. No coverage of the palate required. Minimal noninvasive tooth preparation. More invasive replacement options remain available for the future, including a new adhesive bridge, preparation for a conventional bridge, or provision of an implant. Recent in vivo survival data suggest that adhesive bridges can remain in place for 10 years or more, if designed, executed and maintained properly.	More expensive, significant laboratory fees. Not suitable if there is significant loss of alveolar ridge after extraction. Must be cleaned in place, with more complex oral hygiene procedures.
Conventional bridge	As for the minimal-preparation bridge, a fixed replacement is often preferred by the patient. Additionally, crowning adjacent teeth allows their appearance to be improved if heavily restored. Reasonable longevity approaching 10 years in the absence of primary dental disease and where design is appropriate.	As for the minimal preparation bridge. Additionally destructive of tooth tissue with associated complications including loss of pulp vitailty and reduced options for future replacement.
Implant-retained crown	No abutment tooth preparation needed. Long-term survival rates are good.	Expensive. Involves surgical procedures as well as laboratory fees. Not an immediate result; may take 6–9 months to complete. Patient may require temporary prosthesis while implant integrates. Complications can be significant and costly when they occur.

intact restoration should be replaced, if clinically needed, or resurfaced with new resin composite. Extensively restored teeth leave little natural tooth tissue to supply retention for conventional bridges, whereas, conversely, conventional tooth preparation may be considered unnecessarily destructive where the potential abutments are minimally restored or unrestored. The quality of existing restorations must be known if they are to be used to prepare a core, as well as the amount of coronal dentine that will remain after tooth preparation. It should be remembered that an endodontically treated tooth may have little structural tissue in the core region because of the access cavity, and therefore, axial preparation may significantly further weaken the tooth removing much of the remaining coronal dentine.

Inclination of the potential abutment teeth. A degree of vertical alignment is necessary to eliminate undercuts to create a path of insertion and allow a conventional bridge to be made in the laboratory. Provided the teeth are fairly parallel, this can be achieved with adequate preparation. If the teeth are not parallel, a fixed–movable design is useful because it allows the restoration on each tooth to have a different path of withdrawal. In the case of adhesive bridges, minor preparation/finishing margins within enamel are sometimes considered, although this can risk dentine exposure in the cervical region of the tooth and may not be necessary. Because adhesive bridges will frequently be of a cantilever design, the degree of parallelism of the abutment teeth is not as significant a problem compared with conventional fixed–fixed designs, although it can affect the path of insertion and the size of embrasure spaces.

Reduced height of clinical crown on either potential abutment tooth. Tooth wear or repeated restoration may have reduced the clinical crown height. There may be insufficient crown height for adequate retention and resistance form in the final tooth preparation. In extreme cases, additional retention such as a post may need to be considered. However, post-crowned teeth do not make predictable bridge abutments and using these teeth should be avoided, wherever possible.

Increased height of clinical crown on either potential abutment tooth. Recession makes crown preparation more difficult because it is difficult to prevent undercuts in long preparations without extensive tooth reduction, especially where the roots are tapered. It may be necessary to place the crown margin some distance from the gingival margin, and this might compromise the appearance and adaptation of the pontic to the edentulous ridge.

The dimensions of the alveolar ridge are important if implants are to be considered, although bone grafting may be an option if the deficiency is not too severe. For standard implants, a minimum of 7mm mesio-distal space between the adjacent teeth, sufficient bucco-lingual dimension to accommodate the selected fixture diameter, and sufficient interocclusal space is needed (this may vary, depending on the final vertical positioning of the implant and the specific implant system being used). Particular attention should be given to the buccal contour of the edentulous ridge because a concavity would make implant placement difficult and may compromise the appearance of a bridge as lost tissue cannot be replaced with a flange.

◆ What Investigations Would You Carry Out? Explain Why

Radiography. In this case, radiography of the lower left and right lateral incisors, lower left first premolar and first molar teeth. If implants are being considered, radiographs are essential to assess the feasibility and for care planning. In the case of mandibular implants, a dental panoramic tomogram (DPT) is required to allow the inferior dental canal to be identified, as well as to assess root positon. If roots converge on a potential implant-bearing area, this may preclude implants even though intraoral examination revealed sufficient space between teeth. Cone beam computed tomography (CBCT) may also be helpful for detailed planning, but not generally as part of an initial assessment.

A radiographic assessment of root length is also important, especially in cases where orthodontic treatment has been undertaken, because this can cause root shortening, which may compromise the suitability of a tooth as a bridge abutment.

Periapical radiographic imaging can also provide information regarding the disease status of teeth – including caries, periodontal bone loss or other pathology such as periradicular involvement – requiring attention before a bridge can be provided. It may also be necessary to assess the quality of pre-existing root fillings or for root treatment if either abutment tooth proves to be nonvital on examination (not applicable in this case).

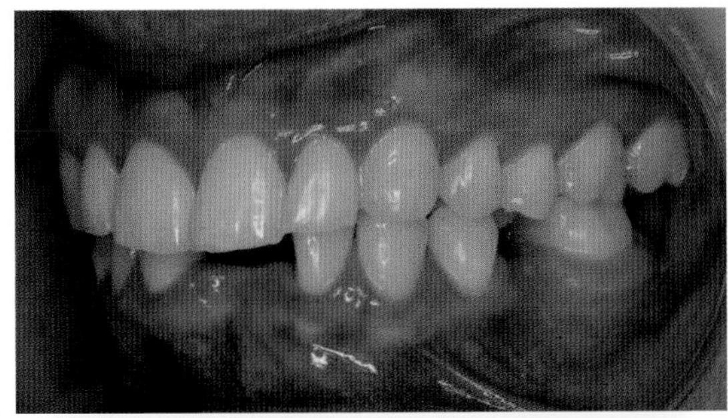

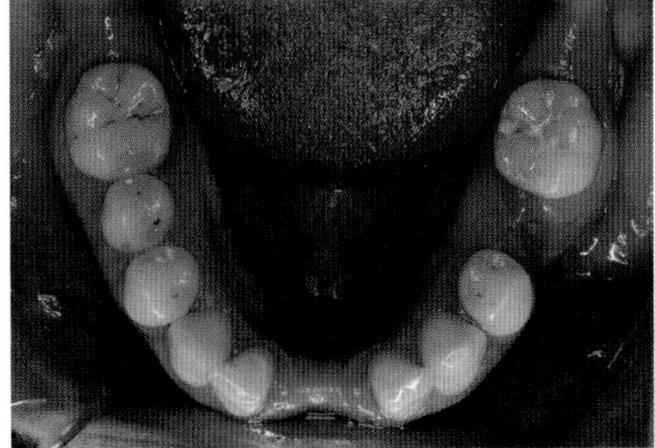

• **Fig. 43.1** The mandibular spaces on presentation, anterior/buccal **(a)** and occlusal **(b)** views.

Sensibility tests of potential abutment teeth. In this case, the teeth are unrestored and asymptomatic, and therefore, sensibility tests are not essential, but in cases where the teeth are restored, or preparations are being considered, the pulp status of the abutment teeth should be checked before any procedure is undertaken. If the teeth show signs of loss of vitality, any bridge design would need to take this into account. If required, endodontic treatment would have to be performed before bridge construction. The bridge should not be made until the definitive root filling has proven successful. A root-treated tooth is a compromised abutment because of its less certain long-term prognosis and the fact that there is reduced tooth structure for mechanical loading of the abutment. The preparation design should take this into account, aiming to preserve as much remaining dentine as possible. Also, it is desirable to root treat a tooth before cementing a bridge, avoiding damage to the retainer whilst gaining access to the pulp and root canal system after the bridge has been placed.

Study models are useful in some cases. They can be used to make a diagnostic wax-up to show the patient the likely shape of the proposed bridge and to mould a former/stent to make a provisional restoration or create an 'intraoral mock-up' to allow the patient to visualize the proposed restoration in situ. The clinician can then assess aspects that cannot be seen on models, for example, lip line and occlusal plane, especially where anterior restorations are planned. Models also allow the clinician to plan treatment, including abutment preparation and pontic size. Articulated models mounted using a facebow could be used to analyze the occlusion.

Treatment Options

◆ What Type of Replacement Appears Ideal?

The patient has indicated a preference for a fixed prosthesis, and there seems no clinical reason to suggest any other option. A minimal preparation bridge is the most tissue-conserving option. A conventional bridge in this region would mean considerable destruction of the unrestored abutment tooth (lower left first molar and/or premolar and both lateral incisors in this case). Minimal preparation bridges are often thought to carry the risk of earlier failure compared with conventional bridges. Recent clinical research indicates this is not the case when careful case selection and appropriate design and maintenance are followed. There would be no advantage in providing a metal-based partial denture. The costs would be similar to those of a bridge, and patient satisfaction is likely to be less. An implant-retained restoration would also preserve tooth tissue and provide an aesthetic, fixed solution but is expensive and requires surgical intervention and there is insufficient bone to accommodate the fixture anteriorly.

The possibility of leaving the gaps unfilled should also be considered. The occlusal stability of teeth should be borne in mind if this is considered. Adjacent teeth might drift into the gap or the opposing teeth might overerupt, creating occlusal interferences or complicating restoration of the spaces at a later date. These changes could be kept under review by using study casts. Examination of the overall occlusion may give an indication as to the likelihood of undesirable movements; for example, a well-interdigitated occlusion may reduce the chances of drifting or tilting. The presence of 'holding contacts' between teeth in opposing arches would mitigate against overeruption compared with those cases where a space leaves teeth out of interocclusal contact. However, even bearing the above factors in mind, a prosthesis remains only advisable and not essential. This is a decision based on appearance, and the final decision must rest with the patient.

◆ What Factors Might Make You Suggest a Removable Prosthesis Instead?

The cost is probably the most common reason for choosing a removable denture rather than a bridge. However, a number of specific reasons might favour the choice of a removable prosthesis:

- Multiple missing teeth requiring replacement on both sides of the arch
- Mobility or significant periodontal bone loss or inflammation around abutment teeth
- In the likelihood of the patient losing more teeth in the short term, easy addition of replacements to an acrylic-based partial denture
- A high smile line with marked resorption of the edentulous alveolar bone in the upper arch – this is most satisfactorily hidden by an acrylic flange. In such cases, a better aesthetic result can be achieved with a removable prosthesis, where soft tissue requires replacement
- Poor oral hygiene or a high caries rate – this would make it unwise to provide a fixed prosthesis, which is difficult to clean and may increase the likelihood of further primary disease. As a general principle, all primary disease should be controlled and evidence of oral health maintenance achieved before any complex restorative work is considered, including indirect restorations. A denture could arguably compromise a larger number of teeth, and neither replacement would be ideal in this instance. However, a carefully designed partial denture is the better option.

◆ If the Patient Opted for a Removable Prosthesis, What Designs Would You Consider?

In this 'bounded saddle' situation, a metal-based tooth-supported design is ideal. Abutment teeth would require small rest seat preparations, and one abutment tooth would require a clasp. A lingual connector would be required. A second clasp on the opposite side would provide sufficient retention.

◆ Should the Study Models Be Mounted On an Articulator To Make the Bridge?

Properly articulated models mounted with the use of a facebow are essential when a bridge:

- Involves many teeth
- Changes the anterior guidance
- Includes occlusal surfaces involved in guidance
- Increases the vertical dimension.

The choice of articulator will depend on the clinician's preference, but in most cases with straightforward restorations, a semiadjustable articulator is satisfactory. For simple crowns and bridges, when the guidance is straightforward such as in the present case, either handheld models or a simple hinge articulator can be sufficient.

◆ What is the Ideal Design of a Minimal-Preparation Bridge?

The ideal design of an adhesive bridge varies, depending on the site and size of the edentulous space. Various possibilities are shown in Fig. 43.2. In the upper anterior region, a simple cantilever design lasts longest. In the lower anterior region, a fixed–fixed design may be more dependable as it is easier to seat at cementation. In the present case, a cantilever design using the molar or premolar as a retainer to replace the lower left second premolar, or fixed–fixed designs are possible.

In this case, a minimal-preparation adhesive mesial cantilever design was selected for the lower left posterior bridge. In the anterior region, a fixed–fixed design was selected. The completed bridges are shown in Figs 43.3 and 43.4.

The following design features are worth noting:

- **Fixed–fixed versus cantilever design.** Research has shown that a cantilever design can be more predictable in general terms because it negates the risk of a silent debonding of one retainer wing. However, where two adjacent lateral incisors are used as abutments, it can be difficult to ensure accurate seating where the lingual morphology of the lateral incisors do not have a defined cingulum to assist positive seating with the pontics perfectly aligned. A fixed–fixed design is generally not recommended because of the risk of a silent debonding of one wing resulting from the differential mobility of the abutment teeth. However, in this site, where the two abutments teeth have similar surface area for adhesion and comparable mobility in both magnitude and direction, the risk of this is reduced. In addition, a fixed–fixed design is more straightforward to cement and does not carry the risk of poor pontic alignment, as described above. Nevertheless, if this design is adopted, it is essential that the patient is warned of the possibility of a unilateral debonding of one of the retainer wings and advised that if he or she feels the bridge may have moved, advice should be sought as soon as possible. Additionally, the dentist should be vigilant in checking this at each review appointment. Conversely, where incisors are being replaced and one canine and one incisor are the abutment teeth, the differential mobility between

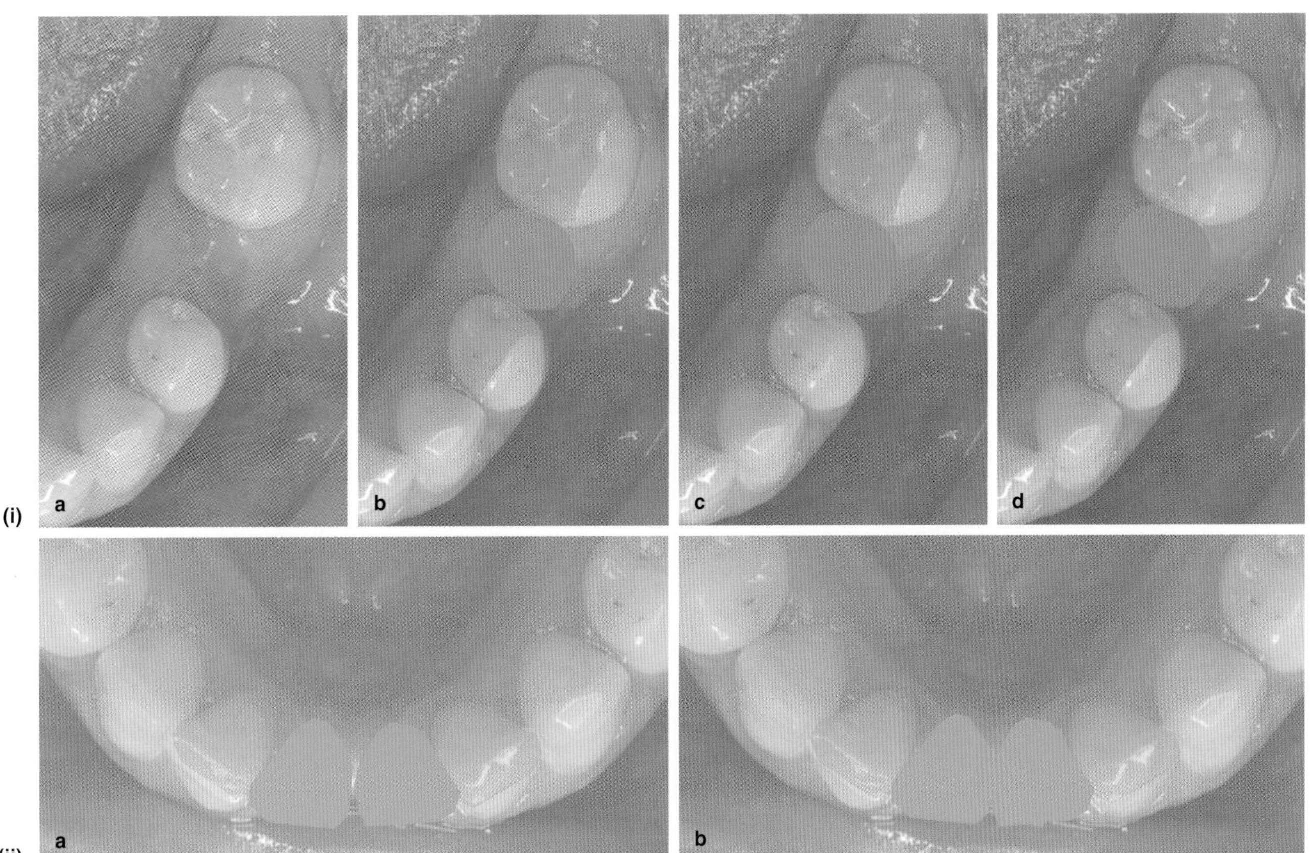

• **Fig. 43.2** Possible bridge designs to fill the left second premolar region **(i)** and lower incisor **(ii)** spaces. **i,** Lower left second premolar space. **a,** The gap can be left and provided overeruption of the opposing dentition does not occur, the existing situation would be stable. In this case, the UL5 is already showing signs of over-eruption (see Fig. 43.1), and therefore, unless an orthodontic retainer is worn, the vertical position of this tooth cannot be guaranteed. **b,** A fixed–fixed adhesive bridge with retainer wings on the lower left first premolar and first molar teeth. **c,** A mesial cantilever design using the LL6 as abutment. **d,** A distal cantilever design using the LL4 as abutment. Distal cantilevers are generally less predictable than mesial cantilevers, and therefore, unless a distal abutment is not present or unsuitable as a bridge abutment, a mesial cantilever would usually be the design of choice. In this case, the LL6 is unrestored and, therefore, is a suitable abutment tooth. The design of the retainers is described in more detail in the text. **ii,** Lower incisor region. **a,** Two individual cantilever bridges can be constructed, cantilevering mesially from each of the adjacent lateral incisors. **b,** A fixed–fixed design utilizing the two lateral incisors. Note the retainer wing design over the entire lingual/occlusal surface of the proposed abutment teeth.

the two abutment teeth is significantly different and a fixed–fixed design would not be advisable.

- **Extension of the retainer wing.** To maximize the rigidity of the retainer and utilize the maximum surface area of enamel available for bonding, the retainer wings are designed to extend over the entire occlusal and lingual surfaces of the posterior abutment teeth. This also means the cement lute is loaded in compression, rather than shear, as would be the case if only the axial surfaces were incorporated in the design, reducing unfavourable forces that might cause debonding. If a restoration is present in an abutment tooth, the retainer wing must be extended to beyond the margins of the entire restoration, such that the retainer margins are in contact with enamel for bonding. A minimum of 0.5–0.7mm retainer thickness is required for rigidity, reducing flexion and thereby reducing the risk of bond failure. For the incisor bridge retainers, the wing is also extended just onto the incisal edge of the abutment teeth to aid in location and to protect the cement lute from shear forces. This design negates the need for an incisal location 'lug', as is sometimes described, which would need to be removed at the fit appointment before the luting cement has fully matured. Vibrations caused during this process may compromise the strength of the cement lute. A location lug may also prevent full seating of the retainer wing, rather than aiding location, and this may compromise bridge retention.
- **Preparation.** No tooth preparation was undertaken in this case, as this is only required if the bulbosity of the axial surfaces of the abutment teeth would create undercuts that might limit the path of insertion or connector height. Maximizing the connector height is, nevertheless, important for ensuring the rigidity and strength of

the connector and to reduce the size of the embrasure space between the pontic and the abutment tooth. Tooth preparation, including rest seats and retention grooves, is not advised because this carries the risk of exposing dentine and compromising bond strength of the adhesive cement and may slightly increase the risk of caries associated with restorations and sealants (CARS – secondary caries) developing if the cement lute fails and leaks. It also constitutes a more complicated procedure, in which the detail of these preparation features must be captured accurately at the impression stage, poured up in the laboratory and cast with a sufficient degree of accuracy so that the restoration fit is not compromised, all for little or no gain with regard to the function and survival of the restoration.

- **Occlusion.** A design extending the retainer wing over part or whole of the occlusal surface, as described, is likely to cause some change in the occlusion. However, if this is cemented 'high', it is not unreasonable to expect dento-alveolar compensation to occur following cementation, resulting in re-establishment of the interocclusal contacts in the weeks following placement (commonly known as the 'Dahl effect'). It would be wise, of course, to monitor these contacts to ensure that this does occur during the review period.
- **Cementation.** A self or dual-cure resin luting cement should be used for cementation, paying careful attention to the manufacturer's instructions or procedural steps. A light-curing cement is not appropriate because the light would not be able to penetrate the metal retainer for a reliable cure beneath the retainer wing. It is also advisable to consider using an opaque cement that blocks the silver metal appearance, sometimes seen as greying through of the abutment teeth, especially anteriorly. It is worth noting, however, that the metal wing prevents light from passing through the abutment teeth, and this change in translucency should be taken into account when shade matching. Patients must be informed of these aesthetic changes during the planning phase before execution to manage their expectations.

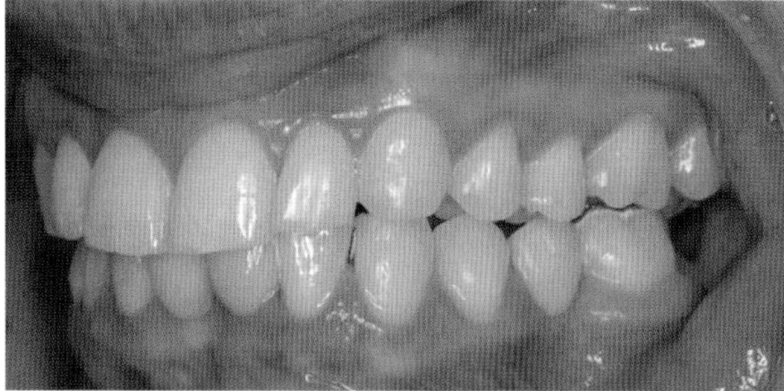
a

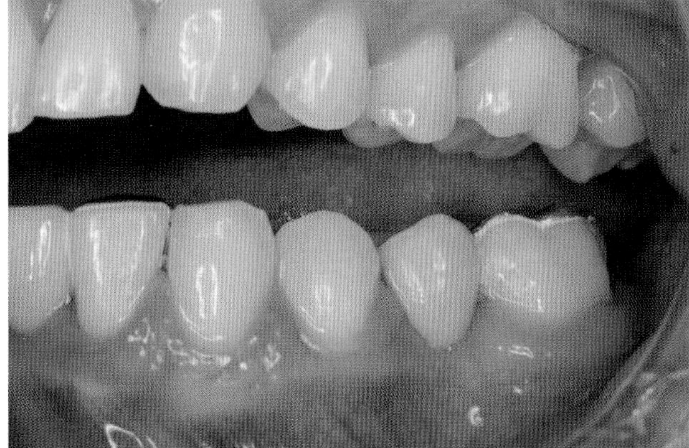
b

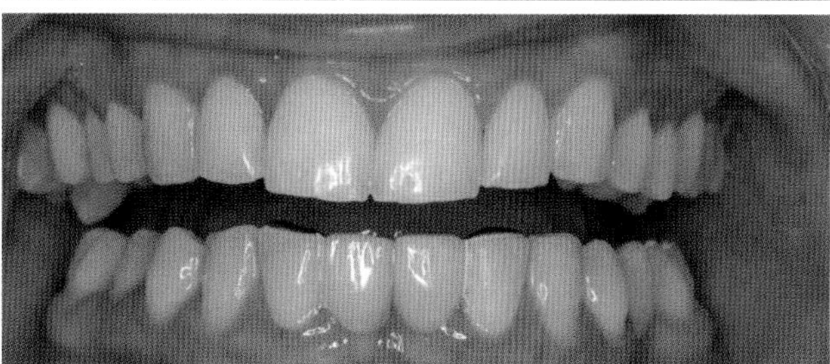
c

• **Fig. 43.3** The completed bridges. Anterior/buccal view in occlusion and two views with teeth apart showing the occlusal appearance of the retainers.

◆ What Would You Do if the Bridge Fails Through Debonding?

If the bridge decements shortly after placement, it is acceptable to recement the bridge and ensure that there is no occlusal interference. If the problem persists, a conventional

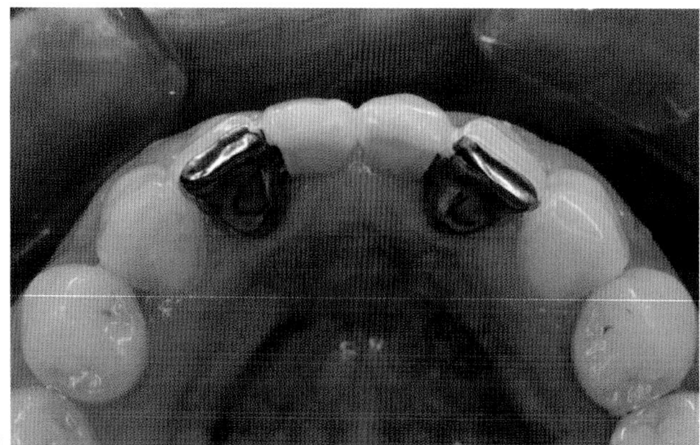
a

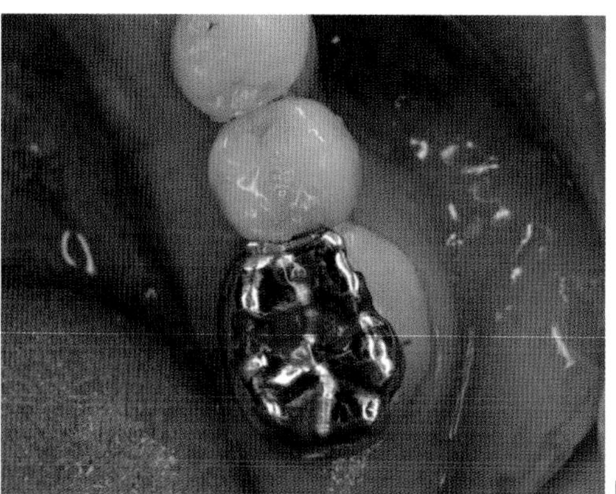
b

• **Fig. 43.4** Occlusal views of the completed anterior and posterior mandibular bridges showing retainer design and coverage.

bridge or an implant may then be indicated. However, if the planning stages have been carried out accurately and thoroughly, this issue may be due to the cementation process, and due care would be required to ensure that all stages of luting were carried out appropriately.

◆ What are the Main Issues with Patient Communication in This Case? What Should Be Explained and Highlighted To the Patient?

As with all cases, it is essential to communicate clearly with the patient from the beginning of treatment and throughout.

In the first instance, it is important to understand clearly what patients' main concerns are and what they hope to gain from treatment. The initial conversation with a patient is important because it is an opportunity to identify and discuss expectations and to ensure that treatment is focused on addressing all their concerns or discussing what is possible or advisable in a situation where their expectations cannot be met. This is also an opportunity to explain to patients what the limitations of the treatment are and what the possible complications may be, as well as the prognosis and maintenance implications. It is important to remember that no prosthetic replacement will last forever. This must be borne in mind during care planning and explained to patients so that they can make appropriate informed decisions with regard to their treatment choices. The diagnostic wax-up may form part of this discussion, with an intraoral 'mock-up' to assist the patient in visualizing the possible result, but it is important to bear in mind that the mock-up can be misleading with regard to what is achievable, and so a critical assessment of this is wise before relying on it too heavily during consultation and planning.

The above discussions form an integral and essential part of the process of obtaining informed consent from a patient, and this should be appropriately documented and discussed with the patient as part of the consent process.

Case 44

Anticoagulation for a Prosthetic Heart Valve

NICHOLAS M. GOODGER

Summary

A 60-year-old man presents at your general dental practice requiring a dental extraction. He is taking oral anticoagulants. How will you deal with his extraction?

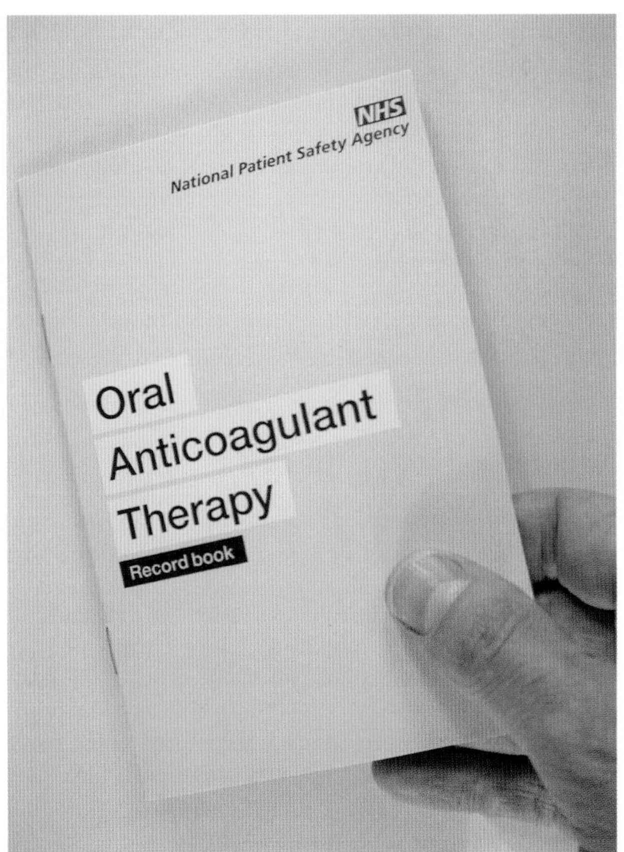

• **Fig. 44.1** Oral anticoagulation record book.

History

Complaint

The patient has a broken-down upper first molar that is tender on biting. The patient points directly at the tooth and requests extraction.

History of Complaint

The tooth has been root filled and crowned but is tender to percussion. There have been several similar episodes of pain in the past year. The crown has been lost from the tooth.

Medical History

The patient reports that he had rheumatic fever as a child, and, as a result of cardiac valve damage, he had received a prosthetic heart valve 7 years ago. He is taking warfarin (9 mg daily) and bendroflumethiazide (5 mg daily). The patient carries an anticoagulation book from his local clinic, showing that his international normalized ratio (INR) prothrombin time (PT) is usually between 3.5 and 4.5 (Fig. 44.1). It was last checked 10 days ago, when it was 3.9.

◆ How Does Warfarin Work, and How is Anticoagulation Monitored?

Warfarin is a vitamin K antagonist. It prevents the liver from utilizing vitamin K to make clotting factors II, VII, IX and X. The patient is usually under the care of an anticoagulation clinic, although some patients are monitored by their general medical practitioner. Blood tests are performed regularly, and the results and drug doses are recorded in a yellow book that the patient should always carry.

◆ What is the INR Test, What is Its Normal Therapeutic Range and How Should the Result Be Interpreted?

The INR is a standardized method of presenting the results of a PT test. The result is the ratio of the patient's PT to that of a standardized control and measures the effectiveness of the extrinsic and common pathways of blood coagulation, those most affected by warfarin. The therapeutic range for patients who have had deep vein thrombosis (DVT) or pulmonary embolism (PE) is 2.5–3.5. For patients with a prosthetic heart valve, it is 3.5–4.5, depending on valve type, at the top of the therapeutic range.

In theory, the INR is a standardized test using an internationally accepted standard. Unfortunately, in practice, accurate standardization of the INR is often not reproducible, and small changes in the decimal places of the result cannot be relied on to reflect small changes in anticoagulation. The test should be regarded as an estimate of anticoagulation, rather than an accurate measure.

◆ Is This Patient At Risk of Infective Endocarditis?

Yes, all patients with the following conditions are considered at risk, and a prosthetic heart valve is a factor that carries a very high risk of fatal outcome if endocarditis develops:

- Valve replacement
- Acquired valvular heart disease with stenosis or regurgitation
- Surgically corrected or altered congenital heart defects*
- Previous infective endocarditis
- Hypertrophic cardiomyopathy.

Examination

Extraoral Examination

No lymphadenopathy is present, and the extraoral examination reveals no abnormalities. However, a large bruise is apparent on the patient's right forearm, consistent with the degree of anticoagulation.

Intraoral Examination

The patient has a number of teeth with large restorations and several crowned teeth. His periodontal condition and oral hygiene are relatively good, with only small amounts of detectable interdental plaque.

The upper first molar tooth is broken down. Root-filling material can be seen in the open pulp chamber and much of the root surface is carious. The tooth is tender to percussion. The second premolar is not tender to percussion but produces a dull percussive note. No draining sinus is present. The periodontal condition seems reasonable, and there is no significant bone loss around the tooth on probing.

There is caries around the distal margin of a crown on the first premolar.

Investigations

◆ What Investigations are Required, and Why?

The premolars and molars should be checked for vitality. *The first premolar is vital, but both the second premolar and the first molar do not respond to testing with an electric pulp tester.* A radiograph is required to determine whether the molar is restorable, that is, to gauge the extent of caries and determine the success of the root filling. If it turns out that extraction is required, a radiograph will be necessary to assess the difficulty of the extraction. This is particularly important in a patient who may suffer prolonged bleeding. The periapical view is the ideal view.

*Excluding isolated atrial septal defect, fully repaired ventricular septal defect or fully repaired patent ductus arteriosus and closure devices that are judged to be covered by an intact layer of endothelium.

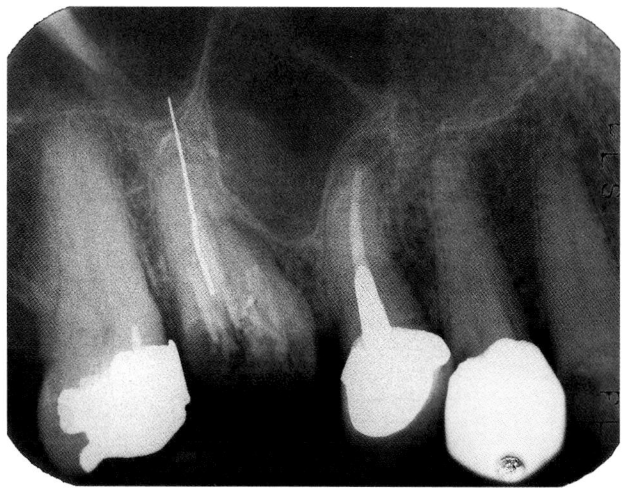

• **Fig. 44.2** Periapical radiograph of the upper first molar.

◆ The Periapical View is Shown in Fig. 44.2. What Does It Show?

The first permanent molar is extensively carious. A root filling is present, but only one gutta percha or silver point is visible in the palatal canal. It extends beyond the apex by approximately 2 mm. The buccal roots are not clearly visible but appear to contain no root filling. The overextended root filling lies close to the antrum, and the antrum extends down between the roots of the first molar and the second premolar. There is no apical radiolucency. The second premolar is also root filled. The root filling appears to stop just short of the anatomical apex at an appropriate point, but a small apical radiolucency is present, surrounded by the lamina dura of the tooth socket. The caries below the crown on the first premolar is visible, and the second molar contains a large pinned amalgam.

Diagnosis

◆ What is Your Diagnosis? Explain Your Diagnosis

The patient's pain is caused by periapical periodontitis of the first permanent molar.

The patient points clearly to this tooth as the source of his pain. This and the tenderness on percussion indicate inflammation of the periodontal ligament, and the overfilled root canal is a likely cause. No radiolucency is shown on the radiograph. However, it is not required for diagnosis in the presence of typical signs and symptoms. There may be either only a small apical lesion or one on the apices of the buccal roots or in the trifurcation, both of which are superimposed on the film.

The second premolar has an unsuccessful root filling and a small periapical radiolucency, almost certainly a periapical granuloma. However, it is not tender to percussion and is not felt to be the cause of the pain by the patient. The first premolar is vital, and the caries would produce pain of the pulpitis type without tenderness on biting or percussion.

Treatment

◆ What Treatment Would You Recommend?

The primary consideration should be that the patient is at risk of infective endocarditis, and potential sources of infection should be eradicated. The first molar cannot be restored without another root filling and extensive preparation. The patient prefers extraction, and this is the appropriate course of action. The first premolar is more problematic. It appears to be symptom-free, and the apical granuloma has probably been present for some time. This lesion is a potential source of infection, and it must be eliminated, either by extraction or another root filling. The success of the new root filling must be monitored to ensure that it is successful, and if not, either apicectomy or extraction will need to be considered. Treatment may be complicated by the anticoagulation treatment, so there must be a comprehensive treatment plan that takes the rest of the dentition into account.

◆ Is the Extraction of the First Molar Likely To Be Straightforward?

No. The tooth is broken down and root filled, and there is little or no bone loss from periodontitis. It will be difficult to grasp with forceps and may be brittle. The roots extend close to the antrum, and there is a risk of creating a surgical oroantral fistula.

A simple forceps extraction may be possible, but the extraction may well require a mucoperiosteal flap and bone removal. A simple forceps extraction would be preferable in an patient on anticoagulation medication because bleeding is more easily controlled when it is limited to a socket and the surrounding gingiva. A surgical extraction would be less traumatic overall, and separating the roots and elevating them singly would reduce the risk of an oroantral fistula.

◆ The Patient is At Risk of Endocarditis. Is Antibiotic Cover Required?

Not necessarily. Before 2008, antibiotic cover would have been routine, and the patient would have been administered oral amoxicillin or an alternative antibiotic regimen. In 2008, the National Institute for Health and Care Excellence recommended that antibiotic cover was no longer recommended for dental procedures, even for the highest-risk patients. However, in 2016, the revised guidance stated that antibiotic cover was **not routinely** required for patients undergoing dental procedures, indicating that sometimes it may be provided.

◆ Why Did the Recommendations Change So Dramatically?

In the past, antibiotic prophylaxis was based on a precautionary principle. It seemed logical because bacterial endocarditis had a high fatality rate, oral bacteria were sometimes implicated and antibiotics could prevent bacteraemia. However, much of the presumed benefit was based on animal models of the disease and the results of those studies could not be extrapolated to humans. There were cases where prophylaxis had been correctly given but had failed. More recent evidence from case control studies suggests that prophylaxis is possibly ineffective.

Although dentistry has frequently been blamed for bacterial endocarditis, there is little or no evidence to suggest that dental procedures were to blame, nor oral bacteria. Low-grade bacteraemias caused by eating and toothbrushing are common enough to be considered normal. There is no evidence to link the level of bacteraemia with the risk of endocarditis, and these normal bacteraemias would appear to be as dangerous as those occurring after dental procedures.

If there is little benefit from antibiotic prophylaxis, there is significant risk. Adverse effects of antibiotics range from fatal anaphylaxis to the development of resistant strains. It has been suggested that death caused by anaphylaxis is five times more likely than death caused by endocarditis. Although this is difficult to ascertain (and anaphylaxis is both avoidable and treatable), it sheds a rather different light on the value of antibiotic cover. A further factor is cost; resources spent on antibiotic prophylaxis are probably wasted and may cause harm.

This UK guidance is not consistent with guidance from Europe and the US. There has been concern about patients who were at the highest risk of endocarditis, and some cardiologists and cardiothoracic surgeons felt that the UK guidance ignored this potentially vulnerable group. Prophylaxis, therefore, remains in use for the highest-risk patients.

◆ How Should Endocarditis Be Avoided?

The emphasis should be on prevention, and patients at risk of endocarditis must maintain a high standard of oral and dental health. They will require effective regimens for the prevention of caries and periodontal disease and must have infections identified and treated promptly and effectively. Patients need to be aware of the signs and symptoms of endocarditis and told to return or seek other expert advice immediately if they do develop. Unnecessary medical and dental interventions should be avoided, and patients need to understand the risks of infection from nonmedical sources as well. Chlorhexidine mouthwash or other topical agents should not be offered as prophylaxis against infective endocarditis. They are not effective.

In patients who might be at high risk of endocarditis such as those who have had previous episodes of endocarditis and those with prosthetic valves, the dentist should discuss the risks and benefits of prophylaxis with the patient's cardiologist.

◆ If the Patient Requested Antibiotic Prophylaxis, What Would You Do?

National Institute for Health and Care Excellence guidance states that practitioners must be able to give clear and consistent information about endocarditis and explain the risks and benefits of antibiotic prophylaxis. If a patient insists on receiving antibiotic cover, support from the patient's medical practitioner or cardiologist may assist in the decision making. A disagreement over antibiotic cover, however, cannot be allowed to delay treatment of infection in a patient at risk of endocarditis. Changes in guidance could place you in a difficult situation; you would be found liable if a patient developed an adverse reaction to antibiotics administered for no better reason than the patient's request. If either the patient or the cardiologist considers antibiotic cover to be necessary, it would prudent to arrange for the cardiologist to determine the antibiotic regimen.

◆ Would You Expect This Patient To Suffer Prolonged Bleeding After a Dental Extraction?

Potentially yes, and if untreated, such bleeding could necessitate hospital admission. The mouth is a highly vascular site, and saliva has fibrinolytic activity. Untreated prolonged haemorrhage could be fatal, although the risk is low.

◆ Does the Patient Require Reduction of the INR To Enable Minor Oral Surgery?

Until recently, it was accepted that the INR had to be reduced for procedures such as intramuscular injections, minor surgery and dental extraction. The INR was reduced to 2.5 or below for inferior dental (ID) nerve block, simple extractions and soft tissue surgery. However, it has recently been demonstrated that the incidence of bleeding after a dental extraction performed without reducing or stopping warfarin is less than has been thought and that any bleeding may be relatively easily controlled. Current UK guidance is available from the British Committee for Standards in Haematology, British Dental Association, National Patient Safety Agency and the Scottish Dental Clinical Effectiveness Programme. The guidance recommends that oral anticoagulants should not be stopped for outpatient oral surgery, including extractions, provided the degree of anticoagulation is stable, with an INR between 2 and 4. Additional procedures to reduce the risk of bleeding such as suturing sockets with an oxidized cellulose (Surgicel) dressing and use of tranexamic acid mouthwashes, are recommended.

◆ Why Did These Guidelines Change?

For two reasons. Firstly, clinical research has shown that it is safe to extract teeth without reducing or stopping warfarin if the INR is below 4.0 and when the sockets have been packed with a haemostatic agent and sutured. Secondly, it has been realized that stopping anticoagulants places patients at risk of thrombosis, embolism or both. Clearly, these complications are of major importance and potentially fatal. The risk of thromboembolism after withdrawal of anticoagulants for a day or two is debated, but it is clear that significant complications can arise when anticoagulants are stopped for a few days. To ensure patient safety, the decision has been made to maintain the level of anticoagulation, if at all possible.

◆ Suppose More Extensive Surgery Were Planned?

For more major surgery, the risk of haemorrhage would rise significantly. The patient would then have to be treated in a hospital setting because he or she would need to be switched from warfarin to heparin. Heparin is given as a daily dose using low-molecular-weight heparin preparations such as enoxaparin (Clexane), avoiding heparin infusion. These have a half-life of only a few hours, allowing anticoagulation to be readily reversed in an emergency with the use of antagonist drugs. Anticoagulation with heparin is monitored by the activated partial thromboplastin time (aPTT) and is usually kept at 1.5–2.5 times the normal level.

◆ Do You Still Need To Check the INR? How Recently Should the Last INR Test Have Been Done?

Yes, you still need to ensure that the INR is 4.0 or less. The more recent the test, the better. In the past, it was suggested that a result less than 24 hours old was required to adjust the warfarin dose.

Because the warfarin dose is not adjusted, a test result up to 72 hours old may be accepted. However, if the INR result on the patient's anticoagulation record card fluctuates without change in dose, only a test performed on the day of treatment should be accepted. If there has been no recent test, one should be requested, or the appointment may be postponed until the next test result is available.

◆ The Patient Says He Tests His Own INR. Is That Acceptable?

Coagulation testing can now be performed by using small handheld, battery-operated devices, allowing coagulation testing to be performed by medical practitioners or the patients themselves ('point of care' testing or 'near-patient' testing). Results from a medical practice can be considered reliable because machines are checked and calibrated regularly. Some patients opt to test their own INR at home, and some evidence suggests that their anticoagulation is managed very well. Selected patients are trained to interpret their own results and are able to adjust their own doses. Provided the patient's coagulometer is monitored under a quality assurance scheme, the results can be relied on. However, patients cannot take the responsibility for adjusting their dose for a medical procedure but can do so only for routine dosing. With approximately 1 million UK patients taking warfarin, and the total rising, this type of testing is likely to be encountered more frequently.

◆ How Can Warfarin Anticoagulation Be Reversed in an Emergency?

Warfarin is a vitamin K antagonist, and administering vitamin K intravenously can reverse its effects (oral dosing is effective but much slower in action). Vitamin K takes some time to become effective because the liver must synthesize the necessary clotting factors. For a more rapid effect, Beriplex, which is a soluble powder containing human prothrombin complex, can be given for rapid reversal in emergency situations. Alternatively, the missing clotting factors can be replaced immediately by transfusing fresh frozen plasma.

◆ **What Additional Precautions Might You Take To Ensure Haemostasis?**

In general, warfarin is associated with oozing of blood from soft tissues, rather than bleeding from bone. Current guidance recommends no reduction in warfarin dose, a single interrupted or mattress suture across the mouth of the socket and an oxidized cellulose (Surgicel) pack for all extractions. Haemostasis must be achieved, usually by applying gentle pressure on the gingiva. Tranexamic acid is an antifibrinolytic agent that inhibits conversion of plasminogen to plasmin, stabilizing clots once formed. It can be administered as a 5% mouthwash and must be used four times a day for several days after extraction.

If there is severe periodontitis, then treating this first, even if only around a few teeth, significantly reduces postoperative bleeding.

In this case, a further test was required, and the INR had fallen slightly to 3.7. The tooth was extracted and the socket sutured. Haemostasis was achieved after a slightly prolonged period.

◆ **What Postoperative Instructions are Necessary Regarding the Patient's Bleeding Tendency?**

No specific instructions are necessary. The patient should be warned not to eat or drink or rinse the mouth for a few hours after extraction. A little blood in saliva is to be expected but should vanish over a few hours. If there is bleeding from the socket or fresh blood in saliva, then biting on a damp gauze swab (provided for the purpose on discharge) should stop the bleeding. Pressure must be maintained for at least 5 minutes at a time to stop the bleeding. If this fails, the patient should not hesitate to contact your practice or a local hospital accident and emergency (A&E) department. The patient may rinse with hot salt mouthwashes on the following day.

◆ **What Postoperative Instructions are Necessary Regarding the Risk of Endocarditis?**

All patients at risk of endocarditis must be warned to be alert for signs and symptoms of endocarditis. Unfortunately, these are relatively nonspecific in the early stages. The symptoms may be of acute onset and progress rapidly or persist for weeks or months before cardiac signs develop. Endocarditis caused by oral streptococci is usually of this latter subacute type. Patients with endocarditis of prosthetic valves progress to heart failure more rapidly. Low-grade endocarditis is often a diagnostic challenge in the early stages, and patients and dentists need to have a high index of suspicion. Patients should seek advice if they develop:

- Influenza-like symptoms of malaise and fatigue
- Fever or night sweats
- Weight loss and loss of appetite
- Rash
- Vague and poorly localized pains
- Splinter haemorrhages beneath the nails
- Painful red nodules in finger tips (Osler's nodes)
- Haematuria
- Joint pains
- Signs of heart failure
- Change in heart murmur
- Transient ischaemic attacks and strokes.

Postoperative

◆ **The Patient Returns 3 Hours Later Reporting That Bleeding Has Continued Throughout Most of This Period. Why Did the Bleeding Restart?**

Bleeding in the immediate postoperative period is stopped by platelet plugs forming in the vessels. This mechanism is unaffected by warfarin, which inhibits only coagulation. After the initial haemostasis, coagulation fails to consolidate the platelet plugs. When the vasoconstrictor in the local anaesthetic wears off, there is a period of hyperaemia as a result of inflammation, and bleeding may start again.

◆ **How Would You Manage This Postextraction Bleeding?**

Initially, check that the socket is only oozing because rapid bleeding would necessitate immediate measures. Then, take a history and assess the degree of blood loss, which, to the patient (and sometimes the dentist), always seems worse than it actually is. Examine the patient by using a good light and suction to remove the old socket dressing and poorly formed blood clots, and identify the bleeding area.

If only soft tissue is bleeding, pressure and a new dressing will probably be all that is required. However, bleeding after packing and suturing may be arising from bone. If a bleeding point can be identified, it can be crushed with a hand instrument. Electrocautery should not be used on or near bone. Bone wax should only be used if all else fails because it delays healing in the longer term. Replace the Surgicel pack, or place a Whitehead's varnish pack, and resuture the socket over the pack to provide pressure to the gingival margins and to keep the pack firmly in the socket. Bleeding from the surgical incision may require additional sutures and deeper sutures to compress the sides of the incision on to the underlying tissues.

Measure blood pressure and pulse to assess whether there has been serious blood loss.

Reassure the patient, who is often very worried and well aware of the problems of the anticoagulation treatment. Observe for 15–30 minutes, and reinforce the usual postoperative instructions. It should be emphasized that the patient not rinse until the next day. It is unlikely that these measures will fail.

◆ **What Would You Do if There Were Tachycardia and Lowered Blood Pressure?**

This would indicate significant blood loss, and as mentioned above, the patient should be speedily admitted to hospital for intravenous fluid administration to prevent circulatory collapse.

◆ **What Would You Do if These Steps Did Fail?**

In a practice setting, the patient should be transferred to a hospital casualty or specialist unit or to an anticoagulation clinic. This should be arranged speedily, and the patient will require an escort. There, the INR and the platelet count would be checked. Antifibrinolytics such as aprotinin and tranexamic acid can be used in conjunction with packing and suturing. If the bleeding persists or if the INR is above the therapeutic range, the patient will need to be admitted for reversal of the anticoagulation by infusion of fresh frozen plasma or prothrombin complex concentrates (a more effective preparation of concentrated dried factors II, VII, IX and X) and vitamin K. The vitamin K injections will not reverse the action of the warfarin for 12 hours and so are not effective in such emergency situations, but they aid stabilization of anticoagulation after the bleeding stops. Major bleeding may necessitate a few days in the hospital.

◆ Warfarin Interacts with a Variety of Other Drugs. Which Drugs That Might Be Prescribed in Dental Practice Can Affect Warfarin Anticoagulation?

In all drug interactions with warfarin, there is increased anticoagulation and a risk of bleeding. Aspirin and related drugs also increase the risk of bleeding, not through interaction but through their separate antiplatelet activity. Discussion with the patient's anticoagulation clinic would be prudent if any of the following drugs are required:

- Nonsteroidal anti-inflammatory drugs
- Antibiotics, including erythromycin, metronidazole, tetracyclines and penicillins
- Fluconazole, ketoconazole and miconazole (including topical preparations).

◆ How Can I Keep Up with All These Changes in Guidance?

This case demonstrates how rapidly accepted practice and guidance from national bodies can change. A few years ago, the patient would have had antibiotic cover and adjustment of the warfarin dose before treatment. Guidance can, unfortunately, come from a wide variety of sources, and it is not always clear whether it is generally accepted, recommended or mandatory. Guidelines from the National Institute for Health and Care Excellence apply to the National Health Service (NHS) in England and Wales, but not in Scotland, where a separate institution, the Scottish Intercollegiate Guidelines Network, plays the equivalent role. Guidance or references to it may also be provided by Royal Colleges, the British Dental Association, the General Dental Council and professional indemnity organizations. Overseas bodies such as the American Association of Oral and Maxillofacial Surgery, the U.S. Food and Drug Administration and similar bodies in Europe and in the Southern Hemisphere may also provide useful sources of guidance (see below). Guidance on medications in the British National Formulary or Dental Practitioners Formulary is regularly updated and usually considered definitive. Almost all guidelines first appear in peer-reviewed scientific or professional journals, although it may take some time for them to become accepted and be given the official seal of approval. This demonstrates the importance of continuing professional development to ensure that dentists remain up to date, one of the key principles for dentists of the UK General Dental Council.

◆ What if the Patient Had Been Taking One of the Novel Oral Anticoagulants Instead of Warfarin? How Do These Differ From Warfarin?

Patients with prosthetic heart valves almost never take the 'novel oral anticoagulants' (NOACs) because these are indicated for the prevention of conditions such as stroke in patients with atrial fibrillation. Examples of NOACs are rivaroxiban, apixaban and edoxaban, which are direct inhibitors of factor Xa, and dabigatran, a direct thrombin inhibitor.

Because good evidence on which to make recommendations is not yet available, it is prudent to treat patients taking these drugs with caution. An inhibitor for dabigatran – idarucizumab – is available and can be used in an emergency to control bleeding, but those for the factor Xa inhibitors are still under development.

The INR test is a poor reflection of anticoagulation with use of these drugs, and so alternative tests are required. However, routine monitoring is not required or normally undertaken, and so the dentist may not have a clear understanding of a patient's degree of anticoagulation. Minor procedures such as scaling would not require special tests, but for extractions and procedures with significant bleeding risk, the dentist should consult the patient's physician and current guidance. NOACs have rapid onset of action and short half-lives, and so they may be interrupted for short periods for dental treatment. If NOAC therapy is stopped, the normal procedure is to omit the morning dose prior to dental extractions if taken twice daily and then take the evening dose after treatment. If the patient is taking a morning-only dose, then that dose should be delayed until 4 hours after treatment has been completed.

Further Guidance

For the UK

Anticoagulation: http://www.sdcep.org.uk/published-guidance/anticoagulants-and-antiplatelets/

Antibiotic prophylaxis NICE: https://www.nice.org.uk/guidance/cg64

Index of guidance: http://www.library.nhs.uk

For the USA

https://www.ada.org/en/member-center/oral-health-topics/antibiotic-prophylaxis

https://www.ada.org/en/member-center/oral-health-topics/anticoagulant-antiplatelet-medications-and-dental-

For Europe

https://www.escardio.org/Guidelines/Clinical-Practice-Guidelines/Infective-Endocarditis-Guidelines-on-Prevention-Diagnosis-and-Treatment-of

NOACS: https://doi.org/10.1093/eurheartj/ehy136

Case 45

A White Patch On the Tongue

HELEN McPARLAND AND EDWARD ODELL

Summary

A 52-year-old woman has a white patch on her tongue. Make a diagnosis, and decide on appropriate treatment.

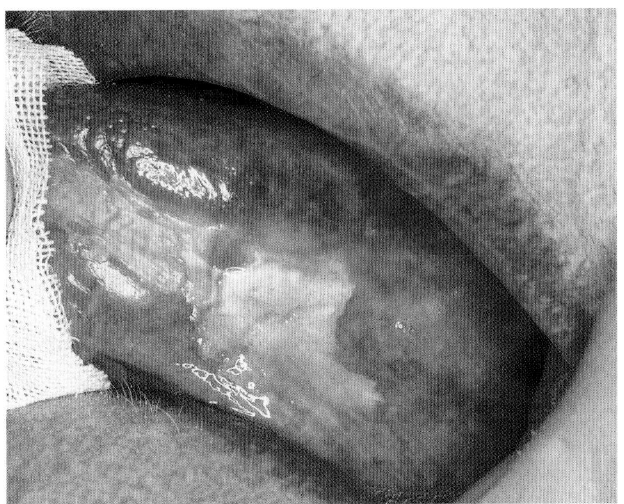

• **Fig. 45.1** The patient's tongue.

History

Complaint

The patient has no complaint.

History of Complaint

You have just noticed the lesion in a patient attending for the first time in several years. There is no written record of the white patch in her notes. The patient had noticed the lesion but had ignored it. She thinks it has probably been there for several years.

Medical History

The patient is otherwise fit and well. She smokes 4 cigarettes a day and drinks 4–8 units of alcohol each week.

Examination

Extraoral Examination

No lymph nodes are palpable in the neck, and there are no abnormal findings on extraoral examination.

Intraoral Examination

Apart from this lesion, the remainder of the oral mucosa is normal.

◆ The Appearance of the Lesion is Shown in Fig. 45.1. What Do You See?

There is a flat and homogeneous white patch on the left lateral border and ventral tongue mucosa. It is well defined and varies slightly in whiteness.

If you were able to feel the lesion, you would find that it is soft and feels no different from the surrounding mucosa.

Differential Diagnosis

◆ What are the Common or Important White Patches in the Mouth? How are They Caused?

Almost all oral white patches are caused by increased keratinization of the epithelium. Keratin absorbs water and appears white, and it is brighter white where it is thicker. The exception is a chemical burn, where the white surface layer is caused by necrosis or ulceration. Common and important causes of oral mucosal white patches are listed in Table 45.1.

TABLE 45.1 Causes of White Patches in the Mouth

Type of Lesion	White Lesion(s)
Normal mucosal variants	Leukoedema Fordyce spots/granules
Inherited epithelial disorders	White sponge naevus Pachyonychia congenita
Traumatic lesions	Frictional keratosis Cheek and tongue biting Chemical burn
Infections	Thrush (acute hyperplastic candidosis) Chronic hyperplastic candidosis (candidal 'leukoplakia') Chronic mucocutaneous candidosis Hairy leukoplakia Syphilitic leukoplakia
Lichen planus and similar conditions	Lichen planus Lichenoid reaction (topical and systemic) Lupus erythematosus Graft versus host disease (GVHD)
Unknown	Leukoplakia (homogenous/verrucous/nodular/speckled)
Smoking-related	Smoker's keratosis Stomatitis nicotina (smoker's palate)
Neoplastic	Squamous cell carcinoma

Which Lesions Would You Include in the Differential Diagnosis for the Current Lesion?

Likely diagnoses:

- Idiopathic white patch (leukoplakia)
- Smoker's keratosis.

Less likely diagnoses:

- Chronic hyperplastic candidosis
- Lichen planus or lichenoid reaction
- Frictional keratosis
- Squamous cell carcinoma.

What is Leukoplakia?

The literal meaning of *leukoplakia* is 'white patch'. The term is correctly defined as a white patch that cannot be characterized as any other lesion. The use of this term is correct only after all possible known causes have been eliminated through whatever investigations are required. Unfortunately, the term *leukoplakia* is often used very loosely in the clinical context, either for a white patch of any cause or for the small minority of white patches with a risk of malignant transformation. This has led to great confusion. Now that the term has also been incorporated into the names of several lesions for which the cause is known (e.g. candidal leukoplakia, hairy leukoplakia and syphilitic leukoplakia), it is being used inconsistently to the point of being unhelpful.

Justify Your Differential Diagnosis

Leukoplakia or Idiopathic White Patch. Although there are many groups of well-defined white patches, the largest single group is that for which no cause can be identified. This is, therefore, a likely diagnosis for the present lesion because there are no clinical features that suggest a specific cause. The group of idiopathic white patches includes some more specific terms that might be applied to this lesion.

- **Sublingual keratosis** refers to a white patch affecting the floor of the mouth or the ventral tongue, and lesions here are considered to have a high risk of malignant transformation. The typical lesion is bilateral and may be extensive in the floor of the mouth, often with a wrinkled surface of 'ebbing tide' parallel corrugations. However, sublingual keratosis is defined only by its site, and any white patch affecting the ventral tongue or the floor of the mouth could be termed *sublingual keratosis.* The present lesion only just extends to the ventral tongue mucosa.
- **Smoker's keratosis** is a white patch of no known cause and found in the mouth of a smoker. This type of lesion is a flat, homogeneous white patch, sometimes with a finely wrinkled surface, on nonkeratinized mucosa. Smoking is assumed to be the cause, although there is rarely any evidence to support this unless the lesion arises where the smoker habitually holds a pipe or a cigarette. This patient's lesion could be smoker's keratosis, but this is not a particularly useful label and does not imply that it should be treated any differently from an idiopathic white patch. Smoker's palate (stomatitis nicotina) is a separate condition and is discussed below.
- **Frictional keratosis** is common along the occlusal line, on edentulous alveolar ridges and on the lateral tongue. It may be associated with sharp teeth or restoration(s) and be unilateral or bilateral. Frictional keratosis usually merges gradually with the surrounding normal mucosa and is not as sharply defined as the present lesion. Tongue biting also causes keratosis, but the surface is often shredded, and there may be similar lesions on the buccal mucosa, usually just behind the commissure. Unless the lesions are associated with clear evidence of habitual biting or sharp teeth or if they resolve on removing the cause, it can be very difficult to identify them on the basis of their clinical appearance.
- **Chronic hyperplastic candidosis** causes white plaques and is sometimes called *candidal leukoplakia.* These lesions arise most commonly on the postcommissural buccal mucosa and dorsal tongue and may be associated with red areas. These lesions are more common in smokers. Unless the site is typical, it is almost impossible to make the diagnosis clinically. Biopsy and resolution following antifungal treatment are the most useful indications to identify these lesions. The present lesion is not typical, but this cause cannot be confidently excluded on clinical grounds.
- **Lichen planus and lichenoid reactions** may cause homogeneous white patches. This more unusual presentation seems to be more common in smokers, and it is not at all clear whether these so-called plaque-type lichen planus lesions are a genuine presentation of lichen planus or are induced by smoking. To be sure of the diagnosis, it is advisable to find evidence of more typical lichen planus elsewhere – on the skin, in the buccal mucosa or in the form of desquamative gingivitis. There is no evidence to suggest that the current lesion is caused by lichen planus, but the plaque type cannot be completely excluded on clinical grounds alone.
- **Squamous cell carcinoma** diagnosis must be included for any white patch in the mouth without an identified cause. The chances of this particular lesion being malignant appear low. Although it is in a high-risk site, it is a flat, homogeneous lesion without ulceration, red areas, speckling or induration. The patient is a light smoker and is in the risk age group for squamous cell carcinoma. Although very unlikely, this just might be a carcinoma.

Which White Lesions Have You Excluded? Explain Why

- *Leukoedema* and patches of *Fordyce spots* (sebaceous glands) are normal mucosal variants that affect primarily the buccal mucosa. Leukoedema causes a milky white appearance and is usually seen in those of African descent. Fordyce spots are sebaceous glands. They occasionally form clusters that resemble plaques but have a slightly yellow appearance, and individual glands are usually visible within the lesion. Both are present from childhood, and neither affects the lateral tongue.

- *White sponge naevus* and *pachyonychia congenita* are examples of rare, inherited conditions that cause diffuse keratosis or multiple discrete white patches on the mucosa. These possibilities are excluded on the basis of the localized extent of the lesion, age at onset and the absence of other skin or nail abnormalities and family history.
- *An aspirin burn* or other form of chemical trauma is unlikely. Such trauma results from the application of aspirin directly to the mucosa, usually in response to toothache. Lesions are mostly in the buccal sulcus and affect the mucosa on both sides of the site where the tablet was placed. This is an unlikely possibility and may be readily excluded through direct questioning.
- *Thrush* affects larger areas of the mucosa, at least parts of the lesion may be wiped off and the underlying mucosa is inflamed. Chronic candidosis, rather than acute candidosis, could have caused the present lesion, as discussed above.
- *Hairy leukoplakia* usually forms bilateral white lesions along the lateral border of the tongue, usually in immunosuppressed patients. Although the possibility of an undiagnosed immunosuppression, particularly resulting from human immunodeficiency virus (HIV) infection, cannot be excluded, the appearances are not typical of hairy leukoplakia. Lesions remain limited to the lateral tongue in almost all cases.
- *Syphilitic leukoplakia* may also be readily. The patient must have tertiary syphilis, and the site of the white patches is the dorsum of the tongue.
- *Smoker's palate (stomatitis nicotina)* may be excluded because it affects only the hard palate of pipe or cigar smokers and that of heavy cigarette smokers.

Investigations

◆ Should a Biopsy Be Performed? Explain Why

Yes. As a general rule, all white lesions in the mouth require biopsy. Completely typical keratotic lichen planus and typical frictional keratoses are considered exceptions to this rule by some authorities, but this would only be acceptable if the clinician were very experienced in the diagnosis of oral white lesions. Even those with extensive experience can be misled occasionally by a carcinomatous lesion that appears to be an innocuous white patch.

The reasons for performing biopsy are:

- To exclude/confirm squamous cell carcinoma
- If not malignant, to determine whether dysplasia is present
- To identify chronic candidal infection, if present
- To help identify specific conditions and cause(s) for the lesion.

◆ Is This Lesion Suitable for Biopsy in General Dental Practice? Explain Why

Yes. The final decision will depend on your experience and confidence and the position of the lesion and its accessibility; however, there is no reason why this biopsy should not be performed in general dental practice. If you perform a biopsy, you are taking on yourself the responsibility of telling the patient the diagnosis, and so you may prefer to refer the patient to a hospital for opinion and biopsy.

If there is any suspicion of malignancy, the patient should be referred to a specialist centre via an expedited referral pathway, according to local and national protocols. Any lesion that shows clinical features suggesting malignancy should be sampled by the person or team who will manage the patient's care.

◆ What Features of a White Patch Might Indicate Malignancy and Contraindicate Performing Biopsy in Dental Practice?

- Associated red areas
- Speckled areas
- Ulceration, especially if chronic
- Induration
- Enlarged lymph nodes draining the site
- Lesion in a high-risk site.

◆ Is a Biopsy Really Necessary? Are There No Less Invasive Tests That Could Help Identify Risk Lesions?

To those not experienced in oral white lesions, it may seem that immediate performance of biopsy is an excessive reaction. After all, benign lesions are so much commoner than potentially malignant causes. To a degree, this is true because almost 5% of the population over 50 years of age have white lesions of some type. Less invasive screening tests have, therefore, been sought to identify the lesions that require biopsy. A number of techniques have been proposed.

Exfoliative Cytology and Brush Biopsy. A sample of epithelial cells can be removed from the lesion by vigorous brushing with a stiff bristle brush. The smear containing cells is examined by using a variety of techniques, including computer-assisted cytopathological analysis. These techniques have improved and have become more reliable but, to date, have not replaced the need for biopsy.

Toluidine Blue Staining. Toluidine blue (tolonium chloride) staining was described decades ago but its use has recently been revived in the form of new commercial test kits. The dye can be applied to the lesion by dabbing or in a mouthwash, and it is claimed that lesions that retain the blue stain indicate a higher risk of dysplasia or carcinoma compared with those that do not. The predictive value of the test remains unclear, with better results shown in high-risk populations. False-positive reactions are common because the dye binds to ulcer slough, staining ulcers, lichen planus and other benign lesions.

Optical Tests. Autofluorescence. The oral mucosa contains a large number of autofluorescent molecules such as collagen and keratin. It is claimed that this normal fluorescence is lost in dysplasia and carcinoma. Handheld blue light illuminators with filters to detect the green florescence are available for screening, but their predictive value is low.

Chemiluminescent light examination. This technique illuminates the mucosa with white light, with or without an initial dilute acetic acid rinse and/or tolonium chloride staining. It is claimed that dysplastic and malignant lesions are more readily seen.

Both these illumination techniques remain to be proven in well-controlled studies.

All these tests are screening tests, and none is of sufficient accuracy to be used as a diagnostic test for carcinoma or dysplasia. Until such techniques are validated, biopsy remains the safest and only justifiable course of action. Studies show that patients do not find biopsy a traumatic procedure and that healing is rarely problematic. It is an investigation that any dental surgeon should be able to perform, and it should not be delayed.

◆ How Much Would You Remove and From Where?

The ideal biopsy sample of mucosa to assess a white patch or mucosal condition is approximately 10 mm long and 4–5 mm wide. The sample should extend to muscle and provide sufficient deep tissue to support the epithelial sample for the pathologist to inspect microscopically. In the lateral tongue, this is only 2–3 mm depth because the muscle lies near the surface. In buccal mucosa, the ideal depth is slightly more – up to 5 mm. If a lesion is suspected to extend deeply, then a thicker sample will be required. This size of sample is readily removed, the wound is easily closed and healing is quick and without significant symptoms.

The site sampled should comprise mostly the lesion but with a part of the margin and some adjacent normal mucosa. In a higher-risk lesion, any suspicious areas (see the list above) would be included. If several such areas were present, multiple samples might be required.

◆ The Biopsy Specimen is Required To Assess Dysplasia. What is Meant By 'Dysplasia'?

When applied to white or red oral patches, 'dysplasia' means the microscopic changes that indicate a risk of malignant transformation.

◆ What are the Features of Epithelial Dysplasia?

Dysplasia is recognized by combinations of histological features listed in Table 45.2.

◆ How Do These Changes Differ From the Histological Changes Seen in Squamous Cell Carcinoma?

Many, if not all, of these features are usually seen in squamous cell carcinomas. Carcinoma differs from dysplasia only in that it invades underlying tissues, usually as separate islands and strands of epithelium, and may metastasize to distant sites.

TABLE 45.2 Histological Features of Dysplasia

Growth Abnormality	Detected By the Presence of
Failure to form an organized epithelial layer	No well-defined basal cell, prickle and squamous cell layers (and keratin layer, if present) Increased number of layers of basal cells Drop-shaped rete processes Loss of polarity of the cells: vertically orientated rather than flattening towards the surface Loss of cohesion between cells
Disordered maturation and differentiation of single cells	Change in keratin pattern Keratinization of single cells or clusters of cells deep in the epithelium rather than at the surface Cells of bizarre shape (pleomorphism)
Abnormalities of cell nuclei	Darkly staining nuclei (hyperchromatism) Nuclei of varying sizes (anisonucleosis) Cells with bizarre nuclei (nuclear pleomorphism)
Abnormal growth regulation	Increased numbers of mitoses Mitoses in suprabasal cells Abnormal mitoses

◆ How is Dysplasia Assessed?

The scoring of dysplasia is extremely difficult, is not very reproducible and requires experience. Most pathologists categorize dysplastic lesions as mild, moderate and severe dysplasia. Severe dysplasia is sometimes called *carcinoma in situ*.

With increasing severity of dysplasia, there is increasing risk of malignant transformation. Although dysplasia is the best indicator of the risk of malignancy, the relationship between the two is complex. Severe dysplasia nearly always indicates a relatively high risk, but carcinoma will occasionally develop in a white lesion that shows minimal or no dysplasia.

◆ Are There More Accurate Predictors of Transformation That Can Be Applied To the Biopsy?

It has been shown that measuring the total DNA content of the epithelial cells (ploidy analysis) is helpful to predict malignant transformation. Aneuploidy (the presence of an abnormal number of chromosomes in a cell) has shown to be a predictor of malignant transformation.

Loss of one allele of key tumour suppressor genes (loss of heterozygocity) in epithelial cells has also been shown to be helpful in predicting malignant transformation.

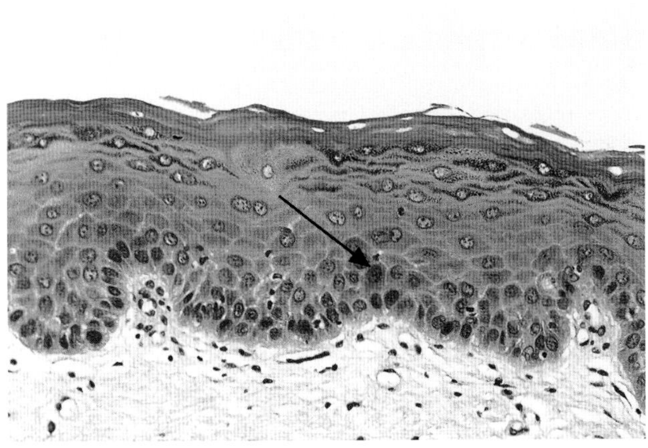

• **Fig. 45.2** The histological appearances of the biopsy sample.

Both ploidy and loss of heterozygocity analysis are an adjunct to supplement histological evaluation but are only available in a few specialist diagnostic laboratories.

◆ Does Dysplasia Always Progress?

No. Dysplasia does not always progress, and in some cases of mild dysplasia, it may regress. Dysplasia indicates increased potential for malignant transformation but does not necessarily mean that this may eventually occur in any particular lesion. Some dysplastic lesions never become malignant, and those that do may not transform into cancer for months or years.

◆ The Histological Features of the Lesion are Shown in Fig. 45.2. What Do You See and How Do You Interpret the Changes?

The surface is covered by a regular orthokeratinized stratified squamous epithelium. The epithelium is abnormal for either the lateral border or the ventral tongue, neither of which shows even orthokeratosis.

There are minimal signs of dysplasia. The epithelium shows good stratification, with well-organized basal, prickle cell, granular cell and keratin layers, each composed of cells at the same stage of maturation. The basal cell layer is slightly disorganized. Instead of a well-defined single layer of small dark cells, there is a slightly irregular layer of cells with nuclei that vary a little in size and staining intensity. Near the centre, there is one darkly staining cell in a suprabasal position (arrowed). *No* Candida *was found in a section stained with periodic acid–Schiff (PAS) stain.*

Changes such as abnormal keratinization and slight basal cell irregularity are not very marked. The epithelial cells form a well-organized epithelium; there are only occasional abnormal single cells, minimal nuclear abnormalities and no evidence of increased growth. These signs might be graded as either nondysplastic or mildly dysplastic, depending on the pathologist. *The final diagnosis given in this case was keratosis with mild dysplasia.*

Diagnosis

◆ What is the Final Diagnosis? Is This a Lesion with a High Risk of Malignant Transformation?

The diagnosis is idiopathic white patch (leukoplakia) with mild dysplasia. This is a lesion with a risk of malignant transformation.

Treatment

◆ What Treatment is Indicated?

The following principles of treatment apply to all idiopathic white patches. The patient should stop smoking and moderate her alcohol intake. If candidal infection had been detected, it should be treated and periodically checked for recurrence. In this case, and others in which dysplasia is mild or absent, it is appropriate to monitor the lesion closely for changes in appearance, initially at 3-monthly intervals and then extending to annual review, provided the lesion does not change significantly. The aim is to detect any change in the severity of dysplasia or malignant transformation, and this may require biopsy from time to time, depending on the changes noted. Photographic or digital images aid recognition of changes and are a valuable adjunct to the long-term review of white patches.

Lesions with moderate or severe dysplasia may be removed through knife or laser excision. Occasionally, patches are too large to treat in these ways, and the only option is close monitoring to detect malignant transformation as early as possible.

In addition, it is important to remember that dysplasia may affect any mucosal areas exposed to tobacco smoke and alcohol. There is a risk of carcinoma arising in the pharynx and in the respiratory tract, and symptoms arising from these areas indicate a need for endoscopy.

Prognosis

◆ What Features Would Indicate That a White Patch Might Become Malignant Over the Coming Years?

The features associated with increased risk of malignant transformation are listed in Table 45.3.

In this case, the lesion remained unchanged, and the patient was reviewed at 3-monthly intervals for 1 year and at 6-monthly intervals for 2 years, and she remains under annual review. Four years after presentation, a second biopsy was performed, and the degree of dysplasia was still mild. Excision was considered because the lesion is relatively accessible and in a site that is at high risk of carcinoma, but it was not carried out because the dysplasia remains mild and the patient prefers not to have surgery. The patient is also maintaining close observation of her white patch and will return for an earlier appointment if she feels it has changed.

TABLE 45.3 Features Associated with Risk of Malignant Transformation

Feature	Risk of Malignant Transformation
Dysplasia	The degree of dysplasia is the best predictor, and it may change, either progressing or regressing, with time.
Genetic status	Aneuploidy and loss of heterozygocity indicate increased risk.
Site	White lesions in the floor of the mouth, posterior and lateral tongue and retromolar area carry the highest risk. Those on the hard palate and dorsum of tongue carry no significant risk except in some cases where plaque-like lichen planus has been present for many years and becomes verrucous. Verrucous lesions on the gingivae can also be high risk for malignant transformation.
Colour	Development of red areas or speckling carries a high risk and is usually associated with severe dysplasia histologically.
Surface	Development of verrucous, nodular areas or ulceration indicate high risk.
Tobacco use	Smoking increases the risk. However, smoking also causes many white patches with no dysplasia, and so statistically, patches in nonsmokers carry the higher risk.
Age	The risk of malignant transformation rises with age.
Gender	Female patients are at higher risk (despite the fact that oral carcinoma is more common in men).
Size	Larger lesions have a higher risk of malignant transformation.
Duration	Patches present for a longer time have a higher risk of malignant transformation.
Multiple areas of leukoplakia	Patients with multiple areas of leukoplakia and those who have had a previous oral cancer are at higher risk.
Family history of carcinoma in upper aerodigestive tract	Indicates increased risk.
Candidal infection in presence of dysplasia	Indicates a small increase in risk.
Change in clinical appearance	Changes apart from that in colour such as changes in size or nodularity or the development of a verrucous surface, indicate a higher risk.
Underlying conditions	Conditions that predispose to oral carcinoma such as submucous fibrosis, raise the relative risk of malignant transformation.

Case 46

Another White Patch On the Tongue

EDWARD ODELL AND SELVAM THAVARAJ

Summary

A 39-year-old woman has a white patch on the lateral margin of her tongue. What is the cause, and what are the treatment options?

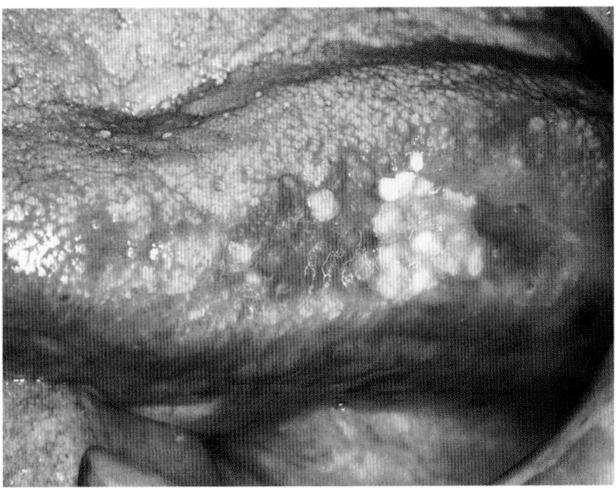

• **Fig. 46.1** The patient's tongue.

History

Complaint

The patient has no symptoms.

History of Complaint

The patient is an infrequent dental attender and has not been to the dentist for at least 5 years. After participating in a week-long oral cancer awareness programme, she inspected her mouth and became nervous about her tongue. She would like to have it checked.

Medical History

She is otherwise fit and well. She has smoked 40 cigarettes daily since the age of 18 years and drinks 14 units of alcohol (wine) per week.

Examination

Extraoral Examination

She seems to be healthy, with no obvious skin, nail or eye lesions present on visible skin. No lymph nodes are palpable in the neck.

Intraoral Examination

The oral mucosa appears normal, except for the tongue, as shown in Fig. 46.1.

Site	Left lateral border of tongue
Size	1–3 cm approximately
Shape	Ill-defined ellipse
Colour	Mixture of white and red components
Surface	Appears nodular or irregular

◆ Describe the Appearance of the Tongue Lesion

Palpation reveals the lesion to be firmer than the adjacent mucosa. The white component of the area cannot be rubbed away. The tongue is freely mobile.

Differential Diagnosis

◆ What are the Causes of Mixed Red and White Patches in the Mouth?

The causes of white patches are discussed more fully in Case 45. Several may also be associated with red areas.

Cause	Red and White Lesion(s)
Trauma	Chemical burn Cheek biting
Infection	Thrush (acute hyperplastic candidosis) Chronic hyperplastic candidosis (candidal 'leukoplakia')
Lichen planus and similar conditions	Lichen planus Lichenoid reaction (topical and systemic) Lupus erythematosus
Idiopathic or smoking	Idiopathic keratosis (leukoplakia) including: Sublingual keratosis Smoker's keratosis Speckled leukoplakia Stomatitis nicotina (smoker's palate)
Neoplasia	Squamous cell carcinoma

◆ Which of the Above Lesions Would You Include in the Differential Diagnosis for This Particular Lesion?

1. Squamous cell carcinoma
2. Idiopathic white patch with or without dysplasia, including speckled leucoplakia
3. Chronic hyperplastic candidosis
4. Lichenoid reaction.

◆ Justify This Differential Diagnosis

The most important consideration in the differential diagnosis of all oral white patches is that squamous cell carcinoma or an oral potentially malignant disorder may be the cause. This is especially so when lesions are red and white or speckled.

Squamous cell carcinoma is a likely diagnosis and the most significant one. Although this patient is young for squamous cell carcinoma, cases are seen in the fourth decade of life, and the incidence in younger patients appears to be increasing in the UK and elsewhere. The patient drinks and smokes heavily, and these are the main risk factors for oral squamous cell carcinoma. She drinks 14 units of alcohol per week, which is the maximum recommended intake. The maximum intake is considered 'safe' in terms of liver and cardiovascular disease risks, but no safe limit is recognized for cancer. There is no safe intake for tobacco, and the combined relative risk of carcinoma for this patient is at least 5–10 times higher than that for a nonsmoker or an occasional drinker. Regardless of the patient's age, the presence of the lesion in a high-risk site, its speckled appearance and association with smoking are very worrying. This lesion should be considered carcinoma until proven otherwise.

A potentially malignant disorder would be the next most likely diagnosis. Option 2 in the differential diagnosis covers all white patches of unknown aetiology, some of which carry a risk of malignant transformation and show dysplasia on microscopic examination. The risk of malignant transformation is higher in those with a red component, which may be seen either in a speckled area or in a separate, usually adjacent, site. The risk factors are the same as those for carcinoma, and if this lesion is not carcinoma, it is almost certainly at risk of malignant transformation.

◆ Which Lesions are Less Likely Possibilities? Explain Why

Candidal infection should always be considered a cause of white patches, particularly when red areas are associated. This infection is very common. The combination of red and white is most likely to signify thrush (acute hyperplastic candidosis. However, lesions of thrush are usually more widespread than in the present case, and at least some of the white plaques may be removed by rubbing. Chronic hyperplastic candidosis (candidal 'leukoplakia') forms a discrete white plaque that is sometimes associated with red areas. Although it is normally found on the buccal mucosa and on the dorsal surface of the tongue, it is a possible diagnosis for the current lesion. It should also be remembered that almost any white patch in the mouth may be susceptible to infection by *Candida*, simply because of the increased thickness of keratin on the surface of the epithelium. Thus, the presence of candidal infection does not preclude an underlying carcinoma, dysplasia, lichen planus or similar conditions.

Lichen planus and similar conditions are relatively common causes of intraoral white lesions. Lichen planus, lichenoid reactions and lupus erythematosus are usually readily identifiable by virtue of the presence of lacy white striae, association with atrophic areas and desquamative gingivitis and their symmetrical bilateral distribution. In smokers, both lichen planus and lichenoid reactions may present as discrete white plaques, but these plaque-type lesions are not usually associated with red areas. Localized single white lesions may also result from topically induced lichenoid reactions such as those to dental restorative materials. However, these are all most unlikely to be responsible for the current lesion because their clinical appearance and distribution are distinct.

◆ What Features Might Indicate That This Lesion is Already Malignant? Which are Early Signs, and Which are Late Signs?

Feature	Early	Late
Red or speckled areas	*	*
Nonhealing ulceration	*	*
Rolled everted ulcer margin		*
Induration of surrounding tissues		*
Bleeding from the surface		*
Fixation of the tissues		*
Destruction of adjacent bone		*
Enlarged hard lymph nodes		*
Size	Small carcinomas are probably diagnosed early, but there is great variation in the rate of growth, and this is only an assumption	
Pain	Unpredictable, often absent and sometimes the presenting complaint	

Investigations

◆ What Investigations are Indicated?

Biopsy is generally considered mandatory for any oral white lesion. This is especially important if no cause is apparent. When malignancy or significant dysplasia is suspected, as in the present case, the biopsy should be performed as soon as possible because early diagnosis is a major factor for the successful treatment of oral squamous cell carcinoma.

◆ Would You Perform This Biopsy in General Practice?

No, definitely not. Although removing a sample of the tissue is well within the capability of the general dental practitioner, it would be unwise to do so. The patient will return for the result, and dental practitioners are not usually the appropriate persons to break the news of malignant disease to the patient. There is also a theoretical risk that biopsy of the wrong site or unintentional removal of a small lesion in its entirety might compromise subsequent treatment, but this is a largely theoretical problem. In a practice environment, the patient should be referred urgently, preferably the same day, to a centre where definitive treatment can be provided. This will allow the most appropriate biopsy to be performed. No other investigations are indicated at this stage.

UK treatment centres operate an urgent cancer referral pathway for suspected malignancy. Dentists must make themselves familiar with fast-track referral processes, according to their local cancer network protocols.

◆ Which Part of the Lesion Should Be Removed for Biopsy?

The specimen should include those areas most likely to be malignant – the red and speckled parts. Some normal tissue should also be included, and the sample should be about 1 cm long, 4–5 mm wide, and of an even depth, including underlying muscle. Larger malignancies are often friable, and if the specimen is too small, it may disintegrate on removal. No attempt should be made to excise the whole lesion until a diagnosis is obtained.

◆ The Biopsy Specimen is Shown in Fig. 46.2. What are the Microscopic Features, and How Do You Interpret Them?

The lower power view (Fig. 46.2a) shows the tongue mucosa with underlying muscle. The overlying epithelium is very irregular, and instead of being an even and well-organized layer, it forms an irregular series of rete processes that penetrate deeply into the underlying tissue. The deepest epithelium is breaking off into apparently separate islands and strands, and these extend deeply between muscle bundles. The higher power view (see Fig. 46.2b) taken from the deep surface shows the deepest epithelium invading muscle. The epithelium is disorganized, with cells demonstrating a squamous morphology in the centre of islands and an irregular darkly stained basal cell layer around the edge. This epithelium has lost its ordered maturation and stratification and is invading the underlying muscle. Invasion indicates malignancy, and the malignant epithelium shows squamous differentiation.

Diagnosis

◆ What is the Diagnosis?

The patient has squamous cell carcinoma. It is only superficially invasive and probably an early lesion.

Treatment

◆ What Types of Treatment are Possible, and What is the Prognosis?

This lesion has been diagnosed at an early stage compared with most oral carcinomas. Treatment is likely to be surgery, followed by radiotherapy with or without chemotherapy. The final treatment decision will depend on the results of investigations to stage the carcinoma (to determine its size and the extent of any metastases to lymph nodes and distant sites). The decision to provide postoperative radiotherapy or chemoradiotherapy will depend on the histological features of an adequately excised tumour. If treated in the early stages, a 5-year survival rate of 85% or better can be achieved. If survival reaches 10 years, the patient is likely to

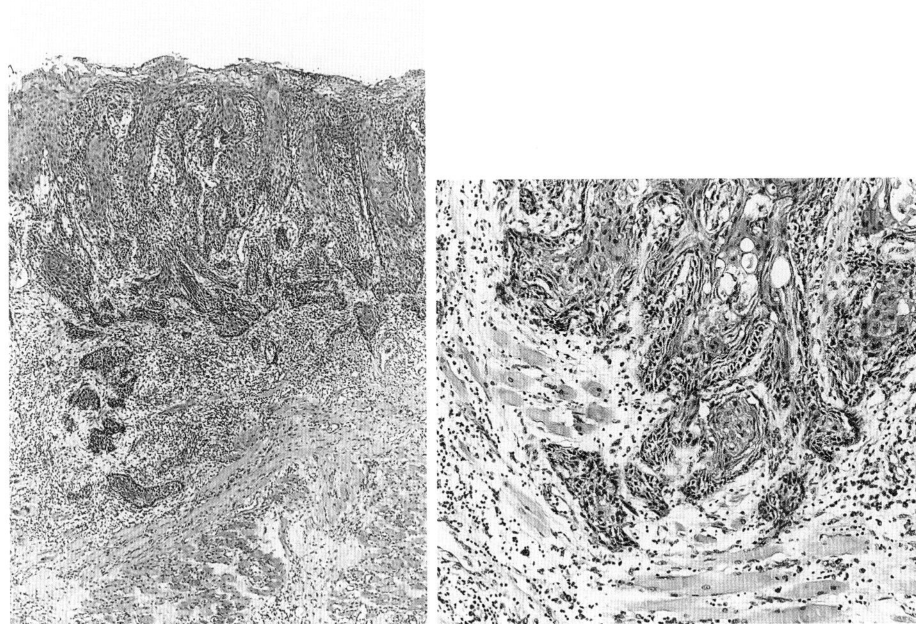

• **Fig. 46.2** The histological appearances of the lesion: **a,** lower power view; **b,** higher power view.

be considered cured. However, 10% of patients with oral carcinoma develop a second primary lesion in the mouth or upper aerodigestive tract. The chances of developing a second lesion may be reduced by stopping smoking, and so the patient should be encouraged to do so. Smoking-associated cardiovascular disease, if severe, may also compromise treatment.

Further details of the treatment of oral carcinoma are given in Case 45.

After the biopsy, further investigations including computed tomography (CT), magnetic resonance imaging (MRI) and fine-needle aspiration cytology (FNAC) showed no cervical lymph node metastasis in this patient.

◆ Should the Patient Have Her Cervical Lymph Nodes Treated?

Although no metastasis has been detected in the cervical lymph nodes, a neck dissection may still be required. This is because malignant cells continually separate from the carcinoma and pass in small numbers into the lymphatics and the bloodstream. The majority of these cells die. However, some could have reached the cervical lymph nodes and be present as very small metastatic deposits not detectable by imaging or FNAC. Approximately 25% of these deposits are not detectable clinically and are termed 'occult metastases'. If left untreated, they would continue to grow, ultimately invading beyond the lymph node and spreading to distant sites.

The following factors are associated with an increased risk of metastasis:

- Large primary tumour
- Long duration
- Poorly differentiated histological grade
- Aggressive pattern of invasion seen histologically
- Depth of invasion
- Vascular invasion at primary site.

Neck dissection performed to remove possible occult metastases is called a *prophylactic* or *elective neck dissection.*

Whether to treat an apparently normal neck when a patient has a small carcinoma is contentious because neck dissection carries significant morbidity. However, the development of metastases later reduces the patient's chances of survival. For this reason, an elective neck dissection is recommended. A neck dissection may also be required for surgical access and to aid reconstruction.

Metastasis from tongue carcinoma is recognized to be unpredictable. When the carcinoma has invaded to a depth of 4 mm, there is a greater likelihood of metastasis. This patient's risk of occult metastasis is compounded by the aggressive tumour infiltration pattern.

◆ Could Neck Dissection Not Be Advised On the Basis of Better Evidence?

Yes, the technique of sentinel node biopsy has been developed to predict lymph node metastasis accurately. In this investigation, a radioactive tracer is injected into and around the carcinomatous lesion on the day before surgery. The tracer drains along the same lymphatic routes to the lymph nodes to which carcinoma cells would travel. At surgery, a radioactivity-detecting probe is used to identify the nodes with concentrated radioactive tracer. These 'sentinel' lymph nodes are removed and sent to the pathology laboratory on the basis that they are the ones most likely to contain metastasis. A thorough and detailed microscopic examination is carried out to examine all the nodes in multiple sections, with the use of special stains.

If the nodes contain no metastasis, no neck dissection is performed. If they contain metastasis, a neck dissection is indicated to remove the rest of the cervical nodes because other metastases may be present.

Further Reading

For guidance on criteria for urgent referral, see: https://www.nice.org.uk/guidance/ng12/chapter/1-Recommendations-organised-by-site-of-cancer#head-and-neck-cancers

For further information on management of the neck in patients with early-stage oral cancer, see section 4.2 of the NICE guidance for the management of upper aerodigestive tract cancer at: https://www.nice.org.uk/guidance/ng36/evidence/full-guideline-pdf-2307980269

Case 47

Molar Endodontic Treatment

FRANCESCO MANNOCCI

Summary

A 52-year-old man presents with pain from a tooth in the lower left quadrant. What is the cause, and how will you treat him?

History

Complaint

This patient complains of pain from a tooth in the lower left quadrant but is unsure which tooth is the cause.

History of Complaint

◆ What Specific Questions Would You Ask With Regard To the History of Pain?

Relevant questions and the patient's answers are shown in Table 47.1.

TABLE 47.1 Questions That Could Be Asked During Anamnesis (Verbal History Taking)

Question	Patient's Answer
When did the pain start?	*About 8 months ago.*
Did anything start or provoke the pain?	*Initially hot and cold foods and drinks brought the pain on.*
How long did the pain last at that time?	*Only for a few seconds.*
What is the character of the pain?	*Initially sharp but now dull and throbbing.*
Other than the change in the intensity of the pain, has it changed in any other way?	*The pain is still brought on by hot and cold foods and now lasts for hours.*
Does the pain start spontaneously? Does it wake you up or keep you awake at night?	*Initially no, but as the pain intensity has increased over the last 2–3 days it has woken me at night.*
Does anything relieve the pain?	*Paracetamol has a mild relieving effect.*
Is the tooth painful to bite on?	*No.*

Dental History

The patient is new to your particular practice but has always attended the dentist regularly.

Medical History

The patient is fit and well.

◆ On the Basis of What You Know Already, What is the Likely Diagnosis?

The pain is almost certainly caused by pulpitis. It is brought on by hot and cold and is poorly localized. It has progressed from intermittent pain, suggesting reversible pulpitis, to a severe pain that lasts hours. The severity and duration now suggest that pulpitis might be irreversible.

◆ What is Irreversible Pulpitis?

Irreversible pulpitis is a concept rather than a well-defined clinical condition. Pulpitis is usually chronic and progresses intermittently and unpredictably with or without acute phases. At some stage, the pulp is irretrievably damaged, probably because pressure from inflammation impedes pulpal blood flow. This causes loss of vitality. The ability to predict pulp necrosis would be useful when deciding possible management options. Unfortunately, the clinical symptoms that accompany pulpitis are variable, especially in multirooted teeth, and pain is a subjective sensation. Severe pain of long duration, spontaneous pain and waking at night are usually taken to indicate the irreversible stage of pulpitis; however, predicting the future course of disease is never reliable, and making this diagnosis involves an element of uncertainty, depending on operator experience.

Examination

Extraoral Examination

The temporomandibular joints appear normal, and there are no palpable submental, submandibular or cervical lymph nodes.

Intraoral Examination

On examination, you discover poor oral hygiene, with gingivitis around posterior teeth. The dentition is moderately restored.

In the lower left quadrant, the second permanent molar tooth has an occlusal amalgam. The premolars appear sound.

◆ **What Parts of the Examination Would Be Most Useful? Why?**

Teeth should be percussed to establish whether any are tender. Adjacent, apparently healthy control teeth should be percussed first for comparison. Tenderness indicates inflammation in the apical periodontal ligament, and causes would include very-late-stage irreversible pulpitis or a necrotic pulp.

Palpation of the mucosa overlying the tooth apices with a fingertip. Tenderness indicates extension of inflammation from the periodontal ligament to the surrounding bone and the activity of any inflammation present. Affected teeth are compared with clinically sound teeth. Lower molar apices are close to the lingual mandibular cortex and must be palpated lingually as well as buccally.

Mobility should be assessed. Mobility is increased slightly if there is inflammation of the periodontal ligament. If a periradicular abscess or acute inflammation is present, the tooth may be raised in the socket. You must exclude increased mobility caused by periodontal disease, root fracture, recent trauma or a premature occlusal contact.

Periodontal probing should be performed to detect loss of attachment or exposed dentine. Dentine hypersensitivity would not cause such severe, long-lasting pain. However, pocketing or previous periodontal treatment could have exposed a lateral canal or canal in the furcation, allowing bacteria access to the pulp.

Search for a sinus would indicate periradicular infection. Sinuses may heal and present as a small fibrous nodule, indicating past or intermittent infection. The search must include the lingual alveolar mucosa because the apices of lower molars lie closer to the lingual cortex than the buccal cortex.

On examining the patient, you find that no teeth are mobile, are tender to percussion or have apical tenderness. There is no detectable sinus. Inflammation appears limited to the pulp. No periodontitis is present.

Investigations

◆ **What Investigations Would You Perform?**

Tests of pulp sensibility are required to increase confidence in your assessment of the status of the pulp. Electric testing and thermal (hot and cold) testing are available, and use of a stimulus that usually provokes the pain is recommended. Ensure that healthy adjacent, opposing and contralateral teeth are also examined to obtain a reference measure of the patient's response. If tests yield equivocal responses, a test cavity without local analgesia should prove conclusive.

A periapical radiograph of the molar teeth is required.

◆ **What are the Limitations of Tests of Sensibility?**

Tests of sensibility do not measure pulp vitality (blood flow) but test for a continuous sensory nerve pathway from the pulp to the brain. For this reason, they are referred to as *sensibility tests.*

It is assumed that pulp without sensory innervation is devitalized, but this is not necessarily so. Inflammation can alter sensation and sensation may be incorrectly localized (see Case 1). Conversely, a positive response does not guarantee the histological health of the pulp.

Tests sometimes indicate a hypersensitive pulp, and this is a more useful piece of information because detection of hypersensitivity is not prone to false-positive or false-negative results.

◆ **What are the Causes of Misleading Electric Pulp Test Results?**

Both false-positive and false-negative sensibility responses can occur. Causes, together with precautions that minimize the risk of a spurious result, are listed in Table 47.2.

On performing these tests, you discover that the lower second molar gives a hypersensitive response to hot gutta percha. The pain lasted until a local anaesthetic was given.

◆ **The Periapical Radiograph of Mandibular Left Second Molar is Shown in Fig. 47.1. What Do You See?**

The mandibular left second molar shows extensive radiolucency under the existing radiopaque amalgam restoration encroaching the pulp horns (most likely to be caries). There is no obvious periapical radiolucency, and an impacted mandibular third molar is visible along with the intact borders of the inferior alveolar canal.

Diagnosis

◆ **What is the Most Likely Diagnosis?**

Irreversible pulpitis in the lower left second molar tooth caused by the large carious lesion. When the pain started 8 months ago, the carious lesion would have been smaller and the pulpitis reversible. If it had been treated preventively and operatively at that stage by the oral healthcare team, it is high likely that any endodontic treatment would now be required for a necrotic pulp.

Treatment

◆ **What Emergency Treatment Would You Provide At the First Appointment?**

The carious lesion is extensive in the second molar. Assuming the tooth is to be retained and conserved, the first priority is relief of pain. Having assessed the pulpitis as irreversible, extirpation of the pulp is the only appropriate treatment, and this will require cleaning and shaping of the root canals to ensure that no remnants remain. Extirpation with barbed broach alone risks leaving fragments of inflamed vital pulp that could cause pain after treatment. A root canal dressing of nonsetting calcium hydroxide will inhibit bacterial growth. This must be sealed from rest of the mouth with a suitable provisional dressing material to prevent bacterial ingress, pending definitive treatment.

TABLE 47.2 Possible Causes of Error in Electric Pulp Testing of Tooth Sensibility and Measures That Can Be Used To Mitigate These

Cause of Error	Possible Precautions To Minimize the False Readings
False-Positive Response	
Patient's anticipation of pain or sensitivity	Test control teeth first, several times if unsure; raise tester level setting slowly and incrementally.
Multirooted tooth, with one or more canals containing necrotic pulp tissue and the remainder vital tissue	Test at several sites, over each root, on exposed dentine, if possible.
Sensation originates in the gingiva because the tooth is not electrically isolated	Ensure teeth are dry, keep electrode away from amalgam restorations that extend subgingivally.
Sensation originates in an adjacent tooth because the tested tooth is not electrically isolated	Keep electrode away from amalgams that contact adjacent teeth, dry teeth, isolate teeth with a small piece of rubber dam.
C nerve fibres within the pulp tissue can still function for some time after loss of their blood supply	None possible.
False-Negative Response	
Poor contact between electrode and tooth	Ensure good contact surface area, and use conductive jelly to couple the two surfaces together.
Inadequate electrical access to tooth tissue because of insulating nonmetallic tooth coverage	None possible unless restoration is to be replaced and access can be cut in crown.
Advanced age – pulp insulated by thick physiological secondary dentine deposition	None possible.
Heavily restored or worn tooth with a pulp insulated by thick reactionary, tertiary, dentine deposits	Place electrode close to root canal rather than occlusally if this is suspected.
High pain or sensation threshold	None possible, not usually a problem.

Pulpotomy, with removal of the coronal pulp, or partial pulpectomy, with removal of pulp from the widest canal, is sometimes advocated in multirooted teeth but should be avoided. The apical extent of inflammation in the pulp is unknown, and pain relief cannot be guaranteed.

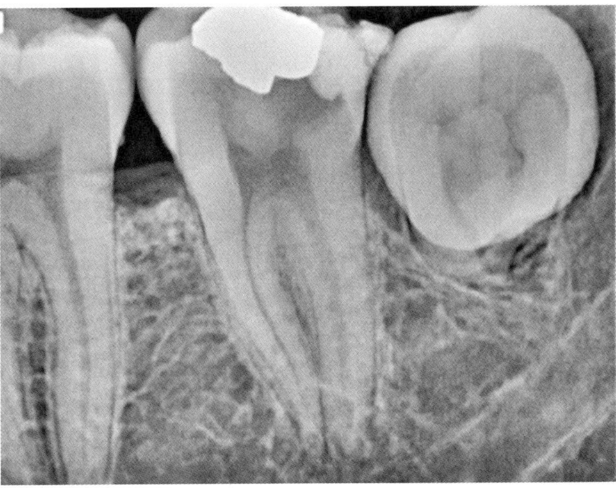

• **Fig. 47.1** Periapical radiograph of mandibular left second molar on presentation.

◆ What Definitive Treatment Does the Patient Require for the Second Molar?

The patient should return for cleaning, shaping and obturation of the root canals and a definitive coronal restoration. A cuspal-coverage indirect restoration, either an onlay or a core with a full-coverage crown, should be considered for protection against occlusal forces. Post crowns in molar teeth are to be avoided because of the incidence of perforations and root fractures. Retention should be sufficient from the undercut shape of the pulp chamber and the remaining coronal tooth structure (see Case 1 and Case 9).

After discussing the possibility of restoring or extracting the second molar, the patient opts for root canal treatment. All options, including the normal advantages and disadvantages of each, need to be discussed. These conversations need to be fully documented in the notes and time given to the patient to understand his responsibility and consequences of the care provided. By managing patient expectations at this stage, later medico-legal issues can be avoided.

You carry out the first stage of treatment successfully. However, the patient fails to return to complete the treatment. When he returns after 6 months, you discover that the tooth has remained asymptomatic but the coronal temporary restoration has been lost and the lingual cusp has fractured off. The pulp chamber is open to the oral cavity, but the tooth is still restorable.

◆ What Effect Will This Have On the Long-Term Prognosis for This Tooth?

Loss of the coronal seal allows microbial invasion of the root canals and dentine tubules. Bacteria and their metabolic and breakdown products are irritants and penetrate apically and along lateral canals to induce or maintain periradicular inflammation. In addition, the flora in the canal change, and a more mixed oral flora with anaerobes become established in the canal. This may be more difficult to eradicate and is more likely to penetrate through the apex and induce an acute abscess. Fracture of the lingual cusp further weakens the tooth and complicates building up a core to support the definitive coronal restoration.

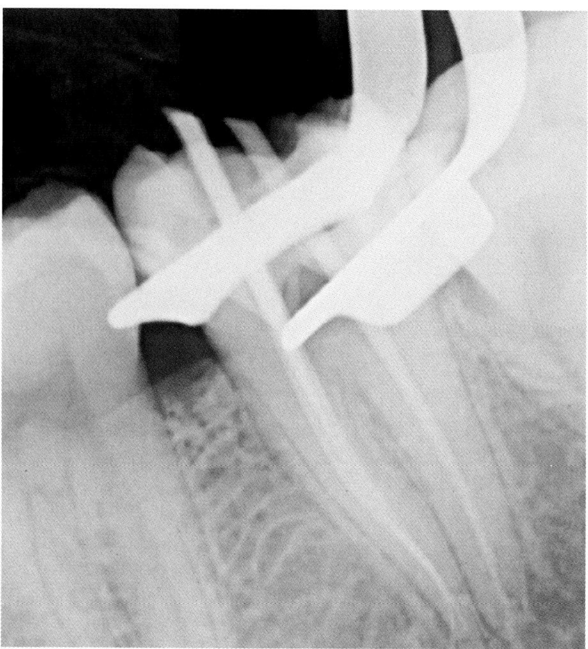

• **Fig. 47.2** The gutta percha master point try-in periapical radiograph.

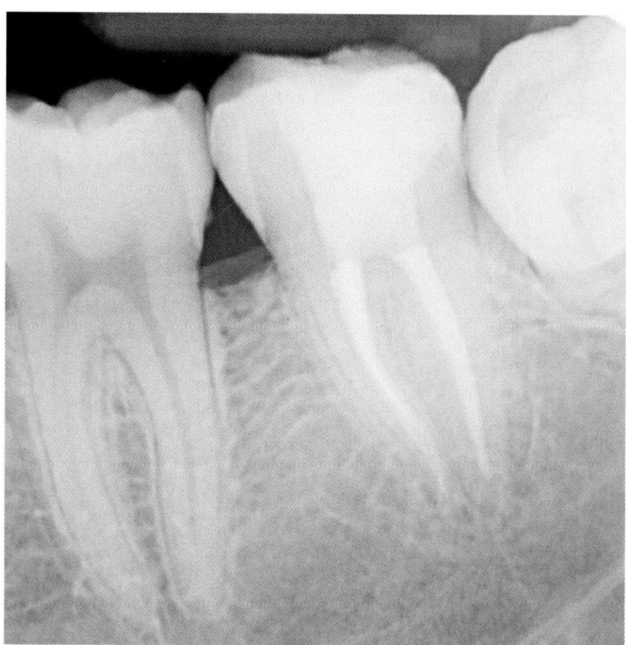

• **Fig. 47.3** Periapical radiograph of the completed root canal filling of the mandibular second molar. The tooth was restored with a resin composite restoration and should be subsequently restored with a full cuspal-coverage restoration.

◆ What Should Be the Next Stage of Treatment?

Root canal treatment must be recommenced as soon as possible. The tooth should be isolated with rubber dam and the root canals cleaned and shaped with use of appropriate files and copious irrigation with sodium hypochlorite. Sodium hypochlorite is antibacterial, but some bacteria may survive in the lateral canals and dentine tubules that are blocked by the smear layer produced by instrumentation. The smear layer must be removed by occasionally irrigating with 17% EDTA (ethylenediaminetetraacetic acid) solution. Hypochlorite will then be able to penetrate dentine and the lateral canals. It is important that coronal root canal preparation is carried out first to reduce the bacterial load and improve access to the apical portion of the root canal. The gutta percha master point try-in radiograph shows the multiple curvatures of the mesial canals (Figs 47.2 and 47.3).

◆ How Long Should This Tooth Be Monitored After Completion of Root Canal Treatment? What are the Criteria for Success?

Root canal treatment should be reviewed after 1 year, as suggested in the guidance of the European society of endodontology (2006). Outcome must be evaluated clinically and radiographically. The radiographic assessment must be made by comparing the appearances with previous films, taken under conditions that are as near standardized as possible. Criteria for success and failure are shown in Table 47.3.

TABLE 47.3 Criteria Used To Assess the Outcome of Root Canal Treatment

Success	No symptoms No tenderness on percussion or increased mobility No sinus Width and contour of periodontal ligament normal Slight radiolucency around excess filling material allowable
Uncertain	No symptoms No tenderness on percussion or increased mobility No sinus Smaller residual radiolucency at 4 years than seen on completion of root canal filling; some authorities suggest that under these circumstances a further period of 3 years' healing time should be given
Failure	Symptoms Tenderness on percussion or increased mobility Sinus Unchanged or enlarged periradicular radiolucency Development of new radiolucency at another site on the tooth

Case 48
An Endodontic Problem

FRANCESCO MANNOCCI

Summary

A 60-year-old female patient has pain from a root-treated tooth. What will you do?

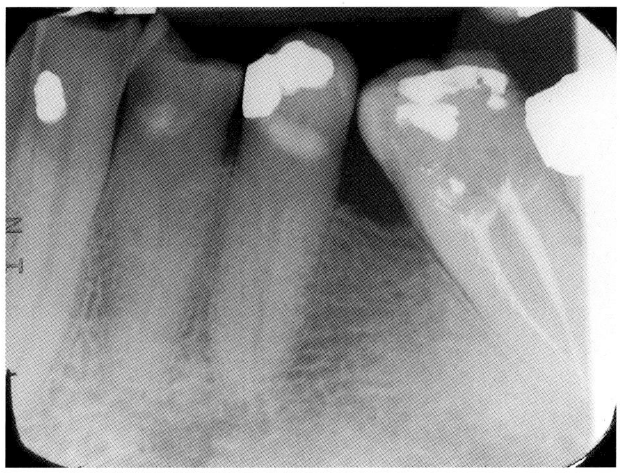

• **Fig. 48.1** The preoperative periapical radiograph of the lower left quadrant.

History

Complaint

The patient presents complaining of discomfort from a lower left posterior tooth. The filling was lost from the tooth about 4 months ago.

History of Complaint

She has suffered intermittent problems since the tooth was root canal treated 2 years ago. Pain is triggered by biting on the tooth, and changes in temperature have no effect. The symptoms have remained similar in intensity ever since the root canal treatment was completed.

Dental History

The patient has always attended regularly for dental treatment, requiring occasional treatment for failed restorations over the last 10–15 years.

The lower left second permanent molar was originally treated endodontically because the patient developed acute pulpitis. Two attempts at root canal treatment were carried out before the intense pain subsided, with the root canal filling being placed at a third appointment. An endodontic instrument separated in one of the root canals at the second appointment; the patient was informed of this by the dentist, and this was documented in the notes. A temporary restoration was placed to allow a period to assess resolution of symptoms, but the patient preferred not to return to the same dentist, feeling that the treatment had gone wrong.

◆ How Do You Assess the Case So Far?

Several features of the history are significant.

Pain on biting and well-localized pain indicate periapical periodontitis, and the cause is almost certainly failure of the previous root canal treatment.

There was a separated instrument which probably means that an inadequate apical seal would have been achieved in that canal, reducing the chances of a successful outcome. The extraction of the tooth, which may or may not be followed by an implant-supported fixed prosthesis, needs to be mentioned as an alternative to the root canal retreatment.

The provisional restoration was lost 4 months ago. This indicates complete loss of coronal seal to the root canal system, allowing microleakage of bacteria and their toxins along the length of the root filling. The extent to which this occurs is time dependent. As a general rule extrapolated from experimental data, if the root canal filling has been exposed to the oral cavity for 3 months or more, retreatment may be considered, even in the absence of clinical signs or symptoms.

Examination

Extraoral Examination

There is no facial swelling or tenderness associated with the tooth.

Intraoral Examination

You examine the patient, following the protocol outlined in Case 47. The lower second molar has a large cavity distally with obvious caries and exposed gutta percha root filling in the pulp chamber. It has tilted mesially and is tender to percussion. The third molar has a large, poorly contoured amalgam restoration.

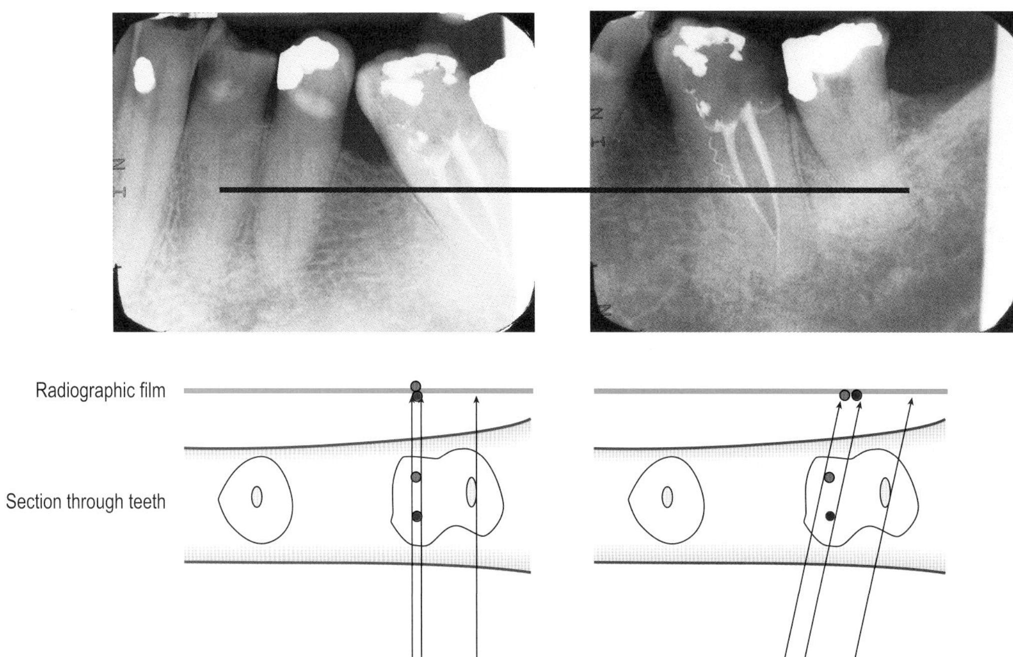

• **Fig. 48.2** The original periapical radiograph, top left and parallax view, taken from the mesial aspect, top right. The black line across both films shows the level of the cross-section shown below from the occlusal aspect. On the left, the beam angle superimposes both mesial molar root canals. On the right, the angled beam produces separate images of the two canals. This describes the parallax technique.

Investigations

A radiograph is necessary, and a periapical view of the teeth in the lower left quadrant is the most appropriate.

◆ What Information Do You Wish To Obtain From the Radiograph?

- **What do you think of the nature and quality** of the previous endodontic treatment?
- **Are any root canals detectable?** Failure of treatment may have been caused by failure to detect or fill all canals. Any remaining canals in teeth that have large carious lesions, restorations or marked tooth wear or have suffered trauma may be sclerosed as a result of tertiary dentine formation.
- **Is there periradicular radiolucency?** This would indicate persistence of infection or inflammation.
- **What is the estimated working length?** This can only be estimated from a periapical radiograph, which is always slightly magnified even when taken using a paralleling technique.
- **What is the root morphology?** The number of roots and their orientation can be identified. Root curvatures and diameters can also be observed; however, it is important to remember that radiographic images are two-dimensional representations of three-dimensional structures. Canals are often much wider bucco-lingually than can be appreciated on a conventional radiograph.

◆ The Preoperative Periapical Radiograph is Shown in Fig. 48.1. What Do You See?

The canine and premolars have been restored, and no caries is present, although there is significant tooth wear anteriorly. The tilted second molar has been root treated, and the fractured instrument is visible in one of the mesial canals.

The film is not of adequate diagnostic quality and must be graded in the notes as such using the updated guidance. The packet or sensor has not been placed far enough posteriorly to include the third molar, and the periapical tissues are not visible. The collimator has coned off the distal part of the film because the tube head has been positioned too far anteriorly. Use of a paralleling technique with a film holder has produced a true parallel projection, but this has superimposed the mesial canals. It is not possible to determine which of the two canals contains the fractured instrument, and it will be necessary to determine exactly where the instrument is, if an attempt is to be made to remove it.

◆ How Will You Locate the Separated Instrument Fragment?

By using the parallax technique. A second radiograph must be taken at the same vertical angulation, but at a different horizontal angle, usually from the mesial aspect.

◆ The Original and Second Parallax Views are Shown in Fig. 48.2. What Do You See, and Where is the Instrument?

The image on the left in Fig. 48.2 is the original radiograph and that on the right is the radiograph taken from the mesial aspect. The second radiograph is better positioned and clearly shows the presence of the fractured instrument and that there is no periapical radiolucency. The poorly contoured amalgam in the third molar can now be assessed.

Using the MBD (mesial, buccal, distal) rule, when the x-ray beam moves to the mesial, the buccal canal will appear

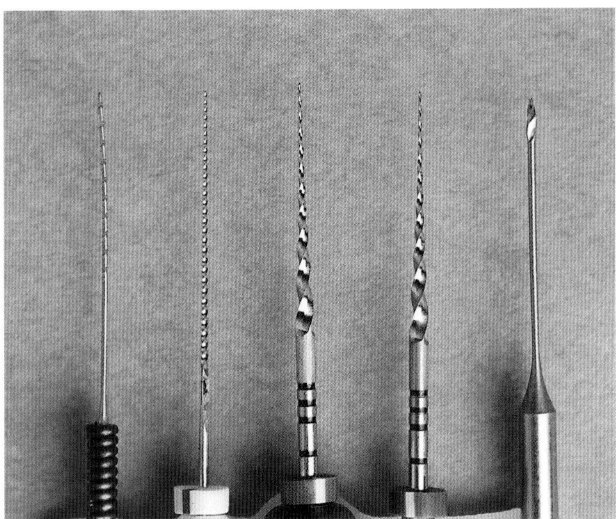

• **Fig. 48.3** Root canal instruments more prone to fracture in root canals. From left to right: a barbed broach, used to extirpate pulp tissue; stainless steel, hand and rotary nickel titanium files used to prepare and shape the root canal; and a Gates–Glidden bur, used for preparation of the coronal root canal.

to move to the distal. The separated instrument appears to move mesially, and so it must be in the mesio-lingual root canal.

◆ What Endodontic Instruments are Prone To Fracture, and What Has Fractured in This Tooth?

The broken instrument is a spiral root canal filler, recognized by its tapering helical shape and broad pitch.

Instruments prone to fracture are shown in Fig. 48.3.

◆ How Can Instrument Separation Be Prevented?

In the past, reuse and heat sterilization of instruments weakened them, but the current guidance recommending single-use instruments largely has overcome this problem. Instruments that jam in a root canal during use may become distorted, thus becoming weakened, and should be immediately discarded. All files should be inspected during use for signs of distortion, as shown in Fig. 48.4.

Otherwise, the most important factors are correct use of instruments and correct access cavity design. Rotary nickel titanium files, in particular, must be used in an electric torque-controlled motor at the correct setting and with minimal apical pressure.

Correct access cavity preparation underpins the success of root canal treatment. The cavity should allow straight-line access for instruments to the root canals. If not, the instruments will be overstressed in use and develop weak points. Fig. 48.5 outlines the ideal access cavity preparation for all tooth types.

Use of some instruments that are prone to fracture can simply be avoided. Gates–Glidden burs can result in over-preparation, and nickel titanium orifice shapers are a better option. Spiral root fillers are mainly used to place nonsetting calcium hydroxide paste between appointments. However, this is largely unnecessary because alternative applicators are available, as shown in Fig. 48.6.

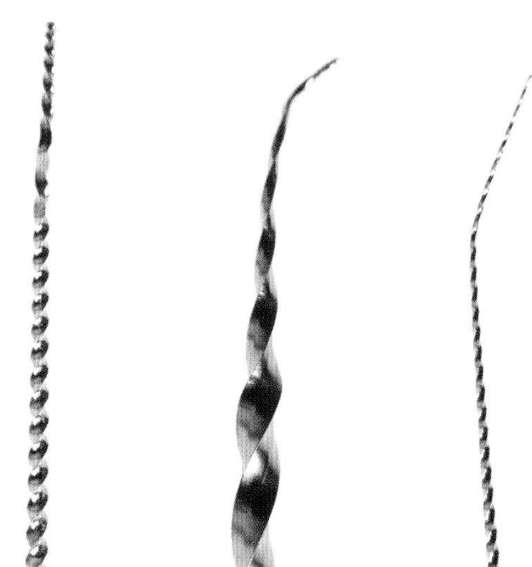

• **Fig. 48.4** Examples of distorted files that should be disposed of to avoid fracture within the root canal.

Treatment

◆ How Will You Remove the Fractured Spiral Filler Fragment?

Magnification is an essential aid to treatment, both to locate the canals and to identify the fragment.

Initially, try simple techniques. Sometimes, an ultrasonic scaler tip applied to the fractured instrument can transmit sufficient energy through the instrument to break down the dentine jammed against it and loosen it. The main disadvantages are the potential for excessive root dentine removal and disintegration of the end of the fractured instrument. Where there is space alongside the instrument, it may be possible to bypass it by using a small Hedström file. On the outward stroke, the flutes may engage with the instrument and pull it out.

Alternatively, specially designed instruments are available. Instrument Removal System (IRS, Dentsply) and Masseran kits both adopt the same principle. Fig. 48.7 shows how the IRS system is used. It consists of two components. The outer part is a colour-coded hollow tube, made in a series of internal and external diameters to accommodate different sizes of root canals and fractured instruments. Inside the tube is a rapidly tapered titanium wedge that locks to the outer tube with a screw thread. The end of the hollow tube is bevelled and has a window cut on one side. The tube is slipped over the head of the fractured instrument and the internal tapered wedge is screwed down until it grips and wedges the fractured instrument against the tube so that it can then be rotated and pulled out. A gutter of root dentine may need to be removed from around the head of the fractured instrument to allow the tube to slip over it.

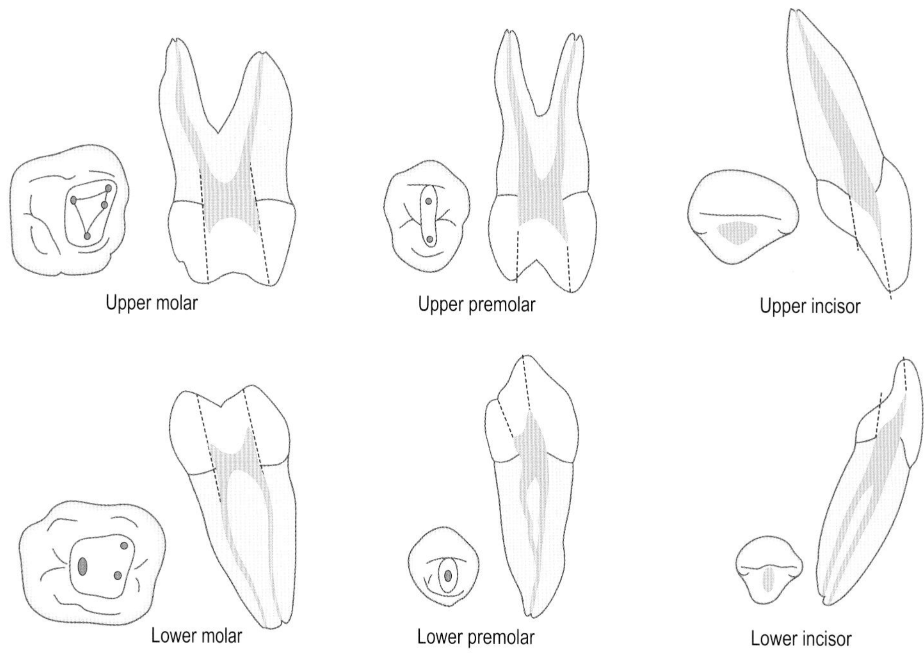

• **Fig. 48.5** Correct outline for pulp chamber access cavities.

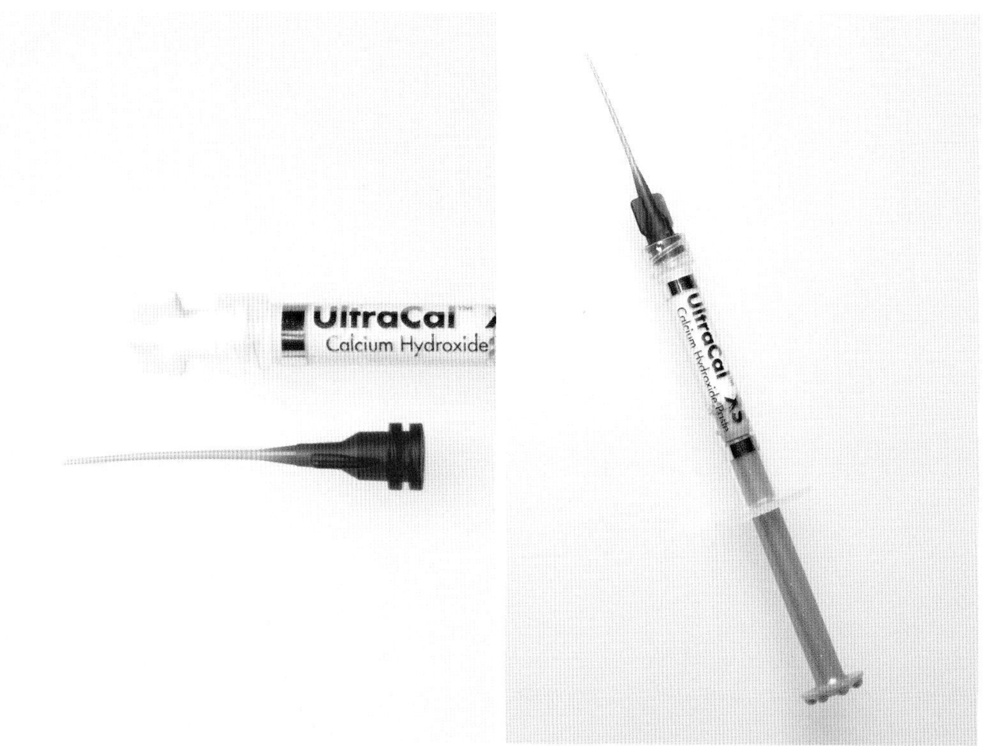

• **Fig. 48.6** Nonsetting calcium hydroxide paste with fine capillary tip (left) and assembled (right) for passive injection into the root canal.

◆ How Easy Will Its Removal Be?

Removal of the separated instrument fragment is always unpredictable and referral to an endodontic specialist needs to be considered. However, the following factors may indicate the likely outcome.

Location within the root canal, coronal, middle or apical third. If the instrument is present in the coronal third and visible using magnification there is a much greater likelihood that it can be removed. Instruments that have fractured apically in curved canals present the greatest challenge. Obtaining access to them in a straight line is often impossible without removing excessive dentine, and there is a risk of perforating the root. It is usually advisable to leave such fragments in situ.

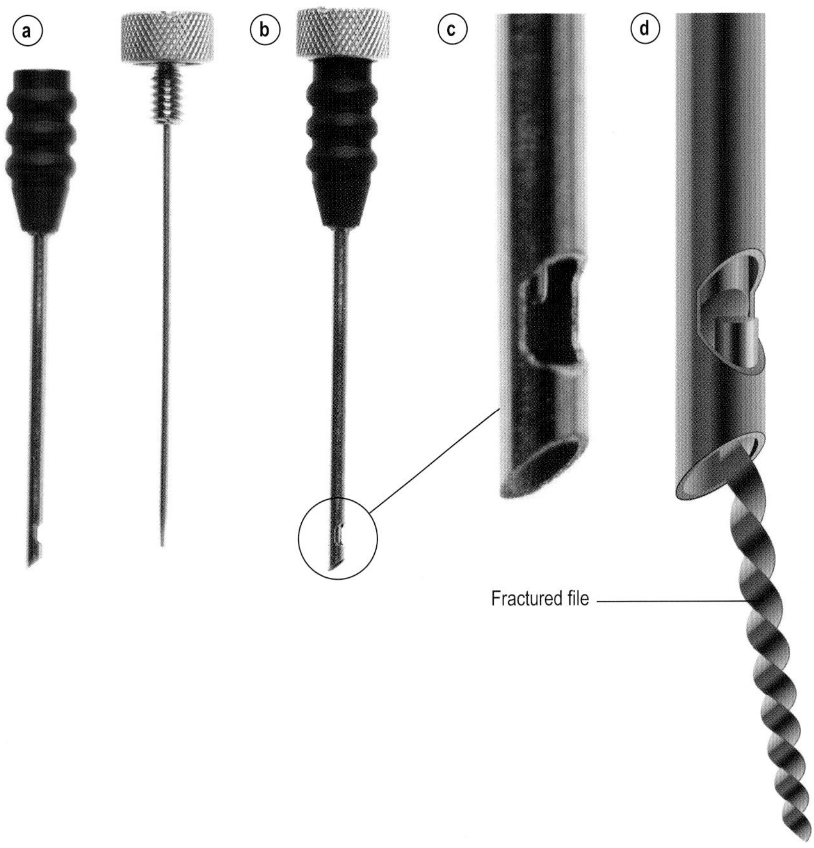

• **Fig. 48.7** Components of the Instrument Removal System for removal of fractured instruments in root canals. **a,** The two components; **b,** assembled; **c,** a high-power image of the instrument tip; **d,** diagrammatic representation showing how the instrument is used to grip and remove the fractured instrument.

Type of instrument. Most stainless-steel files can be removed if they are accessible. These are now commonly used to create an initial guide path prior to nickel titanium instrumentation and, if used correctly, should not have engaged the root canal dentine excessively. Instruments that are designed to cut dentine are more likely to be embedded into it if used incorrectly. For this reason, nickel titanium files and Gates–Glidden burs are usually difficult, if not impossible, to remove.

Width and length of fragment. Wider and more rigid instruments are more difficult to remove, as are longer segments of instruments. Both are more likely to have a large surface area in contact with dentine and bind dentine with greater friction.

Anatomy of canal. It is easier to bypass and remove instruments from an oval canal than from a round one.

◆ What Options are Available if a Separated Instrument Cannot Be Removed?

This partly depends on when the instrument separated. If this happened in the early stages of canal preparation, it is likely that the canal remained infected and treatment was compromised. Fracture during the finishing stages of preparation, after adequate irrigation with sodium hypochlorite, might have reduced the numbers of bacteria sufficiently to allow obturation to the level of the instrument, leading to a successful outcome.

Retreatment of the remaining canals and the canal up to the separated instrument may be sufficient to eliminate residual bacteria from the root canal system and create an adequate seal coronally and throughout the root canal system.

Alternatively, or if retreatment fails on that root alone, root resection or hemisection will allow the affected root to be removed. This is only possible if the roots are not fused and so would not be possible in the present case. Periradicular surgery may also be a possibility but would be difficult in a lower molar tooth because of the density of the buccal bone and the proximity of the inferior dental nerve canal. Unfortunately, extraction may be the only possible option.

In this case, the spiral root canal filler was removed easily because it was possible to bypass the instrument and remove it with a Hedström file. Subsequent root canal preparation with nickel titanium rotary instruments produced a more tapered root canal preparation, allowing excellent shaping, debridement, irrigation and obturation. The final retreatment periapical radiograph is shown in Fig. 48.8. The tooth was definitively restored with a full-coverage gold crown to ensure a good coronal seal and provide cusp reinforcement and a good contact point with the adjacent tooth.

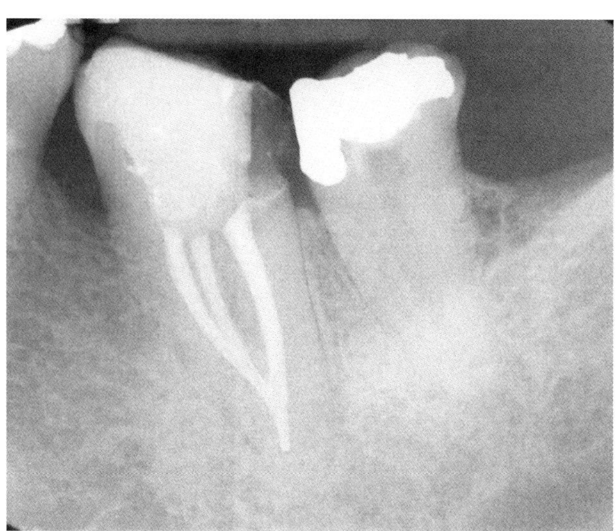

• **Fig. 48.8** Postoperative periapical radiograph of the completed root canal treatment, prior to final restoration.

As for all endodontic treatments, a 1-year recall, including a periapical radiograph and clinical examination, is indicated to assess healing.

In summary, the dentist must always inform the patient if instrument separation occurs during endodontic treatment, with a full explanation of the management options and possible outcomes. This conversation must be contemporaneously recorded in the patient notes. Indeed, the risk of instrument separation should be discussed as part of the initial consent procedure for endodontic treatment – assessment of treatment complexity, curvature of root canals and so on should be taken into consideration before a decision is made as to treat or refer the patient to a specialist.

Acknowledgement

Radiographs courtesy of Dr Suzanne Blacker.

Case 49

A Swollen Face

TARA RENTON

Summary

A 30-year-old man is referred to your dental hospital by his general practitioner with a painful swelling of the right side of the face. What is the cause, and what treatment would you provide?

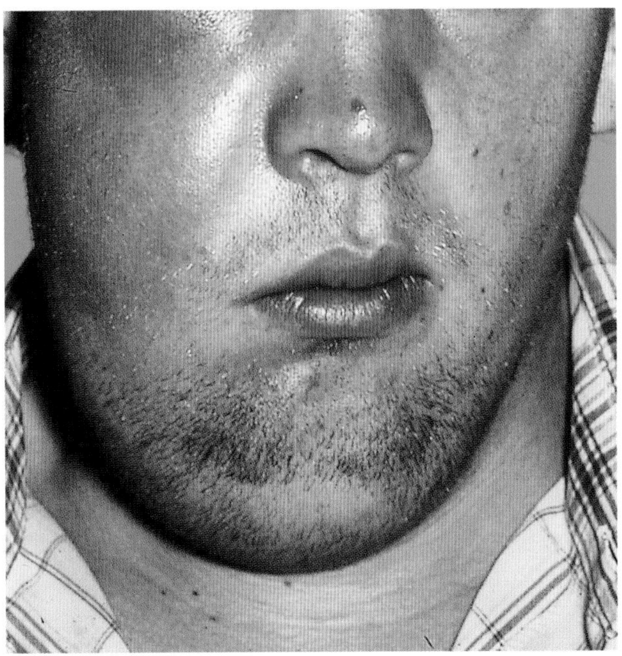

• **Fig. 49.1** The patient on presentation.

History

History of Complaint

The patient has had toothache intermittently for many months. A few weeks ago, the pain became excruciating and did not respond to analgesics. Then, suddenly, it reduced in severity, and the patient thought it had resolved.

However, about 10 days ago, a different pain developed. A tooth on the upper right has become very tender, and he has not been able to bite on it. The swelling suddenly enlarged yesterday.

Over the last few months the patient has been prescribed several courses of antibiotics, and he finished a course of oral erythromycin 2 days ago.

Medical History

The patient is otherwise fit and well.

Examination

Extraoral Examination

The patient is shown in Fig. 49.1. The swelling is hot, tender and firm centrally, but peripherally, it is almost painless and softer. It extends from the nose to the anterior border of the masseter, and the lower eyelid is very oedematous and contains blood pigment, as if bruised.

The swelling is not pointing extraorally. There are palpable tender lymph nodes in the upper deep cervical chain.

Intraoral Examination

The patient has slight limitation of mouth opening, but this does not significantly hamper examination. The sulcus adjacent to the upper first molar and both premolars is tender and slightly reduced in depth by a firm swelling. The upper first and second premolars and the first molar have large amalgam restorations. However, the patient indicates clearly that the second premolar is the cause of the pain, and this tooth is slightly mobile and raised in its socket. It is very tender on percussion and nonvital on testing with ethyl chloride. The first molar and the first premolar appear vital.

Investigations

◆ Which Additional Investigation is Critically Important? Why?

Taking the patient's temperature. This gives a good indication of the systemic effects of the infection and reflects the amount of pus in abscesses and/or the tendency of the infection to spread. The patient has a temperature of 37.2°C.

◆ Would You Take a Radiograph?

In this case, a radiograph is not a useful investigation. Tests of vitality are much more likely to identify the causative tooth and, in any case, there appears to be no doubt about the diagnosis.

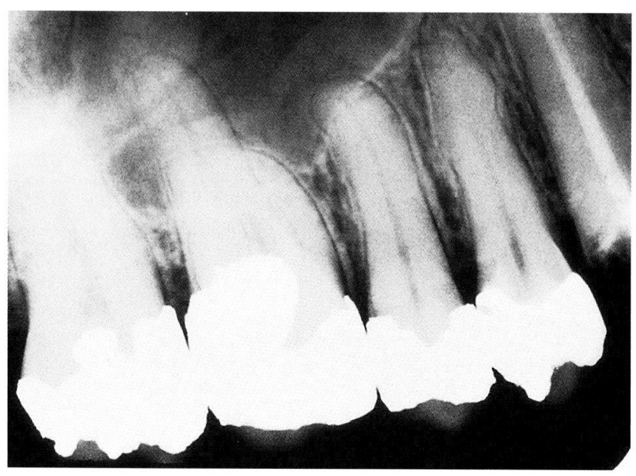

• **Fig. 49.2** Periapical radiograph showing the causative premolar.

However, there are good reasons why taking a radiograph may not help or even be counterproductive:

1. It takes up to 3 weeks for radiographic changes to develop at the root apex after pulp necrosis.
2. The radiographic features may be misleading if you attempt to use them to diagnose loss of vitality. When root apices are radiographed with the maxillary antrum superimposed, the normal periodontal ligament appears wider. This may be confused with early apical changes of infection.

Both these problems are appreciated in Fig. 49.2, the periapical radiograph of this patient, which is completely normal.

Diagnosis

◆ What Do These Findings Tell You?

The combination of inflammation, the nonvital tooth and the adjacent probable abscess indicates an odontogenic soft tissue infection. The history of severe toothache that suddenly resolved suggests pulpitis that was subsequently relieved by necrosis of the pulp. The subsequent pain of a different character with a tender tooth suggests an apical abscess. The patient points clearly to the second premolar, and this is almost certainly the cause of the pain because pain involving the periodontal ligament is well localized.

Trismus is an important sign, indicating that infection or inflammation has spread to involve the muscles of mastication. However, trismus is not severe and probably results from inflammation and oedema of the buccinator and the anterior fibres of the masseter, which lie at the posterior border of the swelling.

The infection has induced minimal systemic effects, and the patient is not significantly pyrexic. Luckily, the infection appears to be localized. The firm centre to the swelling and the swelling in the sulcus will contain pus.

◆ What Types of Soft Tissue Infection Arising From Teeth Cause Facial Swelling? How May They Be Distinguished, and What is the Relevance of Doing So?

Facial swelling may be the result of oedema, abscess formation, cellulitis or a combination of these.

It is important to determine which of these types of infection is present because the treatment and sequelae of each are different. *Abscesses* require drainage. *Cellulitis* requires aggressive treatment, usually including antibiotics, and *oedema* requires no direct treatment but resolves when the causative tooth is removed or the pulp treated.

Despite the fact that the use of the terms mentioned above is convenient, in practice, most odontogenic soft tissue infections are caused by mixed microbial flora and do not fall neatly into one category or another. It is not unusual to find an abscess with a surrounding zone of cellulitis, and a degree of oedema is always present. Which type of infection develops is determined by the virulence of the pathogens (and the synergy between the species in the mixed flora), the resistance of the host and the anatomical constraints on the infection.

Cause of Swelling	Features
Oedema	Soft, not very red or hot, not tender on palpation and not painful. Compressible with slow continuous pressure. Often accounts for much of the facial swelling in children with odontogenic infection.
Abscess	Localized collection of pus, which, if small, feels hard, tense or covered by a thick layer of tissues. If large, it may be softer and exhibit fluctuance. Pointing to the skin or mucosa indicates abscess formation.
Cellulitis	Brawny, poorly localized swelling with marked tenderness and dusky redness. May contain small collections of pus but no large localized abscesses. Spreads, sometimes rapidly, through tissues. Usually associated with systemic symptoms, pyrexia, malaise, leucocytosis and lymphadenitis.

◆ If Infections are Not Easily Characterized, What are the Important Features On Which Treatment Must Be Based?

The critical factors that must be determined are whether:

- an abscess cavity is present (palpation, eliciting fluctuation)
- there is evidence of systemic effects (malaise, pyrexia, a toxic-shocked appearance)
- the infection is spreading rapidly (judged by the history and observation during treatment)
- the patient is predisposed to infection (from the medical history).

◆ Which Type of Infection is This?

This appears to be primarily an abscess with surrounding oedema.

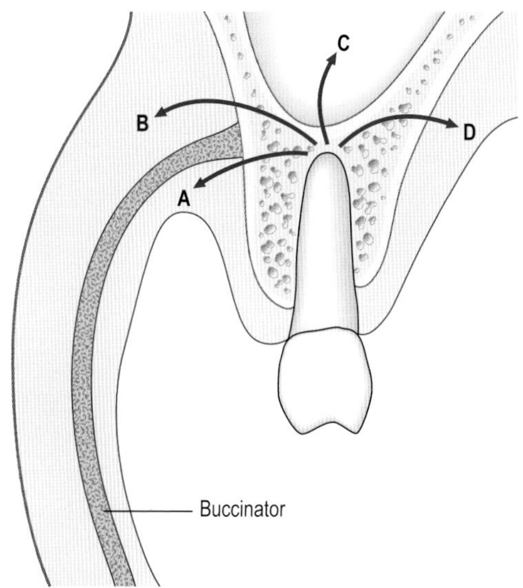

• **Fig .49.3** Coronal section showing the paths of spread of infection from upper molars and premolars. Infection may pass buccally below the buccinator muscle into the sulcus or cheek intraorally (A), above the buccinator into the buccal space (B), into the sinus (C) or into the palate (D).

◆ In What Tissue Space(s) is the Infection Tracking or Localizing? What are the Boundaries of This Space?

This abscess appears to be in the upper part of the buccal space. This is a potential space between the buccinator and facial muscles and the parotid fascia, filled normally with loose connective tissue. Posteriorly, it communicates with the masseter muscle and around the front of the ramus to the pterygoid space. Oedema spreads beyond the buccal space to involve the lower eyelid and anterior cheek in the canine fossa. The abscess is not yet pointing to the skin.

◆ Why Has the Infection Localized Here? Will It Remain Localized Here?

Abscesses arising from the canine, premolar and molar teeth and perforating the buccal plate of the alveolar bone will spill out into the soft tissues either above or below the attachment of the buccinator. The attachment of the buccinator usually runs below the apices of the upper teeth, so the infection is likely to pass superficially to the buccinator and into the cheek. If it passes below the attachment, an alveolar abscess or sinus will develop. Paths of spread of infection from an upper premolar are shown in Fig. 49.3.

Despite being a thin muscle, the buccinator is a significant barrier to the spread of infection. It is unlikely that the infection would be able to perforate the muscle and develop a sinus into the mouth. Several sequelae are possible. Pus would be most likely to gravitate and spread through the whole buccal space down to the lower border of the mandible; it could point and then drain to the skin or spread laterally around the buccinator to involve other areas of the face, tissue around the masseter muscle or the pterygoid space. Its future course cannot be predicted.

◆ Is This a Potentially Life-Threatening Infection? If So, Why?

Not yet. In this case, the infection appears localized, the spread is not particularly rapid and there are no significant systemic symptoms. If the infection spreads more, the situation would change.

Involvement of the tissues around the eyelid is worrying. At present, the swelling here is caused by oedema, but if infection were to spread to the upper lid or the medial canthus of the eye, the patient would be at risk of cavernous sinus thrombosis. This is a very rare, but potentially fatal, complication.

It would also be possible for the infection to spread posteriorly into the pterygo-mandibular space and the infratemporal fossa. From here, the infection could spread to the cavernous sinus or the middle cranial fossa through the veins.

◆ What is Cavernous Sinus Thrombosis, and What are Its Features?

Thrombosis of the cavernous sinus results from spread of odontogenic infection along two main venous pathways. Bacteria and infected emboli travel posteriorly from the upper lip and face via the anterior facial vein. This connects via the ophthalmic veins to the cavernous sinus without valves, which might otherwise prevent this retrograde flow. Alternatively, infection may spread from the pterygoid space via the pterygoid plexus of veins that connect directly to the cavernous sinus via the foramen ovale.

The local features are seen on one side at first, but the signs become bilateral as the thrombus grows. The features are listed below:

Local effects	Marked oedema of the eyelids
	Pulsating exophthalmos caused by venous obstruction
	A dilated facial vein
	Inhibition of movement of the eye
	Papilloedema and retinal haemorrhage
Systemic effects	Rapid pulse
	Marked pyrexia
	Severe malaise

In addition to treatment for the infection, anticoagulation is required for thrombosis. The mortality rate is high.

Treatment

◆ What are the General Principles of Treatment for All Odontogenic Infections of Soft Tissues?

Treatment Should Be Started Immediately. Infection may spread quickly and, in some cases, progress to a life-threatening situation. Identify patients with a risk of significant complications. Those at risk of airway obstruction, cavernous sinus thrombosis or toxaemia and present malaise or a high temperature should be treated immediately, possibly even with parenteral antibiotics while awaiting definitive diagnosis, and admitted to hospital for treatment.

Pus Must Be Drained As Soon As Possible. With most infections causing facial swelling, the only treatment required is effective drainage of pus and removal of the cause. To ensure success, a drain may need to be placed in the incision.

Remove the Cause As Soon As Possible. Removal of the causative tooth both prevents continuing infection and also drains the intraosseous abscess. The exception to this rule is when the cause is pericoronitis. In this case, the soft tissue, rather than the tooth, is the cause, and extraction can be detrimental (see Case 32).

Provide Antibiotic Treatment, if Necessary. Antibiotics provide little benefit over drainage and removal of the cause but are often used and occasionally required. Pus should be collected on drainage and submitted to microbiology for culture and sensitivity investigation, in case a change of antibiotic is required subsequently.

Provide Supportive Measures. Ensure that the patient eats, maintains good fluid intake and rests. Consider admission to hospital until recovery has started, and provide appropriate analgesia.

Review Progress Regularly. Daily review of those patients treated on an outpatient basis is appropriate. Those whose infection is serious enough to merit admission to hospital require more frequent review, between every hour and 6 hours, depending on their status. If signs and symptoms do not improve progressively, further investigation and treatment are probably required.

◆ What are the Principles of Obtaining Drainage? How Will You Drain the Pus in This Case?

The principles of incision for drainage are:

- Take the anatomy into account, and avoid incising near important structures.
- Incise only when pus has localized, unless rapidly increasing swelling is threatening the airway, in which case it should be drained as quickly as possible.
- Incise where the abscess is pointing or at the point of maximum fluctuation.
- Incise along the most direct route to the pus.
- If incision does not release pus, deepen the incision by using blunt forceps, not a scalpel. Open the forceps blades to break open the abscess wall (Hilton's method).
- After incision, explore, identify and open all locules of pus.
- Provide dependent drainage, if possible.
- Place a drain if the abscess is large, is deep or if the incision might close before the abscess resolves (e.g. if the incision penetrates layers of muscle, fascia or skin that can move independently). Leave the drain in place for at least 12–24 hours, or until drainage stops.
- If possible, drain intraorally to prevent facial scarring and skin contraction.
- On the skin, incise along Langer's lines or in a skin crease.
- On the skin, try to incise healthy skin. It will scar less.

In this case, the pus lies between the buccinator muscle and the skin. It is not pointing and is palpable in the upper buccal sulcus. Incision at this site under ethyl chloride spray anaesthesia is perfectly appropriate. However, the incision must extend through the buccinator to be effective, and some might prefer to obtain drainage, with the patient under brief general anaesthesia.

◆ Should Drainage Ever Be Delayed?

Occasionally, drainage must be delayed until pus is properly localized into an abscess. If no pus can be identified on examination, incision will be futile. Waiting a day and providing antibiotics may result in pus localizing. Therefore, such a decision must be carefully considered.

◆ Will a Drain Be Required?

Quite probably. The abscess is not very deep, but the incision must pass through a muscle. However, drainage will be dependent: the incision is being made below the pus, and gravity will favour drainage. It may not be possible to decide in advance. If pus drains freely on incision and a cavity in the tissues is present, it would be sensible to place a drain, preferably a strip of corrugated rubber or, as a second choice, gauze. This should be sutured to the edge of the incision to prevent displacement. In this case, a drain would be as easily placed under either local or general anaesthetic.

◆ Can the Tooth Be Conserved After Soft Tissue Infection? How Might You Remove the Tooth?

A soft tissue infection does not mean that the tooth has to be extracted, and almost all teeth could, in theory, be preserved. However, most such cases arise as a result of neglect; the tooth is often badly broken down and is best extracted. Occasionally, when infection is spreading rapidly or if the airway is compromised, the tooth is extracted to avoid delaying treatment, but even these severe complications do not mandate that the tooth be extracted. The critical factor is that drainage is obtained.

If the tooth is to be conserved, it must be opened and drainage effected through the pulp chamber, in addition to draining pus by incision. Ideally, the pulp chamber can be closed again fairly quickly. As soon as drainage ceases, the pulp chamber can be cleaned and a dressing placed. If pus continues to drain for some time, the chamber may be left open for up to 24 hours. After this period, there is a risk of oral flora entering tissues, reducing the chances of subsequent successful root treatment. Many clinicians prescribe antibiotics because they consider drainage to be less effective when the tooth is retained.

Extraction is the more usual treatment. If local anaesthesia can be obtained and trismus is not severe, the tooth may be extracted at once. Infiltration anaesthesia is often difficult to achieve because of the low pH of inflamed tissues. Injection into infected tissue also carries the risk of wider dissemination of bacteria. Block anaesthesia is required.

General anaesthesia may be necessary. If so, it will be convenient to admit the patient to hospital and complete all the surgical treatments at the same time. General anaesthesia may take some time to organize, and in the meantime, it would be appropriate to try to extract the tooth under local anaesthesia. General anaesthesia should not be used in an attempt to overcome trismus. Forcing the jaws open will spread the infection.

If a surgical extraction is required, it may be delayed. As a general principle, surgery should be avoided if the surgical field is infected. However, this rather old rule is often not followed now because of the availability of very effective antibiotic treatment. Some operators will perform a surgical extraction immediately, and the risk of spreading infection or inducing osteomyelitis seems to be extremely small.

In this case, anaesthesia could not be obtained, and so drainage and extraction were performed under general anaesthesia. A short, corrugated rubber drain was inserted.

◆ When Should Antibiotics Be Prescribed for Odontogenic Soft Tissue Infection?

The attitude to antibiotic treatment varies among different centres. Antibiotics are unnecessary for the treatment of the majority of localized soft tissue abscesses, and this is particularly so when pus collects superficially in the buccal sulcus or on the palate. Drainage and removal of the cause are much more important. However, in practice, many patients who require incision and drainage tend to be prescribed antibiotics by clinicians, without a clear rationale.

Antibiotics should be prescribed if:

- the patient is prone to infection (e.g. because of diabetes or immunosuppression)
- there is spreading infection (cellulitis)
- the airway is compromised
- there is significant malaise, pyrexia or toxaemia
- the tooth is to be preserved rather than extracted (the cause is not immediately eliminated)
- cavernous sinus thrombosis is possible.

Antibiotics prescribed for spreading infection may cause pus to localize, and drainage of abscesses may only be possible a day or so later.

Antibiotics should never be provided as an alternative to draining pus.

◆ What Microorganisms Cause Odontogenic Soft Tissue Infections?

Odontogenic soft tissue infections are mixed infections. The microbial flora usually contains about 25 species derived from oral flora, of which about half are cultivatable. Anaerobes outnumber aerobes by 10 or 100 to 1, and the commonly isolated species are *Porphyromonas* sp., *Prevotella* sp., *Peptostreptococcus* sp. and *Fusobacterium* sp.; however, facultative anaerobes are usually present, often members of the *Streptococcus milleri* group. Although numerically a minor component of the flora, these organisms are important when selecting antibiotics.

◆ If You Decided To Do So, Which Antibiotic Would You Prescribe Initially? Explain Why

Almost all the organisms in odontogenic soft tissue infections are sensitive to penicillins. There is a small, but increasing, proportion of resistant strains, but these do not seem to contraindicate the use of penicillins. It is not necessary to prescribe penicillinase-resistant drugs just because one member of the microbial flora shows resistance and they are of no proven benefit in odontogenic infection. Penicillin V or G is sufficient, provided drainage can be achieved.

Metronidazole is effective against the anaerobic species and is often prescribed. However, metronidazole should be used as an adjunct to a penicillin and never alone. It will kill the anaerobes but leave facultative anaerobes such as the *S. milleri* group unscathed. These organisms are capable of causing a spreading soft tissue infection as a monoculture. Removing their anaerobic microbial competitors with metronidazole risks turning a relatively well-localized, mixed infection into a spreading streptococcal infection. In the wrong site, this could be fatal.

In this case, the patient received a single dose of 500 mg amoxicillin and 400 mg metronidazole intravenously during administration of the anaesthetic. The same doses were prescribed for oral intake three times a day for 5 days afterwards, and this is an appropriate regimen for most odontogenic soft tissue infections. However, as noted above, it may not have contributed greatly to the patient's recovery.

◆ Why Bother To Take a Specimen for Culture and Sensitivity Testing?

As noted above, empirical treatment with penicillin with or without metronidazole is almost always effective. However, in some cases, the infection stabilizes but fails to resolve. This may result from inadequate drainage, but a change of antibiotic may be considered a sensible precaution. The result of sensitivity testing may be helpful in selecting another antibiotic and identifying any unusual pathogens present. As culture and sensitivity testing takes about 3 days, it must be requested as soon as a sample of pus can be obtained and before antibiotics are administered.

To be useful, the sample for culture must be taken in such a way as to favour the growth of anaerobes and fastidious organisms. Ideally, it should be taken directly from the abscess through a needle or through a sterile skin incision and transported anaerobically to the laboratory. Samples on swabs contaminated by oral flora are unlikely to be useful and may even provide a misleading result.

When interpreting the results of culture and sensitivity tests performed on a simple swab of pus, it must be remembered that the organisms isolated are unlikely to be representative of all oral flora. Routine culture methods in most hospitals will detect only a few species, probably not the main components of oral flora. Unless a change to a different antibiotic is clearly justified, it would be better to consider changing the dose and route of administration.

◆ How Quickly Should the Swelling Resolve?

Patients may often feel much better within a few hours, and a noticeable reduction in swelling, trismus, pain and pyrexia should be observed within 24 hours. By this time, drains do not usually show pus and are removed and dressings placed over the site, if extraoral. If there has been no resolution, the diagnosis, antibiotic treatment and effectiveness of drainage must be reviewed. Almost complete resolution should follow in 3–6 days, as in the present case.

Further Guidance

http://www.sdcep.org.uk/ and search 'bacterial infection'.
https://www.fgdp.org.uk/ and search 'antimicrobial prescribing'.

Case 50

Missing Upper Lateral Incisors

SOPHIE WATKINS

Summary

A 17-year-old girl presents to you at your general dental practice requesting restoration of the spaces between her upper front teeth. What is the cause, and how can a better appearance be achieved?

History

Complaint

The patient does not wish to have gaps between her upper front teeth.

History of Complaint

The patient's permanent teeth erupted at a normal age, but with large spaces between them. The primary predecessors had all been present and were exfoliated normally. None of the permanent teeth have been extracted. She has recently completed orthodontic treatment planned to facilitate replacement of the lateral incisors.

Medical History

The patient is fit and well.

Family History

The patient's mother had a number of teeth missing. They had been replaced with a partial denture at an early age.

Examination

Extraoral Examination

The patient has a skeletal class I appearance without facial asymmetry. There is a slight deviation of the mandible to the patient's left-hand side on mouth opening, but without limitation of mouth opening, temporomandibular joint clicks or crepitus or masticatory muscle tenderness.

Intraoral Examination

The patient's soft tissues are healthy, and her oral hygiene is good, with no calculus deposits, gingival inflammation or bleeding on probing. The teeth appear sound, with the exception of slight mobility associated with the upper right central incisor. The spaces in the lateral incisor regions are currently filled with teeth added to her removable orthodontic retainer.

The clinical appearance on presentation is shown in Fig. 50.1.

◆ What Features are Relevant To Treatment?

Both upper lateral incisors are absent. There is a mild class III incisor relationship, with a normal overjet and a reduced but complete overbite. The teeth are well aligned and upright after orthodontic treatment with appropriate dimensions of space for the lateral incisor teeth that are missing.

◆ What are the Possible Causes for the Absence of Lateral Incisors? What is the Most Likely Cause in This Case?

See Box 50.1.

In this case, the most likely cause for the missing lateral incisors is developmental – hypodontia. Excluding third molars, the reported prevalence of hypodontia ranges from 1.6 to 6.9%, depending on the population group studied. The teeth most commonly missing are, in descending order of frequency, the third molars, the mandibular second premolars, the maxillary lateral incisors and the maxillary second premolars. The maxillary lateral incisors are lost in about 1–2% of the population. The fact that the patient's mother wore a denture to replace missing teeth from an early age suggests a possible familial aetiology. Trauma or extraction and the related sequelae are readily excluded by the history (anamnesis).

Investigations

◆ What Investigations are Required?

The reason for each investigation is outlined in Box 50.2.

◆ The Dental Panoramic Tomograph is Displayed in Fig. 50.2b. What Does It Show?

The dental panoramic tomograph confirms the absence of the upper lateral incisors, with no evidence of supernumerary teeth or other bone lesions in this region. All other teeth, including the unerupted third molars, are present.

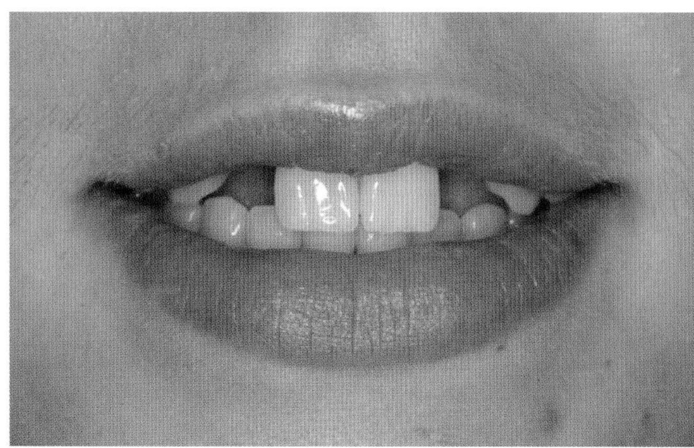
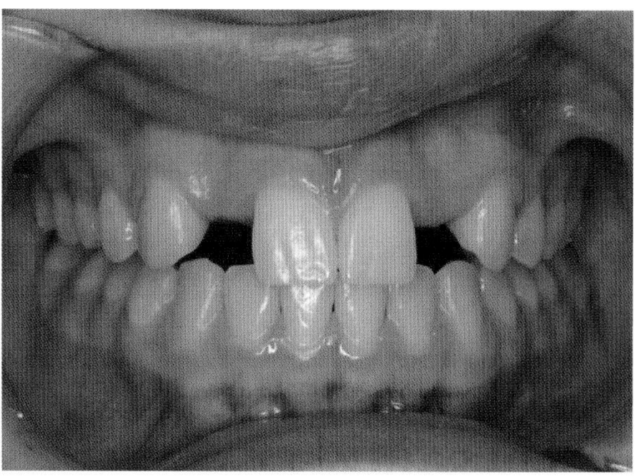
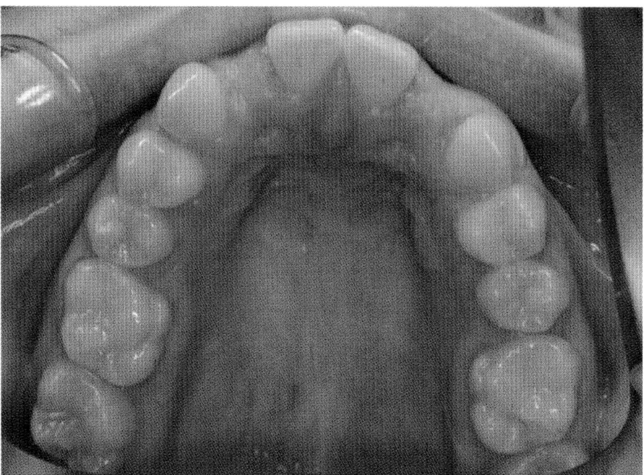

• **Fig. 50.1 a,** Extra oral view, **b,** anterior labial view and **c,** maxillary occlusal view of the patient on presentation.

• BOX 50.1 Possible Causes for the Absence of Lateral Incisors

Missing	Developmentally absent; Hypodontia, possibly associated with cleft lip or palate or other craniofacial syndrome
	Extracted
	Avulsed
	Decoronated
Failure to erupt	Ectopic position
	Dilaceration and/or displacement as a result of trauma
	Scar tissue preventing eruption
	Supernumerary tooth preventing eruption
	Insufficient space as a result of crowding
	Pathological lesion (e.g. cyst or odontogenic tumour) preventing eruption

This confirms the diagnosis that the upper lateral incisors are developmentally absent.

The root of the upper right central incisor has significant resorption, making its prognosis poor. The other central and canine tooth roots are upright, and the root apices of the canines are distally placed. This is important in the planning of orthodontic treatment. Canines can be difficult to move bodily through the alveolar bone because of their bulky root form, and therefore, the position of the root apex prior to orthodontic treatment is important. In this case, the pre-treatment distal positon of the root apex made distalization of the canines to open spaces for the lateral incisors more predictable. This is beneficial, especially if implants are planned as a treatment option in the future, when the roots of the teeth need to be clear of the potential implant-bearing edentate area.

◆ What Might Have Caused the Root Resorption of the Upper Right Central Incisior Root?

There are several possible causes, including:

1. **An ectopic Upper Right Lateral Incisor.** A mesially impacted lateral incisor can cause root resorption. It is, therefore, important to take radiographs as soon as it is noted that a tooth has not erupted at the expected age. Lateral incisors usually erupt at 8–9 years, and therefore, if the patient reaches 10 years with no clinical sign of a lateral incisor, radiographic investigation is essential, or earlier if the contralateral tooth has erupted successfully.

• BOX 50.2 Reasons for Investigations

Investigation	Reason
Tests of sensibility of the upper anterior teeth	To exclude incidental loss of sensibility, to ensure that endodontic treatment is not required and that unsuspected loss of sensibility does not compromise the subsequent care plan. It should be stressed, however, that a negative sensibility test is not necessarily indicative of a loss of vitality and should not be used in isolation when deciding whether to undertake root treatment.
Radiographs	To determine whether the lateral incisors are present and unerupted and to exclude underlying lesions such as supernumerary teeth or cysts. To assess root position of the canines and central incisor teeth to assist in treatment planning: This will be discussed in more detail later. Examination for this patient should include a dental panoramic tomograph (DPT) to provide an overall survey, including root position, to exclude significant periodontal bone loss and to confirm the presence or absence of third molars. Intraoral periapical views or an upper standard occlusal view may assist with detailed analysis of the incisor region, which suffers from cervical spine superimposition in the panoramic film. Further films may be required to define caries status.
Mounted study models	To assess the occlusion, aid in care planning and produce a diagnostic wax-up, if required. Also an essential part of the clinical record for medicolegal purposes, especially in relation to orthodontic planning and treatment.

2. **Trauma.** A traumatic injury to a tooth such as avulsion, intrusion or subluxation, in which the injury damages the periodontal ligament.
3. **Orthodontic forces.** Excessive orthodontic force/rapid orthodontic tooth movement can cause resorption of the root apices. It is, therefore, important to monitor the tooth roots radiographically during orthodontic treatment, especially where the roots are particularly narrow/tapered. However, this is unlikely to occur at a single root. Nevertheless, if a root is severely resorbed, it is unwise to attempt orthodontic movement.
4. **Lesion such as a cyst or a tumour.** In this case, the radiographic appearance was not indicative of a pathological lesion.

Whatever the aetiology of the resorption, it is very important to ensure that the patient is made aware of this as soon as it is identified and that the doubtful prognosis, the possible consequences and the management options are discussed. In this case, orthodontic movement was undertaken with great care, and careful clinical and radiographic monitoring was undertaken; after having made the patient and her parents/guardians aware of the doubtful prognosis of the upper right central incisor, including the risk of further root resorption during orthodontics, which could result in mobility and loss of the tooth as a consequence.

Having been given these warnings both verbally and in written form, including all the options for treatment, the potential consequences and the options for management if the tooth was to be lost, the patient and her parents/guardians were then able to give their fully informed consent. It is very important medico-legally that informed consent is documented in cases such as this, taking the compromised tooth into account in the current treatment planning and with regard to future options. The findings and discussion with the patient must be documented contemporaneously.

Care Plan

◆ What are the Main Treatment Options? What are Their Advantages and Disadvantages?

See Box 50.3 and Fig. 50.3.

◆ The Patient's Main Concern Was Her Appearance. What Other Treatment Options Might Have Been Available, and How Would You Demonstrate the Possible Results To Her?

If the patient is considering committing herself to a long and complex (and potentially expensive) treatment, the potential result of each of the treatment options should be considered carefully. Possible outcomes can be assessed by using study models and diagnostic wax-ups. The feasibility of the orthodontic treatment options can be visualized by using Kesling set-up – cutting the teeth to be moved off duplicate study casts and fixing them in an orthodontically achievable position. The patient and the dentist can then see what might be achieved with each treatment option. There are also computer software programmes that can show on images of the patient's face the effects of altered tooth positions.

In this case, after discussion, the patient opted for the third treatment option outlined in Box 50.3, that of space opening and prosthetic replacement of the missing lateral incisor teeth.

◆ How Would You Carry Out the Orthodontic Treatment?

The tooth movement demands fixed appliance treatment. Tooth tilting with use of a removable appliance would result in a poor appearance in the midline and may produce spaces that are difficult to fill with a prosthetic replacement. Fixed appliance therapy allows the incisors to be moved bodily, and derotation and distalization/uprighting of the canines is

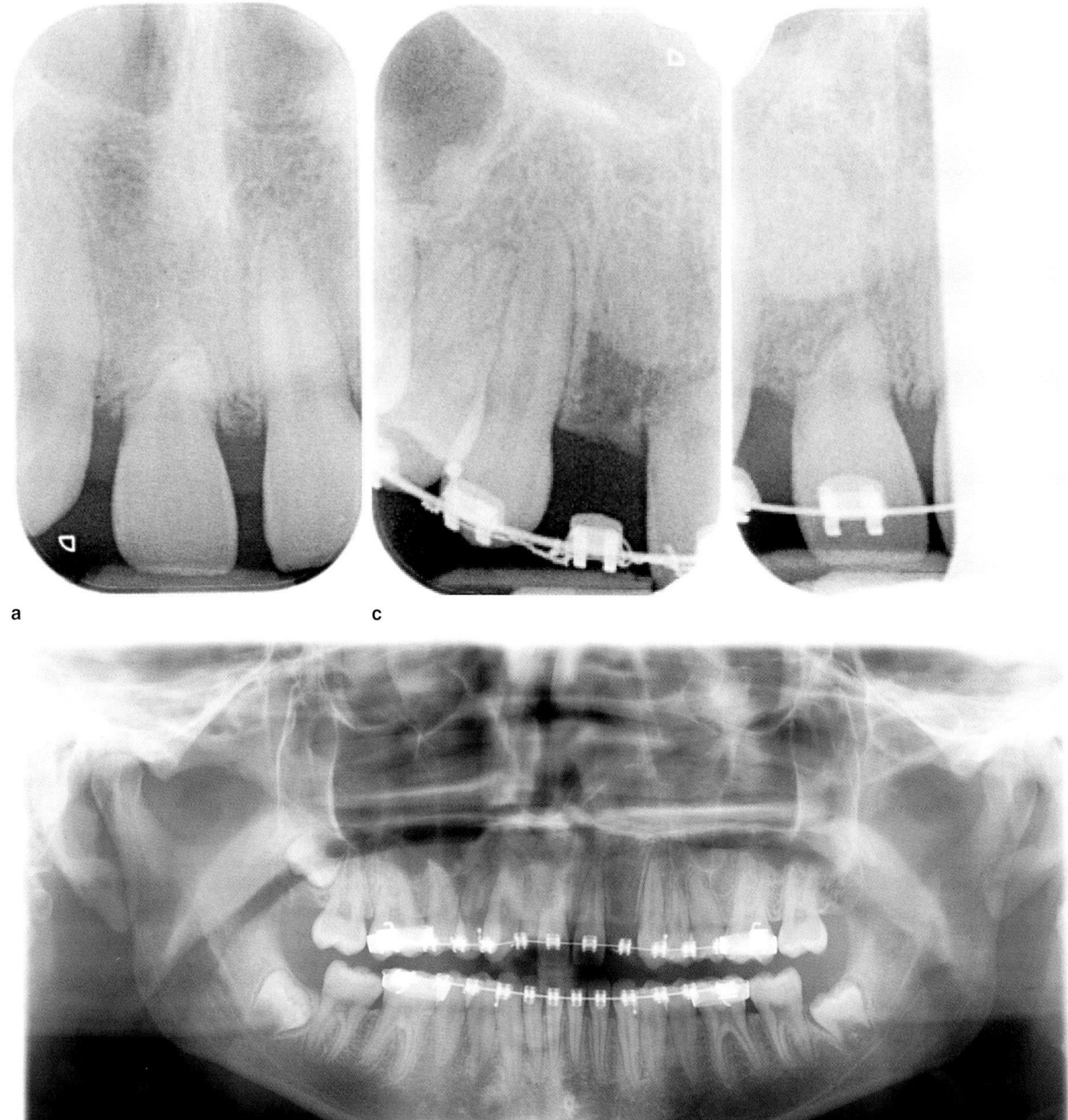

• **Fig. 50.2** **a,** Periapical view of the maxillary anterior teeth prior to orthodontic treatment. **b,** Dental panoramic tomograph. **c,** Periapical radiographs taken at the end of orthodontic treatment.

• BOX 50.3 Advantages and Disadvantages of the Treatment Options

Option	Advantages and Disadvantages
Space closure with adhesive resin composite restorations	Resin composite restorations added to the proximal surfaces of the central incisors and canines can be successful in reducing spaces. This is the least invasive option, technically straightforward and can produce an excellent aesthetic result in selected cases. It also conserves the tooth structure. Complete closure without orthodontics cannot always be achieved without each tooth looking unacceptably wide when build-ups have been placed. Mild microdontia is commonly a feature of hypodontia, and therefore, this is not an uncommon problem. Build-ups to the correct width incisally remain narrow at the cervical margin if unhealthy gingival overhangs are to be avoided. This can result in large, unsightly embrasure spaces.

• BOX 50.3 Advantages and Disadvantages of the Treatment Options—cont'd

Option	Advantages and Disadvantages
Orthodontic space closure	This would bring the canines into the position of the lateral incisors. A good result can often be achieved in this way because the appearance is symmetrical. This option would need to be discussed during preorthodontic planning by those undertaking the orthodontic and restorative treatments, bearing in mind the predictability of space opening or closing and the root positions of the teeth present. The added advantage is that there is no need for prosthetic tooth replacement and the inherent maintenance that will be required in future. Therefore, in cases where orthodontic considerations make space closure preferable to space opening, this can produce an excellent result (see Fig. 50.3) However, the canines frequently require morphological modification to look like lateral incisors. This may involve the addition of resin composite to create a mesio-incisal angle as described above and sometimes grinding of the cusp tip. The darker chroma of the canine can sometimes be conspicuous but can be addressed by selective bleaching of teeth in adult patients. Some are concerned by the gingival contour because of the canine eminence, creating a gingival zenith more apical than that of the adjacent central incisors, but because this would be symmetrical where both laterals are missing, there is evidence that many patients are not concerned by this. The palatal cusp of the first premolar tooth may be visible unless orthodontic movements have incorporated a tilt to mask this and prevent occlusal interference in lateral excursion. Therefore, space closure needs to be carefully planned in discussion with the orthodontic team and, of course, the patient and/or the carers, with appropriate explanations of the pros and cons of each option. This needs to be carefully transcribed in the patient's notes.
Create space for prosthetic lateral incisors	Space creation by orthodontic treatment, followed by provision of lateral incisors with a prosthesis, also involves a protracted phase of orthodontic treatment. A good result can be achieved where the presenting tooth and its root position are favourable for orthodontic space creation. This depends on factors such as the position of the root apices and the interocclusal relationship. Again, case selection, in consultation with the orthodontic team, is key to success when deciding whether to open or close spaces. This was the choice in the current case.

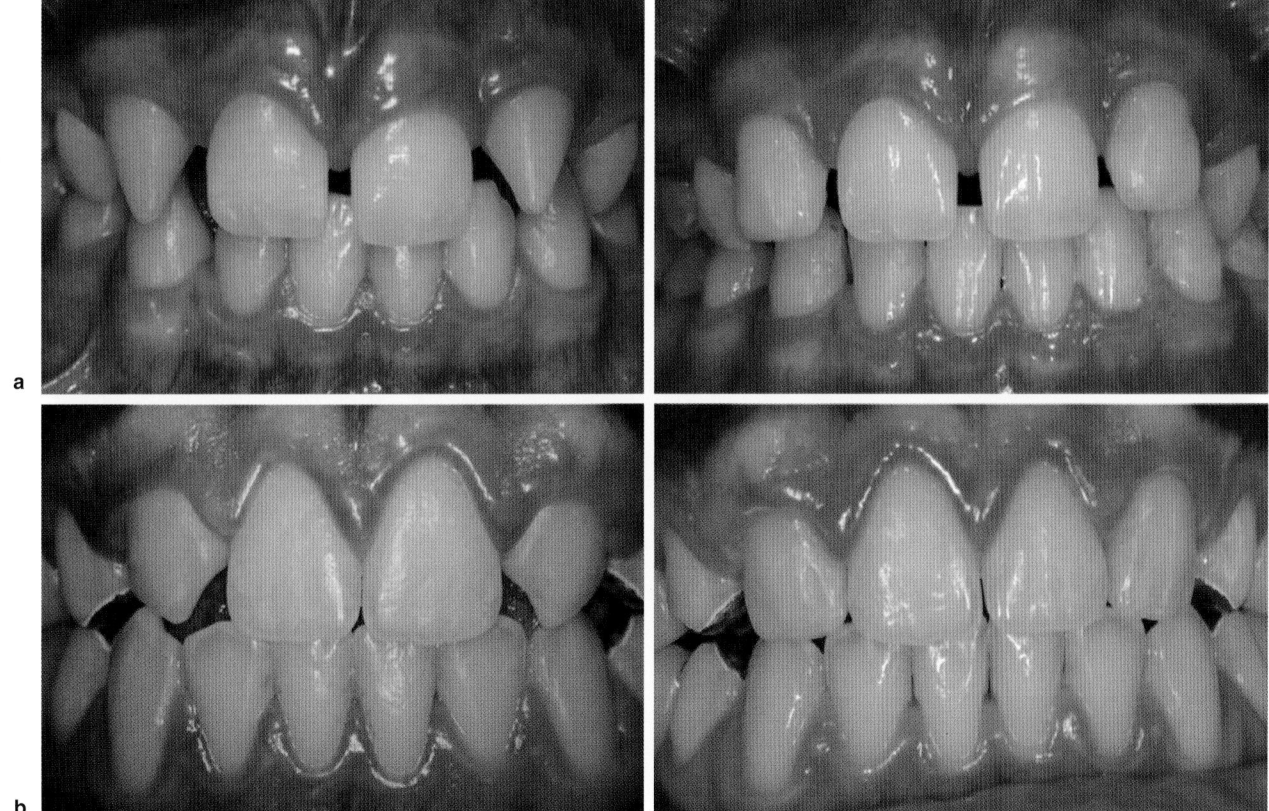

• Fig. 50.3 Canines can sometimes be successfully camouflaged to masquerade as lateral incisors using resin composite direct restorations: **a,** shows a case with residual spacing; **b,** the masking is completed after orthodontic movement to close the spacing. The composite build up shown in illustration **a** was undertaken prior to planned orthodontic alignment to assist in appropriate space closure as the correct tooth dimensions have already been created prior to orthodontic treatment.

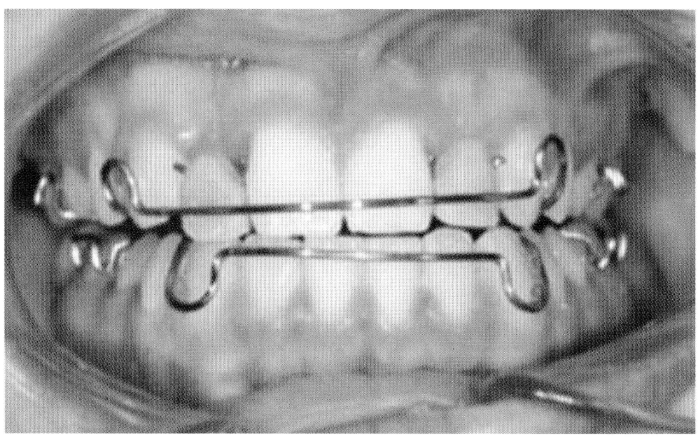

• **Fig. 50.4** The final orthodontic result after orthodontic debond with a Hawley retainer in situ. **a,** Maxillary occlusal view and **b,** Labial view. Note that in a Hawley retainer design has been provided, with teeth in the lateral incisor position and wire stops to prevent space closure until the prosthetic replacements can be provided. A Hawley retainer was selected in preference to an 'Essix' vacuum-formed retainer because a Hawley retainer can be more easily adjusted when adhesive bridges are placed by removing the lateral incisor additions, so there is no break in retainer wear. If implants were planned, an 'Essix' retainer design with replacement teeth incorporated in it would be preferable because the fit surface of the replacement tooth pontics in this design can be more easily relieved to make space for implant healing abutments, with reduced risk of fracture compared with the pontics in a Hawley design which can break off if the acrylic is made too thin.

possible. This option, of course, would need referral to a specialist orthodontist and his or her team for multidisciplinary planning and treatment execution. It is also important to remember the risks associated with the root of the compromised upper right central incisor, and great care is required in moving this tooth with fixed orthodontics. The treatment plan should take into account a possible need to replace this tooth as well as the missing lateral incisors.

The orthodontic result for this patient can be seen in Fig. 50.4.

◆ If the Resorbed Root Had Been an Absolute Contraindication To Orthodontic Treatment, What Other Option Might Have Been Appropriate?

If orthodontic space opening had not been possible without compromising the prognosis of the central incisor tooth, the canine teeth could have been built up to resemble the missing lateral incisor teeth instead of providing orthodontic treatment, accepting some anterior spacing or to assist in correct space closure. An example of this can be seen in Fig. 50.3a. The preoperative periapical view in Fig. 50.2a indicates that the tooth position at initial presentation might have lent itself to this approach, but only if the patient was happy to accept some spacing.

◆ How Would You Now Replace the Missing Lateral Incisors?

Initially, the spaces are filled with teeth added onto the orthodontic retainer. After a period of settling, definitive restorations can be considered.

In this case, definitive prosthodontic treatment had to be as conservative as possible because the upper anterior teeth were vital and sound and the patient was young. The doubtful long-term prognosis of the upper right central incisor was an important consideration. These teeth could be replaced with fixed or removable prostheses; however, in most circumstances, a fixed restoration would be the patient's strong preference. The options, therefore, would include the following.

Adhesive Bridgework. This is a conservative option because it requires little or no tooth preparation. Adhesive bridges, when appropriately designed, can be an option with a very predictable outcome but require sufficient enamel for bonding of the retainer wings. Because the teeth in this case were unrestored, there was ample enamel for bonding, making this a viable treatment option. Conventional bridgework would be contraindicated here because it would be unnecessarily destructive of the abutment teeth.

Implant-Supported Restorations. Implants are now a widely used treatment option for tooth replacement and can produce predictable aesthetic and functional results. It is important to ensure that there is sufficient space between adjacent teeth and sufficient bone volume to accommodate the implants. This will, therefore, need to be planned as part of any orthodontic treatment.

For dental implants to be an option, even if this is not the initial care plan, radiographs are necessary to ensure the tooth roots adjacent to the spaces (upper canines and central incisors in this case) are not encroaching on the potential implant-bearing area and that the mesio-distal space is sufficient to accommodate the size of an implant both at the gingival level and also between the root apices (usually approximately 7 mm). It is also worth considering that because hypodontia is frequently associated with microdontia, it is not always appropriate or, indeed, possible to open the spaces to this dimension; therefore, it is important that the patient is made aware of this before any treatment is started. In this case, the tooth movements were quite extensive; in such a situation, it is wise to warn a patient that it may not be possible to move the tooth roots sufficiently to create space for an implant before orthodontic space creation is started. Managing patient expectations regarding treatment outcome is critical in such cases.

Implants involve one or more surgical procedures and can be costly and, therefore, are not always the most appropriate option. They are also not indicated for patients under the age of 18 years because of the continuing growth of the jaws. Indeed, some would suggest that growth continues for some time after this age and would advocate delaying implants until patients are much older, especially in single tooth sites, because this can result in infraocclusion relative to the adjacent natural teeth.

It is advisable for the dentist who is going to undertake the restorative treatment to review the case prior to orthodontic debond to ensure that the dimensions of the spaces and the tooth/root position are optimal for the most predictable outcome of the restoration to be provided. This includes ensuring that the spaces are symmetrical and that appropriate occlusal guidance is available, as well as radiographs to assess root position, as mentioned above.

In this case, in view of the doubtful prognosis of the upper central incisor, implants were considered a good option to avoid loading the compromised tooth. However, in view of the patient's age and the fact that the incisors were not showing significant mobility at this stage, the recommended treatment of choice was adhesive bridges, maintaining the central incisors for as long as possible and considering an implant-supported restoration to replace them if and when problems occur in future.

Possible bridge designs are shown in Figs 50.5 and 50.6.

Bridge Designs. Normally, a fixed–fixed design in a minimum-preparation bridge (as shown in Fig. 50.5) should be avoided. This is because the differential mobility of the abutment teeth can result in debonding of one retainer, creating an area of stagnation below it and, thus, an increased risk of development of a carious lesion. For this reason, a typical minimum-preparation bridge design to replace a lateral incisor would be a cantilever design retained on either the canine or the central incisor (as shown in Fig. 50.6a and b).

It was important to consider orthodontic retention. The canines were originally mesio-labially rotated, and the orthodontic result would, therefore, be potentially unstable. Relapse would result in the pontics swinging out labially if bridge design option a were chosen in the absence of orthodontic retention. Option b does not include the canines, but because one of the central incisors had a poor prognosis, it was not appropriate to use the incisors as bridge abutments. In cases where a midline diastema has been closed, retention can be incorporated in the adhesive bridge design such as a cantilever design retained on linked central incisors (option c), but, again, because of the condition of the roots of the central incisors, this option was contraindicated in this case.

A fixed–fixed bridge extending from canine to canine (Fig. 50.5) or canine to incisor (Fig 50.6 option d) would include fixed orthodontic retention of the positions of the canines and central incisors, but once again, this involves the questionable incisors. A potentially unstable orthodontic result may in itself favour debonding of one or more of the wings, and so if a linked or fixed–fixed design is used, regular recall will be

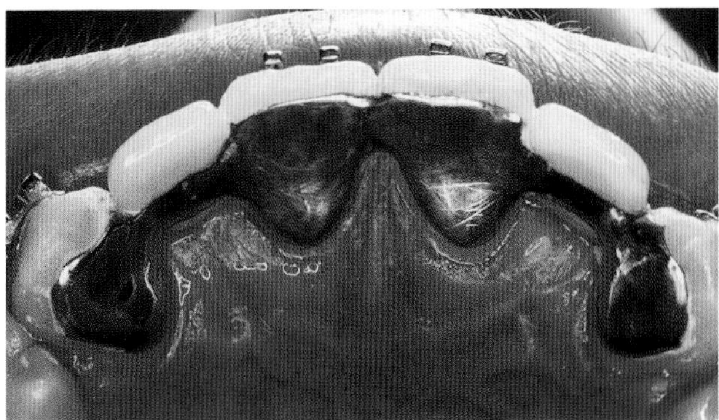

a

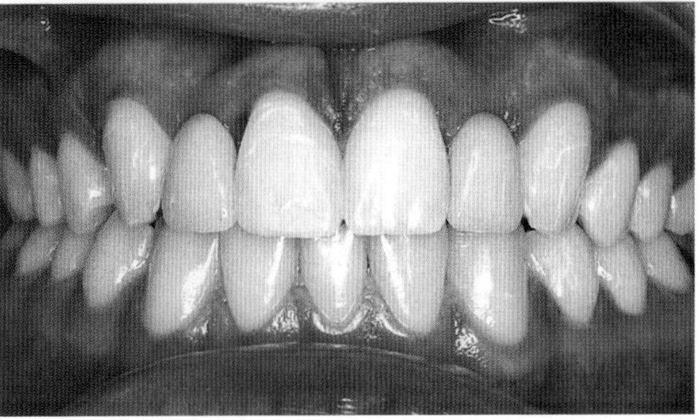

b

• **Fig. 50.5** Possible designs for minimum preparation adhesive bridges to replace missing maxillary lateral incisors. **a,** Occlusal view, **b**, labial view.

essential to detect this early. In case of debonding, the bridge must be removed and either replaced or recemented, if considered appropriate. If this is planned, an assessment of the reason for the debonding must be made to ascertain whether this is an appropriate course of action or whether an alternative design or a different restoration is indicated. Prior to recementation, the abutment teeth and the retainer wings must be cleaned thoroughly. Intraoral air abrasion is useful for this, if available.

Therefore, in this case, option a was the most appropriate bridge design, and orthodontic retention was maintained by making a new retainer fitted simultaneously on the day the bridges were cemented. The patient was given clear instructions to wear the retainer every night and warned clearly, both verbally and with written instruction, that orthodontic relapse is a risk if she does not comply with this advice. It would be wise to ensure that patients read and fully understand the consequences and that they sign the form indicating they have done so. A copy of this form should be retained in the patients' records for future reference.

The final bridge design and appearance are shown in Fig. 50.7. Note how the metal retainer wing is extended over the entire palatal surface of the canine tooth to utilize the maximum available enamel for bonding. Box 50.4 shows a suggested wording and diagrams which can be used in a laboratory prescription for this design of bridge. The orthodontic care plan should take into account the occlusal clearance required to cover the palatal surfaces of the canines, although if there is insufficient interocclusal space, alveolar compensation (the 'Dahl effect') is likely to occur as part of post orthodontic vertical settling if the

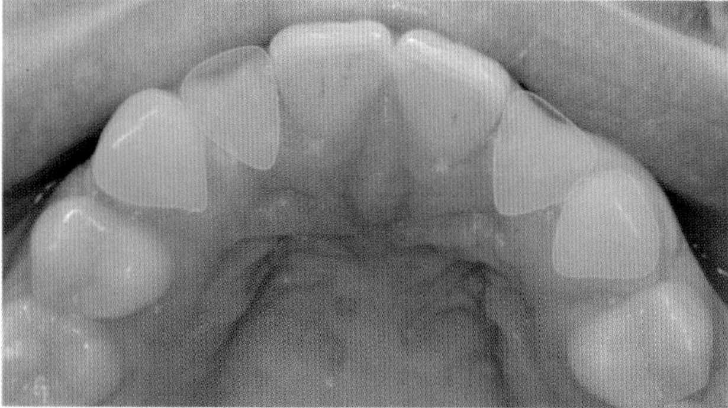
a

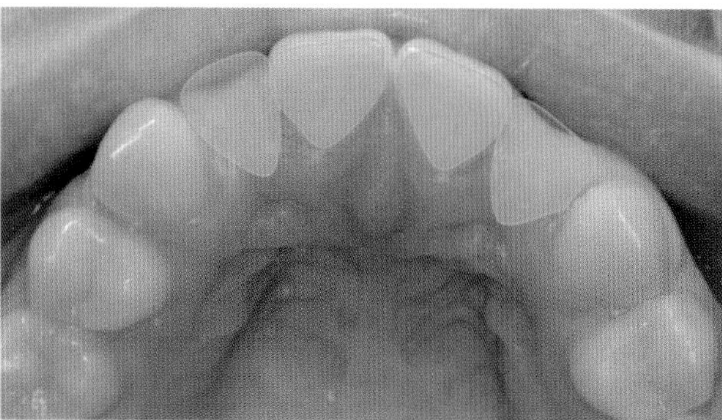
b

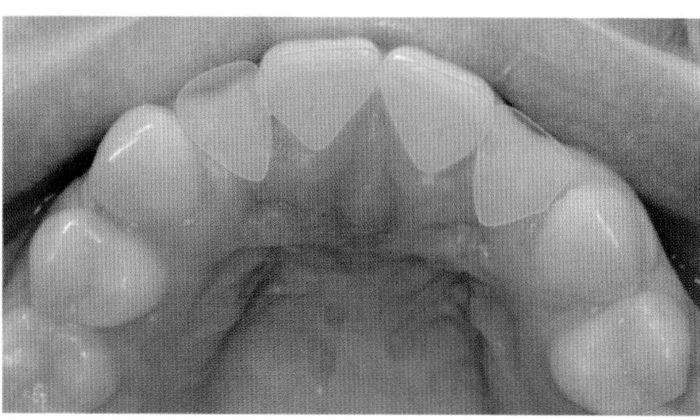
c

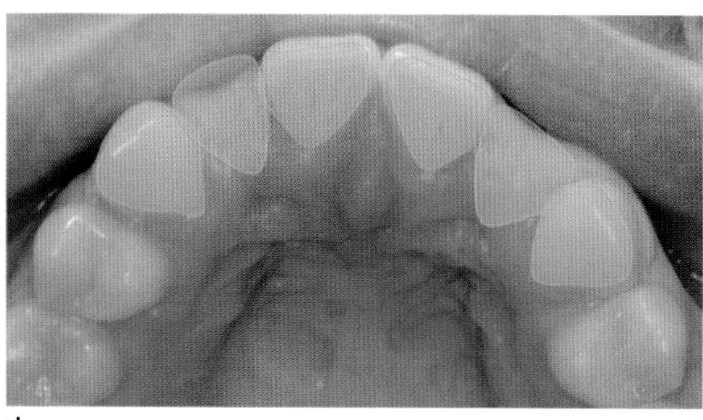
d

• **Fig. 50.6** Possible designs for adhesive bridges. **a,** Mesial cantilever from canine abutment teeth; **b,** Distal cantilever from incisor abutment teeth; **c,** Distal cantilever from incisor abutment teeth, linking incisors for fixed orthodontic retention; **d,** Fixed-fixed bridges from canines to incisors, providing fixed orthodontic retention.

bridges are cemented 'high' in occlusion. In this instance, the occlusal contacts should be monitored at review.

The bridges were cemented by using an opaque resin cement to obscure the colour of metal retainer wings showing through and to prevent 'greying' of the abutment teeth, as is sometimes described, although this is more commonly a problem where more translucent (incisor) teeth are used as abutments. Although this successfully prevents grey shine-through, the altered translucency can affect the final shade and must be taken into account during shade selection, by holding something (e.g. a gloved finger or a cotton wool roll) against the palatal aspect of the abutment tooth to mimic this change.

• BOX 50.4 Adhesive Bridge Laboratory Request

- Please pour upper and lower casts and mount in ICP using wax record and make adhesive bridges to replace Upper 2/2 cantilevered mesially from canine teeth (shade as indicated).
- Please extend metal retainer wings over maximum available palatal enamel for bonding and just extending over cusp slopes (see diagram) to aid positioning at cementation and protect cement lute from shear forces – high in occlusion if necessary.

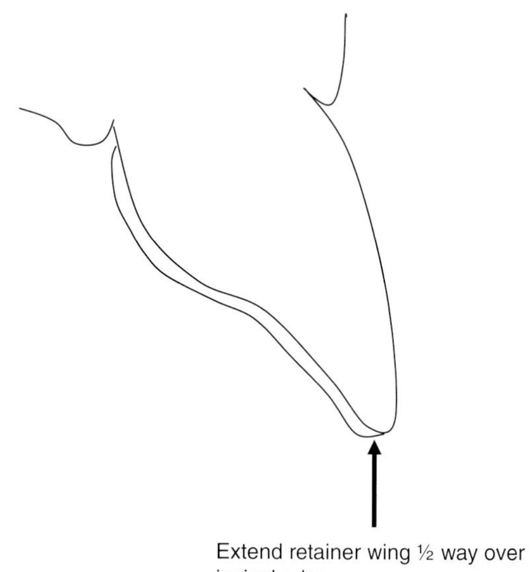

◆ What Warnings Must Be Given To the Patient When Undertaking This Treatment and Obtaining Consent?

The upper right central incisor has a doubtful medium- to long-term prognosis because of the short root evident on the radiograph. It is essential that the patient is aware of this and is involved in the decision regarding choice of restoration, both at this stage and in relation to what options may be available in future. In this case, because the teeth are not excessively mobile and the short root has been monitored over some years, it was decided to maintain the tooth for the time being, rather than extract and replace it as part of the current phase of prosthetic treatment. This decision was based on the acknowledgement that any restoration provided now will require replacement at some stage in the future in view

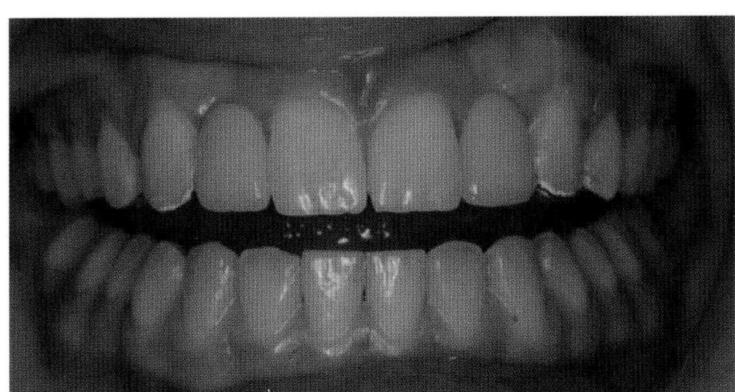
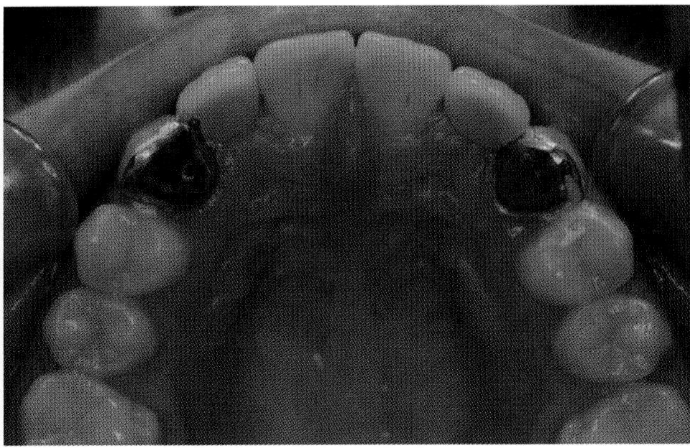

• **Fig. 50.7** The final result. Note the bridge retainer wings are extended over the entire palatal surface of the abutment teeth to incorporate the maximum available enamel for adhesion. In this case, there was interocclusal space for the thickness of the metal retainer wing, but if this is lacking, then it is not unreasonable to consider cementing the bridges high in occlusion and allowing the occlusal contacts to be re-established as a result of alveolar compensation, as described earlier.

of the patient's young age and that hastening the loss of the tooth was not in the patient's best interests. This was discussed with the patient, who was fully involved in the decision-making process, while obtaining informed consent. The decision not to include the central incisors in the bridge design was part of this discussion, as was the associated importance of removable orthodontic retention, and the patient was fully informed and involved in the care planning process. Contemporaneous notes were made throughout this process and the patient's expectations of treatment managed carefully.

◆ Planning for Failure: What Would Be the Options for Restoration if the Central Incisors Became More Mobile and Failed?

In a case such as this, it is important to plan for failure of teeth that have a guarded prognosis because this forms part of the informed consent process during discussions of treatment planning with the patient.

When the incisors do fail, a new adhesive bridge could be considered, replacing all four upper incisors. These long-span adhesive bridges are less predictable compared with shorter-span bridges, but where two canines are utilized as the abutment teeth, the robust nature of these teeth, coupled with the bulky crown and associated area of enamel for bonding, makes this a pragmatic option in this region. If the abutment teeth are significantly different in size, especially with differential mobility, a long-span fixed–fixed bridge is less predictable. An example of this may be where a lateral incisor and a canine are the potential abutments. The greater inherent mobility of the incisor, along with the smaller surface area of enamel for bonding compared with that of the canine, would make the restoration less predictable because it may predispose to retainer wing debonding on the more mobile abutment.

Another option would be an implant-supported bridge. In this case, consideration could be given to providing implants in the lateral incisor regions, subject to bone availability and appropriate space between the adjacent teeth, which could then be used to provide a longer-span bridge to replace all four incisor teeth if this became necessary in future, without the need for further implant surgery or, if the prognosis of the upper left incisor tooth remained good, this could be retained and a cantilever bridge provided, replacing the upper right central and lateral incisor only, as long as a suitably wide diameter implant could be placed in the lateral incisor region to support a cantilever bridge. In this case, the patient elected to delay the treatment with implants and chose the less invasive option of adhesive bridges at this stage. However, it is essential that patients are aware of the consequences of this option so that they can make a fully informed decision.

Case 51

Anterior Crossbite (Class III Malocclusion) with Displacement in the Mixed Dentition

DIRK BISTER

Summary

A 10-year-old male patient presents with a class III incisor relationship, he is in the mixed-dentition. There are signs of tooth wear affecting the front teeth.

History

Complaint

The patient complains about an uncomfortable bite, and the front teeth are meeting 'the wrong way around'.

History of Complaint

The parents report that he developed a class III malocclusion after the upper and lower permanent incisors erupted and came into contact.

Medical History

The patient is medically fit and well.

Examination

Extraoral Examination

The patient presents with a mild class III profile when his posterior teeth are in maximum intercuspation. However, his facial features are normal when biting on the incisors (before displacement).

Intraoral Examination

The patient can achieve an 'edge to edge' incisor relationship. There are signs of tooth wear (attrition) affecting the upper incisors, particularly the upper central incisors (Fig. 51.1).

The patient then postures forwards (so-called 'displacement') into a comfortable bite to achieve good contact between the back teeth (maximum intercuspation).

In the UK, the Index of Orthodontic Treatment Need (IOTN) is used to assess eligibility for treatment free of charge at the point of delivery (https://www.nhs.uk/conditions/Orthodontics/).

The IOTN of this patient is 4c, which is defined as 'anterior or posterior crossbites with greater than 2 mm discrepancy between the retruded contact position and maximum intercuspation'. More detailed information on IOTN can be found at: https://www.bos.org.uk/Public-Patients/Orthodontics-for-Children-Teens/Fact-File-FAQ/What-Is-The-IOTN.

Diagnosis

◆ What are the Possible Causes of Class III Malocclusion?

Potential causes of class III malocclusion are:

1. Unusual eruption path of the upper incisors leading to a forward mandibular displacement
2. Underdevelopment of the maxilla
3. Overdevelopment of the mandible

or a combination of any of the above.

Treatment

A dental panoramic tomogram (DPT) or an upper standard occlusal (USO) radiograph should be taken for planning orthodontic treatment. This will enable the practitioner to exclude the presence of supplemental/supernumerary teeth in the upper anterior labial segment. A lateral cephalogram may be considered if a significant skeletal discrepancy is diagnosed clinically (i.e. there is no displacement and a reverse overjet greater than 2 mm and/or a reduced overbite/open bite; this should trigger a referral to a specialist). The DPT and USO radiograph can be taken by the general dental practitioner.

The choice of treatment depends on the underlying aetiology, as discussed below.

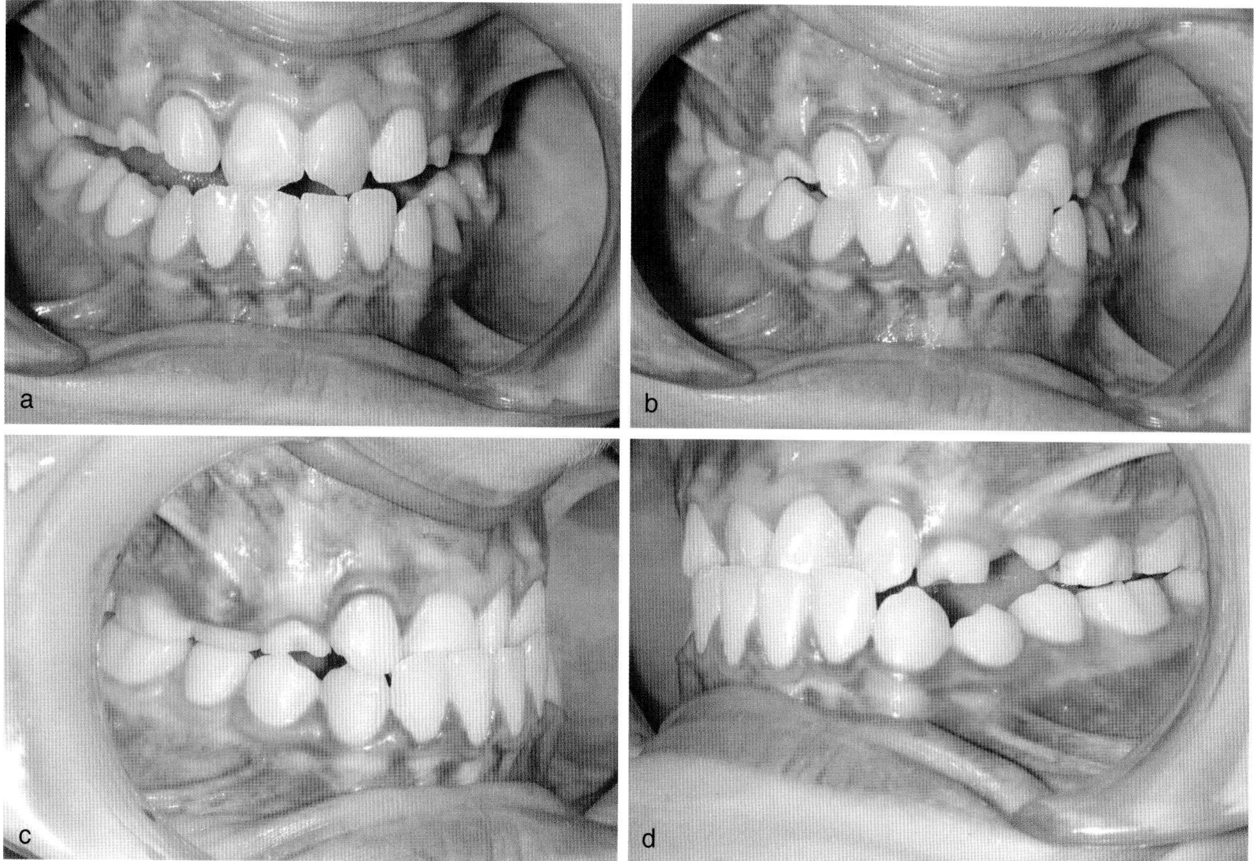

• **Fig. 51.1** **a,** The patient achieves an edge-to-edge incisor relationship when in retruded mandibular position. The patient is asked to roll the tongue to the back of the mouth and close until the anterior teeth come into contact. Alternatively, the mandible can be manipulated manually to achieve the rearmost position. **b–d,** On closure, the patient postures his mandible forwards to achieve maximum intercuspation, as seen on the images on the top right lower right and lower left. There are signs of attrition affecting the upper central incisors in particular.

'Camouflage' Orthodontics

'Camouflage' Orthodontics is defined as leaving the causative underlying skeletal discrepancy untreated. The teeth are moved so that a normal occlusion is established. In case of normal inclination of the maxillary teeth and a minor skeletal discrepancy, opt for tooth movement only. This can be achieved by using either sectional fixed appliances or an upper removable appliance. The latter approach was chosen as a case study here (Fig. 51.1) and does not necessarily require treatment by a specialist orthodontist.

Partial upper fixed appliances are also known as 'two-by-four appliances': The upper first molars are usually banded, and the four incisors are bonded. This treatment should ideally be provided by an orthodontic specialist.

Treatment, usually of short duration, in the mixed dentition that aims at correcting the aetiology of malocclusion is also known as *interceptive treatment.*

Comprehensive 'Early' Treatment for Class III Malocclusion

Correction of the skeletal discrepancy can be attempted with a facemask in the mixed dentition or by using a fixed appliance in the permanent dentition. Jaw surgery can be considered in severe cases, with multidisciplinary collaboration among the orthodontist, and the oral and maxillofacial surgeon. Correcting a mild skeletal discrepancy in the mixed dentition by using a facemask is successful in approximately 70% of cases.

Appliance Design for the Upper Removable Appliance

The appliance consists of an active component, a retention component and a baseplate. A large 'Z' spring is used to procline the upper central and lateral incisors, thereby eliminating displacement (Fig. 51.2). This is the active component. Alternatively, other types of springs can be used (e.g. T-springs).

Adams' cribs on deciduous molars and molars are used for retention. A posterior bite plane can be useful to open the bite and allow the incisors to move forward without interference with the lower dentition.

When the appliance is fitted and activated, it needs to be noted that it will be 'bouncy': The upper spring will create a downward force. The Z-spring is activated by pulling it mainly upwards (cranial) and only slightly forwards so that it does not come to rest in front of the upper incisors on insertion.

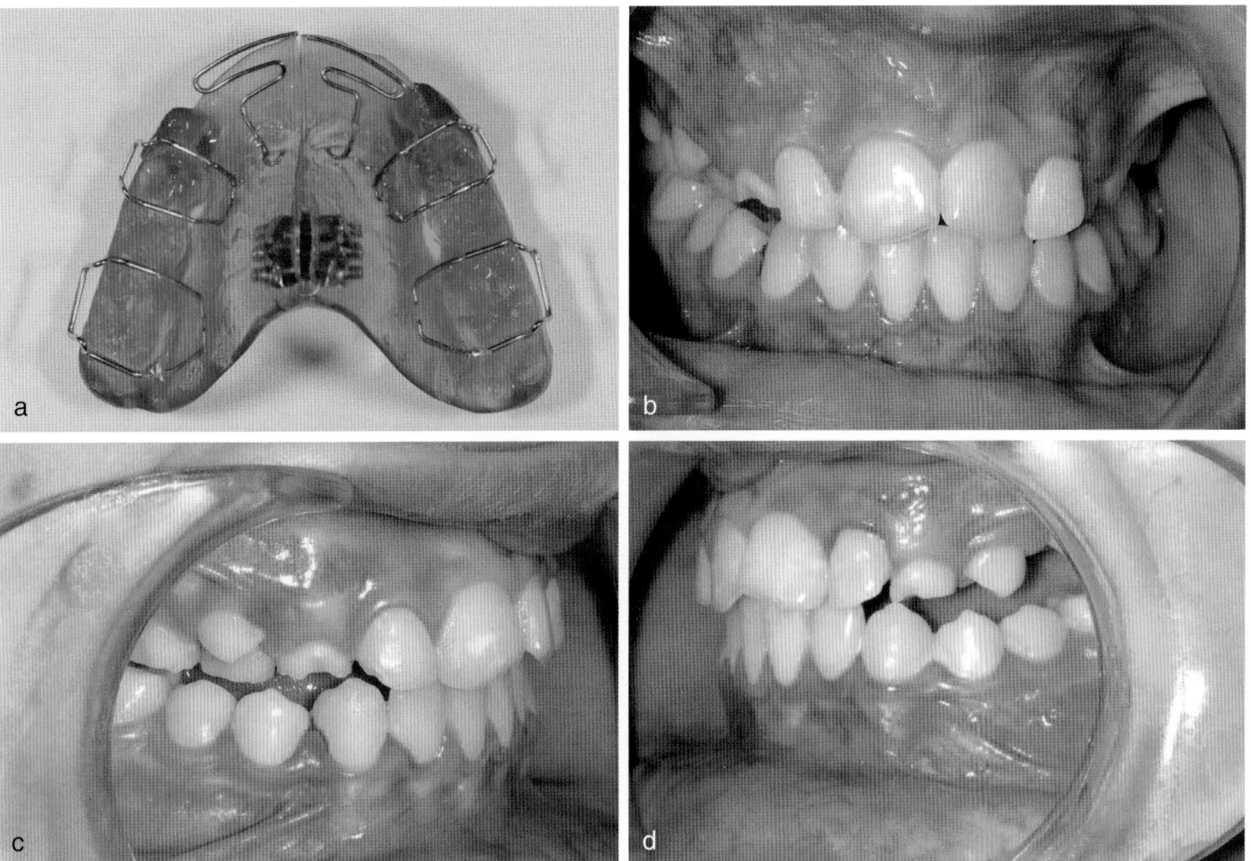

• **Fig. 51.2 a,** Image of an upper removable appliance for proclination of the upper labial segment. Two 'Z' springs are placed on right-hand side and the left-hand side to procline the upper central and lateral incisors. Adams' cribs are used for retention as well a posterior bite plane. An upper midline expansion screw has been added to address the crossbite tendency. **b–d,** Treatment outcome after approximately 8 weeks of treatment. The patient's upper incisors have been proclined and the patient now occludes the anterior teeth but without displacing forwards. At this stage, the appliance is gradually withdrawn and night-time-only wear is prescribed.

The appliance is usually worn full time for a period of 6–8 weeks, followed by nighttime wear for approximately 3 months. There is a posterior open bite once the upper incisors have been proclined, as seen in the images provided (see Fig. 51.2). This settles once the appliance is worn at nighttime only. This is a good example of interceptive orthodontic treatment (Fig. 51.3).

Consent

Obtaining valid consent is one of the nine principles that registered dental professionals must follow at all times (https://standards.gdc-uk.org/pages/principle3/principle3.aspx).

Consent in orthodontics is ideally a two-stage process: In the first stage, the patient and their parents/legal guardian(s) are given the relevant information (often at the stage of orthodontic records: impressions/scan, clinical photographs and radiographs). Information leaflets describing the different aspects of orthodontic treatment are available through the British Orthodontic Society at: https://www.bos.org.uk/Public-Patients/Patient-Information-Leaflets. In this case, leaflets on treatment with a removable appliance, the risks of orthodontics, diet advice, and retention are particularly important.

In the second stage, on the return visit, the patient and parent/legal guardian sign the consent form. It is important to note that consent is an ongoing process and that adherence to treatment (i.e. wearing the removable appliance full time) is paramount to its success.

Potential Legal Issues and Pitfalls

As with all orthodontic treatment, careful note keeping and monitoring of treatment progress are mandatory. The clinical problem is assessing the amount of displacement. The increased displacement will make it easier to treat this patient because his upper front teeth have to move forward less to achieve a positive overjet.

Patient Adherence

Adherence to wearing/maintaining the removable appliance may be an issue in some cases. It is important to remember that most appliances are not worn for the time requested by the orthodontists. Microsensor technology (e.g. TheraMon(R)) can be used to monitor wear, although this technology is not infallible. Patient consent should be obtained when monitoring devices are used.

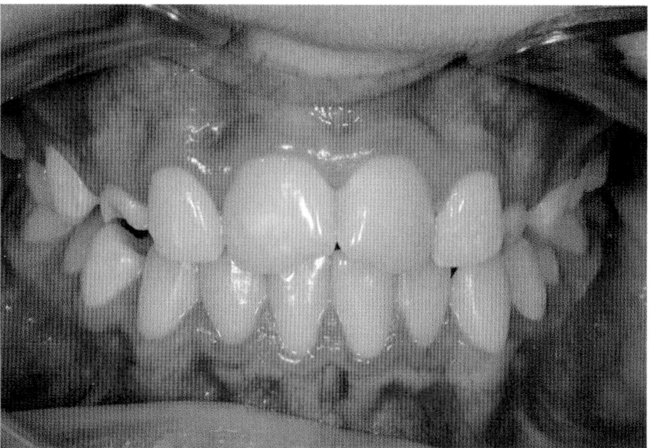

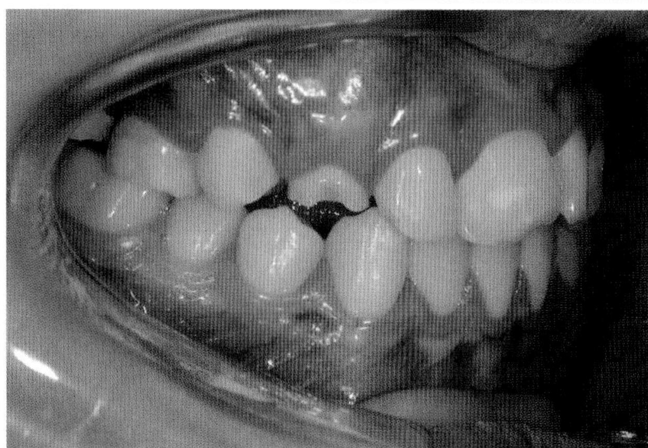

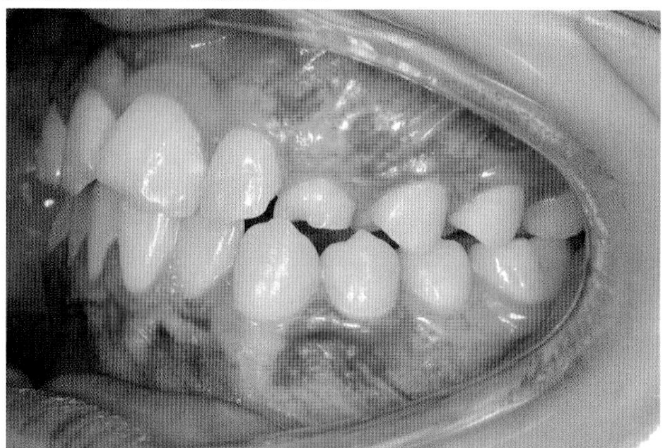

• **Fig. 51.3** Final result after occlusal settling, approximately 2 months later. The patient has discontinued upper removable appliance wear, and the posterior buccal segments have settled.

Prognostic Factors for Treatment of the Upper Arch

A good vertical overlap of the incisors needs to be achieved at the end of orthodontic treatment; otherwise relapse may occur. Ideally, the upper incisors should not already be proclined before commencing orthodontics. Patients need to be advised that continuation of existing growth patterns can jeopardize the orthodontic treatment outcome particularly long-term.

Long-Term Outcome

The bite for this patient remained stable, and no further orthodontic treatment was required.

Summary

Teeth in anterior crossbite can be treated in the mixed dentition by using interceptive orthodontics. This type of treatment can be simple and cost-effective. The need to comply with removable appliance wear needs to be made clear at the start of treatment, and progress needs to be monitored and documented carefully. Obtaining patient consent regarding the long-term prognosis of class III treatment is also important. Growth may not always be favourable – the mandible tends to grow for a longer period compared with the maxilla, and there is potential for the reverse overjet to relapse.

Case 52
Localized Periodontitis?

EDWARD ODELL AND MANDEEP GHUMAN

Summary

A 30-year-old male patient is referred for periodontitis that has not responded to treatment. What is the cause, and how would you proceed?

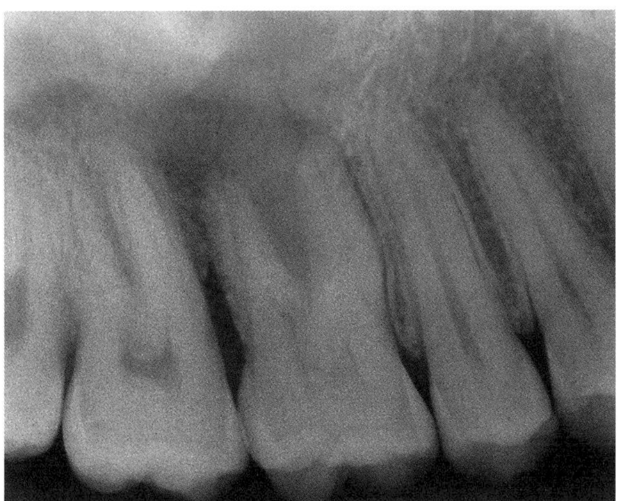

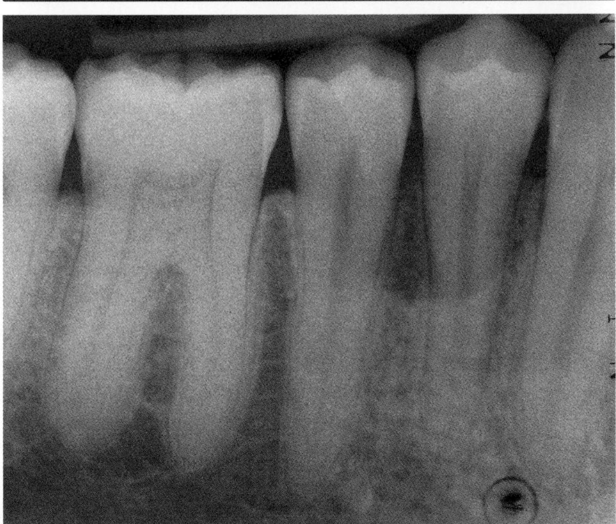

• **Fig. 52.1** Periapical radiographs sent on referral.

History

Complaint

The patient complains that he has been undergoing intensive treatment for gum disease, but with little success. His upper right first molar is slightly loose, and his dentist wishes to extract it. He would like a second opinion.

History of Complaint

He noticed the gum disease 9 months ago. He has never had pain or discomfort from the tooth.

Dental History

The patient is a regular attendee at his dentist's clinic. He has no dental restorations, no caries and no other oral problems. The previous dental practitioner had provided intensive oral hygiene instruction, root surface debridement under local anaesthesia, and reassessment. The patient brushes twice a day with a fluoride toothpaste and uses interdental brushes of two different sizes, as well as flossing daily.

Medical History

The patient is fit and well. He has no allergies and takes no medication. He has never smoked.

◆ What are Your Initial Thoughts?

Periodontitis is often difficult to treat. Many patients are not able to maintain a sufficiently effective oral hygiene regimen or have other risk factors that have not been controlled or are beyond control. It remains possible that this patient is not cleaning effectively regularly despite his efforts, and this must be assessed. Or perhaps previous treatment did not completely remove all the subgingival calculus. Assuming the previous treatment was optimal, there has been sufficient time for non-surgical periodontal treatment to have had some effect.

Examination

Extraoral Examination

The results of the extraoral examination are normal. No lymph nodes are palpable.

Intraoral Examination

One lower third molar is partially erupted; the upper third molars are unopposed and distally inclined. There is no dental caries, and no restorations are present.

The patient's oral hygiene is very good. Only a few flecks of interdental plaque are present. The gingivae in most areas are healthy in appearance and do not bleed on probing.

On full clinical periodontal assessment, three areas of concern are identified:

1. *The upper right first molar is mobile about 1 mm in the bucco-palatal direction. It is grade 2 mobile and is not depressible in the socket. A 9-mm probing depth is present disto-palatally, and the distal furcation has grade 2 furcation involvement. The gingivae appear loose, but they are not oedematous, and there is only slight bleeding on probing. Inflammation appears diffuse, rather than being related to the gingival margin or pocket. The gingiva lifts easily from the tooth.*
2. *The lower right second premolar has a 5-mm probing depth disto-lingually and a 4-mm depth mesio-lingually. The tooth is not mobile. The gingivae are dusky red, not oedematous and relatively firm, although there is slight bleeding on probing.*
3. *There is a 6-mm pocket on the mesio-lingual aspect of the lower left second molar, with no bleeding on probing.*

Root surfaces on all affected areas feel smooth on probing.

Investigations

◆ What Do You See in the Two Periapical Views That the Patient's General Dental Practitioner Sent?

The upper radiograph (Fig. 52.1) shows extensive bone loss distally to the first molar. There is loss of lamina dura around the whole of the distal root, into the furcation and around the apex. No calculus is visible.

The lower film shows a curved area of alveolar bone loss associated with the first and second premolars. The lamina dura and alveolar crest on both teeth appear intact. The bone loss is consistent with the probing depth. No calculus is visible.

◆ What Further Investigations are Required?

The vitality of the upper first molar must be determined. Bone loss extends beyond the apex, and there is a significant risk of loss of vitality. The apical lamina dura is not clearly defined, particularly in relation to the maxillary sinus, giving rise to further suspicion.

A radiograph is needed to appreciate the bone levels around the lower left molars and possibly those around other teeth as well. However, before selecting a suitable view, further thinking is required.

In the meantime, you check the vitality of the upper right first molar. It is vital and not hypersensitive to cold and electric pulp testing.

Differential Diagnosis

◆ What are Your Thoughts Now?

This is odd. The patient is motivated, and his oral hygiene is good; however, there are three areas of localized attachment loss, and these cannot be accounted for by local factors such as overhanging restorations or calculus.

Perhaps the patient has a progressed form of *molar incisor pattern periodontitis*, which is defined as rapid attachment and bone loss occurring mostly at an earlier age, sometimes with a familial pattern. The sites of lesions (on two first molars and one premolar), the age of the patient and failure to respond to treatment suggest this. Would further nonsurgical periodontal treatment with adjunctive antibiotics help?

Perhaps the patient has some systemic predisposition to periodontitis. The most likely cause would be diabetes or smoking. However, diabetes would have to be undiagnosed or poorly controlled to contribute to disease of this severity. Both diabetes and smoking are associated with periodontitis in a more generalized distribution and rarely predispose to localized disease.

Other medical predisposing conditions include neutropenia, Down's syndrome and rare developmental neutrophil defects. These become obvious in childhood and can therefore be excluded in this case.

You decide to take a panoramic radiograph because you are suspicious that there may be more areas affected and because the pattern of disease is unusual. The result is shown in Fig. 52.2.

◆ What Additional Information Do You Gain From the Panoramic Radiograph?

The lower left third molar is missing. The lower second molars have a conical root morphology.

There is a shallow angular bone defect mesial to the lower left second molar. This certainly reinforces the suspicion of molar incisor pattern periodontitis.

Have you missed something? Go back and look again at the periapical and panoramic radiographs and reassess the history.

◆ What Radiographic Features are Inconsistent or Suggest Alternative Causes?

The upper periapical shows a large area of destruction of bone, and it is poorly localized, with the furcation appearing fuzzy. Bone around the apex and the maxillary sinus is not clearly defined, but the tooth is vital. If this were periodontitis, you would expect an endodontic–periodontal lesion, with abnormal results on sensibility testing and an observable corticated sinus margin radiographically.

The same area of the panoramic radiograph shows much more worrying features. You had been concentrating on the periodontal condition and had not noticed that the maxillary antrum above the tooth is indistinct and that the floor of the antrum is eroded over the first and second molars. Compare this area with the contralateral floor of antrum. There is a radiolucency above the molar roots on the right and a poorly defined upper border.

The lower periapical view is also unusual. The lamina dura and the alveolar crest are visible between the premolars despite the smooth, rounded shape of the bone loss adjacent to this. Therefore the bone loss is not interdental, but

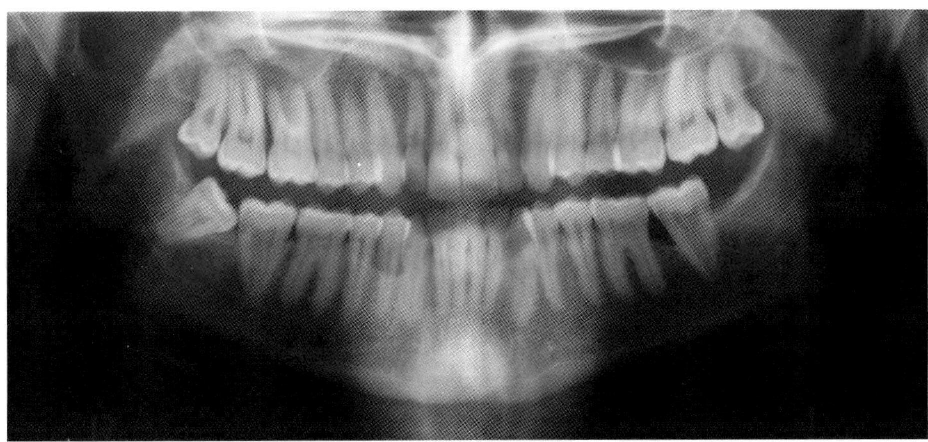

• **Fig. 52.2** The panoramic radiograph.

limited to the lingual cortex and extending across two teeth. The lingual cortex is thicker than the buccal cortex: an infrabony pocket caused by periodontitis could cause such a defect, but more interdental bone loss would be expected because periodontitis is usually initiated interdentally.

Now that you have recognized the extent of the upper molar lesion, your suspicions are confirmed. This is not periodontitis.

◆ What Conditions, Diseases or Lesions May Mimic Plaque-Induced Gingivitis and Periodontitis?

There are many; some mimic gingivitis and others periodontitis. Most are rare. The most significant ones and their characteristic features, as well as useful diagnostic tests, are shown in Table 52.1.

◆ What is Your Differential Diagnosis On the Basis of What You Know So Far? Justify Each Possible Cause

The cause must explain multiple lesions, a predilection for the gingival location and a relatively destructive, poorly defined lesion in a relatively young adult. On the basis of the information presented in Table 52.1, a few causes are likely:

- **Langerhans' cell histiocytosis** is the most likely condition and meets all these criteria. It is rare, but the most common amongst rarities.
- **Squamous odontogenic tumour** also meets all the criteria but is even rarer.
- **Metastatic malignant neoplasm** must be considered. A primary malignancy at a remote site is possible but unlikely at this age. Multiple lesions, particularly in this pattern, would be unlikely.

Further Investigations

◆ What Will You Do Next?

A biopsy is required to achieve the correct diagnosis for any of these diseases. The gingiva is readily sampled under local anaesthesia, and the best site would be soft tissue from the margin of either of the larger lesions – the lower premolar or the upper right molar. A buccal interdental papilla would be ideal.

It would probably be best to extract the affected upper molar tooth. It has lost most of its supporting bone, and obtaining the correct diagnosis is the greater priority. In any case, the prognosis for this tooth is poor, and its removal would allow good access to the deeper tissue to obtain the biopsy sample. The socket could be curetted to obtain additional material from the alveolar bone (keeping in mind the risk of accidentally forming an oro-antral communication).

◆ The Biopsy Specimen is Shown in Fig. 52.3. What Do You See?

The left-hand panel shows the gingival margin. No epithelium is present over the pocket wall, and this ulceration is not compatible with periodontitis. There is a cellular infiltrate in the pocket wall. The second panel shows the infiltrate at higher power. This is not the dense lymphocyte and plasma cell infiltrate of periodontitis. The background cells have prominent pink cytoplasm and large pale lobulated nuclei (cells labelled 'L'). These are typical Langerhans' cells. Bright red eosinophils are also present (labelled 'E').

The appearances are typical of Langerhans' cell histiocytosis. Sheets of neoplastic Langerhans' cells infiltrate the tissues and attract eosinophils, which tend to cluster together and degranulate externally. Bright red eosinophil granules can be seen lying between cells, on the right-hand side of the second panel.

Although the diagnosis is clear, it is necessary to identify Langerhans' cells specifically. Macrophages can also look similar. In the past, this was done by using electron microscopy to demonstrate the characteristic Birbeck's granules in the cell cytoplasm – tennis racket–shaped vesicular organelles. Immunocytochemical staining for the cell surface molecules CD1a and langerin is easier and faster. The third panel shows a low-power view in which a brown stain indicates CD1a on Langerhans' cells. At high power (in the fourth panel), the stain can be seen to be localized around the cell, forming a dark ring at the cell membrane.

TABLE 52.1 Conditions, Diseases and Lesions That May Mimic Plaque-Induced Gingivitis and Periodontitis

Condition	Typical Features	Diagnostic Tests
Conditions That Mimic Gingivitis		
Granulomatous inflammatory conditions (caused by orofacial granulomatosis, oral Crohn's disease, Melkersson–Rosenthal syndrome and sarcoidosis)	Presents from childhood to middle age. Lumpy granular gingival inflammation, more marked in areas of plaque retention. Tags and flaps of redundant gingiva may develop. Shrinks slightly but does not respond completely to plaque control. Tissue contains granulomas. Sarcoidosis may be associated with raised serum calcium, raised serum angiotensin-converting enzyme and lymphadenopathy, especially hilar lymphadenopathy. Bowel disease may be present in those with orofacial granulomatosis or Crohn's disease.	Biopsy. Evidence of bowel, lung or other sites involved. Investigations depend on any associated conditions.
Leukaemia	Usually presents in children with acute myelomonocytic or monocytic leukaemia or in older patients with chronic myeloid leukaemia. May be a lumpy gingivitis with few suspicious features, a very inflamed maroon or greenish gingivitis or one or more ulcerated growths from the gingival margin. Additional infectious signs of immunosuppression, particularly candidosis, may also be present.	Biopsy, blood film, history.
Granulomatosis with polyangiitis	Presents in middle age. The classic gingival presentation is unusual, a rare presentation but striking. Overgrowth of granular or red and white speckled 'strawberry gums'. May grow to cover teeth in a few weeks. Renal involvement may be rapidly fatal. Resembles florid 'hyperplastic' plaque-induced gingivitis.	May be evidence of disease in nose, sinuses or elsewhere, especially kidneys. Circulating antineutrophil cytoplasmic antibodies present.
Hereditary gingival fibromatosis	Presents in childhood or adolescence. Generalized fibrous enlargement of gingiva in presence or absence of infection. May cover crowns of teeth. Solitary or associated with several different syndromes. Family history.	Family history, identification of other features in syndromes. Biopsy.
Autoimmune diseases	Affected areas of fiery red gingivae desquamative gingivitis usually indicative of lichen planus, but also pemphigus vulgaris or pemphigoid. The latter conditions may present with characteristic additional signs of vesiculo-bullous lesions.	Clinical features and biopsy.
Foreign body gingivitis	A rare condition caused by impaction into gingiva of abrasive particles from prophylaxis paste. Occurs if professional cleaning is overzealous and the gingival margin is abraded by brush or ulcerated by heat generated by a rubber cup. The particles elicit a florid foreign body reaction. The gingiva appears duskily inflamed, but plaque control has no effect. Often painful.	Clinical features and biopsy.
Traumatic lesions (mechanical/ chemical/thermal)	May present at any age. Mechanical – tends to occur in those with very frequent or overzealous professional cleaning. May be painful. Chemical – patient use of chlorhexidine, aspirin, cocaine, hydrogen peroxide. Thermal – burns from hot drinks/food. Tends to cause ulcers and unlikely to mimic plaque-induced disease closely.	Clinical findings combined with patient history.
Deposition diseases and inborn errors of metabolism	Presents in newborns or children. Gingiva enlarged by deposition of various metabolic end products such as abnormal glycogen or mucopolysaccharides, producing enlargement rather than inflammation and periodontitis.	Biopsy, biochemical analysis, family history.
Giant cell granuloma	Two forms. Giant cell epulis, resembling fibrous epulis or pyogenic granuloma on the gingival margin and central, a deep cyst-like destructive lesion of maxillary bone less likely to resemble periodontitis. No systemic features.	Biopsy.
Fungal infection	Gingival candidosis presenting as linear gingival erythema with a granular appearance is sometimes associated with human immunodeficiency virus (HIV) infection. South American blastomycosis (paracoccidioidomycosis) causes lumpy granular inflamed gingival swellings but this is an endemic disease and is not seen in the UK. May extend beyond the gingiva.	Biopsy.

TABLE 52.1 Conditions, Diseases and Lesions That May Mimic Plaque-Induced Gingivitis and Periodontitis—cont'd

Condition	Typical Features	Diagnostic Tests
Conditions That Mimic Periodontitis		
Langerhans' cell histiocytosis	Solitary or multifocal destructive lesion that often affects the skull and jaws. May arise at almost any age and often destroys bone around teeth. In late disease, teeth appear to be 'floating in air' radiographically because no bone remains.	Biopsy.
Odontogenic tumours	Occasionally, odontogenic tumours form in the gingiva rather than in bone. Most cause a small mass or erode superficial bone and are easily excised without problems. The commonest odontogenic tumour to occur extraosseously is the calcifying odontogenic cyst. Squamous odontogenic tumour merits special mention because it sometimes arises in the periodontal ligament or gingiva and mimics periodontitis.	Biopsy.
Squamous cell carcinoma of gingiva	Gingiva is a very rare site for carcinoma, which usually presents in those older than 50 years of age. Destroys soft tissue and bone.	Biopsy.
Metastatic malignancy	Most metastatic malignant neoplasms of the jaws grow in the medullary space of the posterior mandible. However, metastases may also seed to the gingiva to produce solitary or multiple masses, often ulcerated.	Biopsy, history.
Hypophosphatasia	Teeth exfoliate with forming roots almost immediately after eruption. No cementum present. Caused by mutation of the tissue nonspecific alkaline phosphatase enzyme required for bone mineralization.	Serum alkaline phosphatase, family history.

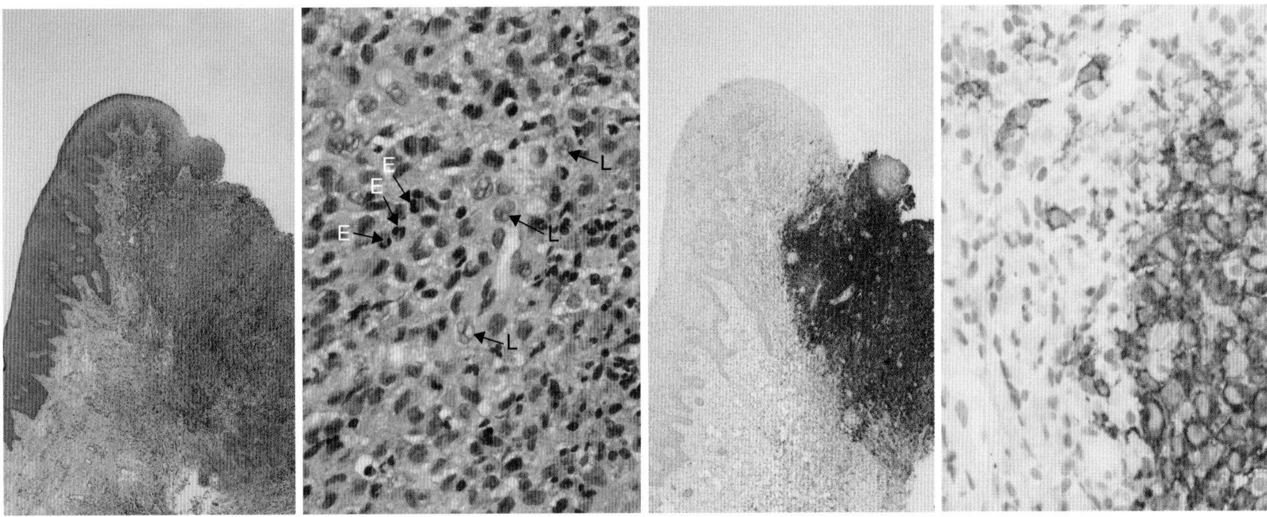

• **Fig. 52.3** The histological appearance of the biopsy. *E*, eosinophils; *L*, lobulated nuclei.

Diagnosis

The diagnosis is Langerhans' cell histiocytosis.

◆ What is a Langerhans' Cell?

A dendritic cell found in epithelium. These cells develop in bone marrow from the monocyte lineage, migrate to the epithelium of the skin and the mucosa and reside there to present external antigens to the immune system.

◆ What is Langerhans' Cell Histiocytosis?

A clonal proliferation of Langerhans' cells presenting as a spectrum of disease severity (Table 52.2).

All types have a predilection for the skull and the jaws. Lesions may be painful or asymptomatic and may be accompanied by soft tissue swelling. This patient has multifocal single-organ-system disease because only bone is affected.

Treatment

◆ What Treatment Would You Recommend?

A radiographic survey of the skull is required, together with a bone scan or skeletal survey to identify any lesions elsewhere. Medical examination and a detailed history are required in case of soft tissue involvement.

TABLE 52.2 Langerhans' Cell Histiocytosis

Presentation	Typical Features
Multifocal multiorgan disease (acute form)	A malignant neoplasm of Langerhans' cells affecting infants and young children younger than 3 years of age. Affects skin, liver, spleen, lymph nodes and bones and requires aggressive treatment with chemotherapy. Bone marrow is involved. Half the patients die before 5 years of age.
Multifocal single-organ disease (chronic multifocal form)	Usually causes multiple bone lesions in the skull and jaws. When the pituitary is involved diabetes insipidus develops and this, with exopthalmos and bone lesions, is called Hand–Schuller–Christian triad or syndrome. Occasionally fatal but usually treatable with curettage of lesions and sometimes with chemotherapy.
Unifocal disease (chronic unifocal form)	The commonest type, usually involves bone. Solitary lesions with a relatively benign course. Curettage is usually curative.

Lesions in chronic multifocal disease and solitary eosinophilic granulomas usually respond to curettage. This will require removal of the upper right first and second molars to gain access and to ensure complete removal. All involved soft tissue must be excised. There is, however, a risk of oro-antral communication.

The lower right premolar lesion may be curetted without tooth loss, but the surrounding presumed affected soft tissue must be removed and may result in tooth loss. A more conservative approach may be possible if the patient accepts the risk of recurrence. Any recurrence could be recuretted.

The lower left molar lesion could have been caused by periodontitis and requires biopsy for treatment planning.

Long-term follow-up is required. Lesions may recur, and new lesions may develop over a period of many years.

From the medico-legal perspective, this case highlights the particular importance of thorough and systematic radiographic reporting to observe any unusual abnormalities, which should prompt referral for specialist investigation and further management. Fortunately, these types of conditions are rare, but delayed referral may have severe consequences, resulting in significant morbidity or mortality, especially in the case of neoplastic lesions.

Case 53

Unexpected Findings

ERIC WHAITES AND EDWARD ODELL

Summary

A 14-year-old boy presents with toothache and a slightly swollen left cheek (Fig. 53.1). What is the diagnosis, and how will you treat him?

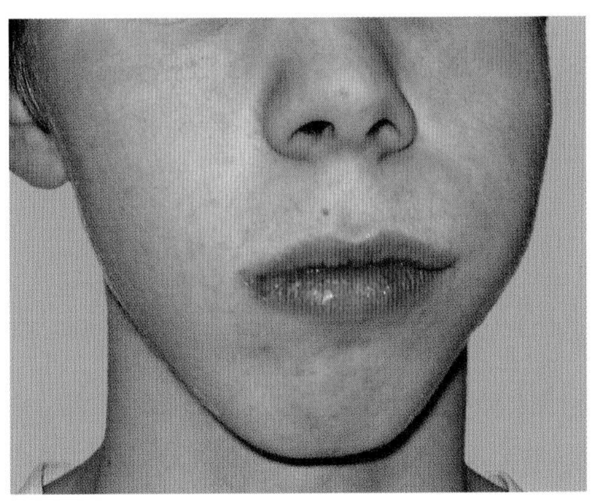

• **Fig. 53.1** The patient's appearance on presentation.

History

Complaint

The patient complains of intermittent toothache on the left side of his face, and he feels the pain is coming from an upper tooth.

History of Complaint

For several months, the patient has been aware of intermittent pain and discomfort from an upper back tooth when eating, especially anything very hot or cold. The pain is gradually getting worse.

Medical History

The patient is otherwise fit and well.

Dental History

The patient has never been to a dentist before.

Examination

Extraoral Examination

The patient is a fit and healthy-looking boy. His left cheek appears slightly swollen, but there is little extraoral asymmetry. The cheek is not tender or inflamed, and both the patient and his parents say that he has always looked like this. No lymph nodes are palpable, and the temporomandibular joints appear normal.

Intraoral Examination

The upper left first molar has heavily stained fissures, and the whole crown is discoloured. The other teeth appear sound. The alveolus in the upper left quadrant is enlarged, with reduction of depth of the buccal sulcus. The swelling affects the buccal and palatal aspects, is smooth, uninflamed and not tender to palpation.

In addition, the upper left second premolar is missing, and there is a small space between the first premolar and the molar. Several supernumerary teeth are evident.

◆ How Do You Interpret the History and the Examination Results So Far?

There could be several explanations for the presentation. The history of pain being exacerbated by hot and cold and poorly localized almost certainly indicates pulpitis. The obvious cause would appear to be caries in the upper first molar. The whole crown is discoloured, and there may be extensive caries despite the intact occlusal surface.

The enlargement of the alveolus has expanded into the buccal sulcus and could account for the slight extraoral swelling. The most common cause of smooth uninflamed expansion of the alveolus is an odontogenic cyst. Further investigation is required.

The absent second premolar may be unerupted or absent. Missing premolar teeth is a relatively common developmental anomaly, but the patient also has supernumerary teeth, and it would be unusual to have missing and supernumerary teeth simultaneously. In addition, if the premolar had never developed, the space between the first premolar and the molar would have closed completely. The tooth is probably unerupted and relatively superficial in the alveolus, holding the teeth apart.

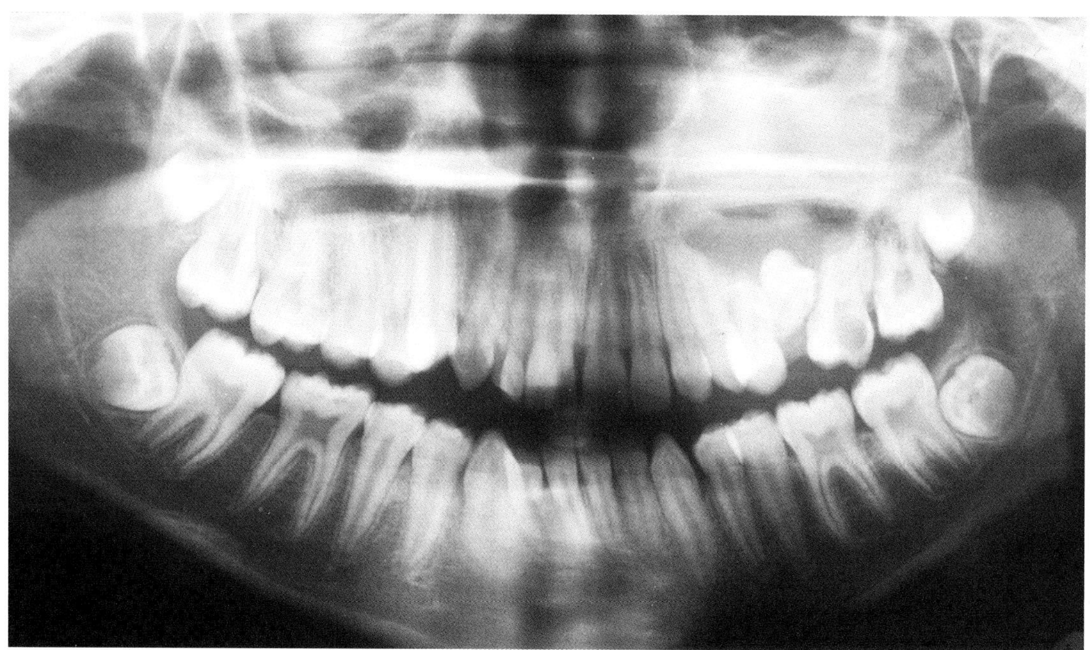

• **Fig. 53.2** Panoramic radiograph.

Investigations

◆ What Investigations Would You Now Undertake, and Why?

Vitality Tests. The vitality of the upper first molar needs to be determined; on testing it, you discover that it appears vital, as are the adjacent teeth.

Radiographs. Right and left bitewings for caries assessment and a panoramic radiograph to assess the overall dentition are indicated. These views should provide sufficient information to explain the missing upper left second premolar, assess any further unerupted supernumerary teeth and investigate the swelling of the left maxilla. If required, further views, including periapicals, an oblique upper occlusal or antral view, may be required later but are not indicated at this stage.

◆ The Panoramic Radiograph is Shown in Fig. 53.2. Look Carefully. What Do You See?

The panoramic radiograph shows:

- Extensive caries in the upper first molar
- Right and left supplemental maxillary canines
- Peg-shaped supernumerary overlying upper right lateral incisor and right canine
- Upper left second premolar present, unerupted and inverted
- Developing third molars in all four quadrants
- Increased opacity in the region of the left maxillary sinus.

◆ What Terms are Used To Describe Extra Teeth? What Do They Mean?

See Table 53.1.

TABLE 53.1 Terminology for Extra Teeth

Term	Definition
Supernumerary tooth	Any tooth over and above the normal complement of teeth.
Supplemental tooth	Supernumerary tooth with the morphology of a normal tooth, usually an additional tooth in a series, for instance additional lateral incisor, third premolar or fourth molar.
Mesiodens	Supernumerary tooth in the upper midline, may be conical (forms early and rarely interferes with eruption of incisors) or tuberculate (with a wide crown with cusps, forms late and often interferes with eruption).

◆ What is the Cause of Supernumerary Teeth?

The cause is unknown, but some clues are available. Supernumerary teeth may be caused by mutations in single genes, for instance, the *CBFA-1* gene. Mutations of this gene cause cleido-cranial dysplasia, in which the presence of multiple supernumerary teeth is a prominent feature. More is known about congenitally **missing** teeth, and only a single gene mutation is sufficient to cause teeth to be absent. For instance, mutations in the skeletal patterning gene *MSX-1* are associated with missing second premolars and third molars, and mutations in *PAX-9* are associated with missing molars and lower incisors. It seems likely that supernumerary teeth in otherwise healthy patients have similar relatively simple genetic causes.

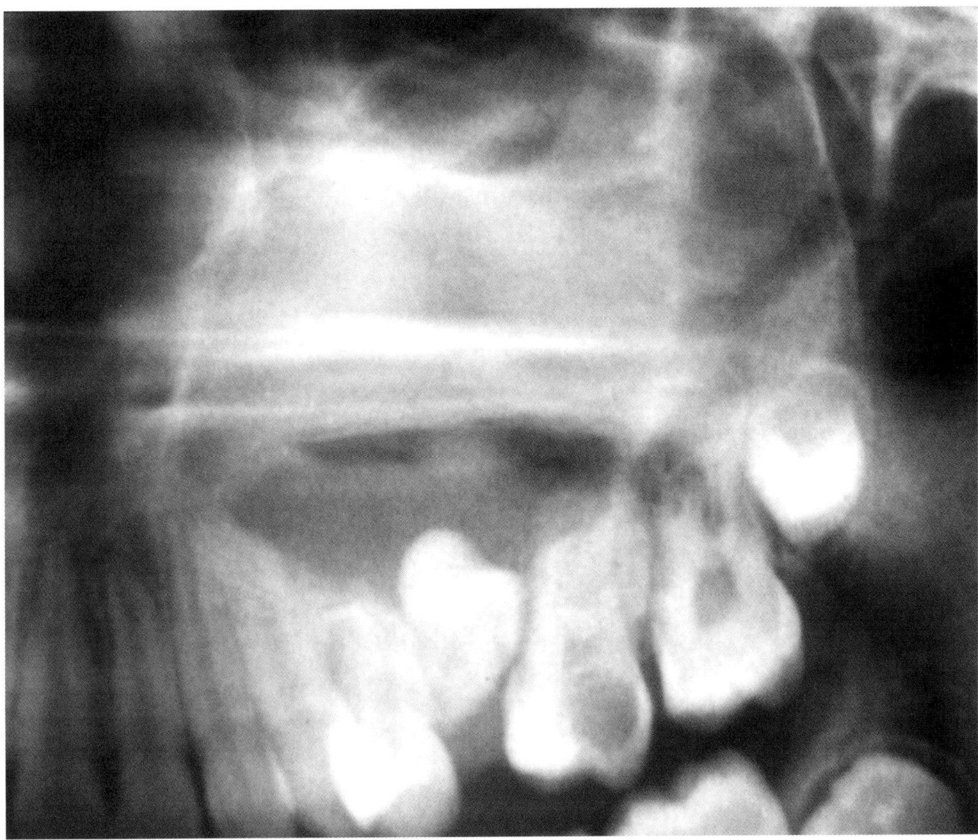

• **Fig. 53.3** Left maxilla enlarged from Fig. 53.2.

◆ The Section of the Panoramic Radiograph Showing the Left Maxilla is Enlarged in Fig. 53.3. What Else Does It Show?

There is loss of the thin radiopaque (white) line of the maxillary cortex forming the bony floor of the maxillary antrum. This is clearly visible on the patient's right side, as evident in Fig. 53.2. A domed, relatively radiopaque lesion occupies most of the maxilla and antrum. It has a very thin radiopaque margin at its upper limit.

The panoramic radiograph is shown again in Fig. 53.4, indicating the supernumerary teeth and the margin of the lesion in the left maxilla.

Differential Diagnosis

◆ What is the Cause of the Patient's Pain?

Pulpitis. As noted above, the symptoms fit pulpitis. The first permanent molar is the most likely source; it is vital and has extensive caries. Periapical periodontitis can be eliminated as a cause because the pain would be well localized and because there are no nonvital teeth in the quadrant.

◆ Give a Differential Diagnosis for the Lesion in the Left Maxilla. Explain Which Cause is Most Likely and Why

The unilocular, dome-shaped lesion with a thin bony margin of expanded periosteal new bone and the overall round shape are highly suggestive of a cyst. The most common cysts in the alveolus and maxilla are odontogenic cysts. There are no radiological features of malignancy.

Dentigerous Cyst. Relatively common and found in children. Dentigerous cysts arise around the crown of an unerupted tooth, and the cyst lining is attached to the tooth at the amelo-cemental junction. This cyst is certainly closely associated with the crown of the unerupted, inverted second premolar, but the radiographic views are not clear enough to see whether the edge of the cyst joins the tooth at the amelo-cemental junction. This information would have led to an almost conclusive diagnosis, but even without this information, a dentigerous cyst is the most likely diagnosis.

Odontogenic Tumour. A less likely possibility. The lesion is not multilocular to suggest ameloblastoma, but in theory, an odontogenic tumour is possible. The odontogenic tumours to consider in children are usually ameloblastic fibroma and ameloblastoma. However, these are solid, are less radiolucent and cause more expansion.

The adenomatoid odontogenic tumour can present as a dentigerous cyst and might be considered if mineralization was detected in the cyst on radiographs. This lesion usually arises on the upper lateral incisors in females but, although unlikely, is a possibility.

Radicular Cyst. The most common odontogenic cyst. However, it would have to arise at the apex of a nonvital tooth. The first molar tooth with caries and all other teeth

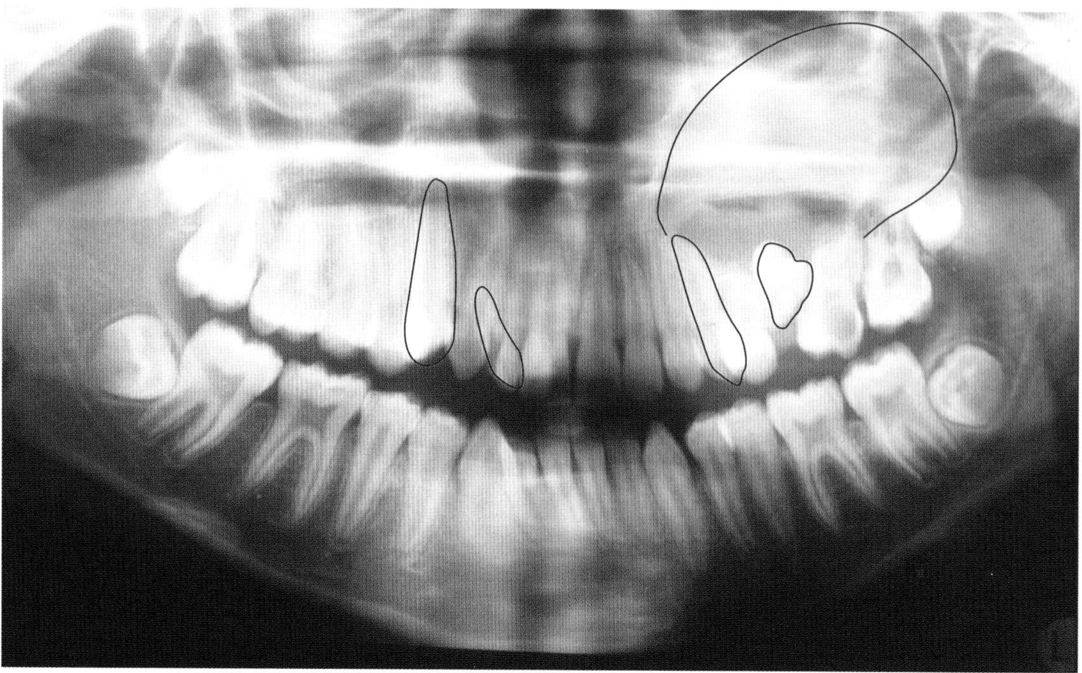

• **Fig. 53.4** The panoramic radiograph with the features outlined.

in the quadrant are vital, excluding this diagnosis. This will only turn out to be the diagnosis if the vitality test result is incorrect.

Antral Cyst. These cysts arise in the antral mucous glands (antral inclusion or retention cysts) but would be unlikely to cause such marked expansion. Also, they would not have a bony margin because they arise within the antral mucosa rather than in bone and so do not expand the alveolus as they enlarge.

◆ Do You Need To Make a Definitive Diagnosis Before Treatment?

No, a dentigerous cyst is almost certainly the cause. Dentigerous cysts and the alternatives can be treated in the same way. Therefore treatment can be planned on the basis of this provisional diagnosis and the final diagnosis confirmed later.

Treatment

◆ What Treatment Would You Recommend for the Pain?

The caries in the first molar should be removed and a temporary sedative dressing placed. The details of the final restoration will depend on the findings after excavation of the caries and the effectiveness of the dressing in reducing pain.

◆ What Types of Treatment are Available for Cysts?

Cysts are usually enucleated; that is, the bony cavity is opened, the cyst lining separated from its inner bony surface and removed and the cavity allowed to fill with blood clot and reorganize.

Alternatively, the cyst may be decompressed and marsupialized. Decompression involves opening the cyst to the exterior to relieve the internal pressure. Radicular, dentigerous and many other cyst types enlarge through hydrostatic pressure, and so decompression prevents further enlargement. Marsupialization is the method by which permanent decompression is ensured. The cyst is opened and the lining is sutured to the overlying mucosa to convert the cyst into a pouch communicating with the mouth (or sometimes the nose or the antrum). Without the internal pressure that causes enlargement, the cavity slowly shrinks and reorganizes from its periphery.

Procedures are slightly different for odontogenic keratocysts because of their risk of recurrence. The lining is thin and easily torn on removal, making enucleation difficult. Access to the cavity needs to be good to ensure that all the lining is removed, and the lining is sometimes treated with a fixative – Carnoy's solution. This can be dabbed onto the lining to make it tougher and also to kill the epithelium so that any small fragments left behind cannot seed recurrences.

◆ What are the Advantages and Disadvantages of Decompression and Marsupialization in the Treatment of Cysts?

See Table 53.2.

Because marsupialization has several disadvantages, it is usually used only for a short period for specific reasons. The cyst can be enucleated when it has shrunk to a more manageable size or away from important structures.

◆ What Treatment Would You Recommend for This Particular Cyst?

The inverted second premolar cannot erupt and needs to be removed. The cyst extends around the apices of the adjacent teeth, and marsupialization would offer the advantage of preserving their vitality. However, after marsupialization, washing out the cavity regularly would be difficult; therefore

TABLE 53.2 Advantages and Disadvantages of Surgical Procedures

Surgical Procedure	Advantages and Disadvantages
Enucleation and primary closure	Complete treatment in one episode. In very large cysts, the clot may break down and become infected, although this is largely a theoretical disadvantage.
Decompression and marsupialization	The cyst cavity reduces in size only slowly, months of follow-up may be required. It is difficult to keep the cavity clean – it requires regular washing. The opening will also shrink, making access difficult. Complete resolution is unlikely. A period of shrinkage may allow enucleation without damage to adjacent structures such as the inferior dental nerve. Shrinkage may allow more teeth to be preserved. Usually ineffective for odontogenic keratocysts because they enlarge by growth of the lining, not hydrostatic pressure.

in a child, it would be better to perform enucleation and complete the treatment in one episode. If the adjacent teeth were devitalized, they would require root treatment unless orthodontic assessment for the crowding suggests gaining space with extraction. In practice, it may be possible to enucleate without devitalizing the adjacent teeth.

A further possibility when enucleating a cyst is to break down the bony wall that separates the cyst from the antrum, remove the cyst lining and extract the unerupted tooth. This effectively re-forms the antrum immediately and marsupializes the cyst into the antrum. A nasal antrostomy (opening from the sinus through the lower part of the lateral wall of the nose) would be required to ensure drainage from the sinus until the antral healing is complete.

Whichever procedure is carried out, a sample, preferably all, of the cyst lining should be taken for histological examination to confirm the diagnosis.

Further Investigations

◆ Fig. 53.5 Shows the Histological Appearances of the Cyst After Enucleation. What Do You See, and How Do You Interpret the Appearances?

The left figure shows a length of the fibrous cyst wall (W) that is lined on its inner aspect by epithelium of regular thickness (E). In the bottom right corner, there is a focus of inflammation, seen as dark nuclei of inflammatory cells (I) and, above it, a large pink mural nodule of cholesterol clefts in loose tissue (C) protruding into the lumen. The cholesterol elicits a foreign body giant cell reaction, and although they are not clear at this magnification, the very dark angulate areas among the cholesterol crystals are foreign body giant cells. Haemorrhage (H) is present in and around the mural nodule, visible most easily as red cells on the left of the nodule between it and the epithelial lining.

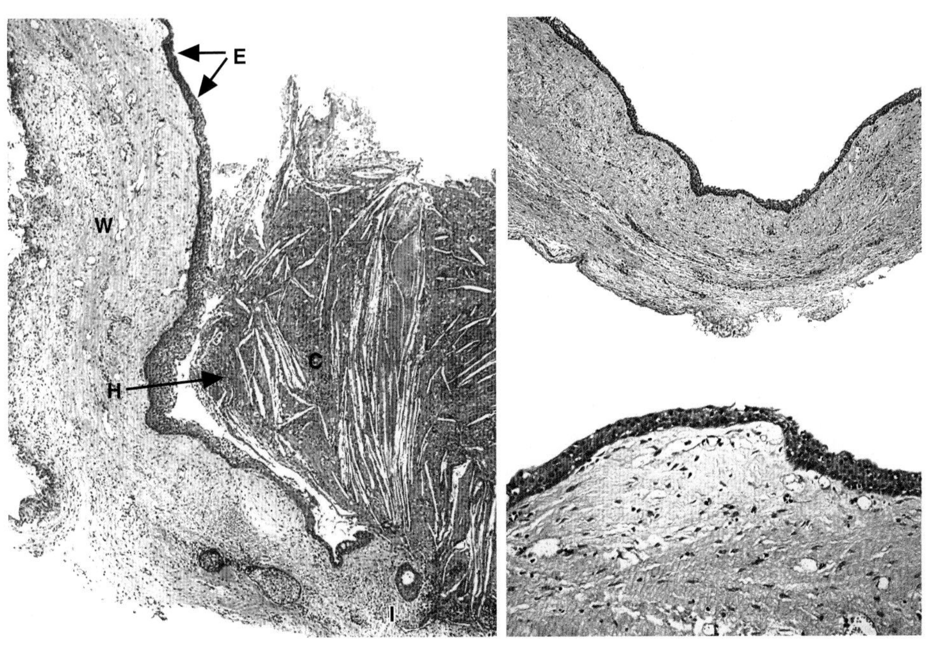

• **Fig. 53.5** Appearances of the cyst lining after removal, sections stained with haematoxylin and eosin. The width of the cyst wall is 1–1.5 mm.

The cholesterol is derived from breakdown of cell membranes of erythrocytes and inflammatory cells that die in the cyst. Two less inflamed areas are shown on the right. The rest of the cyst is lined by similar nonkeratinizing epithelium, often very thin and without rete processes.

Taken together with the radiological features, the appearances indicate a dentigerous cyst. Dentigerous cysts are lined by nonkeratinizing stratified epithelium, although this is not, in itself, a diagnostic feature. In the early stages, the epithelium is characteristically only two cells thick because it is reduced enamel epithelium that has separated from the tooth crown. As the cyst enlarges and impinges on the mucosa or the antrum, it becomes inflamed. The inflammation causes the epithelium to undergo hyperplasia, thicken and develop rete processes. Inflammation causes haemorrhage and release of cholesterol to form crystals in the wall, which ulcerate into the lumen to form the mural nodules. The appearances can then be very like a radicular cyst and the histopathology is not diagnostic. Therefore the main reason for submitting the surgical specimen for examination is to exclude an unexpected diagnosis such as odontogenic keratocyst or ameloblastoma. These alternatives have characteristic histological appearances that are not present here.

The definitive diagnostic criterion is that the epithelial lining and the cyst wall join the unerupted tooth at the amelo-cemental junction. This might be seen only by the surgeon during the surgery.

Case 54

A Gap Between the Front Teeth

JONATHAN TURNER, MANDEEP GHUMAN AND DAVID R. RADFORD

Summary

A 35-year-old man has noticed a gap appearing between two incisors. What is the cause, and how can you treat him?

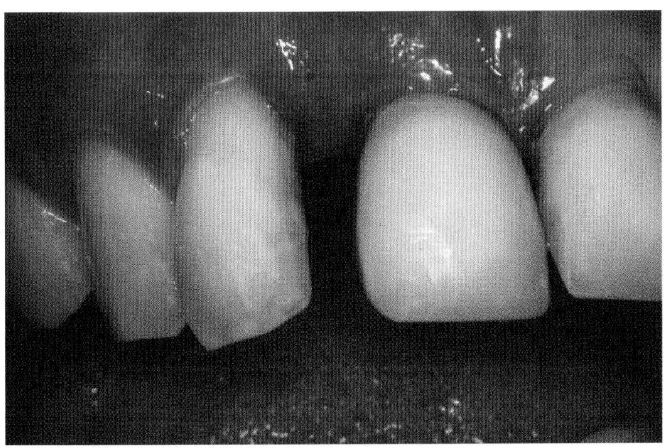

• **Fig. 54.1** The patient's anterior teeth on presentation.

History

Complaint

The patient is concerned about the gap between the crowned upper right central incisor and the lateral incisor teeth.

History of Complaint

He noticed the gap about 9 months ago and feels that it has enlarged, that the teeth have drifted forwards and that the crowns are now loose. He has had no symptoms from these or any other teeth.

Medical History

He has mild asthma, controlled with an inhaled steroid and salbutamol. He does not smoke.

Dental History

The patient is new to your practice. He attended his previous dentist regularly, going every 6 months but now less frequently. The crowns are approximately 6 years old and were fitted to replace some unsightly anterior composite fillings.

◆ The Patient's Anterior Teeth are Shown in Fig. 54.1. What Do You See, and How Do You Interpret the Appearances?

The upper right lateral incisor is rotated mesio-labially and the central incisor disto-labially. There is recession on both the central incisor and the lateral incisor. The gingival tissues have some rounding of the margin and marginal gingivitis. There is loss of stippling and contour. These appearances suggest labial drifting as a result of loss of periodontal support. Pocketing is probably present, even though it is not obvious.

Examination

Extraoral Examination

There is no lymphadenopathy and no temporomandibular joint signs. The two crowns, although prominent and rather light in shade, are under control of the lower lip associated with a competent lip seal. The patient has a broad smile and moderately high lip line.

Intraoral Examination

The oral mucosa is healthy, there is no caries and only a few amalgam restorations are seen, but there is focal marginal inflammation and plaque lying interdentally. The metal ceramic crowns on the two upper central incisors have good margins, but there is 3-mm recession palatally, and both teeth are grade 2 mobile. A further diastema is present in the opposing arch between the lower right canine and the first premolar (Fig. 54.2), and the adjacent lateral incisor has grade 3 mobility.

Basic periodontal examination (BPE) score:

4 /4 /4*

3 / 4 / 4

The gap between the upper central incisor and the lateral incisor is at least 3 mm, and on gentle probing of the area, there is profuse bleeding. The gingival tissue in that area is red and inflamed and has lost any contouring or stippling. There are deep probing depths on several teeth, as well as mobility.

The BPE score would indicate that further periodontal investigations, including plaque and bleeding charts, risk factor assessment and radiography, are necessary. Detailed six-point periodontal charting, including recording of the

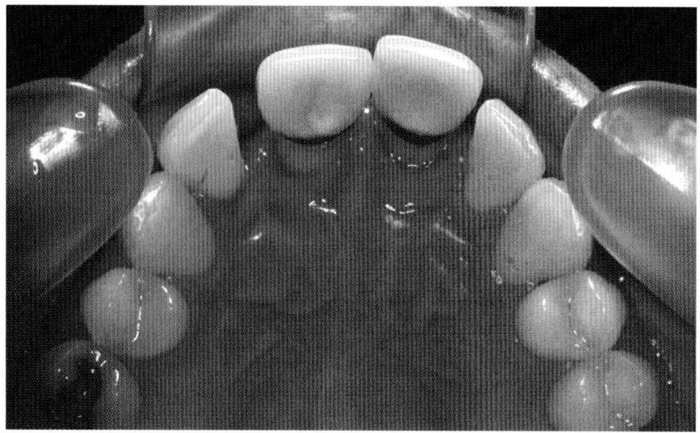

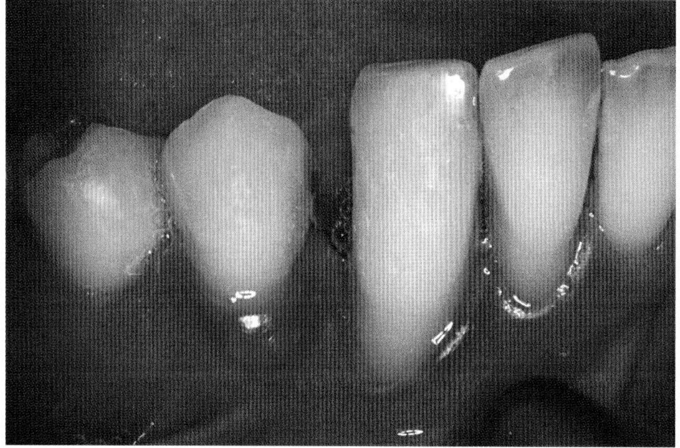

• **Fig. 54.2** Further views showing the appearances on presentation.

bleeding on probing, is required before and after periodontal treatment.

Probing depths and gingival bleeding are shown in Fig. 54.3. For details of indices and periodontal examination, see Case 38.

The crowns of the upper incisors are rather bulky palatally, probably as a result of inadequate tooth preparation. On closing to intercuspal position, the lower teeth occlude on the crowns in premature contact and displace the teeth labially. In both instances, the entire tooth is mobile, not just the crown.

Investigations

All teeth register positive sensibility test results.

The choice of radiographs for periodontal diagnosis is reviewed in Case 38. Periapical radiographs for this patient are shown in Fig. 54.4.

Diagnosis

◆ What is Your Diagnosis?

The patient has generalized periodontitis – stage 4, grade C, and currently unstable. Periodontitis has reduced the bony support for the upper and lower right anterior teeth, which have drifted labially. Bone loss extends close

							1	2	2							Mobility
X	3 2 3	6 8 10	4 2 3	3 2 3	3 2 3	3 5 7	7 6 5	10 2 7	5 2 2	2 2 3	4 2 3	3 2 3	6 3 3	3 2 3	X	Buccal (Attachment loss)
X	4 2 3	7 9 9	3 3 3	3 3 4	3 2 3	3 3 9	9 7 4	8 7 8	5 4 3	3 2 3	3 2 3	3 2 3	7 2 3	2 2 3	X	Palatal (Attachment loss)
8	**7**	**6**	**5**	**4**	**3**	**2**	**1**	**1**	**2**	**3**	**4**	**5**	**6**	**7**	**8**	Tooth
8	**7**	**6**	**5**	**4**	**3**	**2**	**1**	**1**	**2**	**3**	**4**	**5**	**6**	**7**	**8**	Tooth
X	3 2 4	3 3 3	3 2 3	3 2 3	5 5 3	3 2 3	2 2 3	2 3 2	7 3 9	3 3 4	3 2 4	3 2 5	3 2 5	2 2 3	X	Lingual (Attachment loss)
X	3 2 3	3 2 2	2 2 3	3 2 4	7 4 3	4 2 3	2 2 3	3 2 4	6 4 8	2 2 2	3 2 3	3 2 4	4 3 5	3 2 2	X	Buccal (Attachment loss)
									2							Mobility

• **Fig. 54.3** The probing depths (in millimetres) at six points, bleeding sites (ringed in red) and mobility (grade), recorded for each tooth.

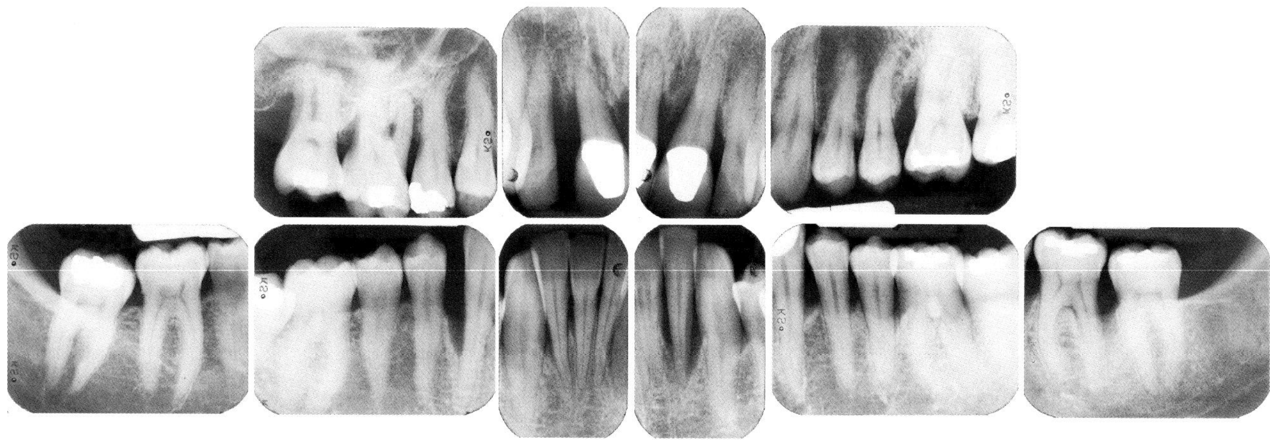

• **Fig. 54.4** Periapical radiographs of the patient on presentation.

to their apices, and they would have drifted further had they not been retained by the high lower lip line and competent lips. Recession is also the result of periodontitis (see Case 4).

However, the pattern of periodontitis is unusual. The patient is only 35 years old but has severe localized attachment loss.

◆ What Predisposes Patients To Localized Attachment Loss?

- Genetic predisposition
- Poor oral hygiene
- Endodontic problems leading to endodontic–periodontal lesions
- Root fractures
- Local factors – food packing and diastemas, overhanging and poorly contoured restorations, high fraenal attachment, oral piercings
- Trauma caused by oral piercings, destructive habits and self-inflicted injury.

◆ Can Any of These Explain This Patient's Pattern of Disease?

Primarily, the incisors and first molars are involved. The pattern of localized destruction and the shape of the deep infrabony pockets suggest that the patient may initially have had a molar–incisor pattern before additional sites become involved. This pattern indicates that the patient is especially susceptible to periodontal tissue loss, in part as a result of a hyperreactive immune response.

Although the crowns have good margins, they are in traumatic occlusion, and the jiggling forces on closing would increase the mobility of the teeth.

Treatment

◆ Is This Patient Suitable for Treatment in General Practice?

The severity of the complaint and the age of the patient indicate that there is a predisposition to periodontitis, which may progress despite treatment. The initial phases of treatment could be carried out in general dental practice, but some teeth already have a poor prognosis. This is a complex case, and unless you have a special interest or are a specialist in periodontology, the case may be best referred for treatment by a periodontologist.

◆ What Would You Include in Your Letter of Referral?

- Patient's current concerns
- Name, title, age and address, including full postcode
- Short dental history, including pattern of attendance and past treatment needs
- Relevant medical history
- Your clinical findings, including BPE score any special test results or study models you have
- Anything else that you feel is relevant or will save time and avoid misunderstanding at the time of consultation
- Whether you are referring for advice, a single aspect of treatment or comprehensive treatment to be undertaken
- Radiographs or digital images, which should be sent with the letter so that repeat radiographs and the consequent exposure to increased radiation dose can be avoided.

◆ What Care Plan Would Be Appropriate?

The prognosis for the three worst affected upper anterior teeth is hopeless because of loss of bony support, drifting and poor appearance. Additionally, if the teeth were to be saved, they would require new crowns. The upper right first molar has furcation involvement and bone loss to the apex and is likely to require either unpredictable complex treatment or extraction. The anterior teeth are symptomless and do not require immediate extraction but should be extracted in the near future to minimize the risk of attachment loss of adjacent teeth and infections/abscesses and to improve appearance. An immediate replacement denture is the treatment of choice because no definitive restorations can be planned until the periodontitis is brought under control and the longer-term prognosis for the other teeth is clear.

In the mandibular arch, the left lateral incisor has bone loss to the apex and probably requires extraction. The long-term prognosis for the lower right canine remains to be determined, but at least initially, it is worth taking a conservative approach and assessing the response to initial nonsurgical periodontal treatment.

The care plan would include:

- patient information and education of the presenting clinical issues and appropriate and achievable goal setting, planning and self-reflection to help the patient manage the situation in the medium to long term
- oral hygiene advice to include instruction in plaque control – tooth brushing and interdental cleaning
- extraction of both upper central incisors, the upper right and lower left lateral incisors and the upper right first molar
- immediate replacement prosthesis
- root surface debridement of all pockets greater than 4 mm under local analgesia, particularly the lower right canine
- periodontal reassessment after 3 months
- regular periodontal maintenance therapy initially on a 3-monthly basis
- continued care of the remaining dentition, including caries prevention
- extraction of further teeth, as required
- assessment for permanent prosthetic replacement.

The details, including the time commitment and cost of treatment, must be discussed with the patient. The patient must be given a written personalized care plan to consider and agree to.

The patient indicates that he would rather attempt to preserve the lower right canine than have it extracted, even though there is no guarantee of success.

What are the Options for an Immediate Replacement Prosthesis in the Upper Arch?

Immediate removable acrylic denture using wrought stainless steel clasps for direct retention. The denture must be kept clear of the gingival margins as much as possible so as to not compromise periodontal health. The patient already has inadequate oral hygiene and has never had a denture before. Once the anterior ridge remoulds, the denture will not fit well in this region and chairside relining will be necessary. Acrylic offers the advantage of ability to add further teeth should periodontitis progress.

Immediate minimum-preparation bridge is much more complex, and success is less predictable. The span is long and the occlusion unfavourable.

Implant solutions With ongoing, unstable periodontitis, there is a significant risk of long-term complications such as peri-implantitis resulting in failure. Again, success would be unpredictable with the complex techniques required. There is little residual bone, and implants would require autogenous bone grafts or guided regeneration techniques with membrane placement. Immediate loading implant techniques have a higher risk of aesthetic complications, including recession, and are not recommended.

What are the Options for an Immediate Replacement Prosthesis in the Lower Arch?

Immediate Removable Acrylic Denture. In the lower arch, this is a less advantageous option. A simple partial denture will be relatively bulky and cannot be designed to avoid the gingival margins. Compared with an upper denture, it would therefore be much more likely to compromise plaque control, and carries the risk of being poorly tolerated.

Immediate Minimum-Preparation Bridge. This could comprise a cantilever pontic retained on the central incisor or the canine. The canine is the obvious choice because of its more favourable crown-to-root ratio, but you will need the maximum wrap-around to maximize retention. The quality of laboratory work will be critical because the restoration cannot be temporized if the fit is not satisfactory; if the immediate replacement does not fit after the extraction, the patient will be left with an unsightly gap. In this immediate option, haemostasis and moisture control will be of critical importance if the adhesion of the immediately placed bridge is to be sufficiently strong. The design of the pontic must be optimized to favour plaque control in view of the patient's susceptibility to periodontitis. It may, however, be the best option if a replacement is required.

No Replacement. In the short term, it is quite possible that the patient would accept the appearance of the gap. This would be the best option for periodontal treatment, and the situation could be reassessed when the prognosis of the lower teeth becomes clearer.

The patient opts for an upper immediate removable acrylic denture, extraction of the lower left lateral incisor and conservative periodontal treatment for the lower canine. He completes the first eight items of your care plan, and no further extractions are necessary. After 6 months, the patient has responded very well to nonsurgical periodontal treatment. There has been marked gingival shrinkage around the lower canine, there is no bleeding on probing, and the pocket depth is 4 mm. The excellent response to treatment is, of course, largely the result of the effort of your hygienist/hygiene therapist, who has motivated and educated the patient and performed the treatment.

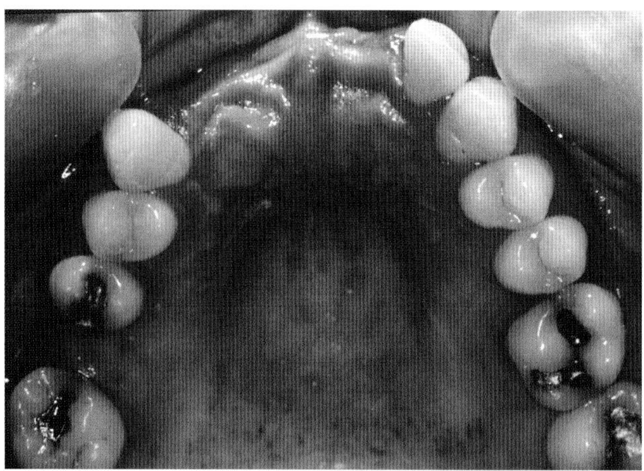

• **Fig. 54.5** The upper arch 6 months after extractions and periodontal treatment.

The patient is 'managing' with the denture but dislikes it. It is now becoming less retentive, and the anterior teeth have dropped on a couple of occasions. He would very much like to discuss options for a more permanent replacement. The lower arch is now stable after periodontal treatment.

The appearances of the patient's mouth after this initial treatment are shown in Fig. 54.5. Bone levels around the remaining teeth are similar to what they were on presentation, as seen in Fig. 54.4.

What are the Options for Definitive Treatment?

A Bridge. This would be possible, but there are some difficulties. The extensive bone loss from periodontitis has resulted in marked shrinkage of the ridge after extraction. This would require the pontic to be placed more palatally than is ideal; this, in combination with the high lip line and the reduced lip support, could make the appearance of a bridge less than ideal. This problem could be overcome by a removable prosthesis with a labial flange.

The span is long, and one of the abutment teeth is a lateral incisor. It is unrestored, but lateral incisors are never abutments of choice because of their small root, thin coronal dentine and angulation. In addition, as Fig. 54.4 shows, there is bone loss of half the root length. Although this tooth is currently stable, doubts about long-term maintenance persist, and this tooth is not suitable to take the load required of a bridge abutment, even if the adjacent canine were prepared as well. If a bridge were to be provided, it might be wiser to extract the compromised upper left lateral incisor and construct a fixed–fixed bridge by using both canines as abutments. This would allow better control of the appearance. Had the tooth been less compromised, it might have been included in a double abutment with the canine. A bridge would also involve considerable expense, and if a

TABLE 54.1 Major and Minor Connectors – Advantages and Disadvantages

Connector	Indications	Advantages	Disadvantages	Key To Clinical Success
Mandibular lingual plate	Commonly used For use where the lingual sulcus is shallow	Teeth can be relatively easily added With prepared rest seats can provide excellent indirect retention	Covers much gingival tissue Has to be fenestrated if diastemas are present	Has to be well adapted to the lingual aspects of the incisor teeth
Mandibular lingual bar	The other most commonly used mandibular connector	Minimal tissue coverage	Teeth cannot be added subsequently Requires minor connectors to connect to rests for support and indirect retention in Kennedy class I and class II situations	Half pear shape in profile Needs at least 8 mm clearance between the gingival margin and the raised floor of the mouth
Mandibular sublingual bar	Where a bar connector is required but the lingual sulcus is shallow	Minimal tissue coverage	Can be bulky due to profile, projects out towards the tongue and risks being poorly tolerated	Very accurate functional impression of the raised floor of the mouth is required
Mandibular continuous bar (cingulum bar)	Where a bar connector is required but the lingual sulcus is shallow	Minimal tissue coverage Teeth can be added	Needs to be bulky on the cingula of the teeth for rigidity Poor aesthetics if diastemas are present	Needs to be well supported and needs good adaptation to the teeth Can be used with a lingual bar (Kennedy connector) and both components can be made with reduced dimensions
Mandibular labial bar	Rarely used Bar is placed in the labial sulcus when the lingual aspect is undercut	Highly retroclined incisor and premolar teeth precluding a lingual connector	Because it is placed in the labial sulcus, this is a long connector and has to be quite substantial to provide rigidity Possibly poorly tolerated by patient	Cannot be used if there are labial soft tissue undercuts in canine and premolar regions
Complete palatal coverage	Commonly used maxillary connector with bilateral free end saddles and large unilateral free end saddles	Support can be derived from the palate where there is lack of tooth support	Difficult to get well adapted to a high palatal vault Patients usually prefer the palate to remain uncovered	Ensure that there is no anteroposterior rock on the major connector before accepting the fit of the casting Ensure good adaptation to posterior border
Palatal strap connector	For use with short bilateral bounded saddles	Reported to be well tolerated by patients, some palate uncovered	No specific disadvantages	Has to include biplanar curves in the palate to ensure rigidity Must be at least 8 mm wide
Anteroposterior palatal bar connectors	Commonly used connector, ideal if there is good tooth support Often loosely called a skeletal pattern connector	Reduced palatal coverage, versatile connector system that can avoid gingival margins Palate uncovered to sense texture, flavour and temperature of food	The connector has a very long circumference (inside and outside the loop), all of which needs to be well adapted to the mucosa Technically more difficult to make than full coverage where only the posterior margin has to fit closely	Ensure good soft tissue adaptation prior to accepting fit of casting
Maxillary U-shaped connector	Not commonly used	Useful if there is a large palatal torus that would impinge on a plate or a bar, otherwise to be avoided	Can be flexible posteriorly if insufficient anterior and roof of palate is not engaged Also this design tends to cover the gingival margins	Ensure good soft tissue adaptation

double abutment is used, there is significant risk of failure of the cement lute on the lateral incisor. This would be difficult to diagnose because the bridge would remain stable and would lead to caries. The double abutment bridge design is no longer recommended.

Implants. An implant-retained bridge is possible. Periodontitis would need to be fully treated and the patient's tooth condition stabilized and maintained, and bone graft would be necessary for ideal placement of the implant and the pontic.

A New Permanent Removable Acrylic Prosthesis. If the periodontitis was not controlled by the patient or the prognosis of the other teeth was questionable, a replacement denture with the major connector constructed from acrylic resin could be considered. This prosthesis would derive some support from the rests on the cingula of the canines and by covering the vault of the palate. Teeth with uncertain prognosis could be added later and, in the meantime, would not be clasped for direct retention. Clasps of either wrought stainless steel or gold could be used on teeth with a favourable prognosis.

Removable Prosthesis with Chrome–Cobalt Framework. This is probably the best option. It is less expensive than a bridge or implants, much simpler and can be designed to favour oral hygiene procedures and addition of further teeth in the future.

The patient was very happy with the appearance of the acrylic partial denture and found it well retained until recently. However, after discussing the other options, the patient opts for a new cobalt–chromium–based removable prosthesis. An additional factor not visible in the figures is that the lower incisors had overerupted as a result of the drifting of the upper teeth. The occlusion makes the option of a bridge untenable without adjustment of the lower incisors.

◆ Who Should Design the Prosthesis – You or the Laboratory? Why?

The design of any denture has to be a team effort between you and the laboratory, with you, as the dentist, taking the final responsibility for the restoration. In an ideal environment, the dentist should have access to a model surveyor and use the skills learnt in dental school to regularly survey and design. However, with increasing emphasis on a team approach, it should be possible to devolve the detailed design to your laboratory technician. At a minimum, you will need to discuss which teeth need to be replaced and identify any teeth with doubtful prognosis.

◆ Could You Refer the Patient?

Yes, you could refer the patient to a colleague who is a specialist or to one with specialist interest. Since 2007, the General Dental Council has registered an additional group of dental professionals – clinical dental technicians (CDTs). These professionals, under their scope of practice, can provide partial dentures on prescription from you, the dentist.

◆ What are the General Principles To Consider When Designing Any Partial Denture?

See box below.

Determine which teeth are to be replaced, and outline the saddles.

Plan support for the denture. Is the denture going to be tooth supported, tooth and mucosa supported or just mucosa supported?

Plan the path of insertion on a model surveyor, identify guide planes and consider their preparation. Because this patient has lost the anterior teeth and has a high lip line, the anterior acrylic flange has to conform closely with soft tissues, so the model will have a tilt to the posterior teeth on the surveyor table.

Plan direct retention normally provided with clasps. Consider engaging 0.25-mm undercuts with cast cobalt–chromium occlusal approaching clasps and 0.5 mm with gingival approaching clasps.

Is there adequate direct retention or will you have to provide indirect retention?

Consider major and minor connectors. These together with proper base extension will help provide stability against lateral and anteroposterior displacing forces. Advantages of different connectors are given in Table 54.1.

Review design for three aspects: simplicity, biological acceptability and appearance. Is as much gingival tissue as possible left uncovered? Are there unsightly anterior clasps or prominent occlusal rests that are really unnecessary?

What tooth preparation is required? This may include rest seat preparation, ideally modifying the profile of existing restorations on the teeth, adding composite resin, preparing guide planes and altering the height of survey lines to allow correctly constructed clasps.

◆ The Final Design is Shown in Figs 54.6 and 54.7. What are the Design Features in this Particular Case?

- The path of insertion was determined by the soft tissue profile of the anterior edentulous saddle. When a large labial undercut is present, the model must be tilted down posteriorly during surveying to ensure that the flange fits well and has the best possible appearance.
- Support was derived from rests placed on the upper right canine, second premolar, first molar, left lateral incisor, canine and first molar. This is probably more than necessary, but the design has not become overcomplicated. The rest on the left canine is necessary in case the compromised lateral incisor is extracted in future. Without it, the denture would have no left anterior support after the extraction. This demonstrates the importance of planning for possible failure and also the need for good communication with the laboratory technician. This rest on the canine might not have been included otherwise.
- Direct retention was provided by cast cobalt–chromium occlusally approaching clasps placed on the posterior teeth because of the patient's high smile line. The clasps face into the main saddle. However, the recurved clasp on the upper right premolar is still visible (see Fig. 54.7). The clasp tips are placed in undercuts relative to the planned path of insertion. There is sufficient direct retention, and so indirect retention is unnecessary.

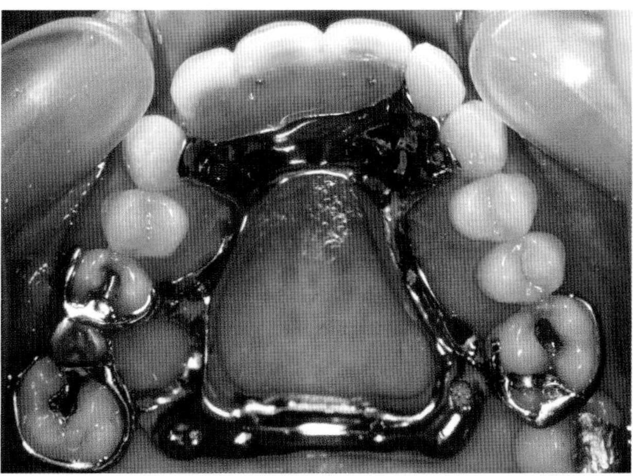

• **Fig. 54.6** Palatal view of prosthesis in position showing the final design.

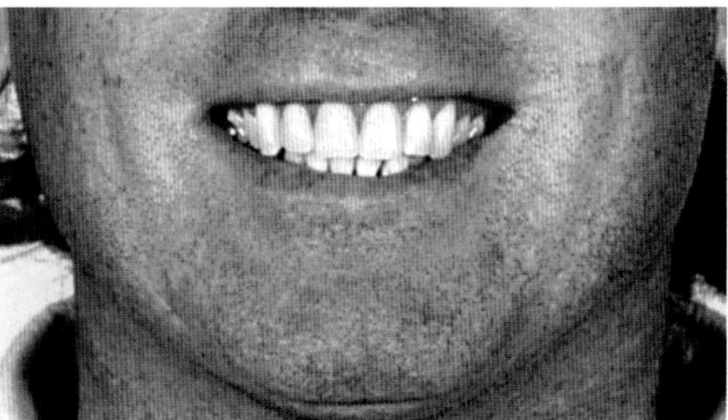

• **Fig. 54.7** The finished result.

- The major connector of anterior and posterior palatal bar connectors has at least 5 mm clearance from the gingival margin (Table 54.1). This type of connector does not provide soft tissue support, and so a fully tooth-supported design is necessary. If the denture had included a posterior saddle as well, an element of tissue support would have been necessary, and full palatal coverage would have been required.
- Minor connectors have been placed to avoid the interdental gingival tissues, which are the areas most susceptible to periodontitis. This has been achieved with midunit minor connectors on the posterior teeth.
- The pontic design chosen for the upper right molar was a metal sanitary pontic. The tilting of the second molar had reduced the space. Use of a sanitary pontic has avoided placing metal tagging and an acrylic tooth in this periodontally vulnerable interdental area.

◆ What is Indirect Retention, and Why is None Required for This Denture?

If a partial denture has two clasps, the denture will tend to rotate away from soft tissues about an axis between the two clasps. Indirect retention is provided by a rigid component placed on the teeth opposite the saddle such that the saddle cannot rotate away from the ridge. Indirect retention is usually required for free end saddles (distal extension) and in Kennedy class IV situations, where direct retention from anterior clasps at each end of the saddle would be unsightly. In a single free end saddle situation, the denture will rotate around the distal clasps, and a rest must be placed on a tooth opposite the saddle and as far away from the axis of rotation as possible. In the present case, direct retention from clasps is sufficient.

Medico-Legal Issues

Fortunately, no medico-legal issues were raised in this case. However, what could the patient have been concerned about? The patient could well have questioned why the periodontal disease was not diagnosed more fully and discussed with the previous dentist about better management, not just treated at 6-monthly hygienist visits. Also, although the patient may have been happy at the time of luting of the upper anterior crowns, he might have just accepted the slightly light shade or felt he had to accept that. Issues regarding management of a patient unhappy with care provided by his or her previous dentist is always difficult and often best handled with advice from your defence organization.

The final result in this case was a restoration that the patient was delighted with and one that you should be pleased with. One posterior clasp is visible, but the overall result is excellent. This case effectively illustrates how a relatively simple care plan produces the most predictable result.

Case 55
A Lump in the Palate

TARA RENTON

Summary

A 32-year-old woman is referred to your hospital's oral and maxillofacial surgery department by her general dental practitioner because of a swelling in her palate. What is the cause, and what treatment is appropriate?

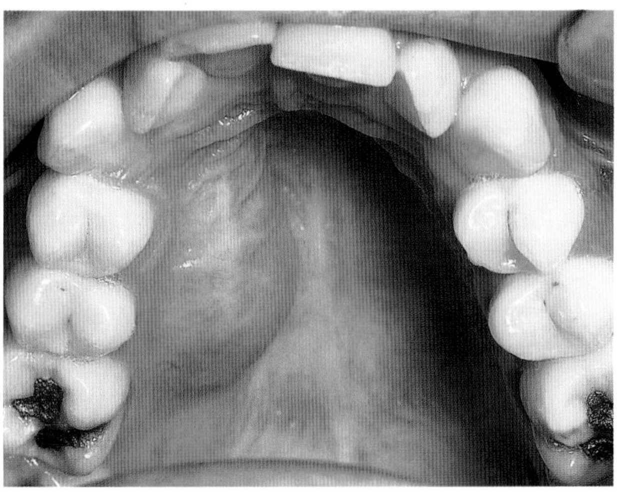

• **Fig. 55.1** The patient's palate on presentation.

History

Complaint

The patient has noticed a lump but has experienced no pain.

History of Complaint

The patient thinks that the lump has been present for at least a year, possibly 2 years. It has enlarged slowly and is now starting to cause discomfort.

Medical History

Her medical history reveals no illness. She has recently given up smoking but previously smoked two to three cigarettes a day.

Examination

Extraoral Examination

She is a fit and well-looking woman. No cervical lymph nodes are palpable, and the temporomandibular joints appear normal. There is no facial asymmetry.

Intraoral Examination

The appearance of the palate is shown in Fig. 55.1. There is a swelling of the right side of the palate and maxillary alveolus. There is no caries and only a few relatively small amalgam restorations.

◆ What are the Features of the Swelling?

The swelling has the following characteristics:

Site	Molar to central incisor region
Size	2 × 3 cm approximately
Shape	Oval
Surface	No ulceration
Colour	Overlying mucosa normal
	Has a slight blue tinge
	No evidence of inflammation, not pointing
Contour	Regular, rounded

If you were able to palpate the lesion and the patient's neck, you would discover the following:

Lesion consistency	Firm, not fluctuant
Lesion mobility	Fixed
Cervical lymph nodes	No submandibular or cervical lymph nodes palpable

Differential Diagnosis

◆ On the Basis of What You Know So Far, What Types of Lesion Would You Include in Your Differential Diagnosis?

1. Benign neoplasm of palatal salivary gland, most probably a pleomorphic adenoma

TABLE 55.1 Selection of Appropriate Radiographic Views

View	Reason
Intraoral views of alveolus	To exclude odontogenic or bony causes.
Oblique occlusal	To see whether the lesion has perforated or resorbed the underlying palate.
Panoramic radiograph or occipito-mental view	To detect changes in the maxillary sinus if there were symptoms of sinus involvement.
Panoramic radiograph	General survey of jaws. The panoramic is not ideal for this lesion because it lies outside the focal trough of the radiograph.
Computed tomography (CT) or cone beam computed tomography (CBCT)	The palate cannot be visualized well by standard views, and you might consider this as an initial investigation. It will give an excellent view of palatal erosion or perforation, if present. However, it does entail a significant x-ray dose, waiting time and expense. A plain film would be a more appropriate initial investigation unless palatal perforation is suspected clinically. CBCT would give a lower x-ray dose, provide excellent definition and may be more readily available as a first investigation in a dental setting.

2. Malignant salivary tumour, and if so:
   - most probably a mucoepidermoid carcinoma, or
   - polymorphous adenocarcinoma,
   - but possibly an adenoid cystic carcinoma
3. Odontogenic causes:
   - either an abscess
   - or an odontogenic cyst, probably a radicular cyst
4. Mucous retention cyst
5. Antral or nasal lesion bulging into the mouth (e.g. carcinoma)
6. Miscellaneous other possibilities, including lymphoma.

◆ Which of These Possibilities are the Most Likely? Explain Why

Benign salivary gland neoplasm. The site of the swelling is compatible with a palatal salivary gland origin, although it is slightly more anterior than is typical. Salivary glands are more numerous in the posterior hard palate or soft palate, and a swelling level with or behind the molars would be more characteristic of a salivary gland origin. If the lesion is arising in a gland, then a neoplasm is the most likely cause of long-standing painless swelling. About 50% of minor gland neoplasms are benign, and 50% are malignant. The most common single benign tumour, by far, is pleomorphic adenoma, and this is a very likely cause in this case. Pleomorphic adenomas are most common in middle age and old age but have a wide age distribution; however, the young age of the patient need not exclude this possibility.

Malignant salivary gland neoplasms are equally common in minor glands, as noted above. If the tumour is malignant, then mucoepidermoid carcinoma or polymorphous adenocarcinoma would be the most likely causes because they are the most prevalent. Adenoid cystic carcinoma is rarer, but clinically significant possibility because it requires more extensive surgery and carries a poorer prognosis. The lack of ulceration and the patient's young age point to a benign neoplasm over a malignant one, but a malignant tumour is a definite possibility because most salivary gland malignant neoplasms are of low grade and can have a benign presentation.

Dental causes must be considered because they are very common. The site would be highly typical for an abscess arising from a nonvital lateral incisor or the palatal root of an upper first molar, but there are no symptoms or signs of acute infection. The slow and painless growth might suggest a cyst as a likely cause. However, the swelling appears to arise in the palate rather than the alveolus, which is not expanded. Dental causes seem less likely than salivary gland causes, but because they are common, it would be prudent to exclude them.

◆ Which of These Possibilities are Unlikely? Explain Why

A mucous retention cyst is the most likely nonneoplastic, salivary gland–related cause, and the bluish tinge to the lesion suggests a cyst. However, this lump is firm and appears to be of long duration. A mucous retention cyst would be expected to burst or fluctuate in size if present over a long period. This lesion is rather large for a mucocoele on the palate.

Antral or nasal causes must be borne in mind but are also unlikely. Any lesion that had eroded through the palate or sinus wall would be expected to be ulcerated or inflamed.

Investigations

◆ What Investigations Would You Perform?

Tests of vitality of all the teeth in the upper right quadrant are required to exclude the possibility that a nonvital tooth is present and is the cause of an abscess or cyst. Radiographs are required for these and other reasons.

◆ Which Radiographic View(s) Would You Select? Explain Why

A selection from the radiographic views shown in Table 55.1 is indicated for the reasons given.

An oblique occlusal radiograph revealed no abnormality in the right palate or alveolus.

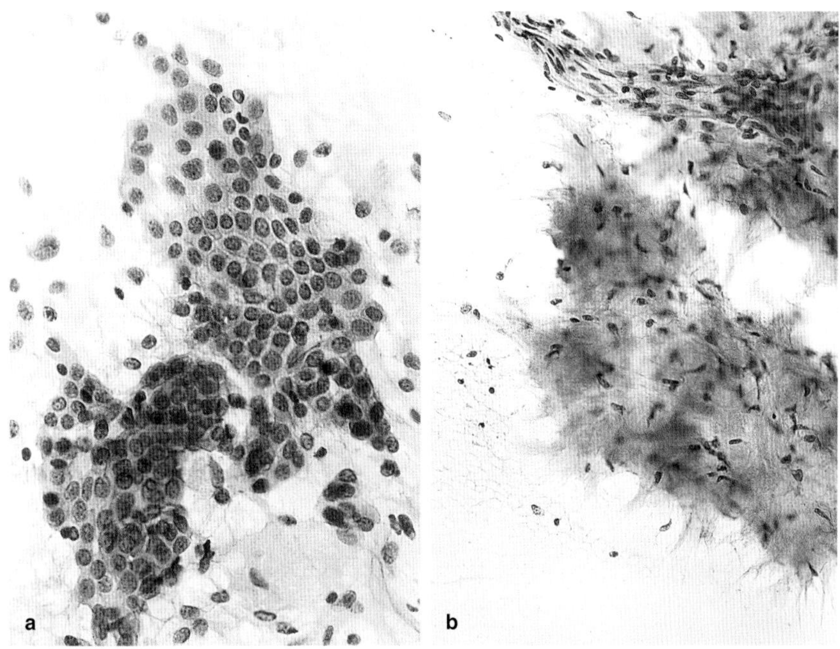

• **Fig. 55.2** The appearances of the smear of cells taken through fine-needle aspiration.

TABLE 55.2 Possible Biopsy Types

Biopsy Type	Advantages and Disadvantages
Fine-needle aspiration cytology (FNA/FNAC)	Quick and accurate in most cases though a minority of such lesions will not be amenable to diagnosis by cytology. Nevertheless, usually accurate enough to give the definitive diagnosis and can be performed in conjunction with other biopsy types, if necessary. Result usually available in 1 day.
Trucut or wide-needle biopsy	These provide a small tissue sample. Wide-needle biopsy is now rarely used because FNA is easier and more accurate. There is a risk of damaging important structures, although this is more of a problem in the parotid gland than in the palate.
Incisional biopsy	As a general rule, incisional biopsy risks spreading salivary neoplasms into tissues. Pleomorphic adenomas, the commonest benign neoplasms, are often mucinous in texture and can spread into the fascial planes of the neck and up to the skull base or down to the mediastinum when incised for biopsy. However, this is only a problem in the submandibular or parotid glands. In these sites, incisional biopsy should not be performed unless the lesion is thought to be malignant. Only then will the specific subtype of neoplasm influence treatment. In the lesion on the palate, tissues are tightly bound down, and spread is not a particular concern. The top of the lesion is accessible, and the entire biopsy site could be excised during definitive surgery if the lesion turns out to be malignant. There is no risk of spread to tissue spaces. An incisional biopsy could be performed and would be appropriate if a FNA failed to provide a diagnosis.
Excisional biopsy	If the lesion were smaller, then excisional biopsy might be considered appropriate. A small margin of normal tissue could be excised on the assumption that the lesion is pleomorphic adenoma. This would not be ideal. FNA or incisional biopsy are readily performed, and it would be better to determine whether the lesion is benign or malignant before excision to ensure that an appropriate margin is taken.

◆ Is Biopsy Appropriate? What Types of Biopsy Might Be Used, and What are Their Advantages and Disadvantages for This Case?

Yes. Only biopsy will help make the definitive diagnosis. However, deciding whether or not to perform biopsy of a salivary gland swelling is not always a simple choice. Inappropriate biopsy could do the patient a disservice. There are numerous possibilities, as presented in Table 55.2.

Either incisional biopsy or fine-needle aspiration should be performed, and the choice will depend on the availability of cytology services in the clinic and the surgeon's preference.

◆ Fine-Needle Aspiration of the Lesion Was Performed, and the Appearances of the Aspirate are Shown in Fig. 55.2. What Do You See?

The cells are stained with Papanicolaou stain, which stains nuclei blue and cytoplasm blue-green, or orange if keratinized. Fig. 55.2a shows a sheet of uniform cells with moderate amounts of cytoplasm. Their cytoplasm, polygonal shape and cohesive growth indicate that these are epithelial cells and their uniform nuclei suggest they are benign. The second field, shown in Fig. 55.2b, shows smaller numbers of spindle cells without significant cytoplasm in a myxoid matrix. Taken together, these appearances are characteristic of pleomorphic adenoma.

Diagnosis

The diagnosis is pleomorphic adenoma.

Treatment

◆ How Should This Lesion Be Treated?

The appropriate treatment is excision with a small margin, at least a few millimetres. Pleomorphic adenoma is benign, but it is often incompletely encapsulated, and simple enucleation would result in recurrence. The defect could be closed with either a temporary acrylic plate or local surgical flaps, depending on the surgeon's preference. Radiotherapy is ineffective as a primary treatment and would not be indicated for a benign neoplasm (although it is sometimes used for widespread recurrences of parotid pleomorphic adenomas).

◆ Would You Like Further Investigations Before Carrying Out Treatment?

Although the pleomorphic adenoma is benign, it can resorb bone by pressure. Before excising the lesion, it is important to know whether the palate has been perforated because any postsurgical oronasal or oroantral fistula would have to be repaired. This lesion is relatively small, and this step might be omitted, but with a larger tumour, it would be an appropriate reason for carrying out computed tomography (CT) or cone beam computed tomography (CBCT) scan.

◆ The Histological Appearances of the Excision Specimen are Shown in Fig. 55.3. What Do You See?

Very different appearances are seen in different areas of the tumour (it is pleomorphic). Fig. 55.3a shows sheets of epithelial cells in which there are small ducts containing eosinophilic material (E). At the edges of the sheets, cells separate and progressively merge with more dispersed cells in a myxoid stroma (M). These sheets and dispersed cells are the same cell types as those seen in the smear made from the fine-needle aspirate shown in Fig. 55.2. Here, they are seen in section, in their correct relationship to each other, whereas the smear is of whole cells spread onto a glass slide, hence their different morphology.

Fig. 55.3b shows numerous small duct-like clusters of cells (D) separated by a hyaline fibrous stroma (F). Many of the ducts have a bilayered structure with a partial outer layer of cells with clear cytoplasm.

Other fields show incomplete encapsulation but a well-demarcated periphery. These features are typical and diagnostic of pleomorphic adenoma. If the lesion appears excised histologically, cure can be expected.

Prognosis

◆ Are There Any Significant Complications of Pleomorphic Adenoma? Are You Concerned for This Patient?

Yes, carcinoma may arise in a long-standing pleomorphic adenoma, and carcinoma ex pleomorphic adenoma carries a very poor prognosis. However, this process takes many years, usually 10 or more, and is therefore seen mostly in older patients. This is an unlikely risk in this young patient with a short history, and complete removal will prevent this complication. There was nothing in the history or the clinical examination to suggest malignancy, and fine-needle aspiration or biopsy followed by examination of the excised specimen has excluded it.

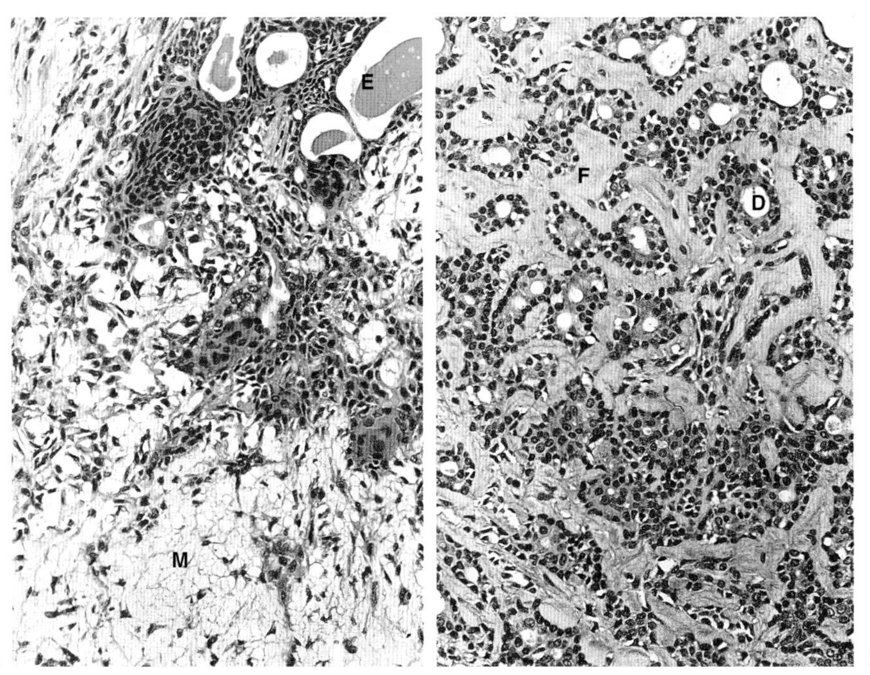

• **Fig. 55.3** The histological appearances of the excision specimen.

Case 56

Rapid Breakdown of First Permanent Molars (Molar–Incisor Hypomineralization)

MIKE HARRISON

Summary

A 7-year-old boy presents with his first permanent molar teeth which, according to his parents, have decayed rapidly, starting immediately on eruption. Identify the cause, and discuss the treatment options.

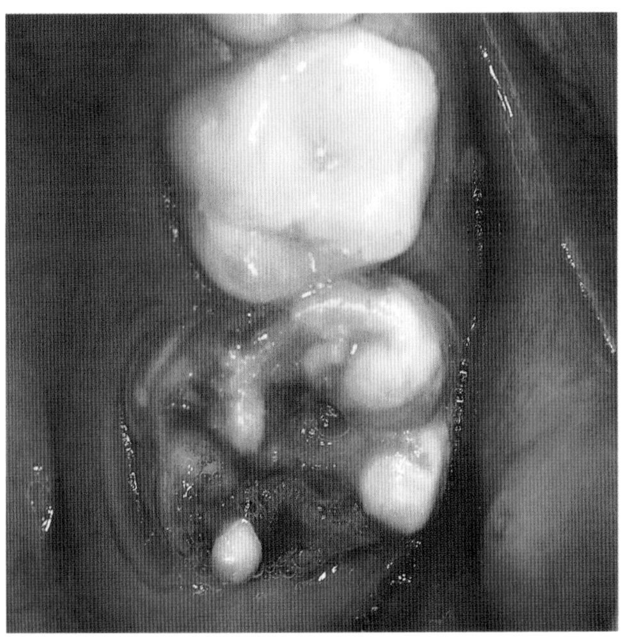

• **Fig. 56.1** An occlusal view of the permanent upper left first molar, on presentation.

History

Complaint

The child complains of pain from his back teeth on both sides. The pain is worse with sweet foods and cold liquids and persists for several minutes after the stimuli are applied. Toothbrushing with cold water is also painful, but the teeth do not cause pain on biting.

History of Complaint

The pain has been present for a few months and has increased in severity over the last month. The child now reports that one of his back teeth feels broken. The first permanent molars erupted on time, and the child's mother noticed that some of them appeared to crumble as soon as they emerged through the gum. She has read in magazines that fluoride can damage teeth and has switched to a toothpaste without fluoride on the assumption that this is the cause.

Medical History

The patient is a healthy child, the only history of note being neonatal jaundice.

Dental History

The child has no experience of operative dental care. The diet history reveals a reasonably well-balanced diet, with limited consumption of refined carbohydrates and carbonated beverages. Toothbrushing has been performed with adult-formula fluoride-containing toothpaste, starting at approximately 1 year and continuing until 7 years of age.

Examination

Extraoral Examination

The child has no facial swelling or asymmetry, and no lymph nodes are palpable.

Intraoral Examination

The child is in the early mixed dentition stage. All four first permanent molars have areas of brown, rough, irregular enamel. Severity varies among teeth, and the worst affected are the maxillary molars, with enamel appearing to be completely absent in some areas. These teeth have soft dentine exposed occlusally. The lower right first permanent molar is the least affected, with only a small localized brown enamel defect on the buccal aspect. This is hard on probing.

In addition, there are areas of white enamel opacity in the incisal third of the labial surface of all permanent central and lateral incisors, and the white enamel opacity is most pronounced in the maxillary central incisors. The remaining primary dentition is caries-free and appears normal in structure and morphology. Oral hygiene appears to be good. The clinical appearance of the dentition at presentation is shown in Figs 56.1 and 56.2.

◆ On the Basis of What You Know Already, What Do You Suspect?

The enamel defects appear to be hypomineralization of the incisors and hypoplasia of the molars. The discrete areas of white enamel opacity on the central incisors are characteristic of enamel hypomineralization, where the contour of the surface is intact and the enamel is of normal thickness. The molars are so severely affected that diagnosis is difficult, and this is consistent with either hypoplasia – where contour is abnormal, leaving it vulnerable to extrinsic staining and caries – or hypomineralization, which has undergone post-eruptive breakdown.

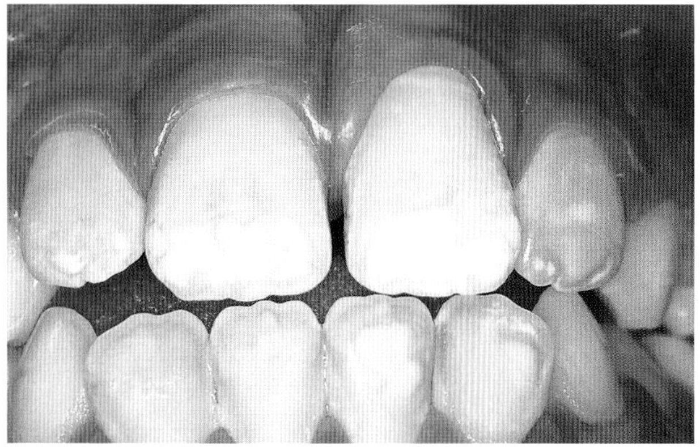

• **Fig. 56.2** Labial view of the central incisors in occlusion, on presentation.

◆ Do the Enamel Defects Follow a Chronological Pattern, and if So, At What Time Was the Affected Enamel Formed?

The incisal and occlusal parts of the permanent central incisors and first molars form almost at the same time, starting to mineralize just before birth. The affected enamel would have been formed after birth and during the first 1–2 years of life. This can be seen in Fig. 56.3.

This distribution of enamel defects is often referred to as molar-incisor hypomineralisation (MIH). There is some evidence that the occurrence of MIH is not completely chronological. The occlusal and buccal surfaces tend to be the worst affected. Canines and premolars are unaffected despite mineralizing at the same time. Defects may be asymmetrical, and enamel loss by post-eruptive breakdown occurs most commonly on affected molars.

◆ What Additional Questions Would You Ask, and Why?

A chronological pattern suggests systemic illness, which may be identifiable in the history. Defining a possible cause may allow other causes, such as fluorosis, to be excluded. You need to ask for further details about the prenatal and perinatal medical history.

The following conditions may be relevant, and information on them should be specifically sought:

- Significant maternal illness
- Preterm birth
- Frequent febrile illness in infancy

These disturbances may manifest as enamel defects distributed along the enamel formed around birth. You should also enquire about all severe systemic disturbances in the first 2 years of life, for example, meningitis, encephalitis, severe measles or pneumonia. Even relatively minor fevers or infections such as ear infections are known to be associated with similar enamel defects if frequent during infancy. There is very little evidence to support medicines being the cause. Fluoride can only cause enamel defects if consumption in infancy is known to be excessive and prolonged.

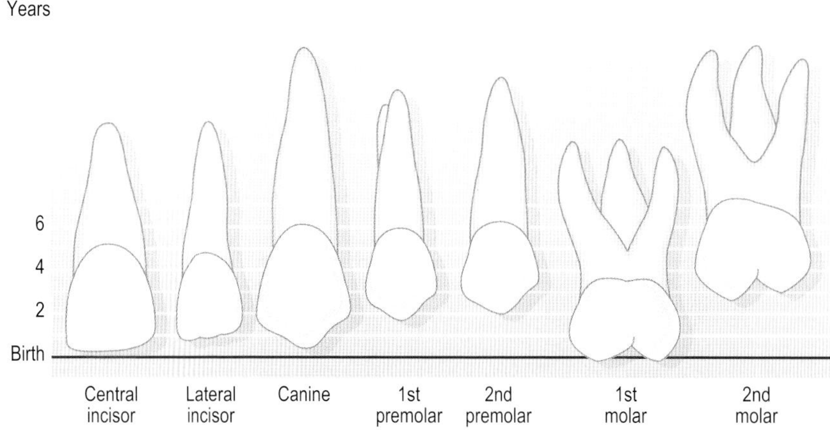

• **Fig. 56.3** Time of mineralization of the permanent dentition.

Differential Diagnosis

◆ What is the Likely Cause of the Child's Pain?

Sensitivity to hot and cold is characteristic of pain mediated by a vital pulp. It could be a result of exposed or more porous dentine or of caries deep in the defects. MIH is frequently associated with pain and sensitivity, and the pulp tissues in severely affected teeth may have chronic low-grade inflammation.

◆ What is Your Initial Differential Diagnosis for the Enamel Defects?

Dental caries is the most common cause of destruction of first permanent molars and should be considered, even though the appearances would be very unusual. The combination of enamel defects on the permanent molars and incisors suggests a working diagnosis of MIH, presuming that the molars had a normal surface contour before eruption but underwent significant posteruptive breakdown (PEB) in the parts where the enamel was very hypomineralized.

Enamel hypoplasia is less likely but should be considered. Developmental, acquired, generalized and localized forms are recognized. Other causes that might be considered are amelogenesis imperfecta, cytotoxic chemotherapy for malignant disease, significant renal disease in infancy or, rarely, fluorosis. In many cases, no cause is found, and the term *idiopathic enamel hypoplasia* is used.

◆ Justify This Differential Diagnosis.

Dental caries is the most common cause of destruction of the dental hard tissues. Newly erupted teeth are particularly prone to dental caries until their enamel maturation is completed in the oral environment. The permanent first molars are also prone to early caries because of their deep fissures. However, the possibility of caries seems unlikely. Although there is no guarantee that the diet history elicited is truly representative of the child's actual diet, there are no restorations or caries in the deciduous dentition. The molars have discoloured or absent enamel over a wide area. This is not typical of dental caries unless carbohydrate intake is excessive or the patient's teeth have some other predisposing factor such as enamel hypoplasia. The soft dentine indicates that some caries is present, but the pattern of destruction suggests that the caries is secondary. The zones of opacity on the incisors look like early 'white spot' demineralization but are present at a site that is almost never affected by caries.

Neonatal jaundice is a very common condition and, in almost all cases, can be excluded as a cause of enamel hypoplasia. In this child, the position of the enamel defects is inconsistent with a short period of jaundice at birth.

Fluorosis is a common cause of enamel opacities and enamel hypoplasia in areas where it is endemic. The deciduous dentition is usually only mildly affected. The level of fluoride required to cause enamel defects depends on concentration, period and age at ingestion.

Fluorosis is almost certainly not the cause of the current problem. The defects in the molars would result from only very high fluoride concentrations, in excess of 25 parts per million (ppm). Such levels do not occur in the UK. In addition, fluorosis of this severity is found only in endemic areas and should not follow a chronological pattern.

Mild fluorosis may be seen as a result of supplementation, and this is presumably what the parent has read. In such cases, there are usually fine opaque white lines following the perikymata and small irregular enamel opacities or flecks with or without staining. Such mild defects are also common in normal teeth and increase in frequency when the fluoride level is lower than 0.7 ppm. Although the severity of the defects and the distribution are incompatible with the diagnosis of fluorosis, it needs to be considered because the child has been using adult-formula fluoride-containing toothpaste from an early age. Ingestion of adult-formula fluoride toothpaste would be the most likely cause of mild fluorosis in those living in the UK.

Amelogenesis imperfecta must be considered, even though it is rare. Amelogenesis imperfecta can cause enamel hypoplasia, hypocalcification or hypomaturation and either of the first two conditions could lead to the appearances seen in the molar teeth in this case. However, several factors indicate that this is not amelogenesis imperfecta. There appears to be no family history, the pattern appears chronological rather than affecting all surfaces of all teeth equally and the deciduous dentition is unaffected. Although these features are not conclusive because of the wide range of clinical presentations seen in the many different types of this disease, they do make the diagnosis most unlikely.

Idiopathic molar–incisor hypomineralization is a convenient term used to describe cases of enamel defects with this distribution for which no cause can be ascertained.

Investigations

◆ What Investigations are Indicated, and Why?

Intraoral radiographs are indicated to assess the proximity of the coronal defects to the dental pulp. A dental panoramic tomograph (DPT) is indicated to ascertain the presence and stage of development of the remaining permanent dentition in view of the possibly poor long-term prognosis of some of the first permanent molars. This patient's DPT is shown in Fig. 56.4.

If there were extensive softening of the occlusal dentine of the molars or if radiographs indicated deep caries, pulp sensibility tests would be required.

◆ What Does the Dental Panoramic Tomograph Show?

All permanent teeth, with the exception of the third permanent molars, are present, and the patient's dental age is consistent with his chronological age. The gross structural defect in the first permanent molars is reflected in their radiographic appearance. The worst affected teeth – the maxillary molars – have irregular enamel outlines, and there is reactionary dentine in the distal pulp horns. The view is unsuitable for detailed examination of the teeth, but no large carious lesions are evident, and the unerupted permanent second molars appear to be of normal shape and to have a normal enamel structure.

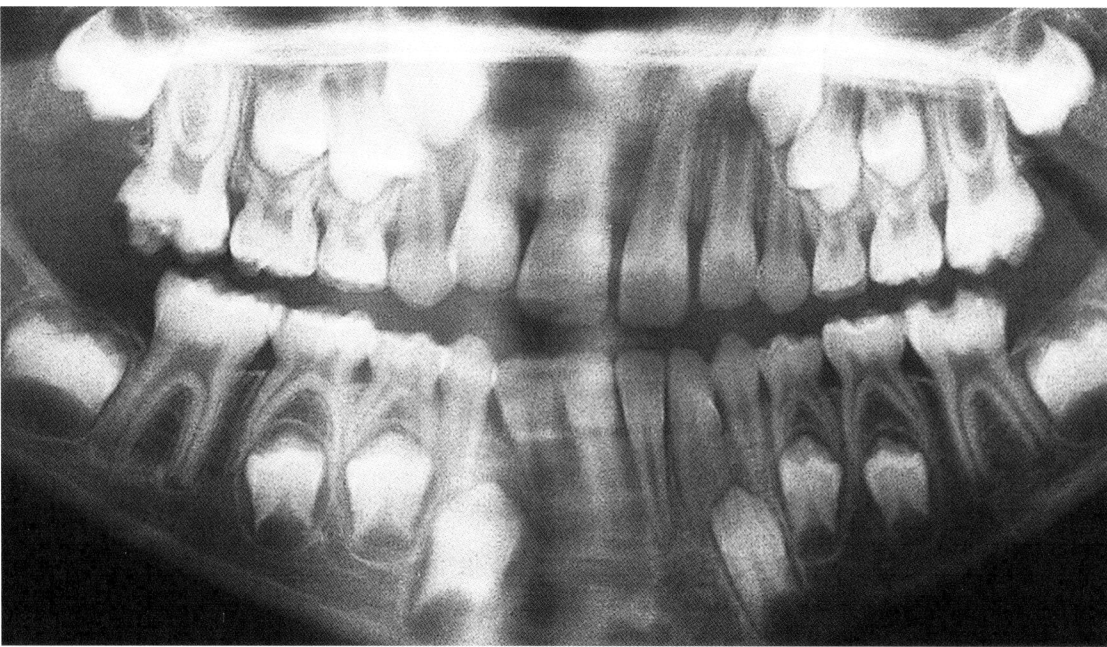

• **Fig. 56.4** The dental panoramic tomograph of this patient on presentation.

Diagnosis

◆ What is Your Diagnosis?

The patient has enamel defects that do not follow a perfect chronological pattern. In the absence of a known insult to account for the defects, idiopathic MIH is the most appropriate working diagnosis. The diagnosis may need to be reviewed if more teeth erupt with similar defects. The diagnosis is sufficiently accurate to help determine the management options.

Treatment

◆ What Treatment Options are Available for the Molars?

Extraction is considered an appropriate treatment for the permanent first molar with a poor long-term prognosis, particularly when, as here, caries is also present. Preservation of these molars through adulthood would require provision of full-coverage crowns. These have a finite lifespan, and their intermittent replacement; the risks of undetected leakage, caries and pulpal involvement; localized periodontitis; and the expense and inconvenience would all cause significant difficulties during the lifetime of the patient.

◆ When Should the Molar Teeth Be Extracted?

Timing of the extractions is important, and several factors must be taken into consideration, as shown in Table 56.1.

TABLE 56.1 Factors Affecting the Timing of Permanent First Molar Extractions

Factor	Reason
Stage of dental development	Permanent second molars are most likely to erupt passively into a favourable position when there is radiographic evidence of calcification of a small crescent of interradicular dentine (mineralizing of the furcation). This is the ideal time to extract the first molar and is generally done between ages 8 and 10 years.
Presence of third molars	This must be assessed radiographically. Hard tissue formation should be visible at age 9–10 years. The crypt may be visible as early as age 7 years.
Orthodontic analysis	A complete assessment must be made. The space gained might be utilized for active orthodontic treatment. Extraction of the permanent first molars is rarely ideal for orthodontic purposes and treatment may be complex. If no third molars are present, the need for orthodontic treatment may be critical in deciding whether or not to extract the first molars.

◆ How Can the Molars Be Preserved Until the Patient is At the Optimal Age for Their Extraction?

Preformed stainless steel crowns offer durable, cheap and relatively simple restoration. Laboratory made nickel–chrome onlays have been advocated as a less destructive option, should it be decided that the teeth are to be retained for full coronal coverage restorations later in life. A preventive resin restoration can be provided for the less severely affected molar in the lower right quadrant.

Molars in MIH are often considered highly sensitive to a variety of stimuli and are known to be difficult to anaesthetize locally.

TABLE 56.2 Possible Restorative Options for the Incisors

Technique	Advantages	Disadvantages
Full resin composite veneers	No destruction of tooth tissue, reversible and generally well tolerated even by anxious children. Excellent aesthetic result possible and easy to maintain.	Discolour with time. Tendency to fracture if placed at/over the incisal edge.
Enamel microabrasion	Minimal destruction of enamel, if carefully performed. Technique well tolerated.	Unpredictable. Teeth may rarely suffer postoperative sensitivity. Accidental exposure of dentine is possible where enamel is thin.
Localized resin composite restoration	Enamel destruction limited to defect, and full thickness need not be removed if opaque resin composite shades are used. Good aesthetic result possible.	Irreversible. Weakens tooth structure and large areas of dentine may be uncovered. Colour change and marginal discoloration with time.
Porcelain veneers	Good appearance.	Contraindicated in this age group because gingival contour not mature and stable tooth position not yet established.
Full-crown restoration	Good appearance.	Inappropriate until late second decade because immature pulp horns may be exposed. Gingival contour not mature and stable tooth position not yet established.

◆ What Treatment Options are Available for the Incisors?

The areas of white enamel on the labial surface of the incisors do not require treatment at this age, and they may become less obvious with time. If an interim cosmetic improvement is required in the patient's teenage years, direct resin composite veneers, requiring no tooth preparation, provide a simple and effective solution. The advantages and disadvantages of the possible minimally invasive restorative solutions are listed in Table 56.2.

◆ What Advice Would You Give the Mother With Regard To Fluoride Use?

The misconception about fluorosis should be dispelled: fluorosis can only develop while teeth are forming. Provided the child can rinse and spit out effectively, it would be appropriate for him to use an adult-formula fluoride toothpaste. This would provide a significant benefit in preventing caries (and the mother would also gain from using it). No fluoride supplement is indicated for this child, who, at least on the basis of a preliminary analysis, eats little sugar and has no caries. There might be a particular advantage in using a fluoride mouthwash during adolescence and early adulthood when a person's diet often changes markedly.

Prognosis

◆ What is the Long-Term Prognosis of Molars with Enamel Hypomineralization Defects?

You need to form an opinion on the likely natural history of each tooth with enamel mineralization defects. Can the affected molars be successfully restored with simple direct resin composite restorations? This is determined by the extent and location of the defect and by the degree of hypomineralization and PEB. Occlusal surfaces with defects surrounded by normally mineralized cusps can usually be restored successfully with resin composite restorations. Defects that involve cusps or that extend over to the vertical walls of the crown can be very difficult to treat with adhesive materials.

If extraction has been considered as an option but maintaining the tooth is still desired, some aspects of future restorative care need to be discussed with the child's parents:

- At what age could a definitive full-coronal restoration be provided? Age greater than 18 years, at skeletal and gingival maturity.
- What material should be used? Gold or porcelain.
- How long would you expect this restoration to last before it needs replacement? A predicted replacement cycle of 15–20 years is reasonable for a full-coronal-coverage restoration if good patient maintenance is achieved
- How would it be most likely to fail, and what would be the clinical consequences? Failure by cement leakage may lead to pulp pathology, requiring endodontic treatment.

It is advisable to document these discussions so that you can demonstrate that the decision to keep a molar of dubious long-term prognosis was a shared one and that the patient and his carers were fully informed.

Further Reading

Lygidakis, N. A., Wong, F., Jälevik, B., Vierrou, A. M., Alaluusua, S., & Espelid, I. (2010). Best clinical practice guidance for clinicians dealing with children presenting with molar-incisor-hypomineralisation (MIH). An EAPD policy document. *European Archives of Paediatric Dentistry*, *11*(2), 75–81.

Case 57

Oral Cancer

NICHOLAS M. GOODGER AND EDWARD ODELL

Summary

A 72-year-old man with squamous cell carcinoma is referred to your cancer treatment centre. How should he be managed?

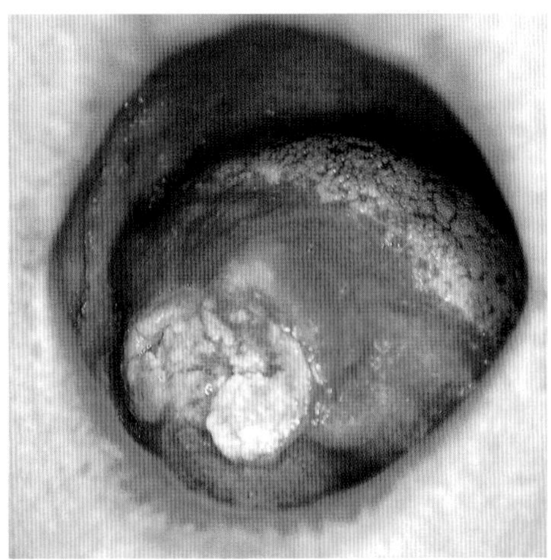

• **Fig. 57.1** The patient's appearance on presentation.

History

Complaint

Despite his large lesion, the patient complains only of discomfort on wearing his dentures and earache on the right.

History of Complaint

The patient first noticed his symptoms 6 weeks ago and has sought treatment because of the earache. He had noticed a 'crack' in his tongue that has not healed for some time, but this has always been painless.

Medical History

He had a small myocardial infarction 7 years ago and has mild hypertension, for which he takes amlodipine and aspirin. He has smoked 20 or more cigarettes a day for the last 55 years and drinks a quarter bottle of whisky per day.

Examination

Extraoral Examination

The examination of the neck is normal, apart from a possible mass just below the right angle of the jaw. It is difficult to ascertain whether or not the mass is hard. It is deeply situated and approximately 15 mm in diameter.

Intraoral Examination

◆ The Appearance of the Tongue is Shown in Fig. 57.1. What Do You See?

There is a large fungating ulcer arising on the right lateral border of the tongue. It is approximately 30 mm in size and has raised everted borders. Towards the dorsal surface, the mucosa bulges, as if there is a mass beneath the intact epithelium, and there is a white patch affecting the mucosa just dorsal to the ulcer margin.

If you could palpate this ulcer, you would find that it is indurated (firm or hard on palpation) and extends down towards the floor of the mouth and up beneath the dorsal mucosa towards the midline. The lesion is clearly much larger than it looks. The patient has reduced tongue mobility.

Diagnosis

In this case, the diagnosis has already been made at the referring hospital. The patient has squamous cell carcinoma, and the appearance and presentation are typical. The patient knows the diagnosis.

◆ Why Might the Patient Have Earache?

Ear pain is thought to result from malignant infiltration (or other damage) of nerves that pass through or supply the ear on their way to the periphery. Thus in the tongue or pharynx, pain may be generated as a result of involvement of the lingual nerve, which contains fibres from the chorda tympani from the ear, and of the auriculo-temporal nerve (branch of the mandibular division of the trigeminal nerve), which also supplies the external auditory meatus. Similar referred pain may result from involvement of the glossopharyngeal nerve.

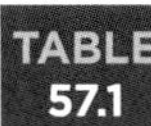

TABLE 57.1 TNM (Tumour–Node–Metastasis) Classification of Oral Cancer

T	T1	Carcinoma less than 20 mm in maximum diameter and less than 5 mm depth of invasion
	T2	Carcinoma less than 20 mm in maximum diameter and 5–10 mm depth of invasion OR Carcinoma 20–40 mm in maximum dimension and less than 10 mm depth of invasion
	T3	Carcinoma greater than 40 mm in maximum diameter OR Carcinoma greater than 10 mm depth of invasion
	T4a T4b	Carcinoma invades through the cortical bone of the mandible or maxillary sinus, or invades the skin of the face Carcinoma invades masticator space, pterygoid plates, or skull base, or encases internal carotid artery
N	N0	No lymph node metastasis
	N1	Metastasis in a single ipsilateral lymph node less than 30 mm diameter, without extranodal extension
	N2a	Metastasis in a single ipsilateral lymph node 30–60 cm in diameter, without extranodal extension
	N2b	Metastasis in multiple ipsilateral nodes, none larger than 60 mm, without extranodal extension
	N2c	Metastasis in bilateral or contralateral nodes, none larger than 60 mm, without extranodal extension
	N3a	Lymph node metastasis greater than 60 mm in diameter, without extranodal extension
	N3b	Metastasis in any lymph node, with extranodal extension
M	M0	No distant metastasis
	M1	Distant metastasis

Principles of Treatment

◆ What are the Principles of Treatment for Oral Squamous Cell Carcinoma?

Patients with oral carcinoma often present too late for cure, and some may not benefit from treatment. Three treatment options are possible:

1. Attempted cure
2. Active palliative care
3. Supportive care only, until death occurs.

If cure is attempted, the highest chances of success are given by multimodality treatment – a combination of surgery, radiotherapy and, more rarely, chemotherapy. In oral squamous cell carcinoma, chemotherapy is always given in combination with radiotherapy. The most aggressive treatment that the patient is able to withstand will be recommended because, if the first round of treatment fails, the chances of survival are much reduced.

TABLE 57.2 Staging of Oral Cancer

Stage	Combinations
Stage I	T1, N0, M0
Stage II	T2, N0, M0
Stage III	T3, N0, M0 Or T1–3, N1, M0
Stage IVa	T4a, N0–1, M0 Or T1–4a, N2, M0
Stage IVb	Any T, N3, M0 Or T4b, Any N, M0
Stage IVc	Any T, Any N, M1

Further Investigations

◆ How Might You Predict the Chances of Successful Treatment?

By using staging and grading. The chances of successful treatment depend on how large the carcinoma has grown and whether it has already spread to other sites in the body. Staging is a standardized method for assessing these parameters and is used to predict survival and also to plan treatment. Accurate staging is therefore essential.

Oral cancers are staged by determining the tumour size and depth of invasion (T), the lymph node status (N) and the presence of distant metastasis (M) (Table 57.1). These parameters are then combined to determine the stage (Table 57.2). Survival decreases with increasing stage. In determining stage and therefore survival, the tumour size and depth of invasion, whether there is spread of the cancer beyond the lymph node in cervical metastasis, and whether there is distant metastasis are important factors to consider.

Staging depends on the fact that carcinomas tend to progress in a predictable way. First, tumours enlarge by invading the surrounding tissues and then the cells break away and travel via the lymphatics to seed metastases in lymph nodes. Blood-borne metastases to distant sites develop last. Although the sequence is usually predictable, the speed at which any individual carcinoma progresses through these stages varies widely.

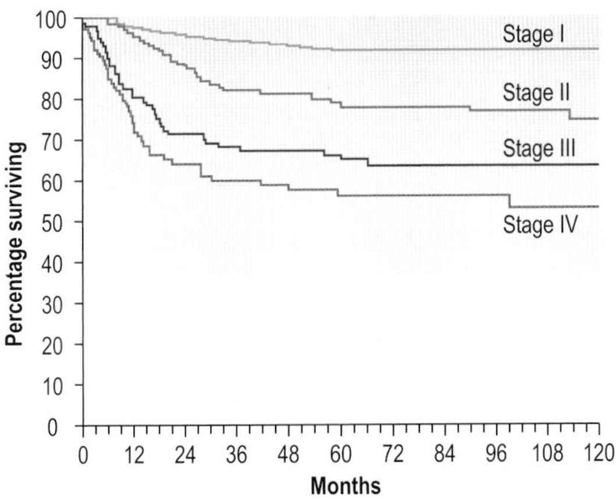

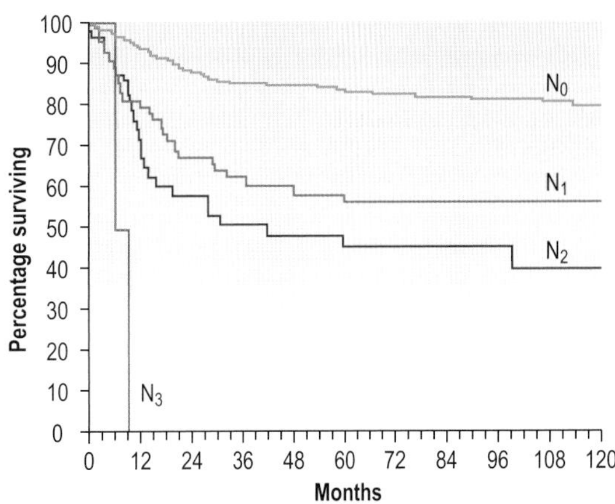

• **Fig. 57.2** Survival curves for oral carcinoma. The left graph shows survival for oral carcinoma of all sites by TNM (tumour–node–metastasis) stage. The right hand graph shows survival for patients with and without metastasis to cervical lymph nodes.

Grading is a histological method to determine how aggressive the carcinoma is and how quickly it is likely to progress (or may already have progressed) from stage to stage. It is a measure of how differentiated the carcinomatous epithelium is – that is, how much it resembles its tissue of origin. Well-differentiated carcinomas grow in tissues as large islands and form keratin. They usually grow slowly and metastasize late. Poorly differentiated carcinomas have more cytological pleomorphism, no keratin and invade more aggressively as small clusters of cells or even as single cells. They are more likely to produce metastases early in their course.

Staging is more important than grading because the size and extent of the tumour determine whether surgery is possible. Grading is useful in deciding which treatments are appropriate and how radical they should be.

◆ How Will You Determine the Disease Stage?

Size (T) can be determined through clinical examination. This is not very accurate and, if the carcinoma is posteriorly placed, may require examination under general anaesthesia. Radiographs must be taken to assess the involvement of bone, because bone invasion automatically indicates a T4 size. Imaging provides a more accurate estimate of size and extent compared with clinical examination.

Presence of lymph node metastasis (N) can be determined through clinical examination. Large, hard, fixed nodes will be obvious, but lymph nodes nonspecifically enlarged as a result of ulceration or infection may also be present. Enlarged lymph nodes may require fine-needle aspiration under ultrasound guidance to confirm whether or not carcinoma is present. Imaging is very useful to detect small lymph node metastases and those in deeply sited nodes. The patient should undergo computed tomography (CT), magnetic resonance imaging (MRI) or positron emission tomography with computed tomography (PET/CT) to detect the involved lymph nodes. Which is used will depend on local circumstances.

Distant metastases (M) should be determined through clinical examination and imaging. The imaging modalities noted above may all be used.

After staging investigations, this patient's carcinoma is staged as T3, N1, M0, making it a stage III lesion. Fine-needle aspiration of the palpable submandibular lymph nodes shows metastatic carcinoma cells. Imaging shows no obvious metastatic spread beyond the submandibular lymph node, and there are no other enlarged lymph nodes. CT scans of the chest and abdomen rule out distant metastasis, and liver function test results are consistent with the patient's alcohol intake. An anaesthetist declares the patient fit for the long general anaesthesia that would be required for surgery. The patient could opt for any of the treatments recommended.

◆ What are the Chances of Cure?

In general, the 5-year survival rate for oral carcinoma is poor. The reason is the late presentation, leading to large carcinomas on presentation, often with extensive lymph node involvement and distant metastases. In addition, many patients are medically compromised by a lifetime of heavy smoking and excessive alcohol intake or are too old or infirm to be able to tolerate aggressive treatment.

The survival rates for oral carcinoma of all sites are shown in Fig. 57.2. These are Kaplan–Meier survival curves; each step in the line represents one or more members of the study population dying of carcinoma at the time indicated on the *x* axis. The graphs show the disease-specific survival, on the left broken down by stage and on the right broken down by presence of lymph node metastases. Note how important metastasis is in determining survival.

In practice, some patients die sooner than this, but of other illnesses that are often smoking induced. The proportion of patients predicted to survive 5 years after diagnosis of **tongue** carcinoma is 75% for stage 1, 60% for stage 2, 45% for stage 3 and only 25% for stage 4. Thus this patient has only a 55% chance of surviving 5 years.

Treatment Planning

◆ What Factors Determine the Appropriate Treatment?

Choosing the appropriate treatment is sometimes difficult, and many factors need to be taken into consideration.

TABLE 57.3 Advantages and Disadvantages of Treatment Modalities

Modality	Advantages	Disadvantages
Surgery	Single episode of treatment Excision of lesion can be confirmed Subsequent radiotherapy still possible	Surgical risks Anaesthesia risks Altered appearance Reduced function Adverse effects at the donor site of flaps
Radiotherapy	No local destruction of tissue Function largely unaffected	Long duration of treatment Scarring and reduced vascularity of treated tissue makes subsequent surgery more difficult Short-term effects: mucositis, candidosis (thrush), difficulty in swallowing, xerostomia, skin pigmentation, mild skin radiation burns Long-term effects: fibrosis of tissues, osteoradionecrosis, caries resulting from xerostomia, poor skin healing, low risk of radiation-induced malignancy 10 years later

- **The patient's wishes.** The patient must decide whether he or she wishes to undergo treatment and which treatment modality is preferred.
- **Medical history.** Major head-and-neck surgery carries a risk of perioperative death of approximately 2–3%. Many patients have coexisting diseases secondary to smoking and drinking alcohol – emphysema, chronic bronchitis, angina, cirrhosis of the liver and a history of myocardial infarction are not unusual. However, untreated oral carcinoma will be fatal, and many patients are prepared to accept the risks associated with general anaesthesia and surgery.
- **Extent of carcinoma.** The primary lesion may be unresectable because of extension to the base of skull, infratemporal fossa, cavernous sinus or across the midline in the pharynx. Metastatic disease in the neck may be unresectable if the carcinoma has invaded beyond the lymph node to involve vital structures such as the carotid arteries. Even if the cancer is theoretically resectable, it may be difficult or impossible to reconstruct the resulting defect.
- **Surgery** causes cosmetic and functional defects that may not be acceptable to the patient. Resection of the tongue base causes complete loss of ability to swallow and predisposes the patient to aspiration of food. Carcinoma in the maxilla may require removal of the eye, and speech is lost after laryngectomy.
- **Home circumstances.** After surgery and during radiotherapy, patients need good support at home. Family, nursing, or social services may provide this. Alternatively, some patients may need to be admitted for a longer period or move to a nursing home.
- **Availability of treatment.** May also need to be considered. In the UK, expertise in surgery and radiotherapy is available throughout the country, but brachytherapy is not offered in all centres. In some developing countries, radiotherapy is the primary treatment modality.

◆ How is the Ideal Treatment Determined?

In the UK, the patient should be under the care of a multidisciplinary team, which usually includes a surgeon, a radiotherapist, a medical oncologist, a pathologist, specialist nurses, a speech therapist, a dietitian, a dentist and a hygienist. Each patient should have an individual treatment plan formulated at a multidisciplinary team meeting, during which all the relevant information is presented. Treatment options are recommended on the basis of evidence-based protocols, but the final choice rests with the patient.

◆ What are the Roles of Surgery and Radiotherapy?

The aim of surgery is to excise the carcinoma, with the largest possible margin. At other body sites, it is usual to attempt to excise a malignant neoplasm by about 3 cm. This is rarely possible in the head and neck region, and margins of only a few millimetres are usual if the lesion is large. Larger margins may be possible, but only at the cost of reduced function and deformity. The head and neck region contains many important structures, and although many can be sacrificed and/or reconstructed, the resulting quality of life may be unacceptable. In some cases, surgery is palliative, designed to remove the bulk of the lesion to reduce the symptoms arising from it.

Radiotherapy may be undertaken as the primary treatment, as an adjunct to surgery or as a palliative measure. Radiation causes cell death through deoxyribonucleic acid (DNA) damage, to which malignant cells are more susceptible compared with normal cells. Cells are most susceptible when they are dividing, and so carcinomas with high rates of cell division, usually the poorly differentiated ones, are most susceptible. The radiation dose is measured in Grays (Gy), and the maximum dose is usually 60–70 Gy given over a 6-week period. Radiotherapy has adverse effects. It causes significantly unpleasant symptoms and therefore should not be seen as a soft option in comparison with surgery.

Chemotherapy may be offered in conjunction with radiotherapy to patients who are relatively fit and have large or late-stage disease. In suitable cases, this may improve 5-year survival by about 10%.

The advantages and disadvantages of surgery and radiotherapy have been described in Table 57.3. However, it must be kept in mind that many patients will undergo both treatments.

TABLE 57.4 Choice of Surgery and Radiotherapy

Treatment Modality	Indications and Contraindications
Excision and primary closure	This is usually reserved for small carcinomas where there is some adjacent tissue that can be mobilized to close the surgical defect. This usually limits primary closure to the lip, tongue or cheek. The advantage of not having to operate on another site to obtain tissue for reconstruction is offset by the resulting distortion of the tissues, risking scarring and poor function. Skin grafting is now rarely used in the mouth. Sometimes the surgical site can be left to granulate. This is usually only the preferred treatment after maxillectomy, when an obturator is placed in the cavity.
Excision and reconstruction	For larger carcinomas and those excised in continuity with a neck dissection, some form of reconstruction is needed. Reconstruction seals the mouth from the tissue planes of the neck and replaces the lost oral tissues to restore function, reduce scarring and improve the cosmetic result. Reconstruction utilizes flaps of tissue grafted into the mouth. The flap of tissue may be local (e.g. nasolabial or temporalis flaps), distant pedicled flaps of muscle from the trunk (e.g. pectoralis major or latissimus dorsi flaps) or microvascular grafts (e.g. radial forearm, deep circumflex iliac artery [DCIA] or fibula flaps). Local flaps provide little tissue. Pedicled flaps are reliable, but the pedicle that provides blood and venous drainage has to reach from the chest to the surgical defect. Microvascular flaps (also known as *free flaps* or *free vascularized flaps*) are a great advance. Blocks of muscle and skin are excised with the arteries and veins that supply them and the vessels are anastomosed to vessels at the surgical site to provide a blood supply and venous drainage. Unfortunately, anastomosis of the vascular supply brings a risk of local thrombosis and vasospasm, which can cause the flap to undergo necrosis. All types of flap may have complications at the donor tissue site.
External beam radiotherapy (teletherapy)	External beam radiotherapy is the most frequently used type of radiotherapy for head and neck malignancy. High energy x-rays are produced by x-ray generators (energy 100 kV) or linear accelerators (energy 20 mV). These more penetrating high energy techniques have largely replaced the older systems based on gamma rays emitted from radionucleotides such as Cobalt-60, which carried a higher risk of inducing osteoradionecrosis. In some centres, particulate radiation using electrons or neutrons may also be available.
Implant radiotherapy (brachytherapy)	Small, localized carcinomas can be treated with implantable radiation sources. These emit gamma rays from needles or pellets of radioactive iridium-192 or gold-198 that are placed into the lesion under general anaesthesia and removed after 6 or 7 days. This type of treatment is useful for T1 or T2 carcinomas of the tongue or cheek. An advantage is that there is a lower dose to external tissues and a very high dose within the lesion. A disadvantage is that a maximal dose of radiation is always given, and no dose can be held in reserve in case of recurrence.
Chemoradiotherapy	Combination of chemotherapy and radiotherapy is used for larger carcinomas. Additional chemotherapy may provide a further advantage over radiotherapy/surgery alone but the patient must be fit and able to withstand the combined adverse effects of both treatments. Various combinations of drugs are used, cisplatinum and 5-fluorouracil being one regimen in use.
Palliative care	Although many patients are anxious to attempt curative treatment, at whatever cost, palliative treatment may be the appropriate choice for good quality of remaining life.

Factors affecting the choice of surgery and radiotherapy are shown in Table 57.4.

Treatment

The recommended treatment for this case was excision of the carcinoma at the primary site and a prophylactic neck dissection en bloc (in one continuous specimen). Postoperative (adjuvant) radiotherapy is planned. The defect in the mouth will be reconstructed with a radial forearm flap. The patient opted for this treatment strategy and made a good recovery after surgery.

◆ What Tissues are Removed in a Block Dissection of the Neck? Why?

In the classic radical neck dissection, the following are removed: the entire sternomastoid muscle, internal and external jugular veins and the contents of the submandibular and submental triangles, including the submandibular gland and all the lymph nodes along the internal jugular vein from the base of the skull to the clavicle. Removing all these tissues in one block ensures complete removal of the carcinoma because the lymph nodes are removed with the surrounding fat or other tissues.

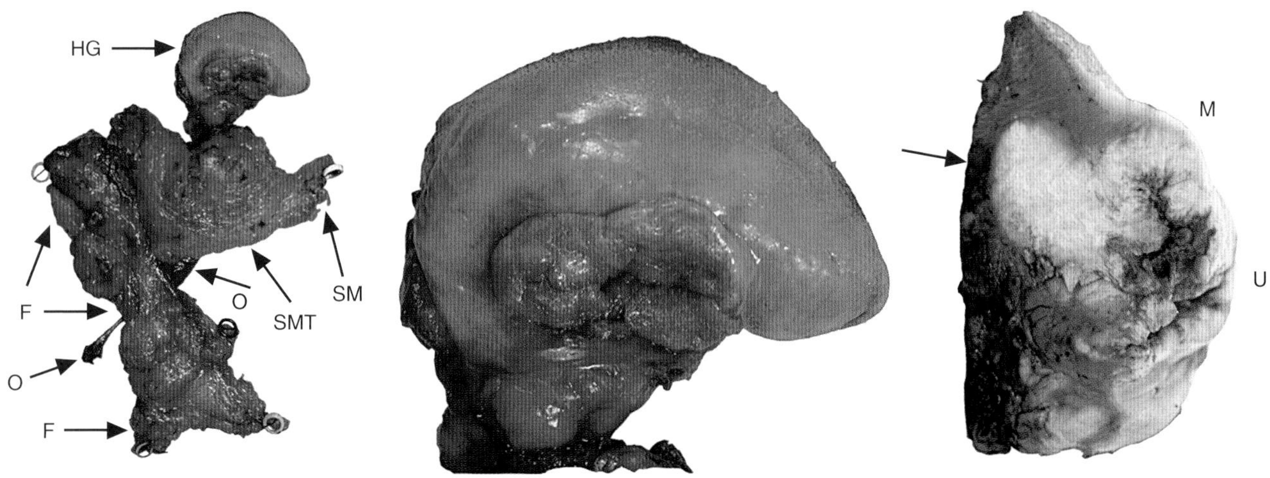

• **Fig. 57.3** The pathology specimen, macroscopic views.

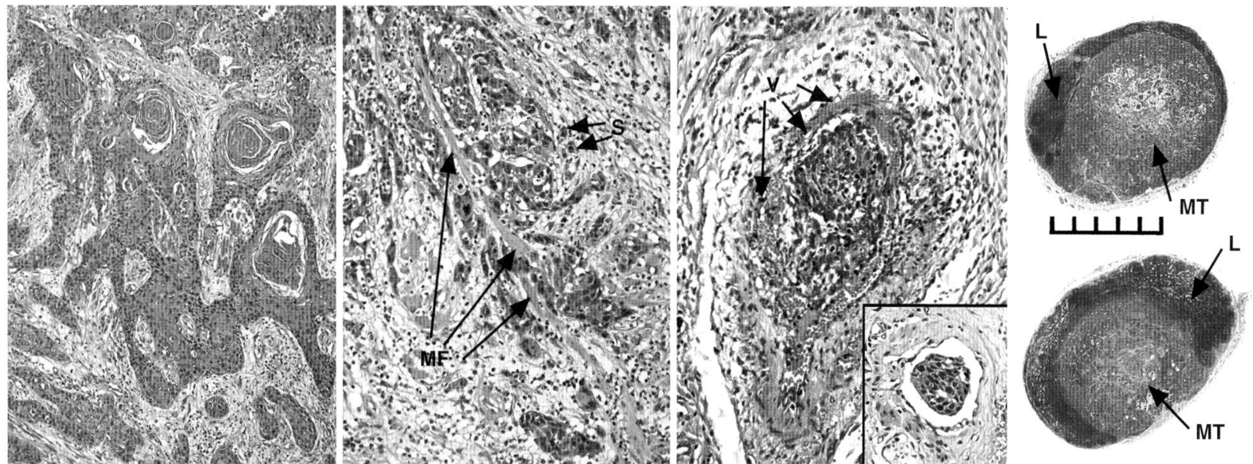

• **Fig. 57.4** The pathology specimen, microscopic views.

Excision of the sternomastoid muscle sacrifices the spinal accessory nerve, which passes through it. This causes postoperative drooping of the shoulder because it supplies the trapezius as well as the sternomastoid muscles. Therefore in most cases where there is no extensive or bulky disease in the neck, either a part or all of the sternomastoid muscle and the internal jugular vein may be left in situ.

◆ Pictures From the Pathological Examination of the Resection Specimen are Shown in Fig. 57.3. What Do You See?

The surgical specimen is shown on the left. At the top is the hemiglossectomy (HG) section, and below it are the contents of the submandibular triangle (SMT) and submental tissue (SM). The sternomastoid muscle has been preserved, and the fat surrounding the jugular vein and cervical lymph nodes is on the left (F). The omohyoid muscle extends across the back of the specimen (O). In the centre, the hemiglossectomy section is shown at higher power. You can see the ulcer with its everted margin on the lateral border of tongue and extending into the floor of mouth. On the right is a vertical coronal section across the tongue, with the midline on the left. The specimen has lost its colour after fixation in formalin. The ulcer (U) and the mass visible clinically toward the dorsum (M) are marked. Carcinoma appears white (because it contains keratin). Note how deeply the carcinoma has penetrated, to within a few millimetres of the midline excision margin (arrowed). Luckily, in this case, carcinoma extends upwards and medially rather than down into the floor of the mouth, where excision would have been more difficult.

◆ The Microscopic Appearances are Shown in Fig. 57.4. What Do You See?

On the left, at medium power, is typical squamous cell carcinoma, comprising islands of epithelium invading around and between muscle fibres. The carcinoma is forming keratin and, in this area, is well or moderately well differentiated. The next panel shows a more poorly differentiated area at high power. Pleomorphic cells with irregular nuclei (anisonucleosis) and darkly staining nuclei (hyperchromatism) are infiltrating along a pink muscle fibre running from top left to bottom right (MF). There is invasion as single cells (S). The third panel, at high power, shows a small vein (V) filled by carcinoma, and the inset shows a cluster of carcinoma cells in a lymphatic vessel. Invasion as single cells and lymphatic and vascular permeation are poor prognostic factors and indicate a high risk of metastasis. Two of the lymph nodes from the neck dissection are shown on the right with a scale in millimetres. Metastases (MT) are seen as round pink areas because of the keratin in them. There is a compressed rim of residual blue lymph node tissue at the periphery (L).

The surgical result was reviewed at a meeting of the multidisciplinary team. The closest margin of excision was 5 mm. Metastatic carcinoma was present in two of the 28 lymph nodes found in the neck dissection, but there was no extranodal extension. The patient is doing well postoperatively.

◆ Are These Excision Margins Adequate?

A margin of 10 mm of normal tissue would be ideal, but in many cases, the excision margins are only a few millimetres. If no radiotherapy had been planned, a margin less than 5 mm would be an indication for postoperative radiotherapy, and the treatment plan would be changed. This patient has poorly differentiated carcinoma, intravascular spread and metastases. Postoperative radiotherapy can compensate for close or incomplete excision, and so a full course of postoperative radiotherapy to the primary site and neck is recommended.

◆ What is the Procedure for Radiotherapy?

Radiotherapy must start within 6 weeks of surgery for the best results. Once the patient has recovered from surgery and the swelling has settled, the preparation for radiotherapy can begin. The radiation will be given in many small doses or fractions to reduce side effects. To ensure that the patient is positioned reproducibly in the x-ray beams, a close fitting acrylic mask, including alignment markers, is made for the patient's face, on a model cast from an impression.

The radiotherapy treatment plan is made on a computer, with calculation of the doses absorbed by the tissues in and around the tumour site. Radiation is delivered by one or more beams of radiation, and metal wedges shield sensitive tissues such as the eyes. In the UK, radiation is usually given at a rate of one fraction per weekday. Recently, hyperfractionation protocols (two fractions per day) have been shown to be equally effective and have fewer side effects. This patient will receive 66 Gy over 6.5 weeks.

◆ After Completing Treatment, What Follow-Up is Required, and Why?

The patient must be monitored regularly for many years. The greatest risk of recurrence is in the first 3 years, and initially, he will be seen every few weeks for a year, gradually extending the review periods to a few months. It must be remembered that in all patients with oral carcinoma, in addition to the risk for recurrence and metastasis, there is a 1-in-10 risk of development of a second primary carcinoma somewhere in the upper aerodigestive tract.

◆ What is the Role of the Dentist in the Care of These Patients?

The dentist in the hospital cancer team will have examined the patient at diagnosis and arranged for extraction of teeth of poor prognosis and for treatment of caries. Teeth in the radiotherapy field used to be routinely extracted. They are now often conserved because advances in radiotherapy have reduced the risk of osteoradionecrosis and because teeth are often restorable with the use of modern techniques. There may also be a need for an obturator or facial prosthesis postoperatively. Ideally, the dentist in the cancer team would continue to care for the patient for a period after treatment.

General dental practitioners will care for patients in the longer term; they need to provide advice on intensive preventive measures, ensure oral health, and prevent infection, particularly around teeth in irradiated bone. There is a need for continued surveillance of the mucosa for recurrence and new lesions and also a need to provide reassurance and support for patients and carers. Support for smoking cessation is important. See also Case 67.

◆ After 21 Months, a Recurrence Develops in the Mouth. What Can Be Done?

If the recurrence is small and accessible, it can be resected. It may be possible to provide radiotherapy, but only if the site has not already been given a full course of radiation.

If no curative treatment can be provided, the patient will require palliative care. Palliative care is the control of symptoms, allowing the patient to end his or her life with dignity. The patient may be cared for at home by family, and community specialist nurses and the local hospice may coordinate treatment and organize short admissions to give some respite to carers. Pain is controlled with strong analgesics, such as morphine, and if the carcinoma fungates and starts to smell, it may be dressed with topical metronidazole. Low-dose palliative radiotherapy or chemotherapy may be possible. The hospice and community palliative care services help the patient with spiritual and physical needs, as well as providing advice on putting affairs in order.

◆ Why is There Such an Emphasis On Early Detection of Oral Cancer?

Oral cancer, like many cancers, is potentially curable if diagnosed early. However, a missed or delayed diagnosis potentially condemns the patient to death. It is therefore imperative that at every dental examination, the mouth is examined thoroughly to ensure there are no lesions of concern. Should such lesions be identified, early and rapid referral should be made by using rapid access schemes, according to local and national protocols. It is also important that general dental practitioners keep themselves up to date regarding knowledge of potentially malignant lesions, which are much more common. Delayed diagnosis is bad for the patient and also for the dentist. Litigation is increasingly becoming a feature of dental practice, and a late or delayed diagnosis could trigger a report to the General Dental Council as well as a legal challenge.

Case 58

A Complicated Extraction

CHRIS DICKINSON

Summary

A 35-year-old man attends your general dental practice surgery requesting extraction of a tooth.

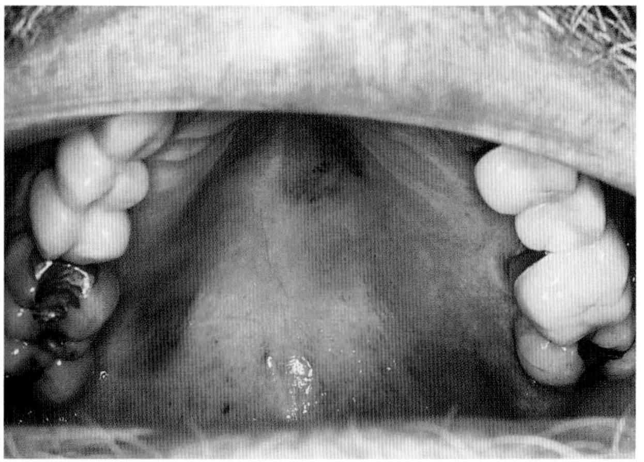

• **Fig. 58.1** The clinical appearance of the patient's palate.

History

Complaint

He points to the lower left second premolar and says that the tooth is very tender to touch and to bite on.

History of Complaint

The tooth has been tender for some months, and root canal treatment at another surgery was initially successful but has proven ineffective in the longer term.

Medical History

The patient's medical questionnaire indicates no relevant medical conditions.

Examination

Extraoral Examination

The extraoral examination is normal except for a few palpable but normal-sized lymph nodes in his right and left cervical chains.

Intraoral Examination

You immediately notice that the patient's oral mucosa is not normal. The appearance of the palate is shown in Fig. 58.1.

The lower left second premolar has a large amalgam restoration and is tender to percussion. A sinus is present in the mucosa overlying the root apex, and the tooth does not respond to a test for sensibility.

◆ What Do You See in the Patient's Mouth?

- The palate appears bruised with two purple-coloured lesions, one on each side of the palate extending from the gingival margin up the sides of the vault. Neither lesion appears to be raised above the surface.
- There is a discrete, sharply defined, slightly red (erythematous) patch in the anterior palate, just to the left of the midline.
- There are a few scattered red spots on the soft palate.

◆ What Do These Changes Tell You?

Individually, none of these lesions can be diagnosed on the basis of the appearance alone. However, in combination, the appearance is almost diagnostic. The purple lesions appear vascular and could be haemangiomas or another blood vessel lesion, including Kaposi's sarcoma. The red patch has the characteristic appearance of erythematous/chronic atrophic candidosis. Both lesions are associated with immunosuppression, and you should immediately suspect human immunodeficiency virus (HIV) infection because Kaposi's sarcoma is extremely rare with other causes of immunosuppression. In this clinical setting, the palpable lymph nodes also support this diagnosis. It is almost certain that the patient is HIV-positive.

◆ What Do You Need To Know? What Would You Say To the Patient?

You need to identify whether the patient is aware of his HIV infection but has chosen not to reveal his full medical history or whether he is completely unaware of it. Almost all patients who know that they are HIV-positive will inform their dentist about it, provided they are asked in an appropriate manner. Patients sometimes withhold this information because of previous insensitive management, refusal to provide treatment or worry that practice confidentiality cannot be relied on. However, your questions need to be carefully phrased, taking into account the fact that the patient may be unaware of his HIV infection. It is very important that you approach this matter with sensitivity. You could adopt the following line of questioning:

- Tell the patient that he has some unusual signs in his mouth and that you cannot easily explain it. Ask whether he has noticed them.
- These changes may be infections. Enquire whether he knows of any reason why he might be particularly prone to infection.
- Point out that there are several possible reasons for being prone to infection and that it would be worthwhile investigating further to find the cause. Provide examples such as anaemia, immunosuppression as a result of steroid therapy or viral infection. Patients who know that they are at risk of HIV infection may often use the mention of a viral infection as a prompt to discuss the possibility.
- If the patient indicates that he or she is HIV-positive, ask whether you might have the address of the patient's clinic so that, if necessary, you may contact the physician for medical advice relating to dental treatment.
- If the patient gives no indication about being HIV-positive, then he or she should be referred to a general medical practitioner or to a specialist in oral medicine or oral surgery unit for further investigation.

It is inappropriate to ask questions about lifestyle or sexuality. Even pointing out that HIV infection is one potential cause of the oral signs may not be well received in a dental setting. It would be reasonable to check the medical history questionnaire, including whether the patient has recorded coming into contact with someone with HIV infection or acquired immunodeficiency syndrome (AIDS).

If the patient discloses having HIV infection, you should respond in a positive manner and acknowledge that you will respect the confidentiality of this sensitive information.

◆ What Other Oral Signs May Be Associated with HIV Infection?

See Box 58.1.

In addition, more rarely, a wide variety of unusual infections may be found.

◆ Which of These Signs are Specific To HIV Infection?

None. All may be seen in other types of immunosuppression and many can be found, albeit rarely, in patients with normal health.

Diagnosis

The patient readily informs you that he is HIV-positive and has only recently been diagnosed. He is aware of Kaposi's sarcoma being the presenting sign of HIV infection. He has just started on antiretroviral drug therapy.

The lower left second premolar has a periapical abscess draining via a sinus.

• BOX 58.1 Conditions, Signs and Symptoms Associated with Human Immunodeficiency Virus (HIV) Infection

Diseases Strongly Associated with HIV Infection

Candidosis
- Erythematous
- Pseudomembranous

Hairy leukoplakia
Periodontal disease
Linear gingival erythema
Necrotizing ulcerative gingivitis
Necrotizing ulcerative periodontitis
Kaposi sarcoma
Lymphoma

Lesions Less Commonly Associated with HIV Infection

Mycobacterial infections
Melanotic pigmentation
Necrotizing (ulcerative) stomatitis
Cystic salivary gland disease
Thrombocytopenic purpura
Nonspecific ulceration
Viral infections, including herpes simplex, herpes zoster and human papillomavirus infection

Treatment

You have decided that extraction of the tooth is indicated.

◆ Is It Appropriate To Extract the Tooth in General Dental Practice?

The General Dental Council (GDC) advocates treating patients with HIV in general practice. Denying this patient treatment on the grounds of his HIV infection alone would put you in breach of the GDC and British Dental Association (BDA) guidance, and might lay you open to a legal case under the Equality Act 2010, UK.

However, when a patient has late or symptomatic HIV infection, his or her medical history may be so complex that a referral to a specialist centre is appropriate. Referral may not be possible in an emergency situation, and treatment, including extraction, may need to be carried out in a general practice setting.

◆ You Will Need Medical Advice. How Will You Obtain It?

People with HIV usually attend outpatient hospital clinics. The patient's general medical practitioner may not have the most up-to-date test results, but clinics are usually very helpful if contacted for information. However, the patient's right to confidentiality must be respected at all times. First, the patient's permission must be obtained to make contact, and second, it is enough to explain to the clinic what you propose to do and to request the results of any tests without mentioning the patient's disease status or irrelevant information.

TABLE 58.1 Further Information Needed From Human Immunodeficiency Virus (HIV) Infection Treatment Centre

Information	Reason
Is the patient prone to infections?	Antibiotics may be prescribed in immunosuppression when they would not normally be considered necessary, but should be reserved for patients with known susceptibility to infections. This is because the risk of adverse effects such as candidosis and diarrhoea resulting from disturbance of the normal flora is increased in HIV infection.
Neutrophil count	Patients may be neutropenic. Neutrophils provide the first line of defence against infection and if the circulating count is less than 1–1.5 × 10^9/L, postoperative antibiotics may be appropriate.
Platelet count	Bone marrow suppression in late HIV infection causes thrombocytopaenia. The normal number of platelets is 150–400 × 10^9/L, but they do not usually fall to a low enough level to cause bleeding problems until late disease. However, this patient has signs of late disease (Kaposi's sarcoma) and the red spots on the palate are probably petechial haemorrhages.
Does the patient have coinfection with hepatitis B or C?	These infections are not uncommon in HIV-positive individuals. Liver damage may cause a coagulation defect that could complicate the extraction. It also disturbs drug metabolism.
The names of the drugs that he is taking	Some of the retroviral drugs have significant interactions with other classes of drugs (see Table 58.2). The patient is taking efavirenz, tenofovir and emtricitabine.

◆ What Additional Information Would You Require From the Patient's HIV Management Clinic? Why?

See Table 58.1.

CD4 T-lymphocyte counts and the viral load – which is a measure of HIV viral ribonucleic acid (RNA) in blood – are often known to the patient or may be obtained from the medical clinic. These indicate the level of immunosuppression and infectivity, respectively, but are not helpful directly in predicting whether a patient is likely to bleed or be at risk of infection after a dental extraction.

◆ Should the Tooth Be Taken Out Without This Additional Information?

No, in a general practice situation, this would be unwise.

◆ Would Any Special Infection Control Precautions Be Required for the Extraction?

No, the patient should be treated normally. It is assumed that all patients have the potential to carry an infectious disease, and dental practices should follow the standard level of infection control ('universal precautions') for all patients. Additional precautions are required for surgical procedures, but not for routine dentistry.

◆ What Antiretroviral Treatment Might the Patient Be Receiving?

See Box 58.2.

There are three main classes of antiretroviral drugs: nucleoside/nucleotide reverse transcriptase inhibitors (NRTIs), non-nucleoside reverse transcriptase inhibitors (NNRTIs) and protease inhibitors (PIs). Recently, there have been developments in entry, integration and maturation inhibitors. These are mainly confined to those patients who have a high degree of resistance to the mainstream antiretroviral drugs.

• BOX 58.2 A List of Possible Antiretroviral Medications

Chemokine antagonist	maraviroc
Fusion inhibitor	enfuvirtide
Nucleoside/nucleotide reverse transcriptase inhibitors (NRTIs)	abacavir didanosine emtricitabine lamivudine stavudine tenofovir zidovudine
Non-nucleoside reverse transcriptase inhibitors (NNRTIs)	delaviridine efavirenz etravirine nevirapine
Integrase inhibitor	raltegravir
Protease inhibitors (PIs)	amprenavir atazanavir darunavir indinavir lopinavir nelfinavir saquinavir tipranavir ritonovir
Maturation inhibitor	bevirimat (unlicensed)

◆ Do These Drugs Interact with Any Other Medications Likely To Be Prescribed in a General Dental Practice Setting?

Yes, they may, and the interactions can be significant (Table 58.2).

TABLE 58.2 Interactions with Antiretroviral Drugs and Drugs Commonly Used in Dental Practice

Drug	Antiretroviral Drug	Effect
Metronidazole	Atazanavir, darunavir, lopinavir, tipranavir, ritonavir	Antiretroviral formulations may contain alcohol, causing a disulfiram reaction.
Clindamycin	Ritonavir	Increase in clindamycin levels.
Erythromycin	Darunavir, fosamprenavir, indinavir, lopinavir, saquinavir, tipranavir, ritonavir	Large increase in erythromycin levels.
Diazepam, midazolam	Protease inhibitors, non-nucleoside reverse transcriptase inhibitors	Oral administration of many benzodiazepines is contraindicated because of their altered metabolism. This leads to an increase in their sedative effects. Oral midazolam particularly is to be avoided. Note that intravenous midazolam, as used in dentistry, is titrated to the patient's response, and this is not contraindicated. However, great care needs to be taken in the titration to avoid oversedation. Proceed slowly. There remains a possibility of prolonged sedation, although this does not appear to be a problem in clinical practice. Reversing the sedative effect with flumazenil may theoretically result in late re-sedation. The recovery time to discharge should be increased to monitor this.
Lidocaine (lignocaine)	Protease inhibitors, non-nucleoside reverse transcriptase inhibitors	There is a theoretical risk of impaired lidocaine (lignocaine) metabolism. The significance of this is unclear in the dental setting but it would be prudent to avoid approaching the accepted maximum dose.
Fluconazole	Tipranavir, nevirapine	Increase in levels of tipranavir, nevirapine.
Miconazole oral gel	Protease inhibitors, non-nucleoside reverse transcriptase inhibitors	Poorly absorbed but may be ingested with saliva. Risk of increase in antiretroviral levels in blood if used to excess.

A useful online tool for assessing the potential for interactions can be found at: http://www.hiv-druginteractions.org/.

The clinic tells you that the patient has a platelet count of 45 × 10^9/L and a neutrophil count of 1.9 × 10^9/L. There is no coinfection with viral hepatitis.

◆ Will You Take Out the Tooth?

No. The platelet count is too low. Bleeding problems would be expected if the count is below 50 × 10^9/L. You should coordinate with the medical clinic to arrange for the patient to be treated in a specialist centre.

◆ The Patient Asks To Return To Your Practice for Routine Treatment. What is Your Reaction?

Yes, he should be able to have routine dental treatment without problems, although further extractions might require referral. Block analgesia is possible, provided the platelet count remains above 30 × 10^9/L.

Antiretroviral combination therapy is usually effective, and this patient's oral signs are likely to disappear with time and as platelets rise in number. Antiretroviral drugs and HIV-associated salivary gland disease may cause dry mouth, and this is a risk factor for caries. People with HIV are also more prone to periodontal attachment loss and gingival recession. The preventive aspects of dental treatment will need to be emphasized, and if there were evidence of continuing attachment loss or excessively high levels of caries, then a referral to a specialist centre would be appropriate. Otherwise, it would be appropriate to reduce the interval between recalls if there are risk factors for dental disease.

Acknowledgement

The editors would like to acknowledge the previous contributions of Guy Palmer.

Further Reading

Further information on HIV/AIDS can be found at https://www.nhs.uk/conditions/hiv-and-aids/.

Case 59

Difficulty Opening the Mouth

ANAND LALLI AND WANNINAYAKA M. TILAKARATNE

Summary

A 40-year-old Indian man presents with limitation of mouth opening. You must identify the cause and institute appropriate management.

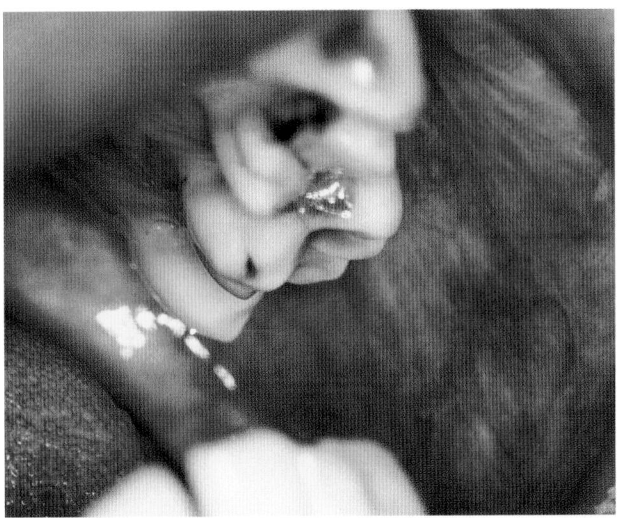

• **Fig. 59.1** Left buccal mucosa, photographed at maximum mouth opening.

History

Complaint

The patient complains of difficulty eating. He cannot open his mouth widely enough to place as much food inside as he could before and also has difficulty chewing.

History of Complaint

He has noticed the reduction in mouth opening over a period of several years but has never sought advice. It has not been overly painful, although during the same period, he has felt an uncomfortable burning sensation in the buccal mucosa on eating.

Medical History

The patient is otherwise fit and well.

◆ What are the Causes of Limitation of Mouth Opening, and How May They Be Classified?

Limitation of mouth opening is most frequently caused by trismus. Trismus is best defined as the clinical sign of limited mouth opening less than 35 mm, which can result from a wide variety of causes. Historically, the definition of trismus was 'spasm of the muscles of mastication', but the broader description of limited opening is more relevant clinically. Trismus is usually reversible and most often results from treatable causes such as trauma or infection. It can be associated with other clinical symptoms such as pain in the jaw and difficulty performing activities that involve opening the mouth, such as toothbrushing or eating. The irreversible causes of trismus, such as oral submucous fibrosis or ankylosis after trauma, may be progressive in their early stages and do not respond to currently available treatment strategies. The causes of trismus are listed in Table 59.1 below. See also Case 8.

◆ What Questions Would You Ask?

The patient should be asked whether there has been trauma or irradiation to the skull, temporomandibular joint (TMJ) or face and whether there have been any episodes of swelling of the face or around the joint. He should also be asked whether he uses betel quid (areca nut or 'paan').

The patient gives no history of trauma, irradiation, inflammation or infection. However, he has been a betel quid chewer for more than 20 years.

Examination

Extraoral Examination

The patient looks mildly anaemic. There is no facial asymmetry or evidence of scars or inflammation around the joint. No tenderness can be elicited from the muscles of mastication. There are no clicks, crepitus or tenderness associated with the TMJ and no mandibular deviation on opening the mouth.

◆ What Measurement Would You Take?

The maximum voluntary mouth opening. The normal interincisal opening in an adult is approximately 35 mm. Measurement will provide a baseline reading against which to judge treatment efficacy or trismus progression. It will also indicate the feasibility of dental and other intraoral treatment.

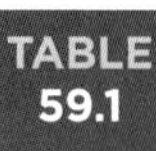

TABLE 59.1 Causes of Trismus (See Also Table 8.1)

Reversible	Inflammation in and around the temporomandibular joint (TMJ) and muscles of mastication (e.g. following wisdom tooth surgery). Soft tissue infection around the jaws or TMJ (usually dental in origin). TMJ myofascial pain dysfunction syndrome (TMD). Trauma (e.g. fractures of the mandible or zygomatic arch and/or soft tissue injury). Tetanus and tetany.
Irreversible	A. Extra-articular causes *Acquired:* Fibrosis caused by burns or irradiation. Oral submucous fibrosis. Mucosal scarring (e.g. in epidermolysis bullosa or scleroderma). *Congenital:* All are rare (e.g. syndromic such as masticatory muscle underdevelopment in trismus-pseudocamptodactyly syndrome, or nonsyndromic such as neurological brainstem digenesis). B. Intra-articular causes *Acquired:* Posttraumatic ankylosis. Ankylosis secondary to septic arthritis. Neoplasms in and invading the TMJ. *Congenital:* Rare abnormalities of the craniofacial structures (e.g. syndromic such as Apert's syndrome, or non-syndromic such as neonatal infections).

This patient can achieve a maximal voluntary interincisal opening of 17 mm.

Intraoral Examination

◆ The Oral Mucosa is Shown in Figs 59.1 and 59.2. What Do You See?

The buccal and soft palate mucosae are paler than normal, although some mucosal pigmentation consistent with the patient's skin colour makes this less obvious. When the mouth is opened fully, thin white hard bands run vertically just below the buccal mucosa. These are just visible in the figure and are much more readily felt as hard ridges. Some of the less pale areas are red and atrophic.

The same changes are found on the labial mucosa, where bands of hard, pale, scar-like tissue are visible below the epithelium when the lip is everted. The gingival mucosa has lost its stippled appearance, and there is oedema and rounding of the gingival contour, consistent with periodontal disease. There is some dark red/brown betel quid stain on the teeth.

If you were able to examine the patient, you would find that he also has some reduction in mobility of the tongue and cannot protrude it very far. Most of the mucosa feels firm.

Diagnosis

◆ What is Your Diagnosis?

The presentation and features are characteristic of oral submucous fibrosis. Gradual limitation of mouth opening and restriction of tongue movements are seen in a betel quid user who shows typical mucosal blanching and fibrosis presenting as bands in the buccal mucosa.

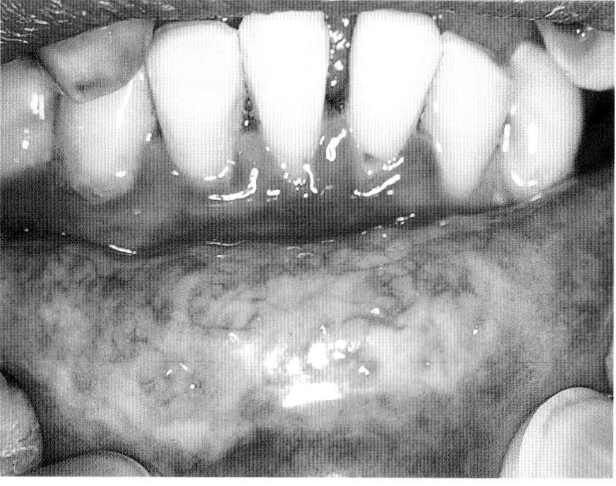

• **Fig. 59.2** The lower lip mucosa.

◆ What Other Features of Oral Submucous Fibrosis Might Be Seen?

In the early stages, some patients complain of vesiculation of the mucosa. In severe cases with extensive tongue involvement, the filiform papillae are lost.

◆ What is Betel Quid Chewing?

A habit practised by many people in the Indian subcontinent, much of south-east Asia and some parts of Africa. The basic quid comprises pieces or paste of areca nut and slaked lime, wrapped and tied into a packet in a vine leaf. A variety of other components is usually added; the combination varies between regions, but tobacco is almost always included, together with flavouring agents such as cinnamon, cloves and ginger. The areca nut contains alkaloids, which have a psychoactive effect and make the habit addictive. The quid is only chewed intermittently and lies in the buccal sulcus for long periods. Many users keep a quid in their mouth all day, and some even sleep with a quid in the mouth. It has been estimated that 10% of the world's population use betel quid, and chewing is a major health problem in many countries, including western societies with significant immigrant populations from endemic areas.

◆ What are the Possible Effects of Betel Quid Chewing?

- Oral submucous fibrosis
- Oral and pharyngeal squamous cell carcinoma
- Periodontitis, recession and root erosion at the site of use
- Tooth staining
- Decreased taste sensation
- Possible worsening of asthma
- Possible association with diabetes and malignancy.

◆ What is the Significance of the Diagnosis? What Else Would You Look For?

Oral submucous fibrosis is a potentially malignant disorder. Tobacco and other carcinogenic agents in the quid make this habit one of the highest known risk factors for oral carcinoma.

The patient's oral mucosa must be carefully examined for carcinoma and potentially malignant lesions. The features of early carcinoma and potentially malignant lesions are discussed in Case 45 and Case 46. Approximately one-third of patients with submucous fibrosis have oral white patches, and dysplasia is present in the mucosa of up to 16%. Malignant transformation to squamous cell carcinoma occurs in 5–8% of cases.

The second significant feature is restricted mouth opening. This is often progressive and responds poorly to treatment. In the late stages of disease, the patient may be unable to open the mouth at all, and incisor extractions may be required to allow feeding. Limited opening is a major handicap in the diagnosis and treatment of malignancy and premalignant lesions. It makes examination, detection and treatment extremely difficult, and the prognosis for oral carcinoma in a patient with submucous fibrosis is very poor, mostly as a result of late diagnosis.

Investigations

◆ What Investigations are Required? Explain Why.

Biopsy is required to assess the dysplasia. If there are lesions that raise suspicions of malignancy, red or white patches or areas of otherwise abnormal mucosa, they should be sampled for microscopy. More than one biopsy may be required. If no particular part of the mucosa is suspect, a sample should be taken from the area where the quid is held in the mouth.

The biopsy will probably also provide evidence to support the diagnosis of oral submucous fibrosis. However, in such a typical case, biopsy for this purpose alone would not be justified. It might be considered in an early case where the diagnosis is in doubt.

◆ Would You Perform This Patient's Biopsy in a General Practice Setting?

No. This patient is at high risk of oral carcinoma, and so biopsy and further recall should be carried out in a specialist centre. Further discussion about when to perform biopsy of potentially dysplastic mucosa can be found in Case 45.

◆ A Biopsy Specimen From the Quid Site is Shown in Fig. 59.3. What Do You See, and How Do You Interpret the Findings?

The mucosa is covered by epithelium that is atrophic, and the thickness of the normal buccal mucosa is about twice the normal thickness from the surface to the dermal papillae in this specimen. It is normally nonkeratinized, except for a thin layer near the occlusal line. The epithelium is largely well organized, and stratification and maturation are not particularly disordered; the epithelial layers are easily differentiated. There is an expanded basal cell layer comprising rather disorganized small and darkly staining cells, which show anisonucleosis (nuclei of different sizes) and irregularly shaped, often angular, nuclei. Towards the centre of the epithelium, there is a cluster of prickle cells between two dermal papillae, showing early and single cell keratinization. These features point to mild dysplasia. Below the epithelium, there is even fibrosis of the connective tissue and scattered lymphocytes.

The deeper tissue shows the fibrosis of the connective tissue more prominently. All the tissue between the epithelium and the underlying muscle is replaced by relatively acellular dense fibrous tissue. The superficial muscle is atrophic and is being replaced by fibrous tissue. Occasional residual muscle fibres lie in the fibrosis. This deeper tissue is uninflamed.

The fibrosis involving deep muscle is consistent with the diagnosis of oral submucous fibrosis, and the overlying epithelium shows mild dysplasia.

Treatment

◆ What Questions Would You Ask the Patient About His Betel Quid Chewing Habit?

You need to know whether the patient includes tobacco in his quid, how many quids he uses each day and whether he sleeps with one in the mouth. In addition, you should check other tobacco-related habits, because many quid users smoke cigarettes as well, and some in India smoke a traditional coarse unfiltered tobacco product, 'bidi' or 'beedi', a rolled uncut tobacco leaf. Some users also practise a form of snuff dipping, placing ground quid constituents ('pan masala') loose in the sulcus.

◆ What are the Available Treatments or Treatment Options? What is the Potential Value of Each?

See Table 59.2.

No treatment regimen yields satisfactory results, and the aim is maintenance of oral health and prevention of complications. If patients are committed to mouth opening exercises, they may be spared the worst effects of extreme trismus. However, if disease is advanced at diagnosis,

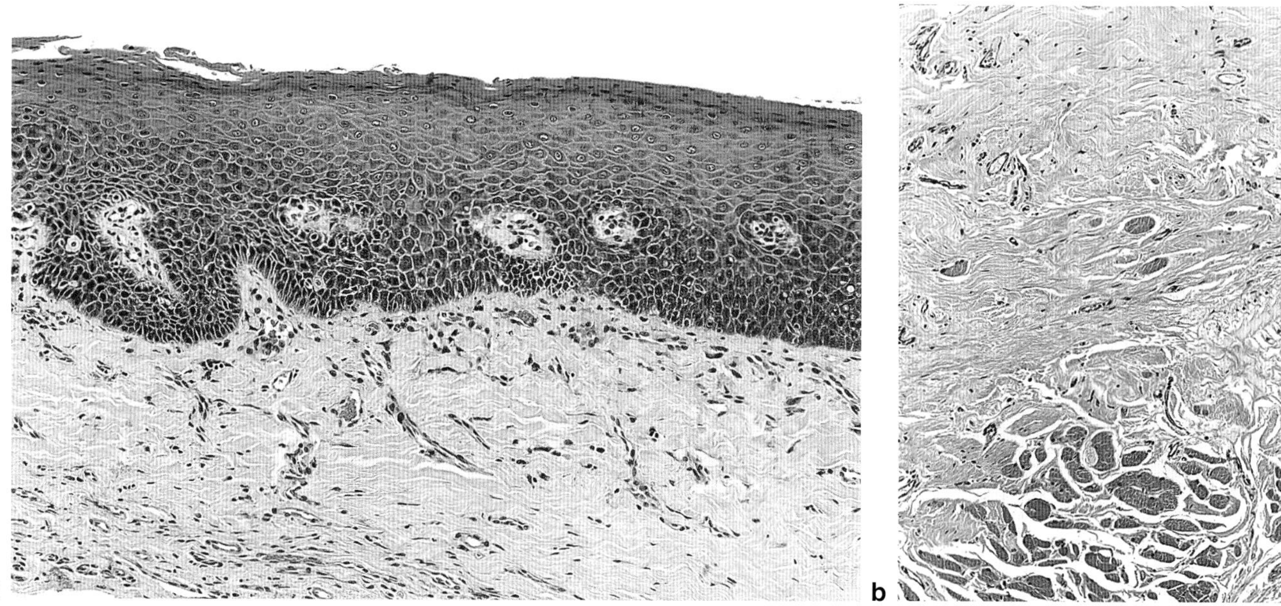

• **Fig. 59.3** Biopsy from the quid site: **a,** buccal mucosa; **b,** underlying tissue.

TABLE 59.2 Treatment Options

Option	Potential Value
Habit intervention	Although areca nut is the main aetiological factor for oral submucous fibrosis, there are a number of other carcinogens. Therefore cessation of the habit rather than altering the composition of the quid should be the aim. As a partial measure, discouraging tobacco in the quid would be valuable. This will reduce the risk of malignancy, but limitation of opening may still worsen. Cessation is best, but there would still be a risk of malignant transformation.
Regular review	The only reliable method for detecting dysplasia and early malignant transformation. Repeated biopsy may be required.
Muscle-stretching exercises	These appear to give good results in some patients. To be effective, muscle stretching exercise must be frequent and prolonged. Bite wedges or a screw appliance may help produce the forcible opening required. Effective exercises are painful, and patients must be highly motivated.
Intralesional steroids	These have been widely used, but the results are not encouraging in most patients and any benefit may not be sustained.
Surgical treatment	Occasionally used as the last resort. The fibrosis extends deeply into muscle, and surgical excision of the scar tissue is rarely possible. Postoperative scarring replaces the original fibrosis, and surgery is usually followed by relapse.
Nutritional supplementation	Many patients are deficient in iron and vitamins. Dietary supplementation with these and carotenes or vitamin A may be helpful in reducing progression, but the effect is not marked.
Experimental methods	The lack of effective treatments has led to trials of many compounds, including interferon-gamma, but none has proven consistently useful.

progressive limitation is likely. The best results are seen in those who have relatively localized disease at diagnosis, perhaps limited to the site of quid placement.

The aims are best achieved by helping the patient with cessation of the habit and by detecting malignancy or dysplasia as early as possible. If suspicious lesions develop, they may be treated by using the same modalities of treatment as in other patients (e.g. surgery and chemotherapy or radiotherapy), as allowed by the degree of trismus. All abnormal mucosa must be regarded with the utmost suspicion and a biopsy performed.

◆ What is the Role of the General Dental Practitioner in Such a Case?

Dental practitioners have an important role in the prevention of betel quid chewing just as in the prevention of smoking. As noted above, most chewers are also smokers, and health workers need to address both tobacco habits.

The majority of those who regularly chew betel quid are from low socioeconomic groups and, at least in the UK, are often poorly informed about the health risks. Health education for chewers is most important and may need to be extended to other family members. The difficulty in convincing patients to give up their habit should not be underestimated. The habit is addictive and is embedded in the cultural, social and religious customs of many ethnic groups. Many justify chewing on the basis of its supposed health benefits that are accepted in their culture. The general dental practitioner can help the specialist centre to modify the patient's high-risk behaviour, reinforcing the message to remove tobacco from the quid and encouraging patients to reduce the areca content and the frequency of chewing. The importance of prompt referral and regular mucosal examination for dysplastic lesions and carcinoma has already been stressed.

In the small number of patients who develop oral submucous fibrosis, dental treatment involves difficult choices and would be best carried out in a specialist centre. Initially, with limited trismus, treatment is not a problem and could be readily performed in a general dental practice. However, some restorative treatment will be rendered impossible as restriction of mouth opening progresses, and a thorough and effective regimen of preventive treatment must be instituted as soon as possible. Extraction of teeth with even small carious lesions or moderate periodontitis may become necessary, although it should be left until the last possible moment. It is still possible to restore and clean some teeth in late disease, although both activities are compromised. Every effort should be made to retain a stable occlusion to prevent progression to permanent overclosure.

◆ This Patient Has a Typical But Late Presentation. What are the Earliest Features?

The earliest features are relatively subtle and nonspecific. There is typically burning of the mucosa and roughness, sometimes described as 'tiny vesicles'. All or part of the lining mucosa may be affected, and these symptoms associated with betel quid chewing should be regarded with the highest suspicion.

Case 60

Erosive Tooth Wear

RUPERT AUSTIN AND DEBORAH BOMFIM

Summary

A 35-year-old policeman presents at your practice after having noticed that his anterior teeth are becoming shorter. Identify the cause, and outline the options for management.

History

Complaint

The patient has become increasingly aware of his shortening front teeth. He is not greatly concerned about the appearance but feels that continued wear will eventually destroy the teeth completely.

History of Complaint

He has noticed that his teeth have become worse over the last 10 years, but first noticed the signs when he was diagnosed with bulimia nervosa in his late teenage years and earlier adulthood. The patient has always attended a dentist regularly and has relatively few, small restorations and maintains regular oral hygiene practices, primarily toothbrushing.

Medical History

The patient is currently in good health, having previously had prolonged medical and psychological treatment for his eating disorder, which was mainly related to food binging followed by purging. He has not had issues with binging or vomiting for over a decade now. He drinks about 10–20 units of alcohol each week. He has noticed some heartburn and indigestion from time to time. This has always been part of his life, and he normally does not pay much attention to the symptoms because he has a very busy work schedule, including working nights and long shifts.

Examination

Extraoral Examination

The patient looks generally well and is of normal body weight. No submandibular or cervical lymph nodes are palpable. No abnormalities of the temporomandibular joints are detected, and there is no evidence of hypertrophy or tenderness of the masticatory muscles on examination.

Intraoral Examination

◆ An Anterior View of the Dentition and the Palato-Occlusal Appearance of the Maxillary Anterior Teeth are Shown in Fig. 60.1. What Do You See?

There are signs of generalized tooth wear, with the palatal surfaces and incisal edges of the anterior maxillary teeth showing marked loss of enamel. The wear generally involves loss of enamel and exposure of dentine; however, there is more extensive exposure of dentine on the palatal aspects of the maxillary anterior teeth. The incisal edges are rough, translucent with small chips of unsupported labial enamel having fractured away. There are multiple white spots associated with the bucco-cervical aspects of the teeth, as well as multiple bucco-cervical restorations, with signs of staining. In addition, the intrinsic discolouration of the mesio-incisal aspect of the upper right central incisor is perhaps suggestive of the presence of caries.

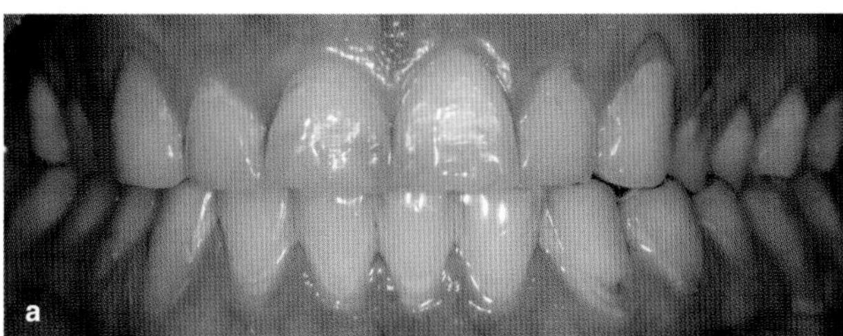

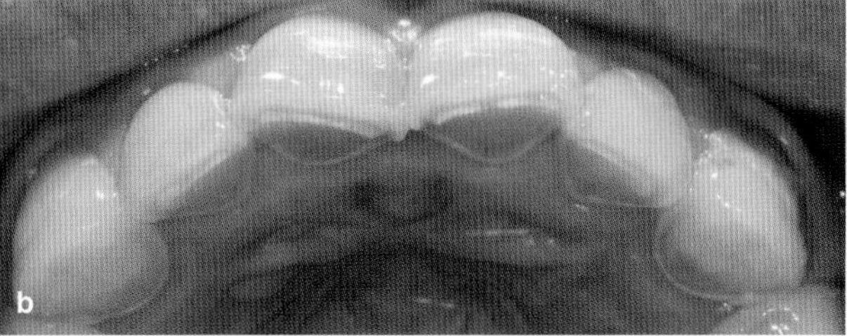

• **Fig. 60.1** **a,** The anterior view of the maxillary and mandibular dentition in maximum intercuspation; and **b,** the palato-occlusal view of the anterior maxillary teeth.

With regard to the periodontium, there are signs of multiple areas of recession and root exposure; however, there are no signs of clinical attachment loss despite the presence of proximal plaque and deposits. Periodontal pocket probing depths range from 2 to 4 mm, with no pocketing greater than 4 mm. Generalized bleeding on periodontal probing is noted.

On occlusal examination, you find that the upper and lower incisor teeth contact in intercuspal and dynamic occlusal relationships (i.e., lateral excursions and protrusion). The occlusal and palatal surfaces of the upper posterior teeth appear relatively unaffected by tooth wear.

◆ What Aetiology of Tooth Wear Would Be Consistent with These Findings From the History and Examination Thus Far?

The tooth wear is consistent in appearance with an aetiology of erosive tooth wear, which is the loss of dental hard tissues through the processes of erosion, attrition and abrasion in combination. Although each process may manifest via separate dynamics, significant clinical tooth wear is usually the result of a combination of these processes, and erosion is often the dominant factor. Therefore the condition is commonly referred to as *erosive tooth wear*.

The history of a previous eating disorder and current symptoms of heartburn and indigestion (most likely from gastro-oesophageal reflux disease [GORD]), suggests that erosion is the predominant factor in this case. Moreover, the distribution of enamel loss further reinforces the suspicion that regurgitation of gastric acid from the stomach may be the primary source of the acid. Erosion from dietary acids is usually associated with more enamel loss on the buccal or labial surfaces of the upper anterior teeth. However, if the patient rinses or swills acidic drinks in the palatal vault prior to swallowing, the pattern of erosion is very similar to that seen when gastric acid is regurgitated. Abrasion and attrition are also likely to be contributing to tooth wear, especially if persistent acid exposure leads to a relative softening of the surface few microns of enamel.

◆ Define Erosion, Abrasion and Attrition.

Erosion is the chemical dissolution of dental hard tissues and is caused by acids.

Attrition is the loss of dental hard tissues and is caused by the physical action of tooth grinding against tooth.

Abrasion is the wear of dental hard tissues and is caused by physical means other than teeth grinding together.

Differential Diagnosis for Erosive Tooth Wear

◆ What are Your Differential Diagnoses for the Cause of the Tooth Wear in This Patient?

1. Tooth wear caused primarily by dietary erosion and secondary abrasion and attrition
2. Tooth wear caused primarily by gastric erosion with secondary abrasion and attrition
3. A combination of tooth wear primarily caused by dietary and gastric erosion, with secondary abrasion and attrition.

◆ What Specific Questions Would You Ask Regarding the Tooth Wear? Explain Why

Tooth wear is often multifactorial, and the patient must be questioned about all causes.

Does the Patient Have a High Consumption of Acidic or Cariogenic Foods or Drinks? Frequent acid intake is a common cause of dental erosion, and the presence of caries, in addition, requires further investigation. The intake of both acid and cariogenic foods and drinks must be ascertained together with the way in which they are consumed.

What is the Patient's Current Oral Hygiene Regimen? There is evidence of poor oral hygiene, which may be complicated by the patient's working patterns. The timings, frequency and effectiveness of toothbrushing, interdental cleaning and choice of oral care products will impact on both periodontal conditions, caries and erosive tooth wear. This is especially the case in terms of the use of fluoride-containing products, such as high-fluoride toothpastes, mouthrinses and gels. Furthermore, agents such as those containing bioavailable calcium and phosphate may be useful for promoting remineralization of white spots, caries and erosion lesions.

How Did the Eating Disorder Manifest Itself Previously, and is It Well Controlled? The history of an eating disorder and the presence of caries suggests that the patient has struggled to achieve a healthy balanced diet in the past. Eating disorders have complex and extensive ramifications on general and oral health. Anorexia nervosa and bulimia nervosa increase the risk of erosive tooth wear for two reasons. First, abnormal dietary patterns can involve either restricted food consumption (anorexia) or excessive binging (bulimia), which can cause dietary erosion, followed by purging (forced vomiting) in both conditions, which causes regurgitation-related gastric erosion. Such eating disorders are lesscommon in males than females, but their incidence is increasing, with current estimates of prevalence rates around 25% among males. Psychological conditions such as these must be handled carefully with the patient and his or her relatives; however, it is important that dental professionals discuss the impact of these conditions on oral health and liaise with appropriate medical professionals.

Does the Patient Suffer Acid Reflux From the Stomach? Regurgitation of stomach acid may be noticed by the patient because of the taste. However, it may go unnoticed if it happens at night and may or may not be associated with symptoms of gastric disease. Occasional mild reflux into the oesophagus or the pharynx is relatively common, for example, during exercise; however, persistent reflux requires medical management. Be aware that patients may have become accustomed to regular, low-level reflux, and so careful questioning during history taking (anamnesis) may be required to elicit this information from the patient.

What is the Patient's Alcohol Intake and Pattern of Consumption? The patient has indicated an intake of 10–20 units of alcohol each week. Patients often underreport their alcohol intake, and it would be worth checking this with the patient. Many alcoholic drinks are acidic, contributing to dietary acid (below), and binge patterns of drinking are often associated with vomiting. The possibility of a history of chronic alcoholism should be considered but dealt with respectfully and with dignity among the patient and their relatives.

Does the Patient Grind or Clench His Teeth During the Day or At Night? Bruxism or other parafunctional habits are common causes of increased wear. Of course, patients may not be aware of grinding habits because they become accustomed to the habit. If nocturnal bruxism occurs, often a partner can help confirm its occurrence and frequency and whether it is associated with a sleep disorder, such as sleep apnoea, or not.

In response to your questioning, the patient denies frequent intake of acidic substances, current vomiting or bruxism. However, he indicates that he does suffer some acid regurgitation associated with his dyspepsia (heartburn) and that alcohol and stress are associated with the attacks. He has had heartburn and regurgitation for 20 years but is not taking any regular medication to relieve the symptoms. He has not visited his medical practitioner regarding these symptoms. His eating disorder is well controlled and has been for at least a decade.

Investigations

◆ What Investigations Would You Perform?

A thorough dietary record should be logged by the patient to determine the true consumption of cariogenic and acidic foods and drinks. Diet analysis sheets need to be filled in for 4 or more days, including a weekend, and it is emphasized that the patient should write down all the foods and drinks taken during that time, including between-meal snacks (essentially, anything that passes between his lips during that period). Both frequency and amount need to be noted, and the patient should be told specifically to note suspect foods such as carbonated drinks, citrus fruits and drinks, vinegar and other acidic condiments, and white wine to ensure that none is missed. It may be wise not to divulge the 'high risk' items prior to asking the patient to complete the diet diary, in case this biases the data recorded.

Impressions or study casts or digital intraoral scans of the patient's teeth should be taken. These will provide a baseline record against which progression of future erosion can be determined. The basic erosive wear examination (BEWE) can also provide a useful, simple scoring system for classifying the risk of tooth wear in more borderline cases; however, this is clearly a high risk case. Tests of tooth sensibility and intraoral bitewing and selected periapical radiographs will be needed to diagnose the extent, location and severity of caries and whether any teeth have compromised pulp sensibility.

Diet analysis confirms the patient's statement that he has a low consumption of acidic foods and beverages. This therefore excludes dietary acid as a cause, leaving gastric acid as the only other erosive source. Regurgitation erosion occurs when the stomach juice passes from the stomach into the mouth. The pH of stomach juice is around 1 or 2, and if regurgitation occurs frequently, the damage to teeth can be catastrophic and rapid.

Further Erosive Tooth Wear Differential Diagnosis

◆ How Might Gastric Acid Enter the Mouth?

1. GORD
2. Eating disorders
3. Chronic alcoholism
4. Rumination.

◆ What Features of These Conditions Might Aid Your Definitive Diagnosis?

GORD is usually associated with heartburn (intermittent retrosternal pain radiating along the oesophagus, worsened by lying down or a recent large meal), or epigastric pain (centred on the xiphisternum). When symptoms are related to meals, the term *dyspepsia* is sometimes used. In most patients, symptoms of GORD are self-limiting, and little or no acid enters the mouth. In others, complete regurgitation into the mouth is frequent and pain becomes persistent, causing patients to seek medical advice. A small proportion of patients treat their pain with over-the-counter antacids and are unaware of the potential of damage to their teeth or oesophagus. A history of taking antacid preparations is a useful indicator for the activity of GORD, and this patient has already indicated that he has noticed some regurgitation. This is the most likely cause.

Eating disorders are a cause of erosion, as discussed above. In 2013, it was estimated that 725,000 people in the UK had an eating disorder. Thus less than 1 in 100 patients in general dental practice are likely to be affected by an eating disorder. Both anorexia nervosa and bulimia nervosa tend to affect adolescent females. Sufferers lose body weight by starving themselves and/or vomiting to lose weight in an attempt to improve their body self-image. A small proportion of patients with severe anorexia die as a result of the disorder. Unlike patients with anorexia, those with bulimia usually have a stable body weight. They eat and drink in binges and self-induce vomiting to control their body weight. There may be an accompanying history of drug and/or alcohol abuse.

Alcoholism is associated with dental erosion, either through vomiting or due to the low pH of some alcoholic drinks.

Rumination is an unusual practice involving habitual chewing of food, swallowing and then regurgitating the food mixed with stomach acid to be chewed and swallowed again. It is considered rare, but there is no accurate information on its prevalence, and it is thought to affect young, healthy and, mainly, professional people. If the habit is continued, it can cause significant damage to teeth.

The patient gives a clear history of regular heartburn and symptomatic regurgitation. He denies rumination and alcoholism.

Diagnosis

◆ What is Your Diagnosis?

1. Generalized plaque-induced gingivitis
2. Generalized severe erosive tooth wear consistent in appearance with multi-factorial erosion, abrasion and attrition
3. Multiple carious lesions bucco-cervically and proximally.

Treatment

◆ How Will You Manage the Patient's Condition?

The patient should be referred to a gastroenterologist or his general medical practitioner for further investigation of his symptoms. Reflux may be caused by a reduction in pressure around the lower oesophageal sphincter (e.g., in hiatus hernia) or abnormal oesophageal motility. Referral is necessary to detect such associated conditions and, if symptoms merit, to consider treatment with drugs that block acid secretion. It is important to ensure the patient's consent to liaising with the medical practitioner, especially if the patient is less than 18 years of age and an eating disorder is suspected; then, careful and sensitive questioning, with involvement of the family, may be required, along with contemporaneous record keeping. Some patients may be reluctant to have dental practitioners raise such concerns with medical practitioners. However, eating disorders are one of the leading causes of mental health–related deaths – whether as a result of the systemic effects of malnutrition or of suicide – and oral healthcare professionals have a clear role to play because they may be the first to spot the early signs, such as poor oral health related to abnormal eating behaviours. If in doubt, medico-legal advice should be sought if a young patient with a suspected eating disorder does not consent to the dental practitioner liaising with parents or general medical practitioners.

A minimally invasive approach to restorative dental treatment of erosion should be taken. No immediate treatment is required if the erosion is relatively minor and the patient is happy with the appearance of his or her teeth. If the cause is identified and treated, erosion will cease or progression will be slowed down. Study models taken at yearly intervals may be compared with those taken at the initial visit to assess progression, and if the tooth wear progresses, restoration may be considered.

In the early stages of erosion, direct resin composite restorations will protect the palatal surfaces from further damage. An example in another patient is shown in Figs 60.2–60.4.

However, the finite lifespan of such restorations requires the patient's commitment to further treatment, with a median time of 6–7 years before revision becomes necessary). This can often be performed with simple minimally invasive revisions, including polishing, surface refurbishment and repair, as opposed to complete replacement of the restoration. Therefore from a consent perspective, it is important that patients are aware, at the outset, of the likely maintenance requirements associated with direct resin composite placement. More complex alternatives for restoring worn teeth, including indirect restorations designed to change the occlusal vertical dimension, are discussed in Chapter 61.

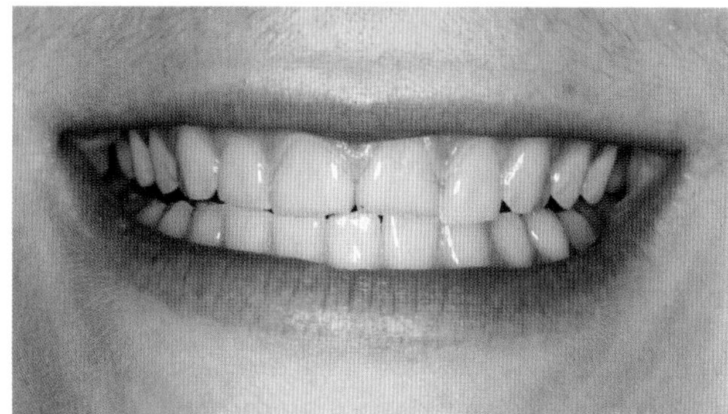

• **Fig. 60.2** Anterior closed-mouth view of another patient with erosive tooth wear requiring restorative intervention with direct composite resin restorations

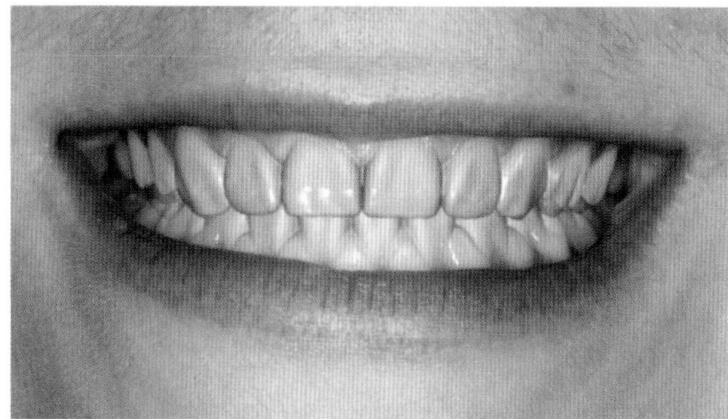

• **Fig. 60.3** 3D Digital smile design showing the proposed additions to the maxillary anterior teeth with use of resin composite restorations in an additive approach.

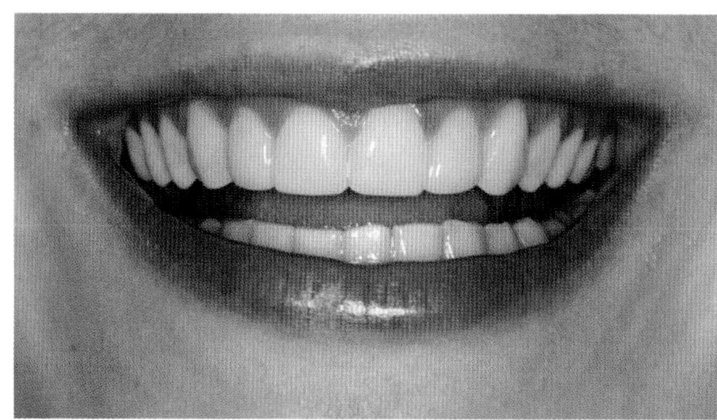

• **Fig. 60.4** Improvement in aesthetics after bleaching with 10% carbamide peroxide to improve the shade of the discoloured teeth and direct resin composite restorations to improve the final shape and aesthetics of the worn teeth,

Case 61

Worn Front Teeth

RUPERT AUSTIN AND DEBORAH BOMFIM

Summary

A 60-year-old man presents at your general dental practice saying that his teeth have worn down. What is the cause, and how should his condition be managed?

History

Complaint

The patient is concerned about his short and discoloured upper front teeth. He is also finding that he has difficulty eating. The appearance of his teeth has recently become more important to him because he has taken a job where he has to deal with the public. He wishes primarily to improve his appearance and seems to be sufficiently motivated to complete a course of complex dental treatment.

History of Complaint

The patient has only recently started to attend his dentist regularly, after a 10-year period without treatment.

Examination

Extraoral Examination

No submandibular or cervical lymph nodes are palpable, the temporomandibular joints appear normal, and there is no tenderness around the muscles of mastication. Despite the anterior tooth wear, there is no clinical evidence of a major loss of occlusal vertical dimension, such as an overclosed facial appearance and increased freeway space.

Intraoral Examination

The oral soft tissues are healthy. All teeth are present. There are deposits of plaque and staining around the cervical margins of his teeth. Despite the plaque, only a few sites display bleeding on periodontal probing, and there are no clinical signs of loss of attachment, with pocket probing depths of 2–4 mm. The appearance of the dentition can be seen inFig. 61.1.

Wear of the upper and lower anterior teeth has resulted in shortened clinical crowns, and the upper incisors and canines are markedly worn. Both the upper and lower incisors and canines have extensive areas of enamel loss and exposure of dentine. As seen in Fig. 61.1, the maxillary tooth wear is localized to the incisors and canines, whereas the premolars and molars show relatively little evidence of wear. The anterior dentition shows signs of secondary dentine formation, with sclerosis of the pulp chambers. All teeth respond normally to cold and electric pulp sensibility testing. When asked to bite his teeth together, the patient adopts a forward mandibular posture, resulting in a class III incisal relationship, as shown inFig. 61.1.

◆ What is Your Differential Diagnosis At This Stage? What Features Suggest Each Possibility?

The patient is suffering from localized severe erosive tooth wear (tooth surface loss). Erosive tooth wear is caused

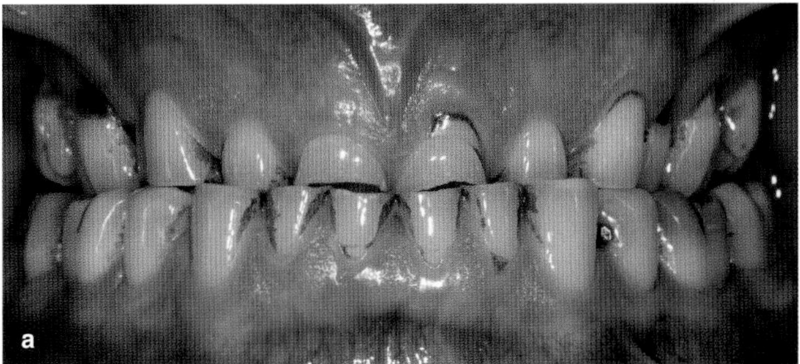

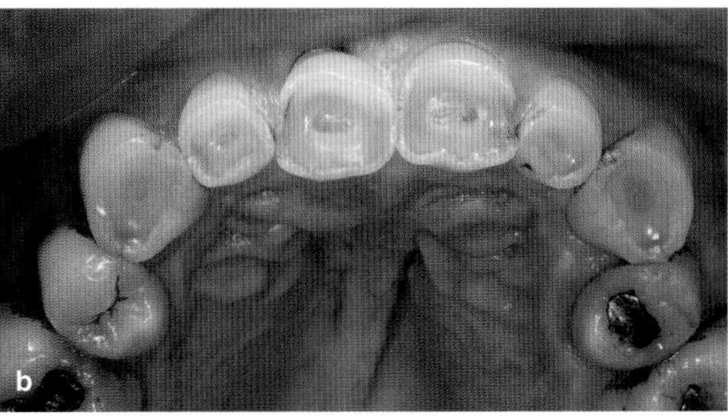

• **Fig. 61.1 a,** Anterior view of patient's dentition in maximum intercuspation; and **b,** the maxillary occlusal view of the patient's anterior dentition at presentation.

• BOX 61.1 Aetiological Factors of Tooth Wear and Their Features

Aetiological Factor	Features
Erosion	Erosion is usually caused by excessive dietary acid or gastric acid regurgitation. Both possibilities must be excluded by careful questioning and dietary analysis (see also Case 60). The appearance of the wear lesions suggests erosion as one of the main causes. Although the teeth interdigitate on incisal enamel, dentine has also been lost from areas that are not in contact with the opposing teeth. However, the presence of staining suggests that the erosion may be inactive because acids normally remove the extrinsic staining. Therefore, this points to attrition being an important factor in this case.
Attrition	Attrition is usually caused by occlusal wear, and a minor degree is normal. Bruxism and other parafunctional habits may have caused increased attrition. The class III incisal relationship also predisposes the patient to wear of the anterior teeth.
Abrasion	Abrasion of teeth is wear caused by an external agent and is seen when a coarse diet is eaten, as in developing countries, or because of abrasive oral care products or habits. There is nothing to suggest an abrasive diet or habits in this case, although the possibility should be excluded by questioning. The pattern is not consistent with a primarily abrasive process.

usually by a combination of three dynamic processes: erosion, attrition and abrasion. In this case, the tooth wear is consistent in appearance with both attrition and erosion as the main factors. See Box 61.1.

Investigations

◆ What Investigations Would You Perform? Why?

Diet analysis is required to determine whether there is excessively frequent intake of dietary acids because the frequency of intake of dietary acids increases the risk of erosive tooth wear.

Referral To the General Medical Practitioner To Investigate the Gastric Causes of Erosion.

Radiographs to assess bone levels, root morphology and possible periapical pathology. Radiographic assessment, by means of either a dental panoramic tomograph (DPT) or full-mouth long cone periapical radiographs, is necessary. Because the patient has not attended a dentist for a decade, the DPT would provide a useful survey of all maxillary and mandibular teeth. Periapical radiographs of all teeth are a reasonable alternative in this case, especially because of the better quality of images of the anterior region, in comparison with a DPT. Periapical radiographs taken with the paralleling technique, as opposed to the bisecting angle technique, would allow a more accurate assessment of bone levels.

Maxillary and mandibular study casts (Fig. 61.2) are required to determine the ideal restorative treatment option, in terms of choosing the best materials and techniques for restoring the teeth. To plan restorations for extensively worn teeth, the casts should be articulated in the retruded contact position on either a fully adjustable or semiadjustable articulator, using a facebow. Obtaining an accurate occlusal record is particularly important in this case because the patient has a habitual forward mandibular posture. The retruded contact position is a reproducible jaw relationship; therefore, study casts mounted to this occlusal record can be used to analyze this patient's occlusion and

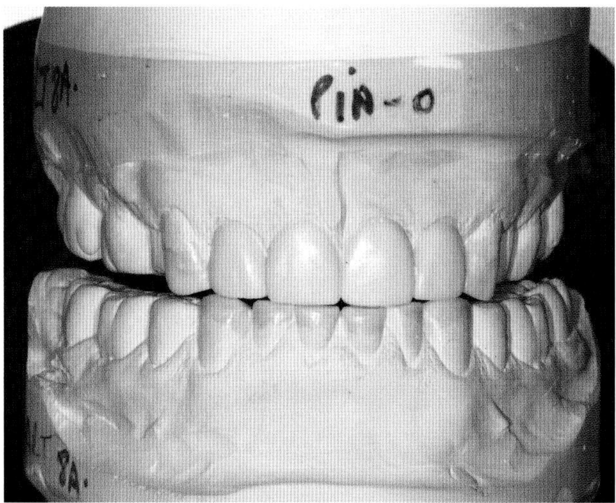

• **Fig. 61.2** Maxillary and mandibular study casts articulated on a semiadjustable articulator and a diagnostic wax-up of the anterior maxillary and mandibular dentition at an increased vertical dimension of occlusion.

to help determine the appropriate occlusal vertical dimension at which the definitive restorations could be provided. The articulated study casts can then also be used to produce a diagnostic wax-up at an increased vertical dimension to provide the proposed shape of the restorations. The diagnostic wax-up can be duplicated in stone and a soft vacuum-formed splint (or silicone matrix) formed around it; this is useful both as a surgical stent for crown lengthening and for constructing provisional chairside crowns suitable for a reorganized occlusion.

Diagnosis

The periodontal diagnosis is plaque-induced gingivitis.

Diet analysis reveals a healthy, balanced diet, with no pattern of intake of erosive foods. The patient is suffering

• BOX 61.2 Advantages and Disadvantages of Options for Managing the Occlusal Relationship

Options for Managing the Occlusal Relationship	Advantages and Disadvantages
Conformative approach	The new restorations are placed, conforming to the existing occlusal vertical dimension and intercuspal position. This means that the patient needs to make minimal adaptation to the new restorations because they will replicate the existing habitual bite (occlusion). However, if teeth are being prepared for full-coverage indirect restorations, the height of the tooth must be reduced further to produce occlusal clearance for the crowns, and this may expose the pulp. The conformative approach is usually appropriate for direct restorations, single crowns and simple bridges, where adequate sound or restored teeth predictably maintain the stability of the existing occlusion.
Reorganized	This is required when the existing occlusal vertical dimension is not conducive to provision of new restorations of adequate shape and size with a predicable outcome. For example, in this case, it is beneficial to reorganize the occlusion when providing multiple restorations that contribute to anterior guidance. In cases of tooth wear, the vertical dimension often needs to be increased and a new occlusal relationship defined to correct the maxillary–mandibular relationships and provide restorations with appropriate crown size and shape. The retruded-contact position is chosen because it is reproducible and can act as the new intercuspal position.

from tooth wear caused primarily by attrition, with an element of erosion. *The extent of the tooth wear may indicate an element of historical asymptomatic gastro-oesophageal reflux disease (GORD), but the patient had consulted a gastroenterologist, who had ruled out the presence of current GORD.*

Care Planning

◆ What is the Main Problem in Providing Restorations for These Teeth?

The short height of the crowns is the main clinical problem. The lack of enamel surface area is likely to result in poor bond strength for resin composite restorations. If conventional crowns were used, reduction of crown length would be required to create space for the crowns, and this would leave short, unretentive preparations, with an insufficient mechanical ferrule effect to retain the crowns (i.e. less than 2 mm of dentine height).

◆ What are the Two Potential Treatment Philosophies That Can Be Used To Manage the Occlusion During Provision of New Restorations in Cases Such As This? What are Their Advantages and Disadvantages, and Which Approach Should Be Chosen in This Specific Case?

One option for an extensively worn dentition is to place restorations at an increased occlusal vertical dimension. This is known as the *reorganized approach* to managing the occlusion. Alternatively, the existing jaw relationship could be maintained (i.e. the habitual occlusion) and short anterior crowns conforming to the existing intercuspal position and vertical dimension could be provided. This is known as the *conformative approach* to occlusal management. See Box 61.2.

◆ Which Approach is Necessary in This Case, and How Would You Manage the Vertical Dimension?

In this case, the reorganized approach should be adopted. This is because the crowns of the worn anterior teeth are very short. If direct resin composite restorations were used, there would insufficient surface area for bonding; in addition, the teeth would have an incorrect height-to-width ratio. If crowns were used, the natural crown would need to be reduced in height to provide occlusal clearance, and this would result in even shorter unretentive preparations and crowns with an incorrect height-to-width ratio.

◆ How Might This Problem Be Overcome?

Therefore, both an increase in the vertical dimension and surgical crown lengthening are necessary to gain space for the new tooth height. Surgical crown lengthening with alveolar bone remodelling is beneficial for increasing the available tooth tissue for retention of restorations. The gingival margin is repositioned apically to create a longer tooth, which provides greater surface area for composite bonding or an increased ferrule for retention of a crown in the conventional manner. Crown lengthening does not alter the occlusal vertical dimension because the additional crown length needed for preparation is obtained by exposing the root surfaces. Surgical crown lengthening is preferable to electrosurgery, which merely alters the gingival contour and is prone to causing a relapse. In this case, the teeth are so short that a combination of both techniques –increasing the vertical dimension of the occlusion and lengthening of the surgical crown – are required. See Fig. 61.3.

◆ How is Surgical Crown Lengthening Achieved?

The diagnostic wax-up is converted to a clear, vacuum-formed stent for guiding the surgical removal of excess gingival soft tissue and bone around the teeth (Fig. 61.4).

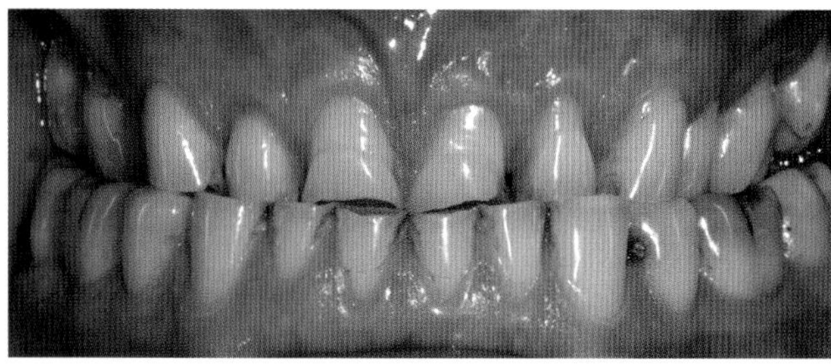

• **Fig. 61.3** The maxillary anterior teeth after surgical crown lengthening. Note the apical repositioning of the gingival margin. This will provide increased surface area for bonding of restorations or an improved axial wall height for subsequent indirect crown preparations.

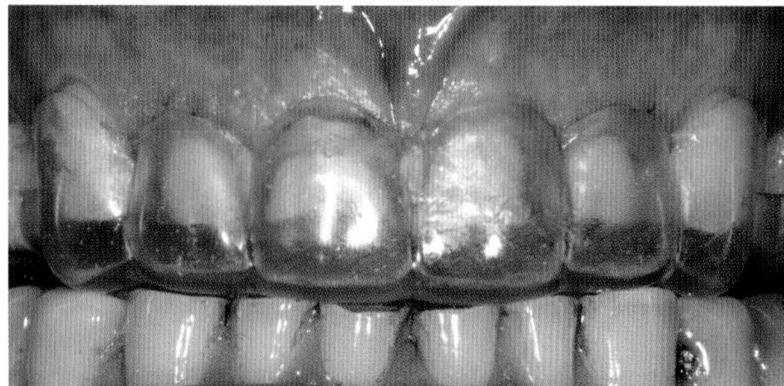

• **Fig. 61.4** The vacuum-formed stent in situ, indicating the level of gingival tissue removal required.

After site preparation and establishment of local anaesthesia, incisions are traced along the stent, and soft tissue is excised to recontour the gingival architecture. Mucoperiosteal tissue flaps are then raised buccally and palatally, and crestal bone is removed with a bur. Both the height of the bone and its width must be adapted, remodelling the alveolar contour so that the soft tissue will return to its new apical position but be able to retain the normal shape of the gingival margin. Bone is removed palatally and buccally. The amount to be removed must be determined to ensure that sufficient crown length is produced to allow a retentive preparation but support from the root is not compromised. The optimal distance from the crest of the alveolar bone to the gingival margin is 3–4 mm, which is also known as the *biological width*. Sufficient bone must be removed to preserve this distance, or the gingival tissues will regrow to their original position.

◆ What are the Disadvantages of Crown Lengthening?

- Crown lengthening results in the crown margins lying on the root surfaces of teeth. The cross-sectional area of the root is smaller than the crown so that the preparation is rather tall and narrow (and, therefore, weaker), and the final restoration is more triangular in shape, with a potentially altered emergence profile of the crown at the new gingival margin.
- Crown lengthening can result in loss of the interdental papilla, which results in poor soft tissue aesthetics, known as 'black triangles'.
- Some patients develop significant sensitivity because of the exposed dentine.
- Part of the periodontium is removed. The support of teeth with short roots may be compromised as a result.
- The procedure is uncomfortable for the patient, and up to 6–12 months may be needed for the new gingival contour to stabilize.

◆ Are There Any Alternatives To Crown Lengthening?

An alternative approach to surgical crown lengthening would be to accept the clinical crown height but gain additional retention by placing a post in the root canal. However, elective root treatment should be avoided whenever possible in cases of tooth wear. This is especially so when there is significant attrition, for instance, that resulting from a parafunctional habit. The additional occlusal loading may result in decementation of the post or fracture of the root.

Secondary dentine formation below the wear may also complicate root treatment by causing sclerosis of the pulp chamber and the root canal system.

Treatment

In this case, the decision was to provide a localized anterior reconstruction at an increased vertical dimension of occlusion by using direct resin composite restorations in combination with crown lengthening of the maxillary anterior dentition.

◆ How Should the Stages of Treatment Be Organized Into a Care Plan Culminating in Definitive Restoration? Why is Each Stage Required?

See Table 61.1.

◆ What Does Relative Axial Movement Mean in Relation To the 'Dahl' Technique?

In patients with localized anterior tooth wear, when there are adequate sound or restored posterior teeth to predictably maintain the existing occlusal relationship, the extra vertical space needed to provide sufficient thickness for the new restorations can be created by using relative axial movement of teeth (i.e. the relative intrusion of the anterior teeth and extrusion of the posterior teeth), which is known as the *Dahl approach* to creating interdental occlusal space for restorations. This is a more minimally invasive option compared to the creation of space by preparing teeth for crowns. The original Dahl appliance was described as an anterior bite plane constructed from cobalt–chrome, similar to a palatal plate major connector, which was cemented to the palatal aspects of the teeth with a relatively weak cement such as a glass–ionomer (Fig. 61.5). This approach allowed the posterior teeth to overerupt and also intruded the anterior teeth so that tooth movement, rather than tooth reduction, provided the additional interocclusal space necessary for direct or indirect restorations. The appliance was worn for approximately 3–6 months, depending on the rate of relative axial movement, with regular recalls to assess axial movement. Once the anterior teeth intruded and the posterior teeth extruded, thus re-establishing the intercuspal

TABLE 61.1 Stages of the Care Plan

Stage	Reason
Diagnostic and care planning phase	To provide study casts articulated in the retruded jaw relationship at an appropriate vertical dimension of occlusion – a diagnostic wax-up and a surgical stent for the crown lengthening. This clear stent shows the proposed new crown margin positions, ensuring that sufficient bone is removed 3–4 mm apical to this. In addition, radiographs, photographs and vitality testing will be carried out as well as nonsurgical periodontal treatment to optimize oral hygiene and to ensure resolution of any periodontal inflammation. This is always the most important phase of care delivery – 'failing to plan is planning to fail'!
Diagnostic try-in/ mock-up	A matrix of the wax-up can be used to do an intraoral try-in by using a bis-acryl composite material, to show the patient the eventual shape and relationships of the planned crowns to the new gingival architecture. Once the patient has approved this, the surgical stent can be constructed. The wax-up can also be used to produce a matrix, which is used to guide the composite bonding or, if crowns are to be provided, as a matrix to guide the preparations and the construction of the provisional restorations, using a bis-acryl composite temporary crown material.
Surgical phase	To gain length for retention of the restorations. Usually, the upper arch is treated first because it is technically easier. The direct composite resin restorations establish the new anterior guidance, which can be copied into future crowns once the occlusion has stabilized or if the direct composites require replacement with indirect restorations.
Healing period	The interval between periodontal surgery and placement of provisional crowns should be in the order of a few weeks because there is some evidence that the tissues can heal back to their original position. Definitive restorations can be provided once the gingival contour is stable, usually around 3–6 months after surgery.
Restorative phase	Provision of direct composite resin restorations at an increased vertical dimension of occlusion. If the 'Dahl approach' is used to manage the occlusal vertical dimension, a further 3–6 months will be required to allow relative axial movement of teeth to re-established posterior occlusal contacts.
Maintenance phase	Once the posterior occlusal contacts have re-established, a hard occlusal splint should be provided to protect the restorations from future wear caused by parafunctional habits such as bruxism.

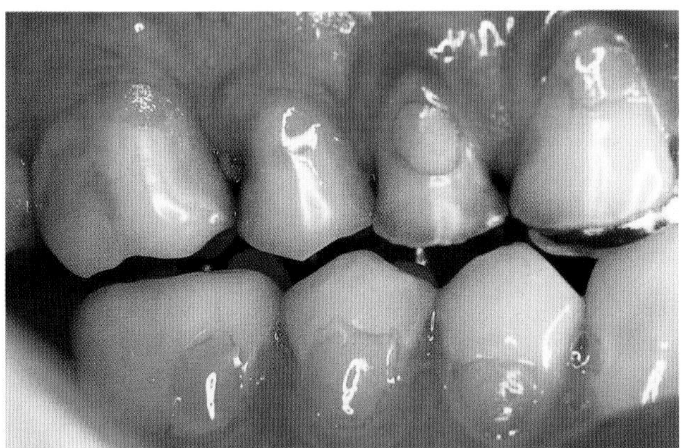

• **Fig. 61.5** A different patient with a conventional Dahl appliance that was used to allow relative axial movement, after which the cobalt–chromium appliance was removed and restorations placed on the anterior teeth.

position, the cobalt–chrome appliance was removed, leaving a space between the front teeth, which was then used to provide interocclusal space for the new restorations.

More recently, direct resin composite restorations are being prescribed as the first restoration of choice for localized anterior tooth wear cases, in order to provide the new definitive restorations at the increased vertical dimension of occlusion and allow the posterior occlusion to re-establish in due course. This avoids the need for a lengthy provisional phase of treatment. However, if the definitive restorations are to be conventional full-coverage crowns, then the direct resin composite restorations are often seen as a provisional treatment to be used whilst the occlusion is being reorganized, and then the definitive crowns can be provided in a conformative approach to the new intercuspal position.

Medico-Legal Issues

As with all cases where potentially lengthy and complex prosthodontic treatment is required, such as those increasing the occlusal vertical dimension to replace missing tooth tissue from erosive tooth wear, it is medico-legally advisable for general dental practitioners to liaise with specialist colleagues to formulate an optimal care plan and to ensure that patients understand all the risks and benefits of the potential options for their oral rehabilitation. A general dental practitioner has a key role to play in case selection and communicating to patients the benefits of either local anterior reconstruction or full-mouth rehabilitations at a reorganized occlusal scheme. The treatment can then be carried out in general dental practice, with frequent liaising with a prosthodontist or restorative specialist and some guidance during the initial phases. Once the provisional restorations have allowed the occlusion to establish a new intercuspal position that is stable and maintainable, provision of definitive restorations conforming to this new occlusal scheme is then straightforward and can be carried out

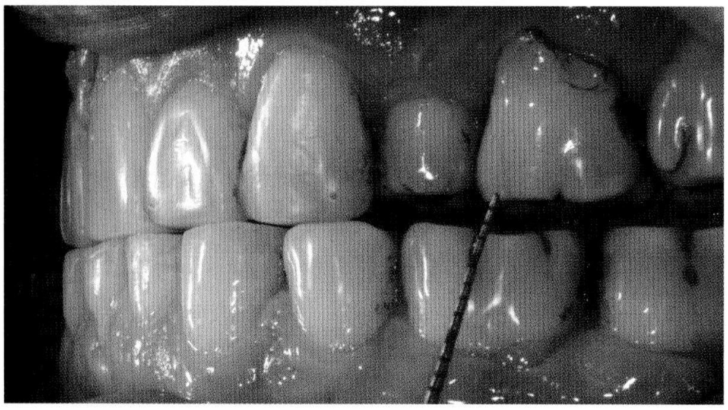

• **Fig. 61.6** Photograph of the dentition at 12 months after treatment, showing a 2-mm space between the maxillary and mandibular teeth that had not been closed by relative axial movement.

in general dental practice. However, on occasion, patients do not respond in a predicable manner when the occlusal vertical dimension is changed. As can be seen in Fig. 61.6, although the patient was comfortable with the new restorations and had satisfactory function and aesthetics, with just the anterior teeth in occlusion, relative axial movement had not occurred at 12 months after treatment and a hard occlusal splint had to be provided for nighttime wear to prevent excessive wear of the restorations. The plans and discussions must be recorded contemporaneously, and keeping clinical photographic records of the different stages is desirable. The patient must be made fully aware of his or her responsibility towards maintaining optimal oral hygiene to prolong the functional life of the definitive restorations placed, as well as attending 6-month recall consultations to ensure that avoidable problems are prevented. This level of care also involves use of a complete oral healthcare team, including hygienists or therapists who can deliver the preventive care required.

Therefore, when multiple restorations, especially indirect conventional restorations, are being used to provide a local or full-arch oral reconstruction at an increased vertical dimension, it is advisable to seek specialist opinion from a prosthodontist or a restorative dentistry specialist. This helps ensure good communication with patients so that they can understand the nature of the treatment and provide fully informed consent after being educated about the maintenance measures required, should the treatment proceed optimally, and about the potential benefits and risks, including the requirement for replacement or further remedial work that may be needed.

Case 62

A Case of Toothache

ERIC WHAITES

Summary

A 36-year-old Nigerian woman presents at your practice for the first time, complaining of toothache.

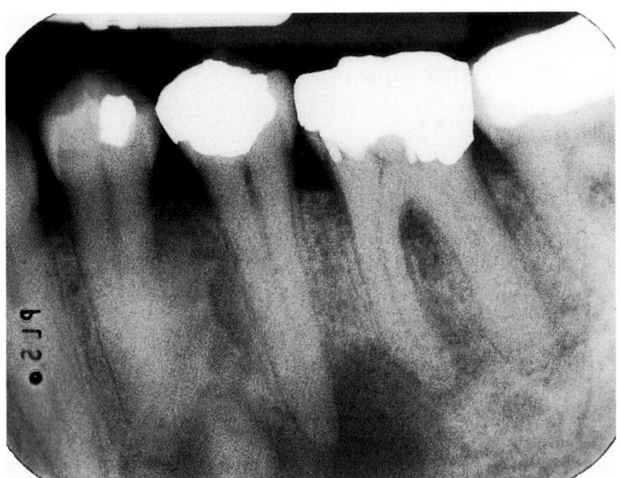

• **Fig. 62.1** Periapical radiograph of both lower left premolars and the first molar.

History

Complaint

The patient complains of toothache associated with her lower left teeth and points somewhat imprecisely to the lower left quadrant.

History of Complaint

The patient has been aware of intermittent pain at this site for several months. Initially, the pain was short lived and brought on by hot and cold drinks, but in the last few days, the discomfort has become progressively worse. She is now suffering a fairly constant and very painful toothache that is no longer closely related to hot and cold stimuli.

Medical History

She is otherwise fit and well, and no positive findings are revealed by the medical history.

Examination

Extraoral Examination

She is a fit and healthy-looking African woman. The submandibular lymph nodes are not palpable. There is no detectable soft tissue swelling, and the temporomandibular joints appear normal.

Intraoral Examination

The lower left second premolar and first and second permanent molars are heavily restored. There is only a small restoration in the first premolar. Several other teeth contain smaller restorations. The surrounding oral mucosa appears normal, and there is no bony enlargement or swelling. No tenderness is elicited on palpation of the lingual or buccal sulcus adjacent to the teeth, and the contour of the tissues appears normal.

◆ How Do You Interpret the History and Examination Results So Far?

The clear history of toothache (which is normally correctly identified by patients) and the large restorations suggest that one or more teeth may be the cause of the pain, probably as a result of caries or complications of restoration. The pain is poorly localized, severe, feels like toothache and has been exacerbated by hot and cold stimuli, almost certainly indicating pulpitis. The recent onset of pain unrelated to hot and cold suggests late or irreversible pulpitis but that the causative pulp remains partially vital. The history does not suggest spread of infection or inflammation to the periodontal ligament, which is normally associated with pain on biting and accurate localization of the causative tooth by the patient.

◆ What Simple Additional Examinations Would You Perform, and Why?

All the teeth in the lower left quadrant distal to, and including, the canine should be percussed. The same teeth should be tested for vitality, together with their equivalent lower right teeth for comparison (provided there are no clinical features, such as caries or restorations, suggesting that these also have compromised vitality).

When this was done, it is found that no teeth were particularly tender to percussion. Both the second premolar and the first molar might be slightly tender (the patient is unclear), but neither gives a dull percussive note. The second premolar is vital. The first molar is slightly hypersensitive, both by electric pulp testing and application of a cold stimulus (ethyl chloride), neither test causing acute pain.

Investigations

◆ What Investigation Would You Now Undertake, and Why?

An intraoral periapical radiograph of the lower left premolars and the first molar should be taken. So far, the examination indicates that the first molar is the most likely cause of the pain. However, the patient is vague as to whether the second premolar is tender to percussion, and it contains a large restoration. There may be two causes for the pain.

A radiograph cannot provide direct evidence of vitality. However, it will provide information on the possible causes of loss of vitality, the presence of caries and inadequate restorations, as well as revealing previous attempted root canal treatment and periapical granuloma or infection (provided there has been sufficient time for apical bone loss to develop). A radiograph will also be required in the event that either extraction or root canal treatment is necessary.

◆ The Periapical Radiograph is Shown in Fig. 62.1. What Do You See?

The periapical radiograph shows:

- A small restoration in the first premolar
- Large restorations in the second premolar and first and second molars
- No radiographic evidence of dental caries
- Early bifurcation bone loss associated with the first molar
- A radiolucent area that is centred on the apex of the second premolar and appears to extend to involve the mesial root of the first molar
- Loss of lamina dura around the apex of the root of the second premolar and the first molar mesial root
- An irregular but relatively well-defined radiopaque zone distal to the first premolar root.

◆ What Would You Do Next, and Why?

Further radiographic views are required. The radiograph has not aided diagnosis of the dental pain because no unsuspected cause for the pulpitis has been identified. However, it has revealed an apical radiolucency on the second premolar and the first molar, and this is not compatible with an uncomplicated periapical granuloma, infection or cyst. The presence of an apical radiolucency on the second premolar is also incompatible with the history and examination results, which indicate that this tooth is vital.

The presence of both radiopacity and radiolucency requires consideration of a wider differential diagnosis, which would include fibro-cemento-osseous lesions, odontogenic tumours and a variety of bone disorders. The margins of the radiolucent lesion are not visible on the radiograph and need to be defined before a more accurate differential diagnosis can be proposed. Because some fibro-cemento-osseous lesions may be bilateral, appropriate views would be a dental panoramic radiograph or right and left oblique laterals. These will also allow all teeth and their supporting structures to be assessed because the patient is being seen in the practice for the first time. Bitewing radiographs to assess caries would also be appropriate in a new patient with several heavily restored teeth if there is clinical suspicion of caries.

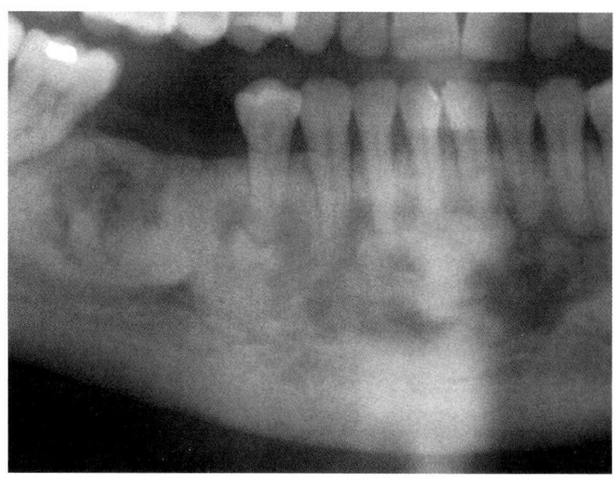

• **Fig. 62.2** Section from the dental panoramic radiograph.

◆ Part of the Dental Panoramic Radiograph is Shown in Fig. 62.2. What Do You See?

The additional radiograph shows several features, including:

- Absent lower right second premolar and first molar, presumed extracted
- A small occlusal restoration in the lower left second molar, which has tipped slightly mesially
- An extensive lesion of mixed radiodensity involving the central body of the mandible from the mesial root of the second molar across the midline to join that shown previously on the left
- The lesion appears to be composed of several radiolucencies, often with a central opacity centred on the root apices
- Little or no expansion of the bone despite the extensive lesion
- The lesion is not displacing teeth or the inferior dental nerve canal

Diagnosis

◆ What are the Causes of a Mixed Radiolucency Such As This in the Jaws?

- Cemento-osseous dysplasias
  - — Periapical
  - — Focal
  - — Florid
- Chronic osteomyelitis
- Paget's disease of bone

- Fibrous dysplasia
- Metastatic malignancy.

◆ What is the Most Likely Diagnosis? Explain Why

One of the cemento-osseous dysplasias is the most likely cause of the patient's jaw lesions. The diagnosis may be made on the radiographic appearances alone. No other condition produces multiple lesions centred on the apices of the teeth, each with a central radiopacity and a variable and poorly defined radiolucent rim. As disease progresses, this pattern may become less distinct, but it is clearly visible in several of this patient's lesions. This patient has the florid form of the disease, with one or more quadrants affected. The periapical form affects a few teeth, usually the lower incisors, and the focal form gives rise to one large lesion, but all are part of a spectrum of disease severity. The diagnosis is supported by the patient's race, these conditions being more prevalent in those of African and Mongoloid races. The lesion(s) are normally asymptomatic.

◆ What Diagnoses Have You Excluded? Explain Why

Chronic osteomyelitis produces a patchy mixed radiolucency but would show symptoms of dull, boring, central bone pain that is quite distinct from those reported. Sinuses or other signs of infection would probably be present. However, this diagnosis should not be completely excluded without further consideration because the sclerotic bone of fibro-cemento-osseous lesions, such as florid cemento-osseous dysplasia, is prone to infection, particularly dental infection, and in the past, the condition was thought to be a form of osteomyelitis. A biopsy to confirm the diagnosis is contraindicated because of the risk of initiating osteomyelitis.

Paget's disease of bone may be confidently excluded because it almost never affects the mandible without producing obvious lesions, signs and symptoms in other bones. If this were Paget's disease, the maxilla would usually be more severely affected. Paget's disease affects predominantly older Caucasians.

Fibrous dysplasia might be considered a cause of patchy and poorly defined radiolucency, but it presents with expansion of the jaw, usually the maxilla, during the first or second decade of life.

Metastatic malignancy might also be considered a further cause. Most cancers cause purely radiolucent lesions, but some, notably prostate and breast cancers, may cause bony sclerosis and 'sun ray' radiopacity. However, the site is usually near the angle of the mandible, and the radiological appearances are sufficiently characteristic of florid cemento-osseous dysplasia to exclude this sinister diagnosis.

◆ How Might You Confirm the Diagnosis Without Biopsy?

Any previous radiographs should be reviewed to determine whether the lesion has been present and slowly progressing for several years. This would confirm the diagnosis.

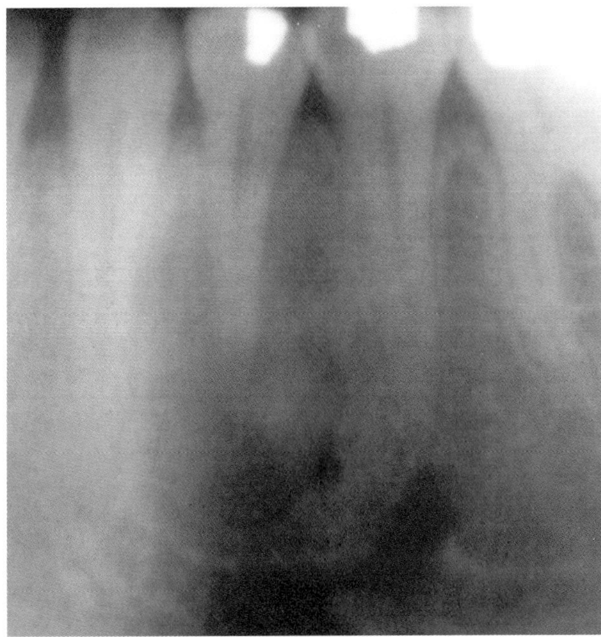

• **Fig. 62.3** Section from the dental panoramic tomograph taken 11 years previously.

A previous dental practitioner was contacted and provided the radiograph seen in Fig. 62.3, which had been taken 11 years previously.

The radiograph shows the lower left quadrant. The lower left second premolar and first molar contain smaller restorations than at present, and there is probable caries in the second premolar. However, the first premolar appears to contain the same restoration as at present, and at its apex, there is a lesion typical of early cemento-osseous dysplasia comprising radiolucency with central opacity at the root apex. This early stage of the lesion provides conclusive evidence for the proposed diagnosis.

◆ What Would You Do About the Patient's Pain?

The causative tooth must be properly identified, and in this patient, the electric pulp test suggested that the first molar is to blame. The increased sensitivity on electric and cold pulp testing may be explained by the presence of pulpitis or small vital pulp remnants in an otherwise nonvital pulp.

When pulp tests fail to identify a definite cause, the most effective method is to perform a test cavity without local analgesia in the most likely tooth. This is not possible (or usually required) in a tooth with acute pulpitis but works well in cases of chronic low-grade pain if a pulp is completely or partially viable or when the patient's response to testing cannot be relied on.

Alternatively, a diagnostic local analgesic injection may be given to abolish the pain, but this is not usually useful for first molars, where a block is required for effective analgesia. Once the anaesthetic is given, no further pulp tests are possible at that visit.

When a test cavity was performed, the first molar was found to be nonvital, with vital pulp in one canal only. Either root canal treatment or extraction was required.

◆ What About the Apical Radiolucency On the Second Premolar?

This was another early lesion of cemento-osseous dysplasia. *Some years later, radiographs revealed that the lesion had developed a zone of radiopacity centrally.*

◆ Does Florid Cemento-Osseous Dysplasia Have Any Significant Complications?

Yes. Precautions must be taken to ensure that the patient does not develop osteomyelitis in the sclerotic bone of the mandible. A regimen for prevention of caries and periodontal disease must be instituted to reduce the risk of future dental infection. In this patient, the periodontal condition of the first molar was poor, so extraction was the preferred option. Other nonvital teeth should also be extracted if there are reasons to suspect that root canal treatment may not be successful. Antibiotics should be prescribed during the healing period for all extractions involving the affected bone. Any surgery in the mandible should be similarly covered and is best performed in hospital rather than in a general practice, unless the practitioner has the appropriate experience.

Case 63

A Child with a Swollen Face

ERIC WHAITES

Summary

A 5-year-old boy has painless bilateral facial swellings. Identify the cause, and recommend a treatment.

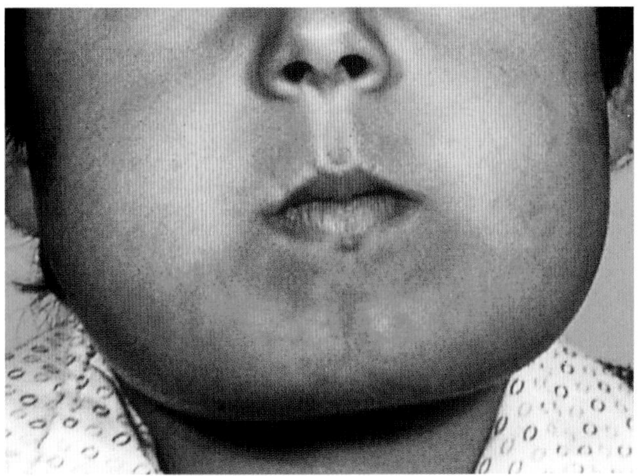

• **Fig. 63.1** The patient's appearance at presentation.

History

Complaint

The patient is brought by his parents, who have noticed that his face has 'become fat'. They are concerned about the child's appearance and say that he is being teased and bullied at school.

History of Complaint

His parents say that their child has had a chubby face since he was a toddler but that the swelling has become more noticeable in the last 2 years. He is in no pain.

Medical History

The boy is otherwise fit and well, has had all recommended immunizations and, amongst childhood illnesses, has suffered only chicken pox. His medical practitioner performed a general examination and found no systemic illness but has referred the boy to you for a further opinion.

Examination

Extraoral Examination

The appearance of the child is shown in Fig. 63.1. He appears healthy but has obvious bilateral enlargement of the sides of the face. The temporomandibular joints appear normal on palpation. Some upper deep cervical lymph nodes are palpable bilaterally. They are only slightly enlarged, are not tender and are freely mobile.

◆ **On the Basis of What You Know, What Types of Lesion Would You Consider?**

From this view alone, it is difficult to tell whether the swelling originates in the salivary glands, mandible or soft tissues. Each site would have different possible causes, as shown in Table 63.1.

Intraoral Examination

Intraoral examination reveals a minimally restored dentition and healthy oral mucosa. Palpation of the mandibular rami shows that they are the source of the enlargement. There is obvious rounded swelling of the posterior body and ramus of the mandible. The lower right second deciduous molar is missing.

Investigations

◆ **A Radiograph is Obviously Required. Which View(s) Would You Choose?**

A dental panoramic radiograph is the investigation of choice as an initial view. The whole of the swellings will be visible, and the left and right sides can be easily compared. A posterior–anterior view of the jaws would also be useful, providing a second view at right angles to the ramus in the panoramic view. It would allow the mediolateral expansion to be assessed.

The radiographic appearance is shown in Fig. 63.2.

◆ **What are the Radiographic Features of the Lesions?**

See Table 63.2.

TABLE 63.1 Possible Causes of Facial Swelling

Condition	Possible Causes
Soft tissue enlargement	Masseteric hypertrophy is possible. Bruxism is common in children, although significant masseteric hypertrophy is rare.
Salivary gland enlargement	Rare in children. Human immunodeficiency virus (HIV) salivary cystic disease is seen in HIV infection. Mumps can be excluded. Mumps is acute, and the child would also have had a mumps vaccine with the rest of the routine childhood vaccinations.
Enlargement of the mandible	A few rare inherited disorders of bone could cause bilateral expansion of the ramus.
A developmental syndrome	Many syndromes have craniofacial signs, and this is a possibility that should be borne in mind. There appear to be no associated features.

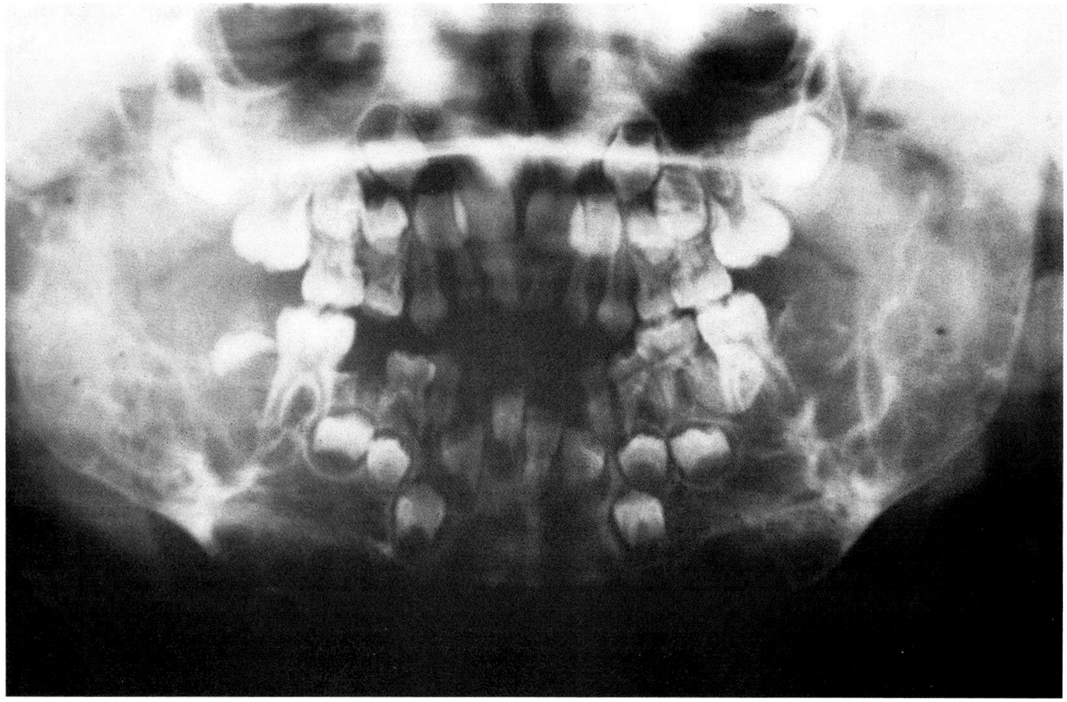

• **Fig. 63.2** Dental panoramic radiograph.

TABLE 63.2 Radiographic Features

Site	Bilateral in the posterior body, angle and rami of the mandible
Size	Relatively large, about 5 × 8 cm
Shape	Multilocular lesions on both sides
Type of outline/edge	Smooth, well-defined and well-corticated
Relative radiodensity	Radiolucent, with internal radiopaque septa producing a multilocular appearance; no dense radiopaque inclusions
Effects on adjacent structures	Gross displacement of the developing permanent second molars; lower right second primary molar has been lost, presumably through exfoliation; extensive expansion of the height of the body of the mandible; condyles not affected

TABLE 63.3 Differential Diagnosis

Diagnosis	Similarity to Present Case
Cherubism	Causes bilateral radiolucencies in the mandibular rami and maxilla. Enlargement starts in children before the age of 5 years. The lesions appear multilocular and radiolucent and disrupt the dentition. The radiographic and facial appearances in this case are characteristic.
Other possible causes	There are a few very rare bone diseases and syndromes that may need to be considered if the most likely diagnosis of cherubism cannot be confirmed. Almost all other causes have prominent signs elsewhere in the body, and none has been noted in this case.

Differential Diagnosis

◆ Give a Differential Diagnosis. Explain Which is the Most Likely Cause, and Why

There is only a very short list of possible differential diagnoses for this case (Table 63.3).

◆ What Further Questions Might Help Confirm Your Diagnosis?

Did Either Parent Have a Similar Problem? Cherubism is inherited in an autosomal dominant fashion. Radiographs of both parents may reveal unsuspected healed lesions, and this would aid in making a definitive diagnosis.

Are Any Brothers or Sisters Affected? For the same reason, siblings would be expected to show similar signs.

How Was the Lower Second Deciduous Molar Lost? Cherubism may cause early exfoliation of teeth.

◆ Would Any Further Radiographs Help Confirm the Diagnosis?

More detailed radiographic examination with intraoral images would be helpful for the following reasons:

- **To demonstrate involvement of the maxilla.** More severely affected patients usually have lesions in the maxilla, usually centred on the tuberosity, but sometimes extending to distort the orbit. These can easily be missed on extraoral images but, if present, confirm the diagnosis.
- **To identify displacement or destruction of teeth.** As noted above, cherubism often destroys tooth germs and displaces teeth.

◆ Is Biopsy Required?

In a classic case of cherubism, the diagnosis may be made with certainty on the basis of family history and clinical and radiographic features. In a new case such as this, or if there were no family history, it would be prudent to confirm that the lesions are histologically compatible with cherubism.

◆ A Biopsy Specimen Was Removed From the Expanded Alveolar Ridge. The Histological Appearances are Shown in Fig. 63.3. What Do You See?

The lesion is composed of cellular fibrous tissue, which appears loose and oedematous, with spaces, rather than dense collagen, between the cells. Scattered in the fibrous tissue are multinucleate giant cells. These are relatively small giant cells and have only 4–8 nuclei each.

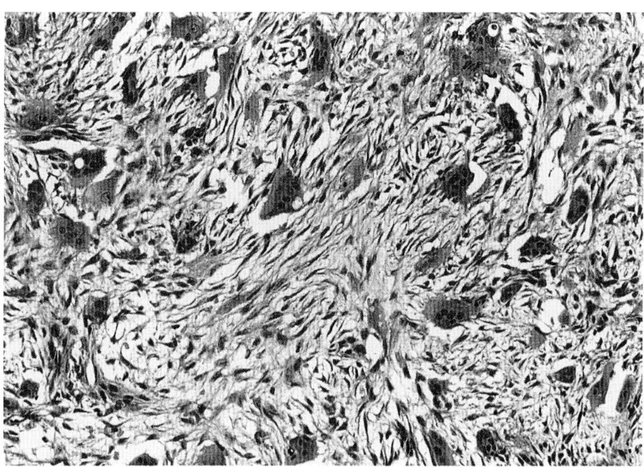

• **Fig. 63.3** The histological appearance of the biopsy specimen.

◆ How Do You Interpret These Appearances? Are They Consistent with Cherubism?

Lesions with many giant cells fall into two broad categories – (1) those with granulomas such as tuberculosis, sarcoidosis and foreign body reactions and (2) giant cell lesions. No granulomas are present, and these appearances indicate a giant cell lesion, the causes of which are:

- Central giant cell granuloma
- Brown tumour of hyperparathyroidism
- Aneurysmal bone cyst
- Cherubism.

These conditions cannot be distinguished from one another on histological grounds alone. However, the only one that matches the clinical and radiographic findings in this case is cherubism.

Diagnosis

Taken together, the evidence supports a diagnosis of cherubism, and this is a typical case.

Aetiology

◆ What is the Cause of Cherubism?

Cherubism is caused by any one of several mutations in the *SH3BP2* gene, a regulator of the *C-Abl* oncogene, a poorly understood signalling molecule involved in the regulation of cell division and many other cell functions.

The condition is usually inherited in an autosomal dominant fashion. It would be expected that one parent would be similarly affected. Females are often less severely affected, and cases may appear to be sporadic.

Treatment

◆ What Treatment Would You Recommend? What Other Advice Would You Give To the Parents?

No treatment is required, although the parents and the child may need reassurance. The parents can be told that lesions of cherubism usually grow fastest before the age of 5 years. Although there will be further growth during the next few years, the lesions will stop growing spontaneously and start to regress around the age of puberty. The swelling should have completely resolved by the age of 25 years, and only radiographic changes will remain into the fourth decade.

Surgical intervention is not usually necessary but may be performed for cosmetic reasons if the lesions are resolving slowly. Some teeth will be lost through the disease process. The parents should also be warned that future children and siblings are likely to be affected. Genetic counselling would be appropriate.

Case 64

Recurrent Neck Swelling

BETHAN THOMAS, NIALL O'NEILL AND MICHAEL ESCUDIER

Summary

A 35-year-old man presents complaining of an intermittent swelling in his neck at mealtimes. What are the possible causes, appropriate investigations and treatment options?

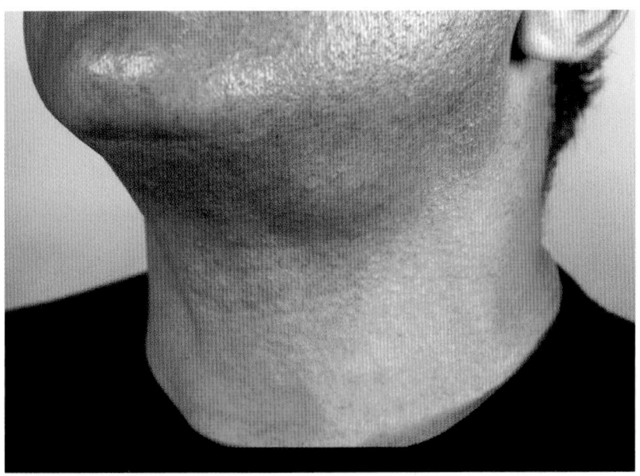

• **Fig. 64.1** The patient on presentation.

History

Complaint

The patient complains of a swelling of the left neck below the angle of the jaw. It appears suddenly on eating and is painful, lasts 30–60 minutes and then subsides slowly. He reports that the swelling is worse when eating certain foods, such as citrus fruit.

History of Complaint

The swelling first appeared suddenly during a meal 3 years ago. It resolved within 15 minutes. In the following month, the patient experienced the same swelling three times and since then has experienced occasional swelling, always associated with food intake. The swelling always resolves quickly and does not cause pain. However, over the last 4 months, the swelling has recurred more frequently and the area has become tender. In the last 2 weeks, the swelling has occurred at almost every meal and takes at least 1 hour to resolve.

Medical History

The patient is otherwise fit and healthy. He is not currently on any medication.

◆ How Do You Interpret the Information You Have So Far?

The patient is describing the symptom known as 'mealtime syndrome', which refers to swelling of a salivary gland associated with eating, the thought of eating or the smell of food. The location of the swelling is important, indicating that the site correlates with a salivary gland. The recurrent nature of the swelling indicates that mealtime syndrome is the most likely underlying process. The cause of mealtime syndrome is obstruction of a salivary gland duct. Between meals, the low flow of saliva can leak around a partial obstruction. When flow is stimulated, the increased volume of saliva is prevented from passing down the duct causing the gland to swell. This can induce pain because the gland is restricted within a capsule. The increase in severity of the symptoms indicates that the degree of obstruction has increased.

◆ Are There Any Specific Questions You Would Ask? Why?

The patient should be asked if he has noticed any abnormality such as a sudden resolution of the swelling following a discharge of saliva or salty fluid into the mouth because this would confirm intermittent obstruction. A report of foul-tasting saliva could indicate infection of the gland.

Examination

Extraoral Examination

◆ The Appearance of the Swelling is Shown in Fig. 64.1. What Do You See?

The patient has a round swelling, approximately 3 cm in diameter, in the region of the left submandibular gland, below the lower border of the mandible on the left side and just anterior to the angle of the mandible. *If you were able to palpate the neck, you would feel no cervical lymphadenopathy and find that the swelling is firm, mobile and tender.*

TABLE 64.1 Important Features of Intraoral Examination

Examination	Rationale
Bimanual palpation	Bimanual palpation of the submandibular gland will allow the gland to be fully examined. Palpation from only one side displaces the mobile gland. Bimanual palpation involves a finger placed at the posterior aspect of the floor of mouth pushing onto the superior surface of the gland, with the clinician's fingers of the other hand palpating the gland extraorally on its inferior aspect. This helps distinguish between swelling of the gland itself, a lump within the gland, or an adjacent enlarged lymph node.
Expression of saliva from the salivary gland ducts	Massaging a healthy gland, with no obstruction, should produce a free flow of clear saliva from the duct orifice. Cloudy saliva indicates infection or inflammation. Lack of saliva on massaging may indicate reduced secretion or blockage. Pus indicates infection, and a sample should be taken for culture and sensitivity.

Intraoral Examination

◆ What Features of the Intraoral Examination are Important?

See Table 64.1.

When you examine the patient, you discover that the oral mucosa and the dentition appear normal. A small amount of clear saliva can be expressed from the orifice of the left submandibular duct but less than that expressed from the right submandibular duct. Bimanual palpation reveals a firm lump, 3 cm in diameter, palpable in the floor of mouth near the posterior free border of mylohyoid muscle and extraorally in the submandibular triangle. The lump is freely mobile vertically and appears to be the enlarged left submandibular gland.

Diagnosis

The patient has mealtime syndrome, probably as the result of an obstruction in the duct. The gland is firm because of fibrosis from chronic sialadenitis caused by repetitive obstruction and possibly intermittent ascending low-grade infection.

◆ What are the Possible Causes of Obstruction?

See Table 64.2.

TABLE 64.2 Causes of Salivary Duct Obstruction

Type	Cause
Intraductal causes (common)	Sialolithiasis (salivary stone, salivary calculus) Ductal stricture Mucus plug
Extraductal causes (rare)	Trauma Pressure or invasion from an adjacent neoplasm (e.g. sublingual gland tumour or anterior floor of mouth squamous cell carcinoma), or other swelling

◆ Are There Any Other Causes of Intermittent Swelling That Need To Be Considered?

Yes. Intermittent swelling may be seen in wind instrument players who force air or liquids back into the gland. This may present as unilateral or bilateral swelling. Several other chronic conditions can cause persistent swelling. These include sialadenitis (usually the result of obstruction), primary Sjögren's syndrome, sialosis, drug-induced salivary gland swelling (caused by iodine-containing compounds, phenylbutazone, chlorhexidine and other drugs). This last group does not generally cause such obvious and short-lived swelling as is seen with obstruction.

Investigations

◆ What Investigations are Required? Why?

The diagnosis is often clear from the clinical history and examination. Investigations are required to confirm the cause of the obstruction and to plan treatment. Radiological investigations will provide information on the cause of the blockage, the site of the blockage and the degree of damage sustained by the gland and ducts from sialadenitis. Useful investigations are shown in Table 64.3.

In this case, ultrasonography and sialography were performed as initial investigations.

◆ The Ultrasound Scan is Shown in Fig. 64.2. What Do You See?

Ultrasonography is a dynamic investigation, and the ultrasound operator may observe the screen for several minutes, altering the angle of the ultrasound transducer (transmitter/detector) to provide views at different angles. Representative images are captured to demonstrate key findings and support the scan report but interpretation of a single image can be challenging for the less experienced clinician. Ultrasound scans are conventionally orientated with the skin surface of the patient (ultrasound transducer) at the top of the image. Objects that reflect ultrasound, such as stones, appear white and cast a dark acoustic shadow because of the inability of the ultrasound waves to penetrate the calcified stone. Dilated ducts, proximal to the stone, appear as dark spaces.

The unlabelled ultrasound scan is shown on the left, and the annotated landmarks are highlighted in the image on the right. There is a calculus in the left submandibular gland. The gland is slightly heterogeneous/mottled in appearance because of sialadenitis. The calculus appears as a

TABLE 64.3 Investigations for Salivary Gland Obstruction

Investigation	Rationale and Role
Ultrasonography	Ultrasonography is noninvasive and does not involve ionizing radiation. It demonstrates the salivary parenchyma, giving an indication of gland status (inflammation, atrophy, enlargement). In the hands of an experienced operator, it can demonstrate stones over 2 mm in diameter and identify enlarged, inflamed lymph nodes, but has limited use in assessing the duct architecture.
Plain radiography	Simple to perform for detection of radiopaque stones in the duct or in the submandibular gland. For the submandibular gland, a lower 90-degree occlusal view, lateral view, oblique lateral view, or panoramic tomography may be considered. A parotid stone may be visualized on a posteroanterior jaw view if the cheek is blown out to reduce superimposition on other structures. Only radiopaque calculi will be detected on plain radiographs. 60–80% of submandibular stones and 20–40% of parotid stones are radiopaque. Radiolucent 'stones' are poorly mineralized masses of inspissated mucin.
Sialography	This is a special investigation carried out by radiologists, involving cannulation of the salivary duct and infusion of a radiopaque contrast medium into the duct. The contrast contains iodine and is, therefore, contraindicated in patients with iodine hypersensitivity. It provides valuable information on the architecture of the duct system and: – Cause of obstruction (whether stone or stricture) – Size and position of stone or stricture – Diameter and length of the duct distal to the obstruction (to assess feasibility of treatment) – Disruption of the duct system within the gland, as an indication of sialadenitis and gland damage – An indirect indication of gland function, by assessing whether there is spontaneous clearance of contrast.
Sialendoscopy	This is an invasive investigation, performed under local anaesthesia. It uses fine endoscopes, ranging from 0.8 to 1.6 mm in diameter placed into the main duct. The endoscopes allow direct inspection of the duct lumen and walls. Sialendoscopy can be used to diagnose the presence of stones, strictures and inflammatory conditions. It can also guide interventional procedures. The technique cannot access the deepest parts of the ductal system, and it is sometimes not possible to view beyond obstructions, thus only providing a partial assessment of the duct.
Computed tomography (CT) or cone beam computed tomography (CBCT)	CT is particularly sensitive for detecting small stones. It is approximately 10 times more sensitive than plain radiography but involves a higher x-ray dose. It has limitations in its ability to assess the details of the duct architecture.
Magnetic resonance imaging (MRI)	MRI provides excellent soft tissue contrast. This is the technique of choice to assess a possible neoplasm within a gland or adjacent to a duct resulting in obstruction. It can distinguish salivary gland disease from an enlarged lymph node. MRI sialography involves the simultaneous use of a sialogogue to fill the ducts with saliva at the time of image capture, thus highlighting the duct system.
Radioisotope scanning	This technique has limited value in assessing salivary gland obstruction because of its very low resolution. It is a functional study mainly reserved for investigation of xerostomia.

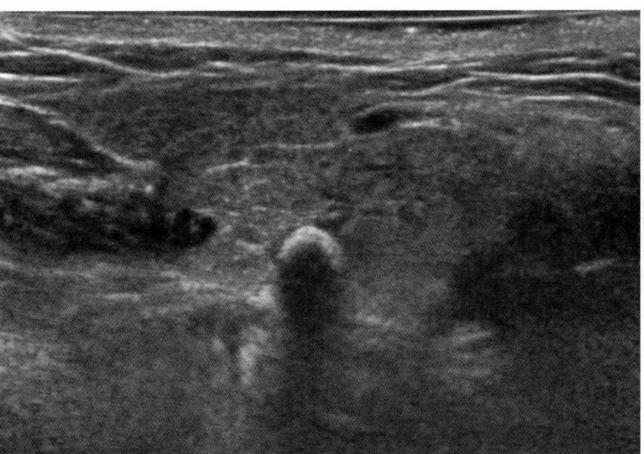

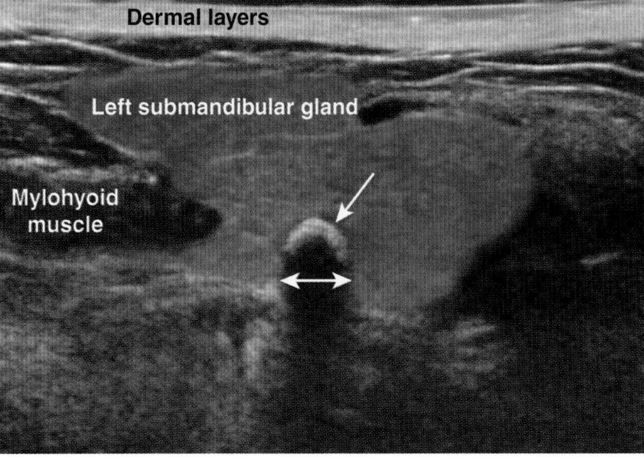

• **Fig. 64.2** The ultrasound scan.

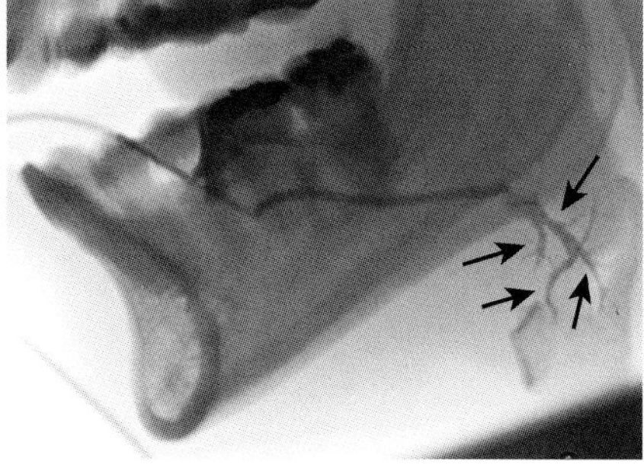

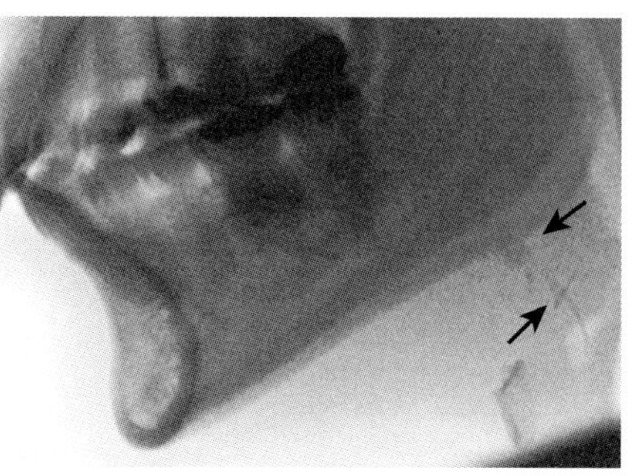

a b c

• **Fig. 64.3** Sialogram of the left submandibular gland prior to infusion of contrast **(a)**, immediately following infusion of contrast **(b)** and 1 minute after removal of catheter **(c)**.

hyperechoic (white) body (white arrow), with a postacoustic shadow (double-headed white arrow). The stone measures approximately 5 mm in length, lying within the left submandibular gland, posterior to the posterior limit of the mylohyoid muscle. The exact location of a stone is assessed by the ultrasound operator with reference to the angle of the ultrasound transducer; however, this information, which is stated in the report, cannot be accurately determined from a single still image.

Having confirmed the presence of this stone, sialography was performed to assess the morphology of the duct and the location of the stone within the duct.

◆ The Sialogram is Shown in Fig. 64.3. What Do You See?

In Fig. 64.3a, the sialography catheter (seen as a curved dark line) is positioned within the left submandibular gland duct opening. Prior to infusion of contrast, the radiopaque calculus can be seen superimposed on the lower border of the mandible, anterior to the angle (arrowhead). In Fig. 64.3b, following infusion of the contrast, the outline of the main duct is clearly visualized, demonstrating a normal calibre within the section lying in the sublingual space. The stone is lying at the genu of the duct and is wider than the duct anterior to it, indicating that simple basket retrieval along the duct would not be an option in this case. The hilar region of the duct is opacified by the contrast, and the secondary and tertiary ducts are demonstrated (arrows). In Fig. 64.3c, 1 minute after removal of the sialography catheter, the contrast has been lost from the main duct distal to the stone within the sublingual space. However, in the region of the stone, and proximal to this, that is, deeper into the ductal system, some contrast is retained (arrows), indicating that the duct is partially obstructed by the stone, preventing outflow.

Treatment

◆ What is the Most Common Technique for Treating Sialolithiasis?

Surgery has been the traditional method to manage salivary gland obstruction. Stones located in the distal-most parts of the submandibular and parotid ducts may sometimes be removed via an intraoral incision. If the stone is within the gland, surgery to remove the whole submandibular or superficial parotid gland has been the traditional way to remove the stone.

◆ What are the Complications of Surgery?

Complications are rare but may be significant, causing distress to the patient. Submandibular gland removal is relatively simple and free of complications, but parotid gland surgery is difficult. The complications are described below.

Frey's syndrome, or gustatory sweating, results when parasympathetic nerves supplying the parotid or submandibular gland are cut to remove the gland. During healing, the nerves regrow and may innervate the sweat glands of the overlying skin. The affected skin then sweats, sometimes profusely, on eating or thinking of food. This is an unpleasant and distressing complication and is difficult to control with anticholinergic drugs. Administration of Botox injections into the affected skin is one means of managing this complication.

Nerve palsy. The facial nerve is at risk during superficial parotidectomy because it passes through the gland. Its mandibular branch, the marginal mandibular nerve, runs along the lower border of the mandible and is at risk if the incision for submandibular gland removal is placed too high. The hypoglossal nerve may be damaged during submandibular gland removal.

Fistula formation. If part or all of the gland is left in situ, saliva may track along the incision, prevent healing and drain permanently to the exterior, facial skin in the case of a parotid fistula. In time, the tract will epithelialize and become chronically infected, resulting in a scar.

◆ Is a More Conservative Approach Possible?

Yes, minimally invasive techniques for the management of salivary obstructive disease are available. These mostly aim to disrupt the stone so that the fragments are washed out by the flow of saliva. It is also possible to remove the stones as a whole and dilate the ductal stenoses. These techniques require careful selection of patients to ensure success, and there is always a possibility that they will fail and surgery will ultimately be required. Methods include those shown in Table 64.4.

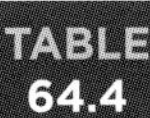

TABLE 64.4 Minimally Invasive Techniques for Salivary Gland Stone Removal

Technique	Details, Indications and Contraindications
Radiologically guided interventional techniques (e.g. Dormia basket extraction of stones)	A Dormia basket can be passed into the salivary duct under the guidance of sialographic fluoroscopy. Baskets are passed closed alongside the stone, opened near the stone and manipulated under x-ray imaging to capture the stone and withdraw it from the duct. The size of the stone relative to the duct and its mobility determine whether this is a feasible option. Dilation of a duct can be performed to stretch it sufficiently to allow passage of a stone. This is performed by using a balloon catheter in a technique similar to that used in coronary angioplasty (Fig. 64.5). An incision at the duct orifice is often needed to allow delivery of the stone.
Endoscopically guided interventional techniques (e.g. Dormia basket extraction or pneumatic stone breaker)	Ultrafine endoscopes (0.8–1.6 mm diameter) are inserted into the duct, with saline flushing to gently dilate the duct for passage of the endoscope. Baskets and balloons can be passed alongside an endoscope if the duct is large enough or down the working channel of the endoscope by using fine instruments. This allows direct visualization of the stone or stricture during the manipulation (see Fig. 64.4). Stones that are too large to be withdrawn intact from the duct can be fragmented into smaller pieces by using a laser or an intracorporeal pneumatic lithotripter, with the resulting fragments captured by basket for withdrawal from the duct (Fig. 64.6).
Extracorporeal lithotripsy	Ultrasonic waves are directed at the stone through the soft tissues of the neck to shatter the stone (Fig. 64.7). The pieces should then pass down the duct and are expelled in saliva. This is suitable for stones up to 7 mm in diameter. It generally requires several treatment sessions to fragment the stone sufficiently. A success rate of approximately 50% has been reported.
Intraoral surgical removal of stones from the submandibular genu region	This is reserved for stones that are too large to be amenable to other more minimally invasive treatment modalities and where gland preservation is desired. The stone should be palpable intraorally to allow localization during surgery. Dissection of the floor of the mouth, identification of the lingual nerve, and careful incision of the duct wall at the site of the stone are required to allow it's safe retrieval. This technique has a high success rate and is generally performed under general anaesthesia.

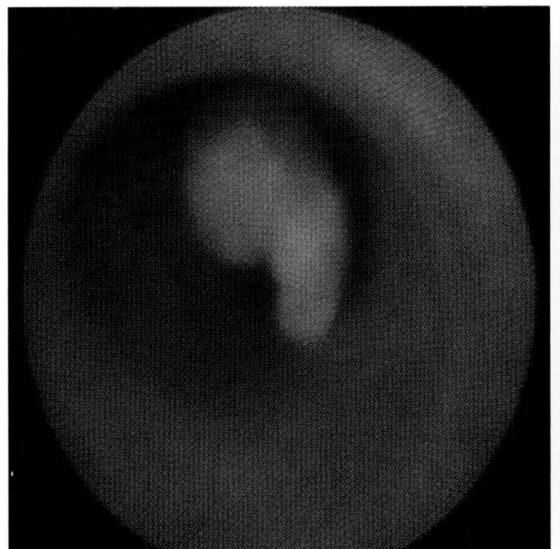
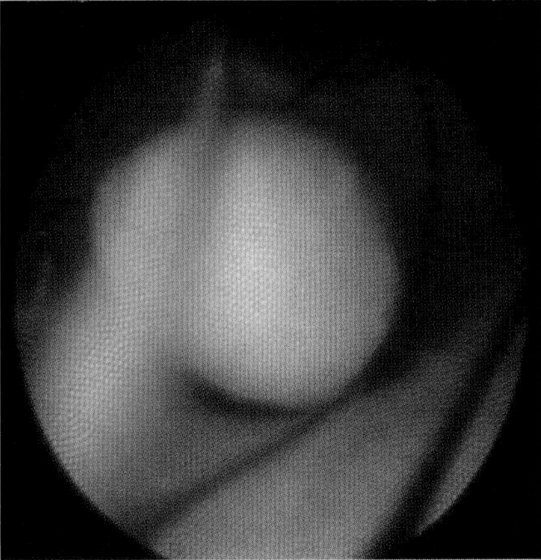
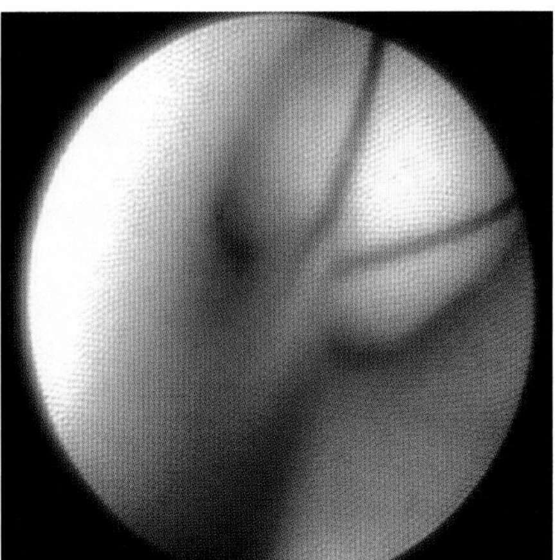

• **Fig. 64.4** Capture of a stone using a Dormia basket under endoscopic guidance. The stone seen through an endoscope (left), the wire basket opened and being manipulated around the stone (centre) and the basket closed around the stone ready for withdrawal (right).

Occasionally, a combination of several methods is used. For instance, a stone may be broken by using extracorporeal lithotripsy, and any fragments that do not wash out may be further broken by using a pneumatic stone fragmentation technique via endoscopy and the remaining pieces removed in a basket.

◆ Is the Present Case Suitable for Treatment with Minimally Invasive Techniques?

Yes, but it is important to note that the stone is wider than the distal part of the duct, and it is located beyond the genu of the duct. *This stone was, therefore, not amenable to removal with the use of endoscopic techniques. Minimal surgery was not*

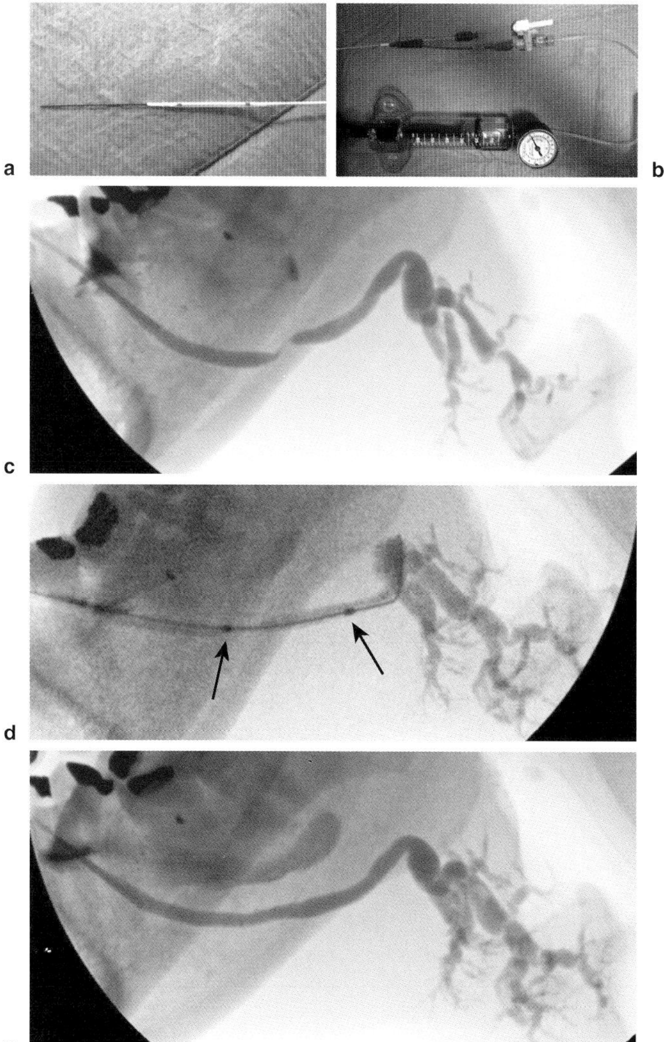

• **Fig. 64.5** Balloon ductoplasty uses the same balloon technology as used in coronary angioplasty. With a guide wire inserted through the balloon **(a)**, and an inflation device **(b)** to accurately inflate the balloon to an appropriate pressure (15 Atm). Under sialographic guidance, a point stricture **(c)** is dilated (the black arrows indicating each end of the balloon) by inflating the balloon **(d)**. A postdilation sialogram **(e)** demonstrates the successful dilation of the tight stricture.

recommended because the stone was not palpable intraorally. The patient, therefore, underwent extracorporeal lithotripsy to fragment the stone first, with basket retrieval of the resultant fragments.

Another Possibility

◆ If the Obstruction Had Been Caused By a Stricture, How Would Your Management Have Differed?

Strictures are caused by inflammatory fibrosis, usually around stones, although the stones may be passed spontaneously, leaving only the stricture. The duct proximal to a stricture often dilates because of back pressure, and a series of strictures and dilatations gives rise to the 'string of sausages' or 'string of beads' appearance on a sialogram. This appearance indicates inflammation around the duct or sialodochitis.

Strictures located at or near a duct orifice may be dilated by introduction of graded lacrimal duct dilators or serial dilators. More proximally located strictures are less accessible and present a more difficult management problem, which has traditionally been treated with surgical resection of the gland. More recently, for the dilatation of strictures with the use of a balloon catheter, an adaptation of the techniques used in angioplasty has been developed (see Fig. 64.5). Although this is often successful, some strictures may relapse repeatedly, requiring alternative treatments such as surgery or medical management to ease symptoms by reducing salivary flow.

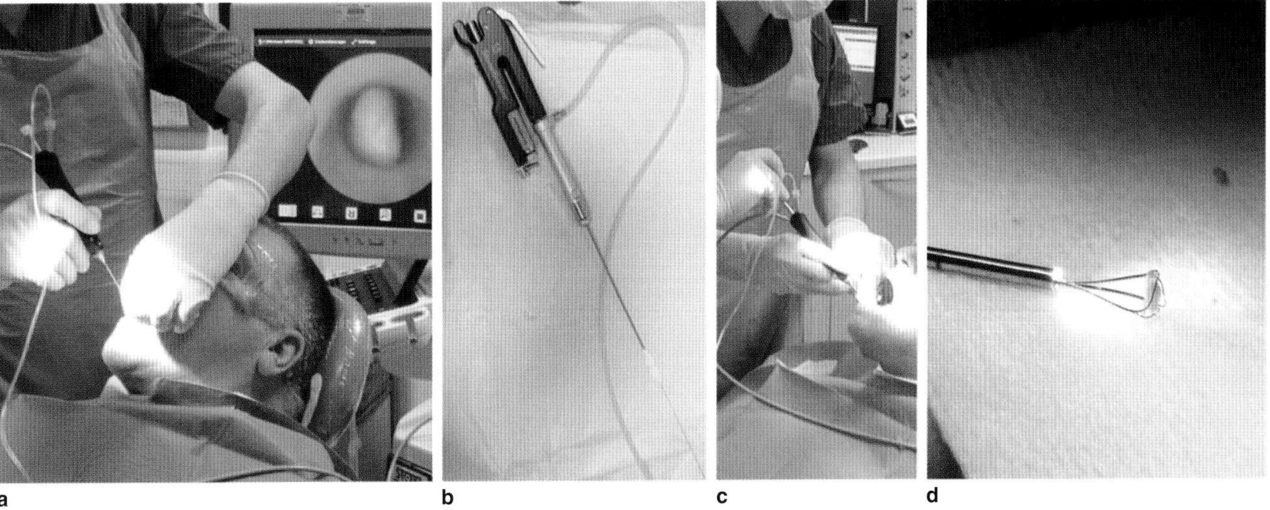

• **Fig. 64.6** Intracorporeal pneumatic lithotripter. Use of endoscopy and pneumatic lithotripter enables fragmentation of stones that would not be amenable to simple basket capture and withdrawal. The stone fragments are then retrieved by basket under endoscopy guidance. This stone in the left submandibular gland is viewed via the endoscope **(a)**, and the pneumatic lithotripter **(b)** is used in the working channel of the endoscope to fragment the stone. The resulting fragments are then retrieved by using a basket **(c, d)**, also via the working channel of the endoscope.

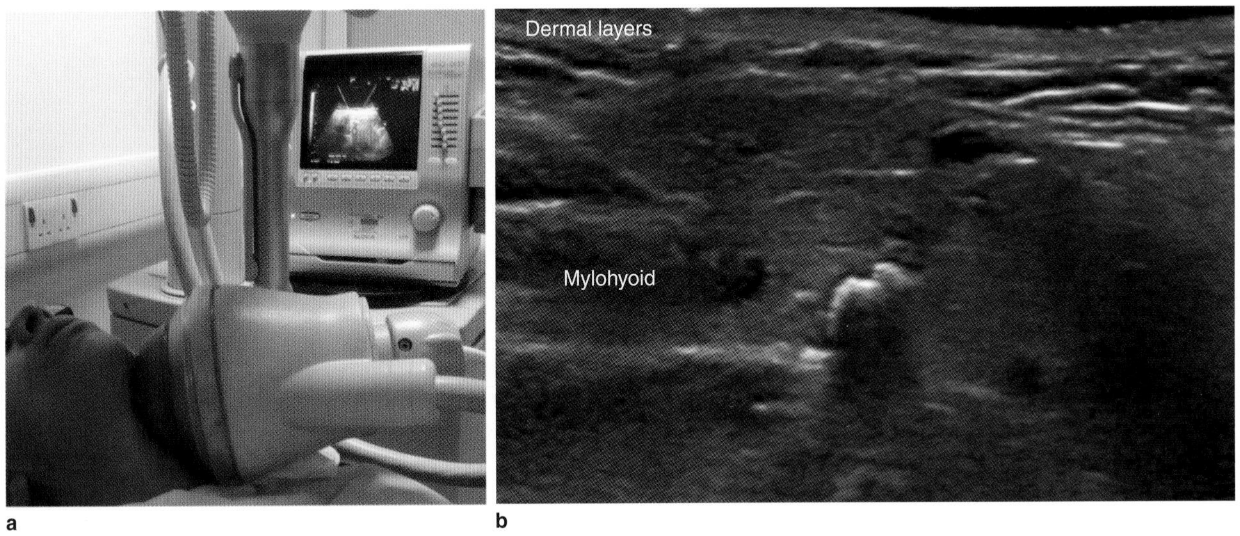

• **Fig. 64.7** **a,** Extracorporeal shockwave lithotripsy to a stone located in the left submandibular duct. The stone is visualized on the ultrasound scanner in the background. Aiming markers on the scan are used to align the ultrasound waves emitted by the transducer head, applied to the neck as close to the stone as possible. **b,** Compared with Fig. 64.2, the appearance of the gland has improved because the stone is seen to have fragmented during the course of extracorporeal shockwave lithotripsy treatment, reducing the obstruction of the duct.

Case 65
Failed Endodontic Treatment

FRANCESCO MANNOCCI

Summary

A 17-year-old female patient presents to you with apical infection on a root-treated maxillary first molar. What are the treatment options and their chances of success?

History

Complaint

The patient, pointing to her upper left first molar, reports that it is tender on biting.

History of Complaint

The tenderness on biting developed 4 months ago.

Dental History

The patient has always attended regularly for dental treatment, and root canal treatment had been carried out 2 years ago.

Medical History

The patient is otherwise medically fit and well.

Examination

Extraoral Examination

The temporomandibular joints appear normal, and no submental, submandibular or cervical lymph nodes are palpable.

Intraoral Examination

The patient presents with an otherwise unrestored dentition. The permanent upper left first molar has been restored with a large occlusal resin composite restoration.

Investigations

◆ What Investigations Would You Carry Out, and Why?

Periodontal examination, including recording of probing depths and gingival bleeding. A wide pocket that can be probed to the apex would indicate a probable endodontic–periodontal lesion. A localized deep pocket would raise the suspicion of a vertical root fracture.

Check the marginal integrity of the resin composite restoration by gently 'drawing' a straight ball-ended probe along and across the filling–tooth interface without pressure (pressure might cavitate any early carious lesions present).

Check the mobility of the upper teeth. *An increased mobility of the upper left first molar would suggest the presence of a periapical abscess.*

Palpation around the buccal and palatal apices of the upper left first molar tenderness to palpation would suggest the presence of acute apical periodontitis.

On performing these investigations, you discover that the upper left fist molar is more tender to percussion and slightly more mobile compared with the adjacent/contralateral healthy teeth.

Radiographic examination of the upper left molars. Periapical radiographs, ideally taken by using the paralleling technique and a beam aiming device, are required to:

- Assess presence and quality of any root fillings and the status of the periradicular tissues
- Aid identification of the source of the sinus
- Detect or exclude caries
- Help eliminate root fracture as a cause. This is difficult as the fracture line would have to be in the line of the x-ray beam (bucco-palatally) to be visible and even then might be superimposed on the root canal or root filling
- Confirm the alveolar bone levels.

Small-volume cone beam computed tomography (CBCT) with high resolution is useful in complex retreatments of upper molars:

- To assess the presence of additional roots and canals
- To assess the presence of unexpected curvatures of the root
- To exclude endodontic–periodontal involvement
- To establish if a reactionary thickening of the mucosa of the sinus is present.

◆ The Periapical Radiograph and CBCT Image of the Upper Left Quadrant are Shown in Fig. 65.1. What Do You See?

See Table 65.1.

Diagnosis

◆ What is Your Diagnosis?

The diagnosis is acute apical periodontitis of the upper left first molar.

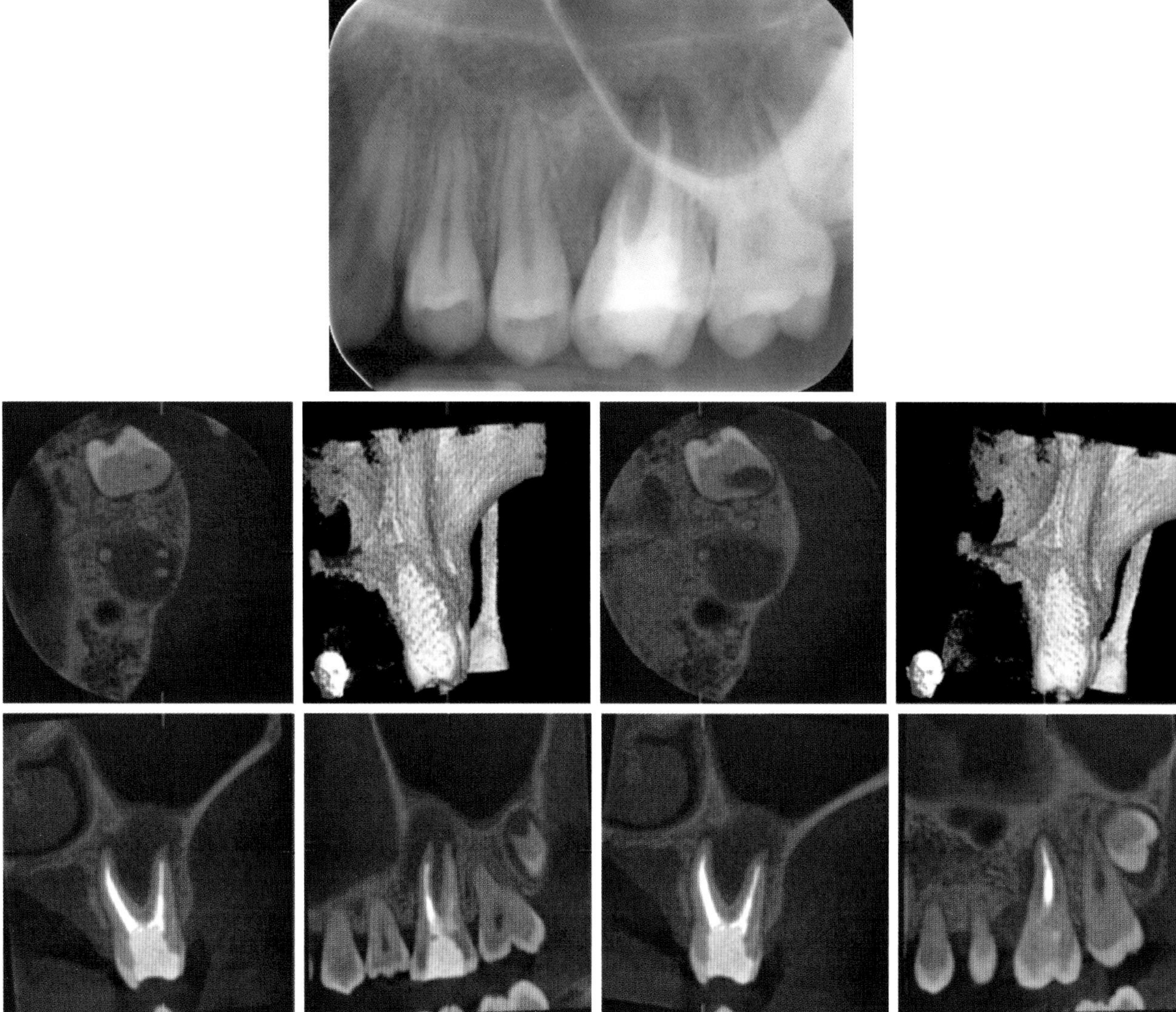

• **Fig. 65.1** Periapical radiographs and small-volume cone beam computed tomography (CBCT) image of the patient's upper left quadrant, taken on presentation.

TABLE 65.1 Radiographic and CBCT Investigations

Upper Left First Molar Periapical Radiograph	Upper Left First Molar CBCT Image
The upper left first molar shows a defective root canal obturation that appears to be short of the apex in the mesial and distal root and not well condensed in the palatal root. A large apical radiolucency appears to be associated with the mesial and palatal root of the upper left first molar.	The buccal view of the CBCT image shows that the radiolucency is also associated with the distal root and that the radiolucency associated with the palatal root is limited in size. There is no evidence of an associated inflammation of the maxillary sinus.

CBCT, cone beam computed tomography.

Treatment

◆ How Would You Manage This Case?

This retreatment case does not present particularly difficult challenges. Both on the periapical radiograph and on the CBCT image, the lumen of the canals is clearly visible beyond the root filling, suggesting that the canal has not been blocked with dentine. Also, the CBCT image clearly shows that the distance between the pulp floor and the furcation is at least 5–6 mm, ensuring 'safe' removal of the resin composite restorative material, which clearly reaches the pulpal floor, minimizing the risk of perforation at the furcation area.

The resin composite material can be removed coronally by using high-speed burs and in the deeper part of the pulp chamber by using dedicated ultrasonic tips, which will aid in selective, minimally invasive removal of the material.

Once a provisional working length is established by using the posteroanterior radiograph or the CBCT image, the gutta percha is removed by gently softening it with a drop of chloroform or other solvent and by using Hedström files size 25 or 30 ISO. Superflexible Ni-Ti files in reciprocation or in continuous rotation can also be used for this purpose. It is essential not to engage the Hedström files in the curves of the canals because such files are easily separated. The provisional working length is essential to prevent extrusion of gutta percha into the periapical tissues while attempting to remove it. This is a risk that is relevant clinically, particularly when the obturation is close to large apices.

Once the existing root canal obturation material has been removed, it is essential to identify the orifice of the second mesio-buccal canal.

◆ The 1-Year Periapical Radiograph and the CBCT Image are Shown in Fig. 65.2. What Do You See?

See Table 65.2.

In this instance, the CBCT image shows that the healing is not as complete as it appears in the periapical radiograph, and the case needs to be reviewed clinically and radiographically annually. It is also important to protect the cusps of the upper left first molar with a metal or ceramic onlay to prevent the fracture of the tooth. A further recall in 1 year is indicated to confirm complete healing.

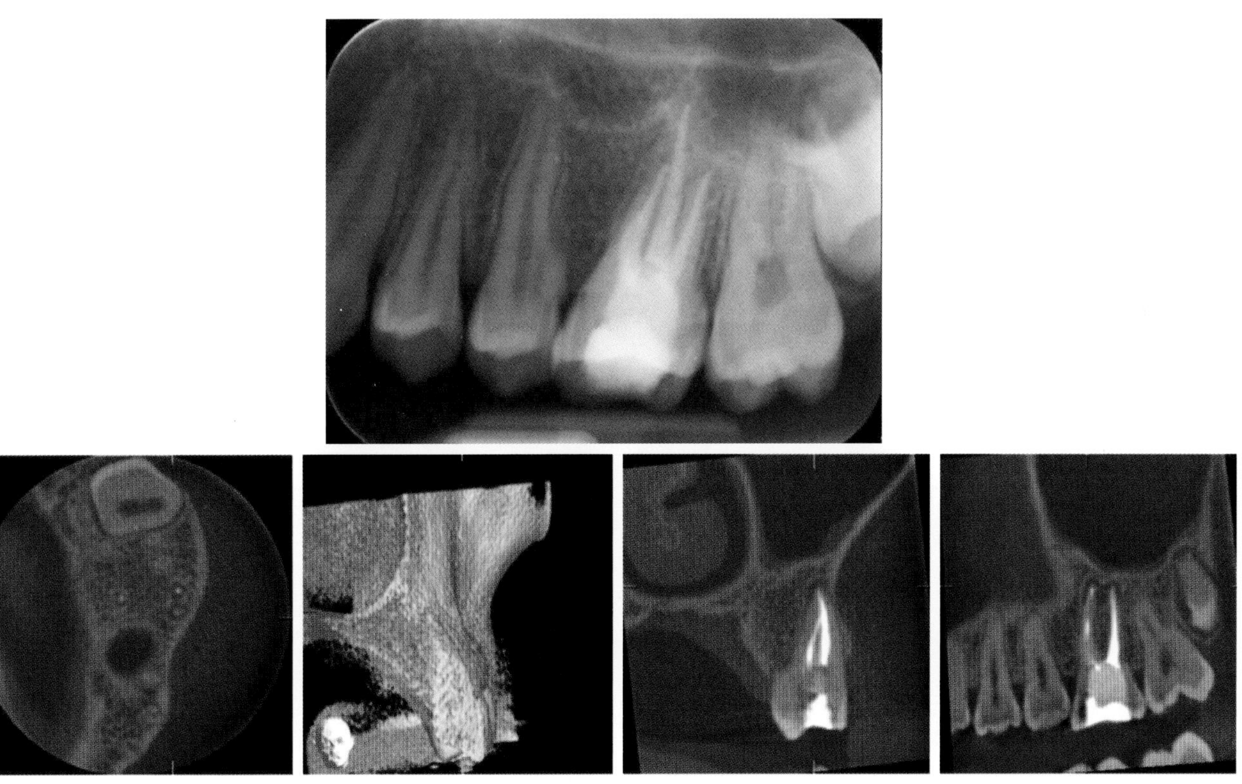

• **Fig. 65.2** Periapical radiograph and small-volume cone beam computed tomography (CBCT) image of the upper left quadrant, taken at the 1-year recall.

TABLE 65.2 Findings From the Periapical Radiograph and CBCT Image of the Upper Left Quadrant Taken at 1 Year Recall

Upper Left First Molar Periapical Radiograph	Upper Left First Molar CBCT
The upper left first molar shows complete healing.	The sagittal image shows incomplete healing of the buccal roots, whereas the coronal view shows clearly that a second mesio-buccal canal has been correctly obturated up to the level of its confluence with the first mesio-buccal canal.

CBCT, cone beam computed tomography.

Case 66

A Pain in the Head

TARA RENTON

Summary

A 58-year-old female patient attending for routine dental care mentions that she has a severe headache and wishes to delay treatment (Fig. 66.1). What should you do?

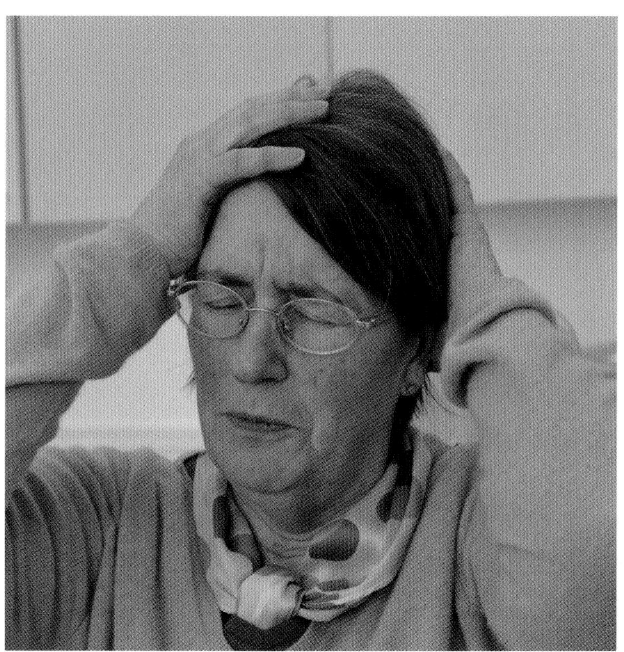

• **Fig. 66.1** The patient on presentation.

History

Complaint

The headaches affect her whole head, are short but severe, causing dizziness, nausea and blurred vision.

History of Complaint

The headaches started only 2 weeks ago. She has not been able to identify any causes. The only way she has been able to manage the pain is to lie still in bed until the pain is over. Over-the-counter painkillers have no effect. The present headache started on the way to your surgery.

Medical History

The patient is overweight, has smoked 15 cigarettes a day for 20 years and drinks 22 units of alcohol a week.

Dental History

The patient attends regularly and has no dental problems. You have noted attrition from bruxism but she has never complained of tenderness in the muscles of mastication.

◆ How Do You Assess the History So Far?

Severe headaches with nausea and visual disturbance on an occasional basis would suggest migraine as a cause.

However, migraine usually has onset in young or middle adulthood and would be unusual as a new diagnosis in a postmenopausal patient. The headache is not described as unilateral, as most migraines are, and there is no typical description of an aura. Dizziness, nausea and blurred vision, however, can be associated with migraine.

Bruxism is irrelevant. It may be associated with masticatory muscle tenderness but is usually asymptomatic.

◆ What is the Role of the Dentist in Headache Diagnosis and Treatment?

It would be wise to consider this question before dismissing the complaint, referring the patient to a medical practitioner or taking on analysis of the problem. A dentist would be expected to have a fairly broad knowledge of the signs, symptoms and causes of craniofacial pain, but mainly for diagnostic and patient referral purposes.

The primary role of the dentist in headache is to exclude pain of dental or local origin. This is most important but not always easy.

The key causes of pain of dental origin that might present as headache are:

- Pulpitis and referred pain of dental origin
- Sinusitis
- Temporomandibular joint/myofascial pain disorders.

In addition, some causes of head and neck pain can be misinterpreted by the patient as pain of dental origin, causing the patient to present to the dentist. The key causes to consider are:

- Trigeminal and other neuralgias
- Trigeminal autonomic cephalalgias (cluster headache-type conditions, including sudden-onset unilateral

TABLE 66.1 Questioning the Patient

You Ask About	The Patient Indicates
The pain distribution	The pain is felt bilaterally, within and on the surface of the head; it is worse at the back of the head
Severity and nature of pain	Extremely painful, immediate onset, crippling pain
Triggering and relieving factors	None identified
Frequency of attacks	Has only had four or five episodes in 2 weeks
Whether pain resolves between attacks	Gradually fades over hours; the patient is normal between attacks
The exact nature of the visual disturbance	Sensitivity to light, blurred vision
Any recent illness?	None
Any recent trauma?	None
Has there been loss of consciousness or confusion?	No
Nausea or vomiting	Nausea accompanies the pain; she has not vomited
Other medical conditions and medication	None

neuralgiform headache, with conjunctival irritation and tearing [SUNCT]).

- Giant cell arteritis
- Persistent idiopathic (atypical) facial pain.

The dentist should be very familiar with these causes of pain and should also be able to diagnose many others. However, it is not the role of the dentist to undertake the primary diagnostic responsibility for other causes of headache or chronic orofacial pain. Orofacial pain is usually managed by a multidisciplinary team, which may well include a dentist, and in such a setting, the dentist may take on considerably more responsibility. In other settings, the dentist will not have the necessary neurological knowledge or access to investigations.

Some dentists extend their care to treatment of headache, migraine and a range of musculoskeletal pains. There is danger of extending beyond one's competence or to nonorthodox treatments without a good evidence base.

Your role in the management of true headache, whether in primary or secondary care, should be limited to:

- Identifying and treating dental causes, or
- Making a provisional diagnosis
- Ensuring appropriate referral
- Informing the patient about possible causes and treatments.

One of the most important factors is to be able to identify any sinister signs that might indicate significant underlying disease.

◆ What Further Information Do You Need?

You will need to question the patient for further details about the features that are listed in the left column of Table 66.1. When you do this, the patient gives the answers shown in the right column.

◆ How Can Pulpitis Be Excluded As a Cause of Craniofacial Pain?

Toothache is the commonest cause of pain sensed by the trigeminal system. Diagnosis of toothache is discussed under several other cases in this book. The key features of pulpitis are that it may be intermittent or constant, sometimes with a dental trigger; exacerbated by hot, cold and osmotic stimuli; and may be poorly localized. Periapical periodontitis, sensed in the periodontal ligament, is well localized and sensitive only to pressure. Pain from multirooted teeth may have both a pulpal and periodontal components.

The main problems in excluding pulpal pain are caused by teeth with cracks or low-grade chronic pulpitis, such as in teeth with leaking restorations or small amounts of caries below restorations. When a cause is not evident, it may be necessary to investigate a number of teeth by performing tests of vitality, replace restorations and place orthodontic bands or copper rings to exclude cracks; this may be quite time consuming and require several visits. Short, stabbing neuralgia-type pain from a pulpitic or cracked tooth can often be detected with cold stimulation or by applying biting pressure on to individual cusps.

One of the most useful diagnostic features of toothache is the patient's interpretation of the pain. In past decades, when dental disease was prevalent, most patients would have sufficient experience to make a clear diagnosis themselves. Now that caries is less prevalent and less extensive, patients may have no experience of either the severity or the poor localization of toothache and so attribute the pain to other causes.

Pain from the pulp is classically poorly localized and may radiate to other teeth, the opposite jaw, the temporal region or any area supplied by the trigeminal nerve. More rarely, pain can be referred to trigeminal nerves from areas innervated by other cranial nerves and even cervical spinal nerves. Referred pain may be as severe as nonreferred pain, but there is usually a component of pain felt locally to aid diagnosis. Dental pain misinterpreted as headache is usually felt on the front and sides of the head. Referred pain will not radiate across the midline.

Referred pain can be a major diagnostic problem. When a dental cause is suspected, a long-lasting Marcain local analgesic may be applied to suspected sources in an attempt to find out whether it blocks the pain. However, response to diagnostic blocks is not necessarily definitive because there is a strong placebo effect.

The character and distribution of the pain in this patient exclude all dental causes.

◆ How May Pain of Temporomandibular Disorders Be Excluded?

This pain originates in the muscles of mastication, is felt there and is referred to the superficial tissues in and around the joint and the ear. It may be identified by its distribution and accompanying signs of abnormal mandibular movement. Because the symptoms can be very variable, a diagnostic appliance may be helpful.

Pain may be unilateral or bilateral and tends to be a dull, constant pain that is worsened on mouth opening, on biting hard foods or on palpation of the joints. There may be wear facets indicating bruxism or another mandibular parafunction.

This pain is often misinterpreted as headache by patients, but it is superficial and should not be confused with intracranial pain.

The character and distribution of the pain in this case immediately exclude this cause.

◆ How Can Sinusitis Be Excluded As a Cause of Headache?

Sinusitis usually follows an upper respiratory tract infection and is accompanied by nasal obstruction or stuffiness. The pain is usually well localized and is more likely to be confused with toothache than with headache. Maxillary sinusitis causes tenderness of the teeth adjacent to the sinus. If the sinus is fluid filled, the pain may alter with posture. Only sinusitis in the sphenoid, ethmoid and frontal sinuses is likely to be confused with headache, but even there, sinusitis is considered a very rare cause of headache.

A high proportion of self-reported and physician-reported chronic sinusitis may be caused by migraine. Sinusitis may be of dental origin if inflammation spreads from the roots of the upper molar teeth. There may then be additional pain of dental origin.

The pain in this patient is predominantly posterior, acute and severe. Sinusitis cannot be the cause.

◆ Are There Other Headache-Like Pains That May Be Mistaken for Dental Pain?

Yes, and the most important is probably temporal arteritis (giant cell arteritis). The pain of temporal arteritis is felt in and around the temporal artery and muscle but is frequently referred to the jaws or teeth and mistaken for toothache. The temporal artery wall is inflamed and gradually destroyed by inflammatory cells, including multinucleate giant cells, and the lumen is occluded. Ischaemia of the temporal muscle is felt as pain on mastication.

The same process affects other branches of the carotid artery, including the ophthalmic artery, and so blindness may result. This can happen very quickly, and a suspected diagnosis of temporal arteritis should be investigated as an emergency. The tender enlarged artery may be palpable. Diagnosis is supported by a raised erythrocyte sedimentation rate; biopsy of the artery is diagnostic, although corticosteroids are often started immediately because of the risk of blindness.

Other causes of referred pain include obstructive salivary disease, earache and joint pain from degenerative disease of the cervical spine.

◆ Could This Patient Have Neuralgia?

Neuralgia is pain felt in the distribution of a nerve and that is not triggered by a normal pain stimulus. It may result from nerve hypersensitivity or central causes and be acute or chronic but is not felt by the patient to be a headache. Trigeminal neuralgia is more likely to be misconstrued as severe pulpitis, and teeth may be unnecessarily extracted or filled before the diagnosis is made. It particularly mimics the pain of a cracked tooth. Atypical trigeminal neuralgia, with its constant pain and wider distribution, is often misconstrued as migraine, dental pain, temporomandibular joint pain dysfunction or atypical facial pain.

The features of cranial nerve neuralgias are shown in Table 66.2.

When a pain of trigeminal or glossopharyngeal neuralgia-type is diagnosed in a patient younger than 50 years of age, there is a possibility that it has a central origin such as a neoplasm or multiple sclerosis and must be investigated. Similar acute or chronic, often chronic burning, nerve pain is also experienced by those suffering from peripheral neuropathy, which may accompany diabetes, chemotherapy, human immunodeficiency virus (HIV) infection and other conditions. Neuralgic pain may also follow nerve damage caused by trauma or surgery. Greater than 70% of patients with lingual or inferior alveolar nerve damage present with neuralgia.

This patient's pain does not follow the sensory distribution of the cranial nerves. The character and distribution are different; this is not neuralgia.

◆ What are the Common Causes of True Recurrent Headache?

The common causes of recurrent headache are shown in Table 66.3. An occasional headache is so common that it is often regarded as normal. In all, 80% of the population

TABLE 66.2 Features of the Main Cranial Nerve Neuralgias

Trigeminal Neuralgia, Classic	Glossopharyngeal Neuralgia	Trigeminal Neuralgia, Nonclassic	Postherpetic Neuralgia
Acute neuralgic pain	Acute neuralgic pain	Constant, less severe than typical neuralgia	Chronic neuralgic pain
Affects older adults	Affects older adults	Affects all ages	Affects older adults
Excruciating short-lasting stabbing pain; may be remissions of years	Excruciating short-lasting stabbing pain; may be remissions of years	Severe aching or burning pain, sometimes with stabbing pain as typical neuralgia is superimposed Remission unusual	Stabbing and/or burning pain; severity varies, may be very severe Lasts months or years; most cases resolve in 5 years
May be elicited by touching a trigger area on the face, on the scalp or in the mouth	May be elicited by a trigger area in the throat, coughing, sneezing, chewing, yawning or swallowing	May worsen with movement, but no typical trigger area	No trigger areas Sensation in the dermatome may also be affected
Sharply defined to area innervated by divisions 1 and/or 2 of the trigeminal nerve, usually unilateral, bilateral in 10% of cases	Affects the oropharynx, posterior tongue and ear Some patients have a hypotensive or fainting period during attack	Often affects all three divisions of the trigeminal nerve, often bilateral	Limited to the dermatome distribution of a nerve previously affected by herpes zoster (shingles). Usually starts as skin lesions heal
Cause usually unknown; some cases related to vascular pressure on the nerve in the skull base	Cause usually unknown; some cases related to vascular pressure on the nerve in the skull base	Cause usually unknown; some cases related to vascular pressure in the skull base or nerve damage	Results from nerve damage caused by herpes zoster
Treated with carbamazepine or similar drugs in the first instance and gabapentin or phenytoin, if necessary; persistent pain may necessitate surgery to decompress the nerve or even to ablate it	Treated with carbamazepine or similar drugs in the first instance and gabapentin or phenytoin, if necessary; persistent pain may necessitate surgery to decompress the nerve or even ablate it, sometimes together with fibres of other cranial nerves	Treated with use of multiple approaches, including high-dose anticonvulsants, tricyclic antidepressants or opiate analgesics; may require surgery to decompress the nerve or ablate it	Prevented by aggressive early treatment of herpes zoster with antiviral drugs, steroids and/or amitriptyline; treatment requires multiple approaches: topical lidocaine patches; anticonvulsants, including phenytoin or carbamazepine, gabapentin and lamotrigine; surgery usually avoided

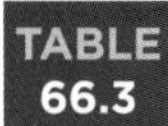

TABLE 66.3 Common Causes of Recurrent Headache

Type of Headache		Main Diagnostic Features
Chronic daily headaches	Tension headaches and chronic tension headaches	The most common type of headache. More frequent in women than men. Usually fewer than 15 days each month but more than 80 days a year. Usually affects both sides of the head. No nausea or other neurological symptoms. Usually wears off after up to 6 hours but may last several days. More frequent during times of stress. Constant ache, tightening of the neck muscles and a feeling of pressure behind the eyes.
	Medication overuse headache	Relatively rare; 1–3% of all chronic daily headaches. Usually greater than 15 days/month for greater than 3 months. Patients using over-the-counter (OTC) pain medication for 10 days each month are much more likely to develop medication overuse headache, and the risk is highest with painkillers containing codeine or ergotamine. Headaches improve after 2 months of withdrawal of analgesics.
Migraine		Common; one in five women and 6% of men have had at least one migraine-type headache in the previous year. The incidence in women rises after puberty. Migraine becomes less frequent in older adults. There may be a family history. Attacks may be precipitated by ingestion of alcohol, chocolate or cheese; menstruation; stress or fatigue in certain patients. In one in five patients, the attack begins with an aura, typically for 20–30 minutes before the headache. This varies among patients, but common features are: • Visual disturbance, usually blurred vision, flashing lights or occasionally a zigzag pattern that moves across the field of vision (fortification spectra). • Tingling and/or numbness affecting the face, lips, tongue, cheek or fingertips. The headache is severe, is usually disabling, may be throbbing and is often made worse by the lightest exercise. In classic cases, the pain is one sided, although it may affect the front, back or whole head. Often accompanied by nausea and/or vomiting and sensitivity to light and/or smells. Less common features include flashing lights, blindness, tingling in the face or speech disturbance. Diarrhoea is not uncommon, and some people pass a lot of urine as the headache is subsiding.
Cluster headache (migrainous neuralgia)		A fairly rare condition affecting around 1 in 1000 people, mostly males and smokers. The pain is excruciating, much more severe than migraine and is often described as a stabbing pain rather than a headache. The pain begins quickly and is not associated with the systemic effects of migraine. Pain is felt in, above, behind or below the eye, strictly on one side of the head. It is steady rather than throbbing and lasts for 20 minutes to 2 hours. During the attack, the eye may water or become bloodshot, and the eyelid on one side droops; the nostril on the same side will run or become blocked. Attacks come in clusters, often several times a day on consecutive days for 2–3 months before disappearing completely for a year or even longer. Often, the attacks occur at the same time early every morning ('alarm clock headache').
Sudden-onset unilateral neuralgiform heading, with conjunctival irritation and tearing (SUNCT)		A trigeminal nerve pain that is like cluster headache but affects the face and is characterized by facial flushing of the affected area, with a red eye and tears.
Low-pressure headache		Caused by low cerebrospinal fluid pressure. It develops over a few days, become persistent and may be associated with neurological symptoms.
Sinister headache		This is rare but important to diagnose because it indicates possible important underlying disease. Features suggesting a sinister headache are: • An acute single headache ('thunderclap headache') • Abrupt onset • Nausea and/or vomiting • Older patient with no chronic headache history • Fever • Neck stiffness • Rash • Head injury • Loss of consciousness • Limb weakness or difficulty speaking • Eye signs: unequal pupils, failure to accommodate, ptosis, which might indicate underlying causes such as cerebral ischaemia or stroke, subarachnoid haemorrhage, ruptured aneurysm, meningitis, brain tumour, hypertension, cerebral abscess.

have had at least one tension-type headache in the previous year. Only intermittent, but relatively frequent, headaches that meet the criteria listed in Table 66.3 are amenable to diagnosis without specialist knowledge and investigations.

◆ Could This Be a Pain of Idiopathic Origin?

In the current classification of headache and craniofacial and oral pain, there are several categories of idiopathic facial pain with defined diagnostic criteria. These include the entities of persistent idiopathic facial pain (atypical facial pain and atypical odontalgia). Useful features are unusual descriptions of pain and distributions that appear anatomically impossible, crossing dermatomes or the midline. Burning mouth syndrome is another type of idiopathic facial pain and is now recognized as neuropathy. All these conditions are characterized by constant pain that may regress spontaneously. These diagnoses should not be applied until all possible causes have been excluded; they are best supported by the results of investigation in a specialized pain centre.

There are no features to suggest that this patient has an idiopathic pain. All other causes must be excluded before this diagnosis can be entertained.

Differential Diagnosis

◆ What is Your Differential Diagnosis? What Would You Do Next?

This is a true headache. Of the other potential causes, only migraine remains a possibility, but as noted above, this is unlikely. No definitive diagnosis is possible, but there are several features that suggest that this is a sinister headache.

- Sudden onset
- Acute, extreme pain
- Few discrete headaches, all severe
- Associated with nausea and visual disturbance.

The patient is overweight, is a smoker, and is likely to have peripheral vascular disease; there must be concern that these unusual headaches might be caused by minor strokes or leakage from a subarachnoid vessel or an aneurysm. There is no muscle weakness and loss of consciousness to confirm the diagnosis of stroke, and these symptoms are usually present when stroke is the cause. However, headache is the commonest preceding symptom of subarachnoid haemorrhage and is seen in about half the cases with a ruptured aneurysm.

◆ What Would You Do Next?

The features are sufficiently worrying to recommend that the patient attend her general medical practitioner immediately. A letter detailing your suspicions and that you have excluded dental causes should be given to the patient. She must be accompanied, and she must not drive.

Case 67

Aggressive Tooth Decay

MARY BURKE

Summary

A 65-year-old man presents to you at your general practice complaining of sharp and discoloured teeth (Fig. 67.1). ***Identify the cause, and plan appropriate management.***

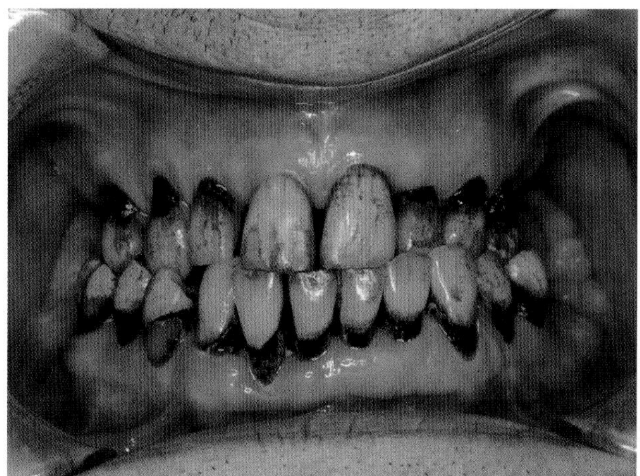

• **Fig. 67.1** The patient's appearance on presentation.

History

Complaint

The patient complains of discoloured and very sharp lower front teeth, with pieces breaking away. There is no pain.

History of Complaint

He has only noticed this in the last 3 months.

Medical History

The patient had radiotherapy and chemotherapy for squamous cell carcinoma of the left tonsil, followed by surgery to the neck. This treatment was completed 18 months ago.

He was a long-term smoker (40 pack-years; 1 pack-year is 20 cigarettes [1 pack] smoked per day for 1 year) but stopped smoking soon after the diagnosis of cancer. He has reduced his alcohol intake to 14 units a week, but his intake was higher previously. He is otherwise fit and takes no medication.

Dental History

The patient was an irregular dental attender, only seeking care when in pain.

Examination

Extraoral Examination

The patient's mouth opening is slightly reduced, with a maximum interincisal opening of 28 mm. No lymph nodes are palpable on either side of the neck.

◆ The Appearance of His Neck is Shown in Fig. 67.2. What Do You See?

The patient has a scar running from below and behind the ear lobe towards the laryngeal prominence and stopping approximately 2 cm before it. The scar runs more or less parallel to the skin creases anteriorly.

◆ What Can Be Deduced From the Site of the Scar?

This is a typical incision to perform a supramylohyoid neck dissection, giving access to lymph nodes in levels 2 and 3. The incision starts a centimetre below the level of the lower

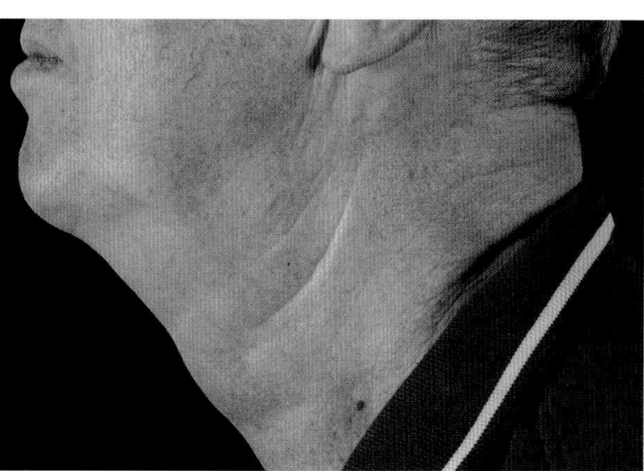

• **Fig. 67.2** The left side of the patient's neck.

border of the mandible and is more vertical posteriorly to avoid damaging the marginal mandibular branch of the facial nerve, which passes forwards and downwards from the parotid gland to supply the depressor labii inferioris, depressor anguli oris and mentalis muscles. This scar is consistent with the history of surgery to remove metastasis or suspected metastasis from tonsil cancer.

Intraoral Examination

◆ The Intraoral Appearance is Shown in Figs 67.1 and 67.3. What Do You See?

The alveolar mucosa in Fig. 67.1 appears dry, matt and 'glazed' and in Fig. 67.3, the alveolar ridge appears matt. There is a small, but less than normal, amount of saliva in the floor of mouth.

There is caries particularly at the cervical margin of most of the teeth. In addition, there is caries at the incisal edges of the lower incisors, and enamel has chipped here.

◆ What Features of the Intraoral Examination are Particularly Important in This Patient?

Examine the whole mouth and the visible oropharynx for carcinoma and potentially malignant changes.

People who have had oral cancer will be under review in their cancer centre, usually for 5 years. They will be checked regularly for recurrence. Although recurrence of oropharyngeal carcinoma may be difficult to see in a routine dental examination, every opportunity to examine for recurrence must be taken.

In addition, the patient is a former smoker and is at risk of a second primary carcinoma. Approximately 10% of patients with oral carcinoma develop a second primary, and so, with this in mind, the mouth must be examined carefully. Second primary cancers are less likely to occur after tonsil and oropharynx carcinomas caused by human papillomavirus, but not all carcinomas at these sites are caused by the virus. A careful examination of the mouth and the visible pharynx is required.

Diagnosis

◆ What is Your Diagnosis?

The patient has radiation caries. This name is given to aggressive caries that occurs frequently after radiation to the head and neck region. Here, it shows the classic distribution of lesions at the incisal edges, the tips of cusps and the cervical margin.

◆ What is the Significance of This Diagnosis?

The whole dentine may be affected, but the enamel shell remains largely intact and pain is not generally reported. Caries may become very extensive and go unnoticed until teeth fracture.

◆ What are the Factors Contributing To Radiation Caries?

Reduced quantity and buffering capacity saliva caused by radiation effects on the salivary gland. Other contributory factors are high-sugar diet; reduced oral clearance of sugars; poor oral hygiene, often compounded by limited mouth opening; and a sore mouth. Changes in the oral flora may be a factor.

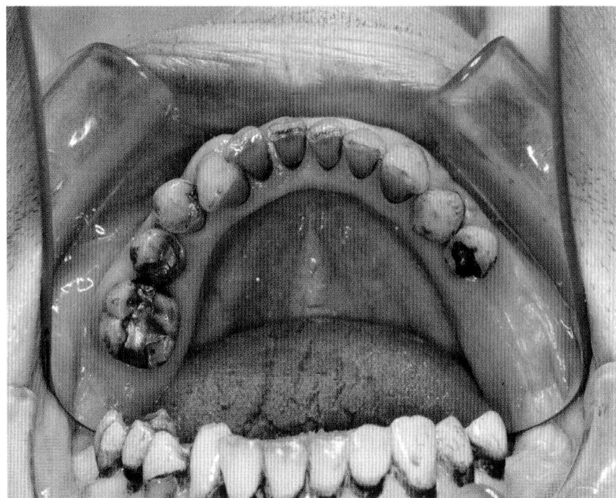

• **Fig. 67.3** The patient's lower dental arch, shown in a mirror view.

◆ Why Can the Salivary Glands Not Be Protected During Radiotherapy?

Radiotherapy (use of ionizing radiation to treat disease, usually x-rays to treat cancer) also damages normal tissue. Because so many important and radiosensitive tissues lie in the head and neck region (particularly salivary glands, eye, spinal cord and thyroid gland), protecting them is difficult, and some compromise often has to be made between effective cancer treatment and its adverse effects.

The full curative dose for most head and neck cancers is 60–65 grays (Gy; 1 Gy is the absorption of 1 joule of radiation energy per kilogram), but mild salivary gland damage can be detected after only 4 Gy, and severe permanent damage occurs with doses above 30 Gy to the glands. Some protection is provided by fractionation, delivering the total dose in small daily amounts or fractions, usually 2 Gy each weekday for 6 weeks. Fractionation allows some recovery time between treatments, thus reducing toxicity to normal tissues. However, if the salivary glands lie in the path of the beam as it passes from skin to cancer, fractionation offers insufficient protection, and complete dry mouth will occur during treatment, with partial and slow recovery afterwards.

Additional protection is provided by using intensity-modulated radiotherapy (IMRT). This method uses multiple smaller 'beamlets' to converge on the cancer from different directions. The intensity and shape of the beams change at each fraction and are calculated to match the size of the tumour from each direction. These features guarantee the necessary high dose to the tumour while greatly reducing the dose to the sensitive normal surrounding tissues. An example of a radiotherapy planning scan is provided in Fig. 67.4, which shows the areas of different radiation intensities colour coded, with the highest dose in red and

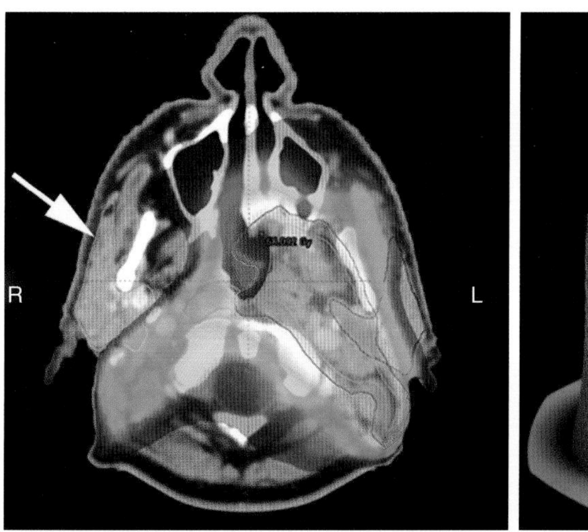

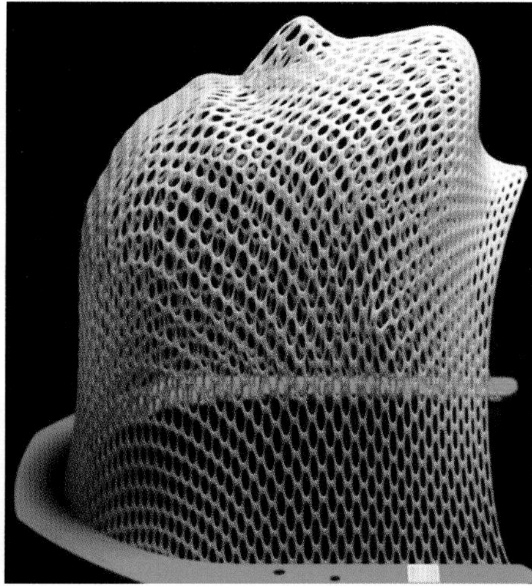

• **Fig. 67.4** Radiotherapy planning scan (left) showing the effective radiation dose to the target volume in red, around the left tonsil and lymph nodes lying posteriorly. The dose is achieved by multiple intersecting beams of x-rays. Note how the right parotid gland, outlined in orange (arrow) has been spared by bringing the beam in from behind its posterior margin. However, the left parotid gland, although not receiving a full dose, will absorb a significant radiation dose, as will much of the oral and nasal mucosae and the left submandibular gland (not in the plane of this computed tomography [CT] slice). Note how the red zone of full effective dose is tightly defined, and only a few millimetres misplacement of the patient's head would allow part of the carcinoma to receive only a partial ineffective dose. To ensure accurate delivery of the x-ray beams, the patient is immobilized in a custom-made mask (right) to prevent any movement.

TABLE 67.1 Adverse Effects of Radiotherapy To the Mouth and Adjacent Areas

Early
• Xerostomia • Oral mucositis • Skin burns • Oral infections, particularly candidosis • Taste alteration
Longer-Term
• Xerostomia • Trismus • Radiation caries • Loss of periodontal attachment • Osteoradionecrosis
General
• Weight loss • Fatigue • Eating difficulty • Swallowing difficulty • Speech difficulty

lowest in blue. You can see two features of importance. The first is that the salivary glands will get irradiated. The second is how closely the effective dose is applied to the carcinoma. If the patient were not correctly aligned in the beams, even by only a few millimetres, part of the tumour might receive an insufficient dose. To ensure accurate beam delivery, the patient must be held immobile under a hard plastic mesh mask (Fig. 67.4), making radiotherapy a very claustrophobic experience. With the use of IMRT, the dose to the salivary gland and the mucosa can be substantially reduced, but not abolished; and a degree of dry mouth always follows radiation to the mouth, nose, nasopharynx and oropharynx.

The minor glands in the mucosa, although only producing 10% of the total volume of saliva, produce the majority of mucins, which serve as lubricants and aid hydration of the mucosa.

Although there may be recovery of salivary function for up to 2 years after radiotherapy, xerostomia is a distressing long-term effect. Generally, patients use sips of water for symptomatic relief; salivary substitutes could also be tried.

◆ What are the Other Adverse Effects of Radiation To the Mouth and Adjacent Areas? Has This Patient Developed Others?

Radiotherapy effects are divided into early, longer-term, and general effects and are listed in Table 67.1.

Oral mucositis – inflammation of the mouth – affects all patients initially. Its features include erythema, ulceration, swelling and atrophy. It causes extreme soreness and can prevent eating, necessitating nasogastric or percutaneous feeding during and for quite a while after cancer treatment.

This patient has limited mouth opening, most likely as a consequence of fibrosis in the masticatory muscles. Similar changes may also result from scarring after surgery. If trismus were of recent onset and progressive, there would be a suspicion that it may be caused by tumour infiltrating the muscles and thus indicate recurrence; otherwise, radiation is the likely cause.

Investigations

◆ What Investigations and Additional History are Required? Explain Why

Clinical and radiological examinations. These are performed to assess the extent of caries, periodontal condition, any periapical disease, alveolar bone levels and restorability of teeth.

Oral care habits. Ask patients whether they are brushing their teeth and about their toothpaste use. Patients may stop brushing during the painful period of mucositis because this condition renders the mouth too sensitive to toothpaste.

Ask about food intake. Many patients have difficulty eating during and after radiotherapy because of painful mucositis, taste disturbance, dryness and muscle fibrosis affecting chewing and swallowing. They may be prescribed high-calorie food supplements to maintain their weight, but these have high sugar content. Some patients with cancer may consume up to 10 sugary supplements a day and continue to use supplements long after active treatment because swallowing continues to be difficult, and preparation of special foods can be time consuming.

Treatment

◆ What are the Treatment Options?

The ideal treatment would maintain the teeth with restorations and periodontal treatment, thus avoiding extractions or periodontal surgery. Treatments, including restorations, root surface debridement and use of local anaesthetic, can be carried out without special precautions. Dentures can be constructed but should be reviewed regularly to check for mucosal trauma, which could precipitate osteoradionecrosis (ORN). For this reason, it is best that the patient manages without replacement of missing teeth, for example, with a shortened dental arch. Dentures are more difficult to manage with xerostomia, and there is greater risk of *Candida* infection and increased caries risk in an already vulnerable mouth. Implant construction after cancer treatment should be done by a specialist. It may be the only option if jaw resection was carried out. Implants in areas of bone that have been subjected to high-dose radiotherapy should be avoided.

◆ What is Osteoradionecrosis?

ORN is osteomyelitis affecting bone after radiotherapy. Most cases of osteomyelitis of the jaws have a local or systemic predisposing factor, and irradiation acts by reducing the vascularity of the bone.

ORN, by definition, is present when there is exposed devitalised bone for greater than 3 months in an area that has been irradiated. It may present with pain, redness, swelling, altered sensation, discharge, skin fistula or a pathological fracture. ORN may arise spontaneously but develops most often after an extraction. Risk factors for ORN are shown in Table 67.2.

TABLE 67.2 Risk Factors for Osteoradionecrosis

Dental Factors

- Extraction after radiotherapy, especially in mandibular molar area
- Extraction before radiotherapy if within 10 days of start of radiotherapy
- Denture trauma
- Implant placement
- Biopsy
- Periodontal surgery

General Factors

- >60 Gy radiotherapy, rare if <40 Gy
- Combined chemotherapy with radiotherapy
- Smoking
- High alcohol intake

ORN is very resistant to treatment. Antibiotics do not penetrate well to the site of infection, and healing is compromised by the reduced vascularity. Patients with suspected ORN should be referred to a specialist oral surgeon. Management may be conservative, but sometimes surgery and bone grafting may be needed.

◆ How Could You Manage Very Broken Down Teeth in the Radiation Field?

Find out from the patient's oncologist the dose of radiation the patient received to the area concerned. If a tooth is on the same side as the cancer and the patient had a full course of curative radiotherapy, extraction would carry a high risk for ORN. Ideally, extractions should be avoided and teeth managed conservatively. Root treatment and decoronation of teeth are preferable if the risk is high.

The risk of ORN is lifelong. Patients should be referred to an oral surgeon if an extraction is required.

◆ Why Has This Patient Suffered Such Severe Complications?

This patient never had a dental assessment prior to radiotherapy. Such an assessment with treatment of pre-existing disease dramatically reduces the risks of oral complications later. The patient should have been given information about the oral complications of radiotherapy and preventive advice. Oral disease would have been treated and necessary extractions performed prior to treatment. Such assessments are usually arranged with specialist dentists attached to the head and neck cancer team.

◆ Which Teeth Should Be Extracted Prior To Radiotherapy?

Teeth that are infected, unrestorable or have pockets of greater than 5 mm depth should be extracted. Extraction of partially erupted third molars, as well as any teeth that are likely to become inaccessible after cancer treatment, is recommended, bearing in mind that there is a high risk of caries needing treatment in the future and of reduced mouth opening.

Other teeth must be assessed, taking several factors into account: the position of the tooth, volume of radiation to the area, strategic importance of the tooth and patient choice and compliance. Extraction of the second and third molars may often be recommended in cases of tonsillar or tongue base cancer, where a high radiation dose is given to the tooth-bearing area.

Any necessary extractions should be done as soon as possible to allow time (minimum 10 days) for healing before radiotherapy is started.

Patients should be given information about the risks of radiotherapy and instructed to always inform their dentist about the treatment they have had. An alert card is useful for this.

◆ What Preventive Advice Would You Give the Patients?

After radiotherapy, the mouth becomes very sore, and brushing is difficult, and so a very soft brush may be necessary. Once the soreness reduces, a medium manual or electric toothbrush should be used twice a day. High-fluoride toothpaste (e.g. Duraphat 5000) should be prescribed and continued lifelong; excess toothpaste should be spat out without rinsing. Sugary dietary supplements should be discontinued as soon as possible in consultation with the patient's dietitian. Taking supplements through a straw will reduce adhesion to teeth, and rinsing with alcohol-free fluoride mouthwash after each supplement may be helpful in reducing caries.

◆ What is the Role of the General Dental Practitioner?

- Do not assume that patients with cancer will receive routine dental care in the hospital.
- Recommend regular recalls at least every 6 months to ensure that any dental disease is identified and treated early.
- Reinforce advice on smoking cessation and moderating alcohol intake.
- Reinforce preventive care, with instructions on oral hygiene, application of fluoride varnish at least twice a year and use of high-fluoride toothpaste.
- Carry out restorative treatment, if required, or refer to a specialist.
- Refer to oral surgery if extraction is considered the only option for a tooth.
- Treat candidosis.
- Be observant for ORN, which may occur after slight trauma, for example, from a denture or spontaneously.
- Be aware of the risk of recurrence or a new primary, and carefully examine the mouth, visible oropharynx and neck.
- Make prompt referral in case of suspicious lesions.

Case 68

Should I Repair or Replace These Restorations? – the '5 Rs'

LOUIS MACKENZIE AND AVIJIT BANERJEE

Summary

A 40-year-old woman presents as a new patient at your general dental practice complaining of two fractured teeth and requesting advice on treatment options. Assess and diagnose the condition of the restorations, and identify the management options that can be presented to the patient.

History

Complaint

The patient recently fractured two teeth whilst eating – the mandibular right first permanent molar, which is uncomfortable on biting and is sensitive to thermal stimuli, and the maxillary left first permanent premolar. The patient also has aesthetic concerns regarding staining around the direct resin composite restorations on her maxillary left central incisor and mandibular left first permanent molar and is also concerned about the appearance of a porcelain-fused-to-metal (PFM) crown restoring her maxillary right first premolar.

Dental History

The patient has not visited a dentist for 7 years. Previously, she was a regular attender and underwent a range of restorative procedures between the ages of 20 and 30 years. She has a healthy diet, good oral hygiene and no medical conditions that would complicate dental treatment.

Examination

Extraoral and soft tissue examinations detected no pathology, but intraoral examination revealed the following positive findings, which are illustrated in Fig. 68.1.

1. Fractured, mobile, disto-lingual cusp on the mandibular right first molar adjacent to an occlusal amalgam restoration
2. Fractured buccal cusp of the maxillary left first premolar adjacent to a mesio-occlusal-distal amalgam
3. Marginal staining of a class IV resin composite restoring the maxillary left central incisor
4. Marginal staining of the occlusal resin composite restoring the mandibular left first molar
5. Open buccal margin on the PFM crown restoring the maxillary right first premolar.

Assessment of Failing Restorations

Failing dental restorations exhibiting minor defects are a common clinical occurrence in everyday dental practice, representing the major part of contemporary general dental practice, with greater than 50% of all operative procedures being carried out for this reason. Caries associated with restorations and sealants (CARS – secondary caries) is the most prevalent reason given for restoration replacements, regardless of the restorative material used. The subjective nature of diagnosing restorative failure presents challenges, and it is widely acknowledged that the unnecessary replacement of 'sound' restorations is common, resulting in a range of negative consequences, including those listed below:

- Every time a restoration is removed cavities become significantly larger regardless of material because of cavity overpreparation.
- Further preparation weakens residual tooth tissue.
- Operative intervention may initiate or precipitate cracks/fractures.
- Operative treatment may cause further damage to the dentine–pulp complex.
- Operative interventions involving proximal surfaces carry a very high risk of iatrogenic damage to the adjacent structures.
- Deepening proximal preparations increases the risk of damaging the periodontal attachment (biological width violation).
- As restorations become larger, there is increased risk of future failure.
- Increased length of restorative margins may increase risk of microleakage and CARS.

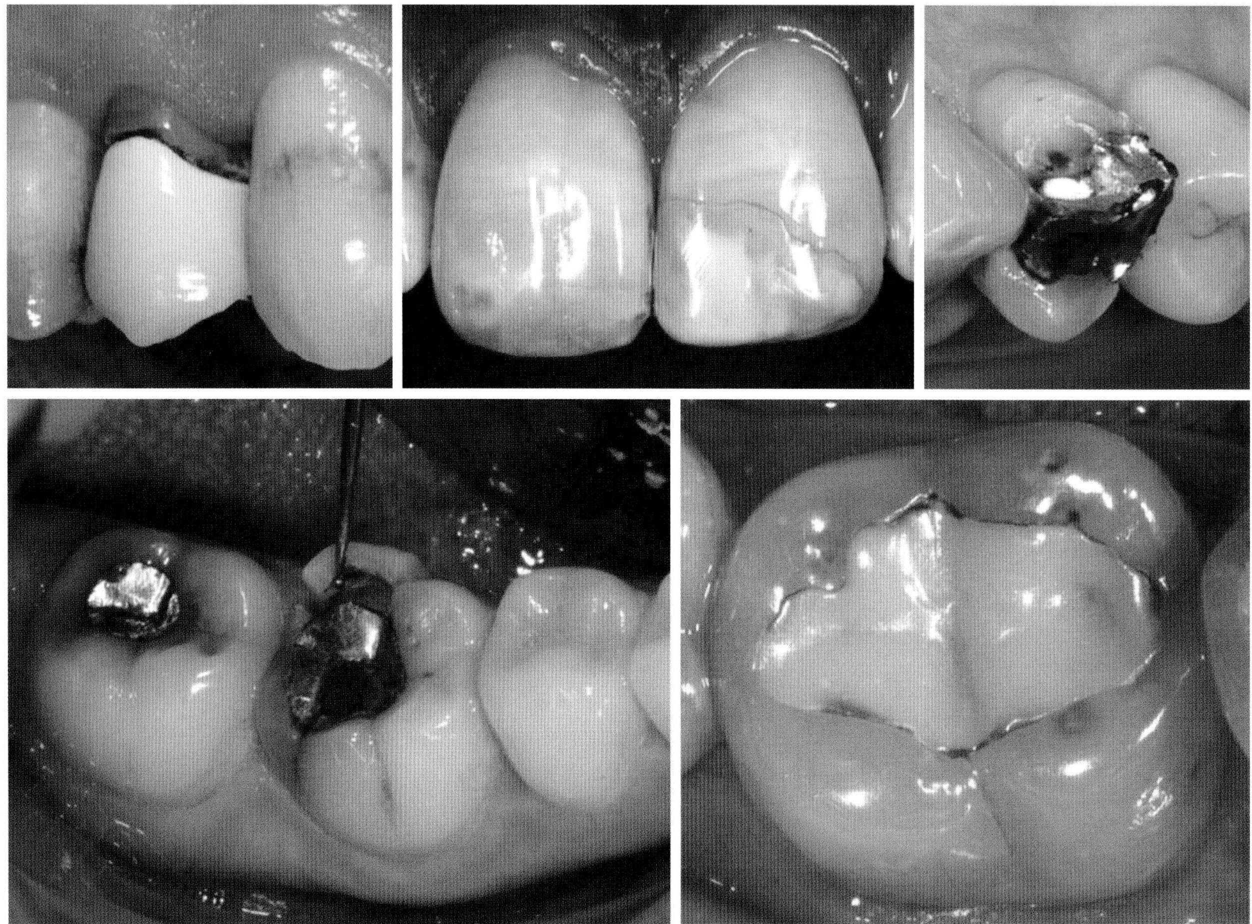

• **Fig. 68.1** Clinical views of the teeth the patient has concerns over.

- Complete removal of restorations increases restorative difficulty and may result in unrestorable clinical conditions.
- The interval to the next restorative intervention may be progressively shortened.
- Unnecessary restorations waste clinical time and resources.

Assessment Training

It is widely reported that when assessing failing restorations, individual clinicians are inconsistent in their decision making and that wide variation exists among dentists in deciding whether or not to replace a restoration. This has a major negative impact on the validity of clinical studies designed to measure restoration longevity.

With regard to the number of existing restorations examined, accuracy of assessment is an important clinical skill. Training in the assessment of existing restorations has been demonstrated to result in significant improvement in clinical performance by offering the following benefits:

- Measuring and describing failure results through clearer thought processes
- Removal of subjective decision making, thus increasing reliability and reproducibility
- Internalization of objective assessment skills, resulting in faster, more accurate diagnoses.

Evaluating the Clinical Quality of Restorations

When assessing existing restorations, the operator's vision is the most important tool, and it may be significantly improved by the use of magnification and good lighting. Clinical photography is an essential skill in contemporary dental practice; in addition to improving diagnostic accuracy and patient communication, high-quality clinical images of the patient's preoperative condition form an important dento-legal record.

After visual examination, further investigations such as the use of measuring probes, articulating paper, pulp testing, shade measurements and radiographs (where justified) may be used to obtain additional information.

Use of high-quality, standardized radiographic images is an important diagnostic and monitoring tool, but training is also recommended for the radiographic assessment of existing restorations to overcome the challenges of diagnosing radiolucencies, superimposition and masking by radiopaque materials.

Classifying Restorative Failure

The Ryge standardized method of classifying tooth–restoration complex (TRC) failures has been available since the 1970s. This well-respected system was designed to help improve the accuracy and consistency of decision making

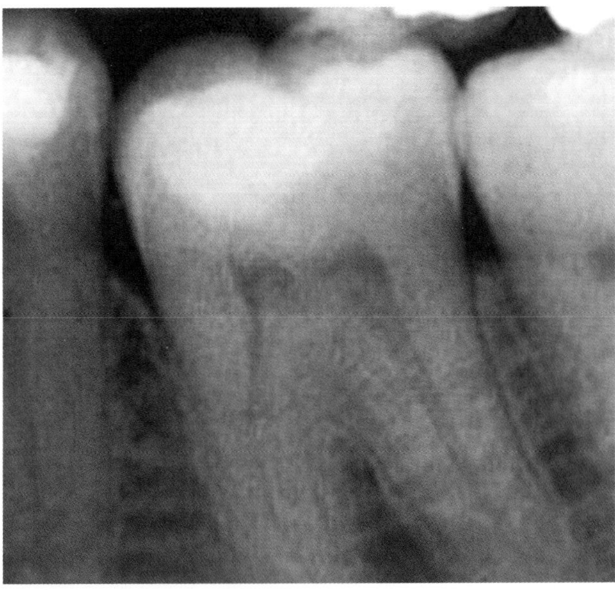

• **Fig. 68.2** Radiographic appearance of the lower left first permanent molar restored with an occlusal resin composite.

and to enhance the reliability and relevance of clinical studies.

More recently, a clinical evaluation system – **Hickel classification system** – has been introduced, and it aims to provide a more sensitive scale that enables the early detection of restorative deterioration and the accurate monitoring of subtle differences over time. This system defines the clinical criteria for the evaluation of direct and indirect restorations and is designed to provide a benchmark to assist practitioners in making accurate decisions, thereby reducing the risk of unnecessary treatment and overtreatment. The classification is divided into three separate indices:

- **Aesthetics** (four subcriteria)
- **Function** (six subcriteria)
- **Biology** (six subcriteria).

Each of the 16 restorative assessment criteria is given a score on a five-point scale. Scores 1, 2 and 3 divide acceptable restorations into three distinct categories, and there are two further categories defining unsatisfactory restorations. See Table 68.1.

The Hickel system provides a standardized classification of the common types of restorative failure and provides guidelines that describe the timing of failure. See Table 68.2.

TABLE 68.1 Clinical Criteria for the Evaluation of Direct and Indirect Restorations

Score	Category	Definition
1	Clinically excellent/ very good	Optimal in all quality assessment criteria
2	Clinically good/highly acceptable	One or more criteria deviate from the ideal but do not necessarily require improvement/restorations; may be renovated to very good/excellent
3	Clinically acceptable/ satisfactory	Minor shortcomings but no unacceptable effects; may not be amenable to renovation or repair because of location, extent, accessibility, risk of tooth damage and so on
4	Unsatisfactory	Suitable for renovation or repair
5	Unsatisfactory	Restoration requires replacement

TABLE 68.2 Timing Definitions for Restorative Failure[10]

Definition	Timing	Examples
Early failures	0–6 months	Postoperative sensitivity severe enough to require immediate removal of restoration, loss of restoration
Medium term	6–24 months	Cracked tooth/tooth fracture/ marginal discolouration/ material chipping/bulk fractures/pulp death
Long term	> 24 months	Secondary caries (CARS – see below)/bulk fractures/ excessive wear/ periodontal complications

Using the Hickel Restorative Assessment System

The assessment system may be employed for each restoration by using the following method:

1. Use Table 68.3 to assess the aesthetic condition of the restoration.
2. Use Table 68.4 to assess the functional condition of the restoration.
3. Use Table 68.5 to assess the biological condition of the restoration.
4. Record a precise diagnosis for each restoration (exact signs/symptoms of failure and scores if useful).
5. Decide which restorations are clinically unacceptable (e.g. discomfort or pain/will impede proper function/ will result in further dysfunction or breakdown).
6. Decide which unsatisfactory restorations require complete replacement (grade 5).
7. Decide which unsatisfactory restorations are suitable for repair (grade 4).

N.B. The location of the defect, extent and accessibility are important factors in determining whether restorations can be renovated or repaired, and a restoration that requires repair should still be considered a failure.

Aesthetic acceptability is inherently subjective, and opinions may differ between the patient and the clinician. The

TABLE 68.3 Aesthetic Criteria for the Assessment of Existing Restorations

Score	1	2	3	4	5
Definition	Clinically excellent/ very good	Clinically good Highly acceptable	Clinically acceptable (satisfactory)	Unsatisfactory Suitable for renovation or repair	Unsatisfactory Restoration requires replacement
Surface lustre	Lustre comparable with enamel	Slightly dull (not noticeable from speaking distance)	Dull (acceptable when saliva-covered)	Rough (not amenable to simple polishing)	Unacceptably rough
Surface staining	No surface staining	Minor staining (easily removable)	Moderate staining (aesthetically acceptable)	Unacceptable staining	Severe staining (replacement necessary)
Colour stability and translucency	Good match	Minor deviations	Clear deviation (acceptable)	Unsatisfactory (repairable)	Replacement necessary
Anatomical form	Optimal	Minor errors	Errors (not aesthetically displeasing)	Aesthetically unacceptable (repairable)	Replacement necessary

TABLE 68.4 Functional Criteria for the Assessment of Existing Restorations

Score	1	2	3	4	5
Definition	Clinically excellent/ very good	Clinically good Highly acceptable	Clinically acceptable (satisfactory)	Unsatisfactory Suitable for renovation or repair	Unsatisfactory Restoration requires replacement
Fractures and retention	No fractures/ cracks	Small hairline crack	≥ 2 hairline cracks/ chipping	Repairable fractures/chipping	Partial or complete loss of restoration
Marginal adaptation	Optimal	Small marginal gap (< 150 μm) (polishable)	Gap/tooth fractures (< 250 μm) (not repairable)	Gap/tooth fractures (> 250 μm) or dentine/lining exposure	Filling loose but in situ
Wear	Physiological	Slight difference to adjacent enamel	Wear within natural variation limits	Significant wear or loss of occlusal contact(s)	Excessive wear
Contact point/ food trapping	Optimal	Too tight (acceptable)	Too weak (acceptable)	Too weak (repairable)	Too weak + complications (replacement necessary)
Radiographic examination (where applicable)	No pathology	Positive or negative step (< 150 μm)	Gap/step (< 250 μm) or poor radiopacity) (no adverse effects)	Gap/step (> 250 μm) or immovable excess	Secondary caries/ apical pathology/ fracture/large gap(s)/restoration loss
Patient's view	Entirely satisfied	Satisfied	Minor criticisms (clinically satisfactory) (difficult/time consuming to repair)	Desire for improvement	Completely dissatisfied or adverse effects

TABLE 68.5 Biological Assessment of Existing Restorations

Score	1	2	3	4	5
Definition	Clinically excellent/very good	Clinically good Highly acceptable	Clinically acceptable (satisfactory)	Unsatisfactory Suitable for renovation or repair	Unsatisfactory Restoration requires replacement
Postoperative (hyper) sensitivity/ tooth sensibility	No sensitivity/ vital	Slight sensitivity (brief)	Sensitive (no treatment needed)	Sensitivity complaints (intervention necessary – without replacement)	Pulpitis or nonvital (treatment/ replacement necessary)
Recurrent pathology (e.g. CARS/ NCTTL)	No pathology	Small/localised defect (no operative treatment required)	Larger defect (amenable to preventive measures)	Cavitated carious lesion/ NCTTL amenable to repair	CARS/exposed dentine (replacement necessary)
Tooth integrity	Complete integrity	Hairline crack (< 150 μm) (Not probable)	Enamel crack (< 250 μm) (No adverse effects)	Large crack (> 250 μm) (Probe penetrates)	Cusp or tooth fracture
Periodontal response	No inflammation/ No plaque	No inflammation (plaque present)	Gingivitis (acceptable plaque levels/ pocket depths)	Unacceptable plaque/ bleeding levels (pocket depth increase > 1 mm)	Periodontitis
Adjacent mucosae	Healthy	Healthy after removal of irritations	Alteration of mucosa (but no cause-and-effect relationship)	Suspected mild allergic reaction	Suspected severe allergic reaction
Oral and general health	No symptoms	Minor transient symptoms	Transient symptoms	Persistent symptoms (intervention required but with no restoration replacement)	Acute/severe local or general symptoms

CARS, caries associated with restorations and sealants; *NCTTL*, noncarious tooth tissue loss

optical properties of restorations are determined by shape, surface texture and colour, and aesthetic properties are related to how well these parameters integrate with the surrounding dentition.

Clinical photographs are useful for documenting aesthetic assessment findings and may be supported by using colour measurements with an appropriate shade guide. Formal written consent is required for clinical photography, and all photographs should be documented and reported, as part of the patient's confidential clinical record.

Although fractures, open contacts and abnormal wear are relatively easy to diagnose, marginal adaptation is much more challenging, and its inaccurate diagnosis probably results in more unnecessary restoration replacements than any other assessment parameter. When assessing restorative margins, it is vital to remember that:

- A discoloured margin is not indicative of CARS
- The majority of restorations present with overfilled (43%) and underfilled (25%) margins
- Gap width, depth and continuity of margins are important considerations when assessing marginal defects
- In easily accessible areas gap widths in excess of 400 μm are necessary for secondary caries to develop.

CARS is identical to primary caries, but it occurs adjacent to the margin of existing restorations. There is general agreement that epidemic levels of overdiagnosis of CARS exists and that many restorations are unnecessarily replaced as a result. Marginal discolouration and localized restoration defects are commonly misdiagnosed as secondary caries. When assessing restorative margins, it is essential to carefully consider that:

- There is poor correlation between marginal appearance and histological findings
- CARS is an infrequent occurrence with resin composite restorations when placed under ideal conditions
- CARS is diagnosed most commonly at proximal cervical margins, but the clinically relevant gap dimensions required for its development are not clear
- Use of the International Caries Detection and Assessment System (ICDAS) is recommended when assessing, monitoring and diagnosing defects at the margins of existing restorations
- Like primary caries, CARS is multifactorial

- Accurate diagnosis of CARS is difficult
- The differentiation between inactive and active caries is fundamental to successful management.

Minimum-Intervention Treatment Options

Prevention is the cornerstone of minimum-intervention management of existing restorations.

- Modifying patient behaviour with regard to maintenance increases restoration longevity by reducing the risk of failure
- Failure to educate and monitor patient adherence to recommended dietary and plaque control protocols will increase the likelihood of premature restoration failure
- In many clinical situations, restorations with minor defects may be maintained successfully for many years through good oral hygiene practices alone

Once preventive patient factors have been optimized, minimally invasive management strategies should be prioritized because improvement in clinical conditions has been demonstrated to result in a significant increase in the functional longevity of restorations. Minimally invasive management options may be classified using the **'5 Rs' system** (Table 68.6).

TABLE 68.6 Minimally Invasive Management Options for the Failing Tooth–Restoration Complex (the 5 Rs)

Option	Definition
Review	Monitoring of minor defects, where there would be no clinical advantage in undertaking treatment
Refurbish	Correction of small restoration defects to prevent further deterioration
Reseal	Application of sealant material into noncarious marginal defects
Repair	Addition of material to a defect in an existing restoration
Replace	Removal and replacement of an entire restoration

Review

Diagnosis. This occlusal resin composite restoration on the mandibular left first permanent molar has a number of small (< 150 μm), interrupted, marginal gaps affecting approximately 50% of the restorative margin (**functional assessment: grade 2**) (Fig. 68.3).

The suspected aetiology is that an occlusal bevel may have been placed around the outline form of the cavity during preparation. Thin extensions of marginal resin composite may then have fractured under occlusal loads and resulted in shallow defects susceptible to extrinsic marginal staining.

Management. It is reported that dentists are more likely to resort to surgical interventions when existing restorations are made of resin composite compared with amalgam. As the clinical images in Fig. 68.4 (taken 8 years apart) demonstrate, it is usually unnecessary to replace restorations solely on the basis of a diagnosis of marginal staining. No treatment was carried out for this tooth. The restoration will be monitored at routine examination appointments, and the patient is reassured that there is no CARS present and that removal and replacement aimed at aesthetic improvement would result in unnecessary cavity enlargement.

Refurbish

Diagnosis. Marginal excess and staining of (possibly unbonded) resin composite has affected approximately 80% of the labial restorative margin of the class IV resin composite restoring the mesial line angle of the maxillary left central incisor in this patient (**functional assessment – grade 2: small marginal gap [< 150 μm], polishable; and grade 4: patient's desire for improvement**) (Fig. 68.4).

Management. The presence of marginal excess beyond the outline form of cavities restored with direct composite is a common clinical finding. Where excess is in accessible locations, it can very easily be removed by using appropriate rotary instruments at negligible biological cost, as was carried out in this clinical example. Recontouring and repolishing surfaces have also been demonstrated to reduce the incidence of unnecessary restoration replacement for amalgam restorations.

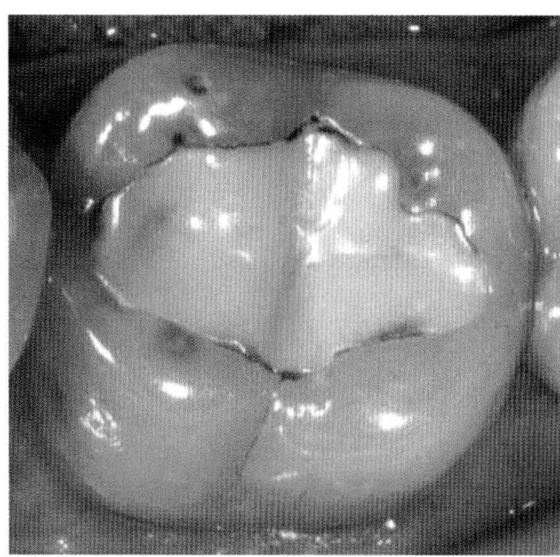
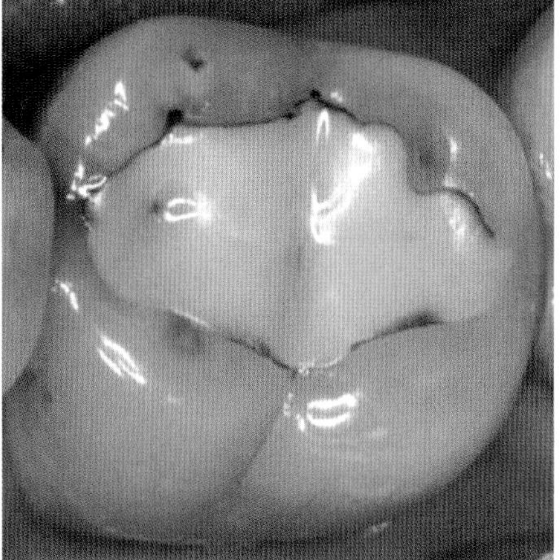

• **Fig. 68.3** Clinical views 8 years apart of the lower left first molar showing little or no change in the resin composite occlusal restoration.

Reseal

Diagnosis. Direct and indirect restorations with defects are common clinical presentations. For example, most crowns are reported to have poor resemblance to adjacent residual dentition, and these differences are obvious to both patients and clinicians.

In this clinical example, the shade and translucency of the PFM crown on the maxillary right first premolar do not match those of the adjacent teeth (Fig. 68.5) (**aesthetic assessment – grade 3: clear deviation, but acceptable to patient in this case**), and a gap (> 250 μm) is present on the buccal margin, with dentine exposure after the dissolution of luting cement (**functional assessment: grade 4**). Although the marginal gap is large and obvious in this example, the presence of small (≈ 100 μm) gaps around the vast majority of indirect restorations is common.

Special investigations revealed that the abutment tooth responded positively to thermal pulp sensibility tests, and no radiographic pathology, other than the radiolucent appearance of the open margin, was detected.

Management. As the patient was willing to accept the aesthetic defects and was keen to minimize the expense of restoration replacement, the open buccal margin was cleaned with hand and small rotary instruments, revealing minimal carious demineralization and no extension into inaccessible proximal areas. The margin was sealed with resin-modified glass–ionomer cement (RMGIC) to reduce the risk of CARS (see Fig. 68.5). The patient has been happy with this minimally invasive resealing procedure, the result of which has now been successful for 3 years. The restoration is being monitored at routine assessment appointments, and radiographic examinations are repeated at appropriate intervals based on the patient's current caries susceptibility.

Repair

Diagnosis. Tooth tissue fractures adjacent to intracoronal restorations are a common finding because tooth preparation weakens the residual tooth structure. In this case, the disto-lingual cusp of the mandibular right first permanent molar has fractured and is retained only by weak attachment

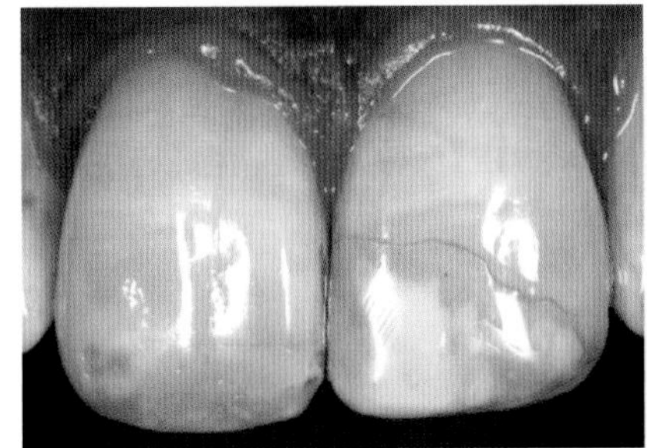
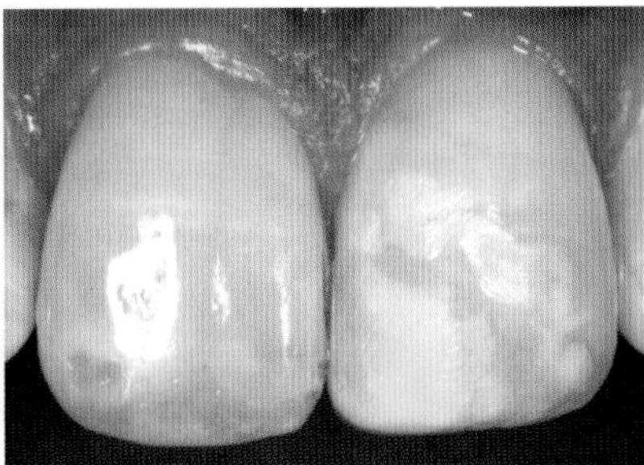
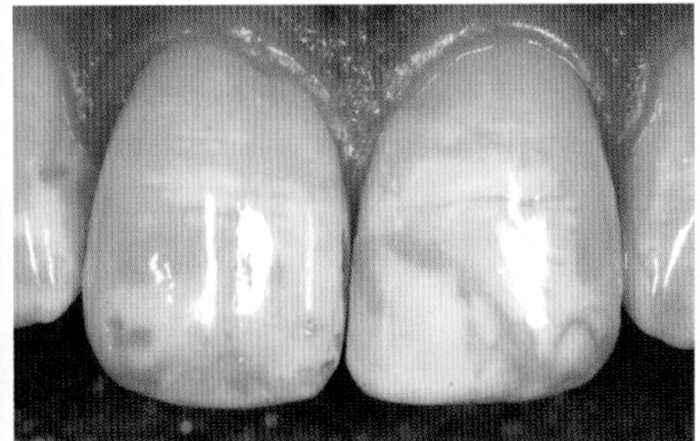

• **Fig. 68.4** Upper left incisor (UL1 or 9) before and after the resin composite restoration surface was polished/refurbished, removing the aesthetically displeasing stained margin.

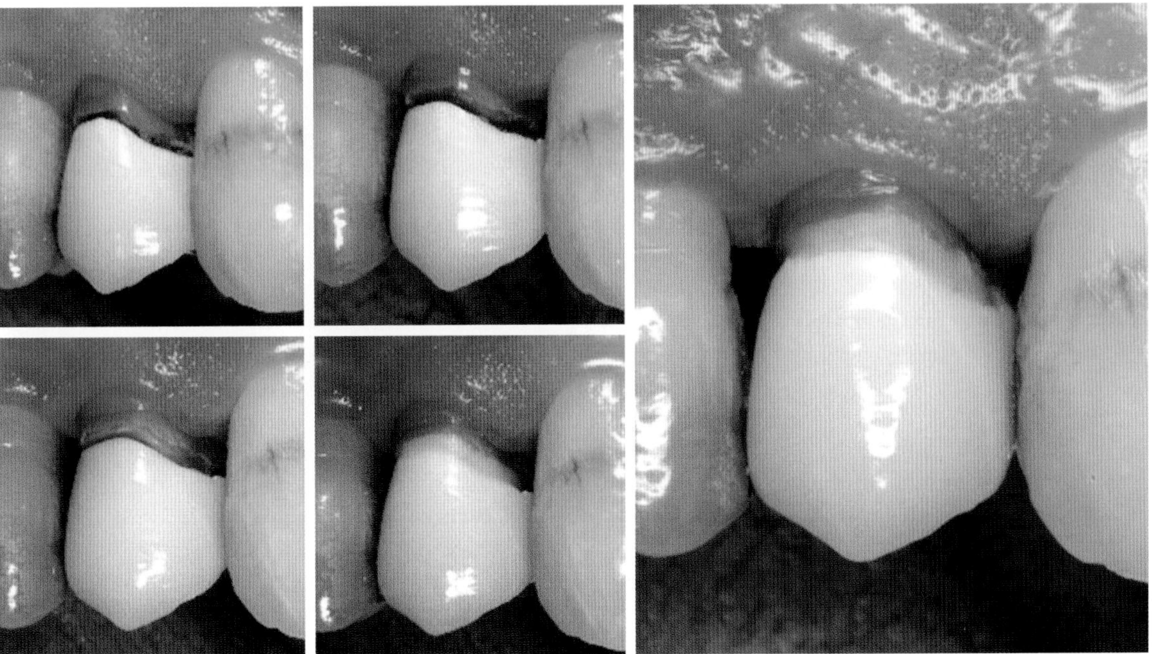

• **Fig. 68.5** Upper right premolar showing defective crown margin that has been resealed with resin-modified glass–ionomer cement (RMGIC) to aid aesthetics and cleansability.

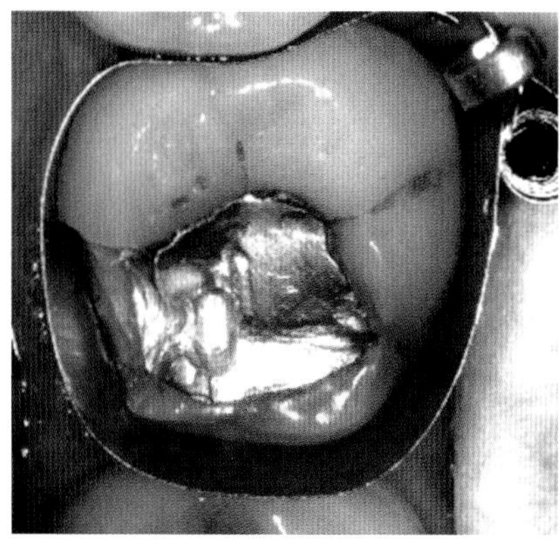
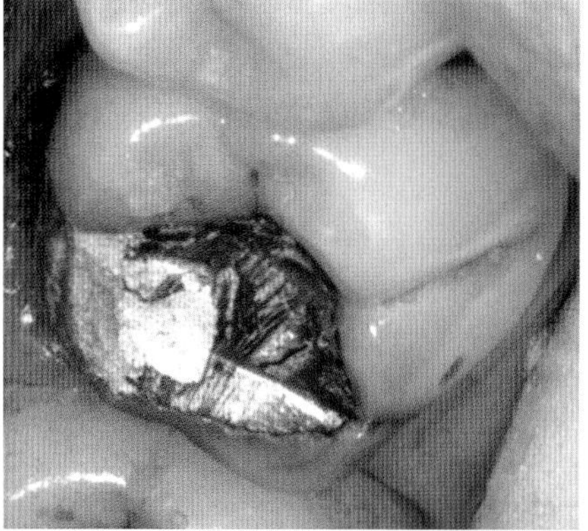
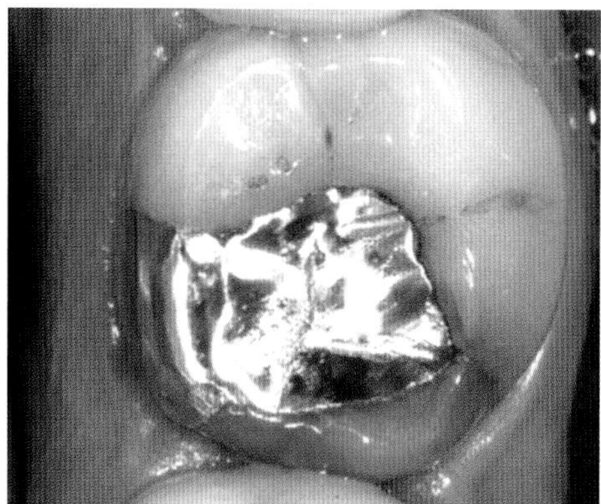

• **Fig. 68.6** Fracture disto-lingual cusp of lower right molar (LR6 or 30), which has been repaired using dental amalgam and finally polished to reduce biofilm accretion.

to the periodontal ligament (Fig. 68.6) (**biological assessment: grade 5**).

Management. Although it is reported to be dentists' least favoured option, **repair should be considered as the first option in contemporary minimally invasive operative practice** because repairs have been demonstrated to be successful, with high bond strengths reported for both amalgam and resin composite repairs. Repairs also reduce the risk of further tooth tissue fracture, which is a common complication of total removal of restorations.

As in this example, repairs may require removal of the localized defective part of the tooth–restoration complex. Cavity shapes may also require modification to increase resistance and retention form by preparation with burs and/or particle air abrasion, and the use of adhesives for resin composite repair. The dovetail preparation used in this amalgam repair technique does not require the use of adhesives because the new amalgam develops high bond strengths with the residual amalgam.

Replace

Diagnosis. When fractures occur in the aesthetic zone, patients will usually request a tooth-coloured restoration, as in this example of the UL4 (Fig. 68.7) (**aesthetic assessment – grade 5: desire for improvement; functional assessment – grade 5: filling loose in-situ; biological assessment – grade 5: cusp fracture**).

Management. Although total restoration replacement may be associated with a range of complications (listed previously), minimally invasive strategies may still be employed, as in this example.

As the retention of the residual amalgam restoration was uncertain, it was removed completely. The colour contrast of amalgam allows this to be done conservatively and the resultant mesio-occlusal-disto-buccal cavity was restored with a direct resin composite restoration, which will be reviewed at routine examination appointments.

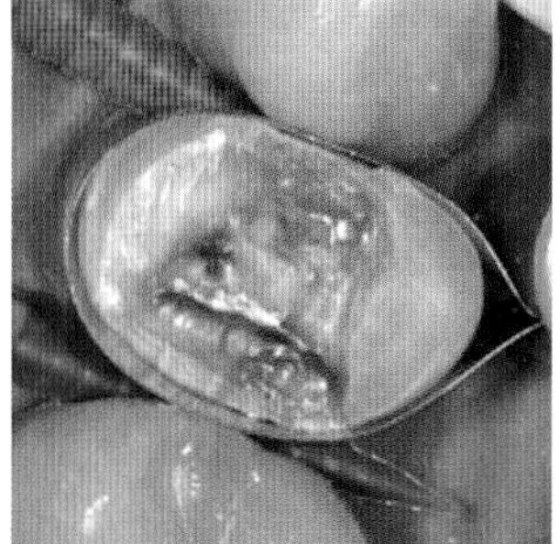
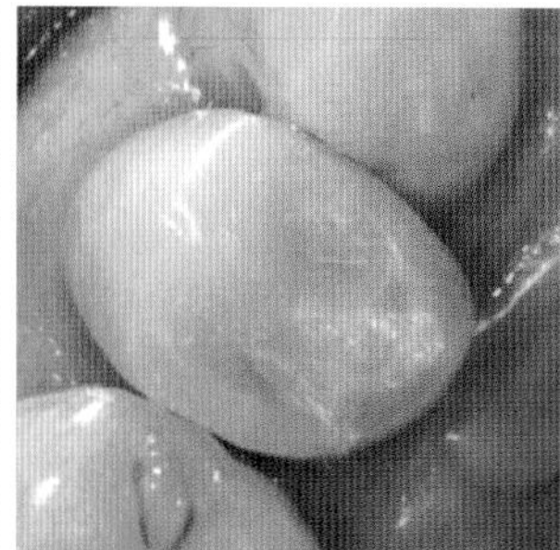
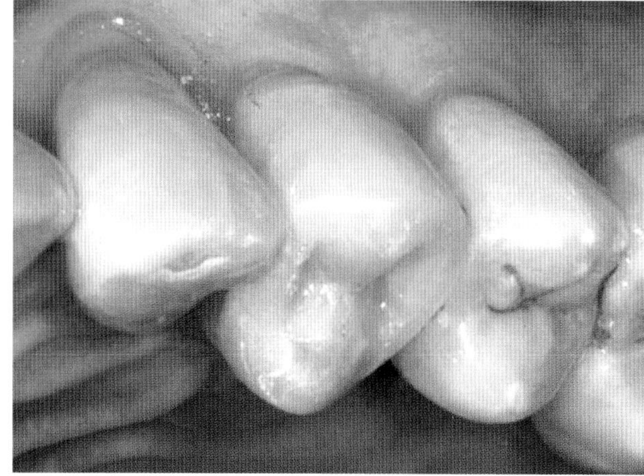

• **Fig. 68.7** Upper left premolar (UL4 or 12), with the old dental amalgam removed and a tooth-coloured resin composite restoration placed.

Medico-Legal Issues

As in all cases, the patient must been taken along the decision-making journey with the dentists and the oral healthcare team. Managing the failing TRC forms a large part of the clinical work carried out by oral healthcare practitioners. Replacing restorations must only be carried out in those clinical situations where no other alternative exists. The consequences of the '5 Rs management' strategy should be fully discussed with the patient and clearly documented in the patient's records, along with the results of all investigations and the clinical photographs taken, with date stamps and annotations, where necessary. Consent must be obtained from the patient, and no operative intervention should be commenced without careful diagnosis of the cause of failure and the successful application of nonoperative preventive regimens by the patient.

Further Reading

Bader, J. D., & Shugars, D. A. (1993). Agreement among dentists' recommendations for restorative. *Journal of Dental Research, 72*, 891–896.

Blum, I. R., Lynch, C. D., Schriever, A., Heidemann, D., & Wilson, N. H. (2011). Repair versus replacement of defective composite restorations in dental schools in Germany. *European Journal of Prosthodontics and Restorative Dentistry, 19*(2), 56–61.

Burke, F. J., Wilson, N. H., Cheung, S. W., & Mjör, I. A. (2001). Influence of patient factors on age of restorations at failure and reasons for their placement and replacement. *Journal of Dentistry, 29*, 317–324.

Cardoso, M., Baratieri, L. N., & Ritter, A. V. (1999). The effect of finishing and polishing on the decision to replace existing amalgam restorations. *Quintessence International, 30*, 413–418.

Dörter, C., Yildiz, E., & Erdemir, U. (2000). Effect of operators' skills on increase in cavity volume of restorations. *Quintessence International, 34*(1), 27–30.

Fernández, E. M., Martin, J. A., Angel, P. A., Mjör, I. A., Gordan, V. V., & Moncada, G. A. (2011). Survival rate of sealed, refurbished and repaired defective restorations: 4-year follow-up. *Brazilian Dental Journal, 22*(2), 134–139.

Gordan, V. V., Garvan, C. W., Richman, J. S., Fellows, J. L., Rindal, D. B., Qvist, V., et al. (2009 Nov-Dec). How dentists diagnose and treat defective restorations: evidence from the dental practice-based research network. *Operative Dentistry, 34*(6), 664–673.

Green, D., Mackenzie, L., & Banerjee, A. (2015). Minimally invasive long-term management of direct restorations: The '5 Rs'. *Dental Update, 42*, 413–426.

Hickel, R., Peschke, A., Tyas, M., Mjör, I., Bayne, S., & Peters, M. (2010). FDI World Dental Federation: Clinical criteria for the evaluation of direct and indirect restorations – update and clinical examples. *Clinical Oral Investigations, 14*(4), 349–366.

McAndrew, R., Chadwick, B., & Treasure, E. T. (2011). The influence of a short training program on the clinical examination of dental restorations. *Operative Dentistry, 36*(2), 143–152.

Moncada, G., Martin, J., Fernández, E., Hempel, M. C., Mjör, I. A., & Gordan, V. V. (2009 Apr). Sealing, refurbishment and repair of class I and class II defective restorations: A three-year clinical trial. *Journal of the American Dental Association, 140*(4), 425–432.

Pitts, N. (2004 Sep). 'ICDAS' – an international system for caries detection and assessment being developed to facilitate caries epidemiology, research and appropriate clinical management. *Community Dental Health, 21*(3), 193–198.

Qvist, V., Johannessen, L., & Bruun, M. (1992). Progression of approximal caries in relation to iatrogenic preparation damage. *Journal of Dental Research, 71*, 1370–1373.

Ryge, G., & Snyder, M. (1973). Evaluating the clinical quality of restorations. *Journal of the American Dental Association, 87*, 369–377.

Setcos, J. C., Khosravi, R., Wilson, N. H., Shen, C., Yang, M., & Mjör, I. A. (2004 Jul-Aug). Repair or replacement of amalgam restorations: Decisions at a USA and a UK dental school. *Operative Dentistry, 29*(4), 392–397.

Case 69
Implant Planning

KALPESH A. BAVISHA

Summary

A 30-year-old man presents to you with missing central and lateral incisors. What are the treatment options and their likely chances of success?

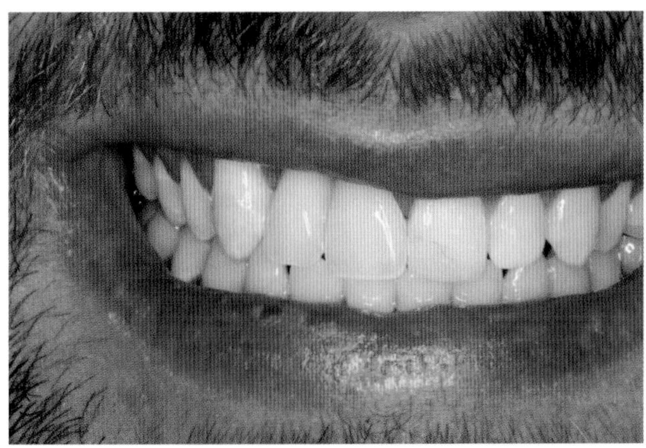

• **Fig. 69.1** An intraoral clinical anterior view of the patient in the intercuspal position with the denture replacing upper right incisor and upper right incisor in place.

History

Complaint

The patient requests fixed replacement of his two front teeth.

History of Complaint

The patient fell 6 months ago and knocked out his two front teeth. He has been wearing an immediate replacement denture since.

Dental History

The patient has attended regularly for dental treatment. He had previous fixed orthodontic treatment as a child.

Medical History

The patient is otherwise fit and well.

Examination

Extraoral Examination

The temporomandibular joints appear normal, and no submental, submandibular or cervical lymph nodes are palpable.

◆ What Can You Deduce From the Clinical Appearances Seen in Figs 69.1 and 69.2?

In the extraoral examination, certain aesthetic considerations should be assessed:

- Extraoral examination of the lips and the amount of tooth and gingiva visible when the patient is in a resting lip position and smiling
- The case becoming more challenging as more gingiva and tooth are visible
- Recording the position of lip in relation to coverage of teeth and gingiva at rest and smiling and noting the lip support a removable prosthesis may provide
- Asking the patient to swallow and to have their teeth slightly apart will give an idea of the amount of tooth tissue visible

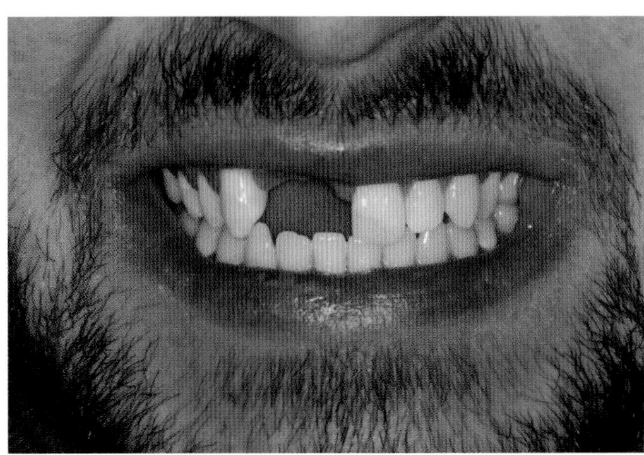

• **Fig. 69.2** Intraoral clinical anterior view in the intercuspal position with denture removed, showing amount of tooth tissue and gingiva visible on smiling.

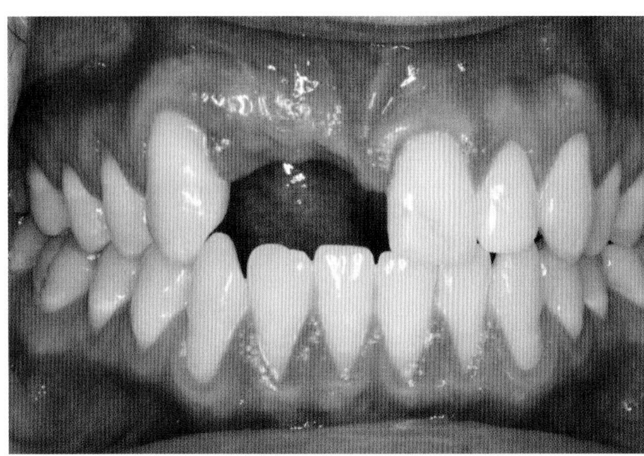

• **Fig. 69.3** Intraoral clinical anterior view in the intercuspal position with denture out, showing interocclusal space and mesio-distal space and amount of vertical tissue loss in the edentulous area.

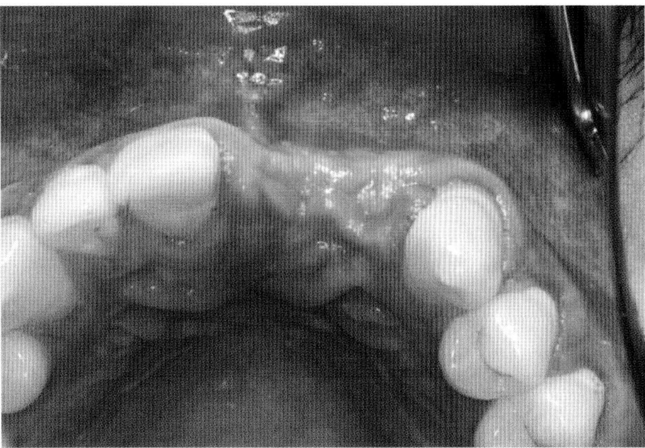

• **Fig. 69.4** Intraoral clinical occlusal view of the maxilla, showing the healthy appearance of the mucosa in the denture-bearing area and the anteroposterior width of the ridge in the edentulous area.

- Observing the patient during routine conservation will give a more accurate lip position
- Asking the patient to smile and then to give a maximum extension smile is also helpful.

Intraoral Examination

A thorough intraoral clinical examination should be carried out to ensure that no primary disease is present. Any existing periodontal disease, caries or endodontic problems should be identified and treated prior to any implant treatment. Preventive protocols should be instituted and checked for adherence before any further complex prosthodontic treatment is advised. Once soft and hard tissues have been examined, focus should be on the edentulous space.

Evaluation of the Edentulous Space

Figs 69.3 and 69.4 show that the upper right central and lateral incisors are missing. The ridge height in this region is irregular. Approximately 3 mm of keratinized tissue band is visible. This is the pale pink soft gingival tissue near the tooth. When smiling, the patient does not show the gingival zeniths (highest point) of the contralateral natural teeth (see Figs 69.1 and 69.2).

The upper left central incisor is restored with resin composite involving the mesio-incisal surfaces. Healthy, sharply defined papillae are visible around the remaining teeth. No gingival recession or loss of papilla is noted.

The patient is wearing a removable, acrylic, mucosa-borne partial denture with no clasps. The palate appears to have healthy mucosa, and no inflammation is present over the denture-bearing region. There is minimal gingival inflammation around the premolars, and oral hygiene seems to be satisfactory.

It is important to keep in mind that susceptibility to periodontitis is associated with increased implant failure and risk of peri-implantitis.

No signs of parafunctional activity can be observed. Any signs of parafunctional activity such as occlusal facets, or worn/fractured cups as a result of clenching or grinding will also factor in the decision regarding treatment option. Narrow diameter implants are contraindicated in patients showing signs and symptoms of bruxism.

The edentulous ridge height and width are assessed by careful digital palpation. Large concavities are usually readily detectable.

An important measurement is that of the available tooth space/dimensions of the edentulous ridge. It is best to measure at the narrowest point between adjacent natural teeth at the level of the crown. A commonly quoted minimum span is 6 mm, allowing a narrow 4 mm implant diameter, with 1 mm of bone surrounding it.

However, it is also important to remember that the selection of the most appropriate diameter of implant has a bearing on the final aesthetics to allow the correct emergence profile of the definitive restoration. As a guide, aim for a head diameter of an implant being similar to the root diameter of the tooth being replaced, provided space allows.

Also, assess if too much space exists between adjacent teeth. If this is the case, you will need to decide whether wider prosthetic teeth or spaces/midline diastema between them will be acceptable. Asses the distance between the edentulous ridge and the opposing dentition to determine if there is sufficient interocclusal space. This can be carried out by using a Williams periodontal probe, with the patient occluding in the intercuspal position.

In examining the edentulous ridge, the assessment of overlying soft tissue is important, specifically the amount of keratinized tissue available. Keratinized tissues will provide a better peri-implant soft tissue architecture compared with nonkeratinized mobile mucosa. As has already been mentioned, there is an adequate 3 mm band of keratinized mucosa available.

Assessment of Prosthesis

If the patient happy with the current denture, aim to copy it. It can, however, be difficult to transfer the aesthetics of a removable prosthesis to that of a fixed prosthesis. Examination of the current prosthesis is also a good indicator of the interocclusal space being sufficient or not. Care should be taken to ensure that the prosthetic teeth are not ridge lapped or set up labial to the alveolar ridge because this will give a false record of the actual space available. In Fig. 69.2, the prosthetic teeth appear longer than the contralateral natural teeth, and there is no papilla between the central and lateral prosthetic incisors.

Any fixed restoration will not have a labial flange, and that may result in poor upper lip support. Is a flange needed for labial support? It is possible to position teeth more labially in a removable prosthesis. It is, however, not possible to allow normal-sized teeth to exist in a smaller span or to have a fixed implant prosthesis placed anterior to alveolar bone. It is possible to create interproximal papillae in a removable denture, but natural papillae are not guaranteed in individual implant crown restorations.

Investigations

◆ What Investigations Would You Carry Out, and Why?

Periodontal examination, including a basic periodontal examination (BPE), probing depths and gingival bleeding. It is necessary to identify if active periodontal disease is present in the remaining dentition.

Examination of the Occlusion

Record occlusal contacts in the patient's retruded contact position, in the intercuspal position and protrusive and lateral excursions. For single implant-retained restorations, it is important that the initial contact occurs on adjacent natural teeth. In this case, there are no signs of wear facets or worn occlusal surfaces, and the teeth interdigitate closely in the intercuspal position, suggesting a stable intercuspal position.

Radiographic Examination

Periapical radiographs, shown in Fig. 69.5, obtained with use of a paralleling technique, offer the clinician information about:

- The overall anatomy of the maxilla in the edentulous space
- Adjacent teeth, root length, shape, angulation and proximity
- Vertical height of available bone
- Normal anatomical features, as well as any anomalies or pathological features.

Avoid placing implants near teeth that are associated with periapical radiolucent areas.

◆ The Periapical Radiographs are Shown in Fig. 69.5. What Do You See?

- Adjacent roots of the upper right canine and upper left incisor are parallel
- Presence of a retained root in the upper right incisor region
- Adequate bone support of upper right canine and upper left incisor

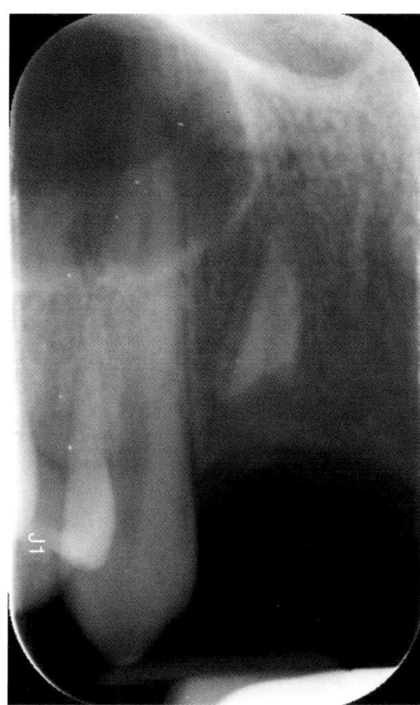

• **Fig. 69.5** A long-cone periapical radiograph showing the upper right canine (UR3 or 27) and the retained root in the upper right incisor (UR2 or 7) position and the edentulous space adjacent to it.

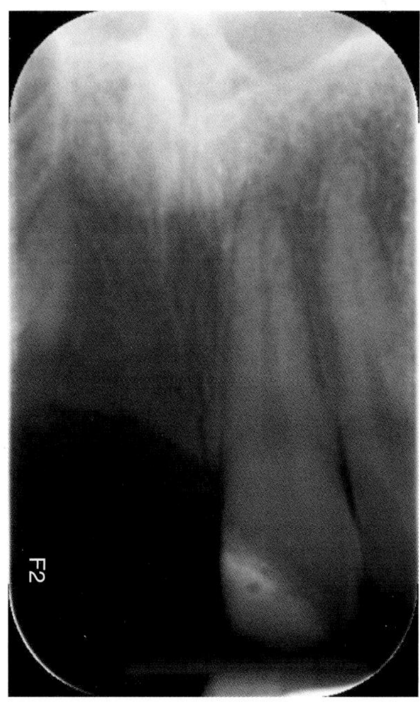

• **Fig. 69.6** A long-cone periapical radiograph showing the upper left incisor Also visible is the retained root in the upper right incisor region and the edentulous space adjacent to it.

In Fig. 69.6, it is also possible to make out the region of the incisive canal.

Cone Beam Computed Tomography

In some complex cases, plane film images may need to be supplemented with three-dimensional (3D) imaging with computed tomography (CT). Cone beam computed tomography (CBCT) allows small volume scans, which are

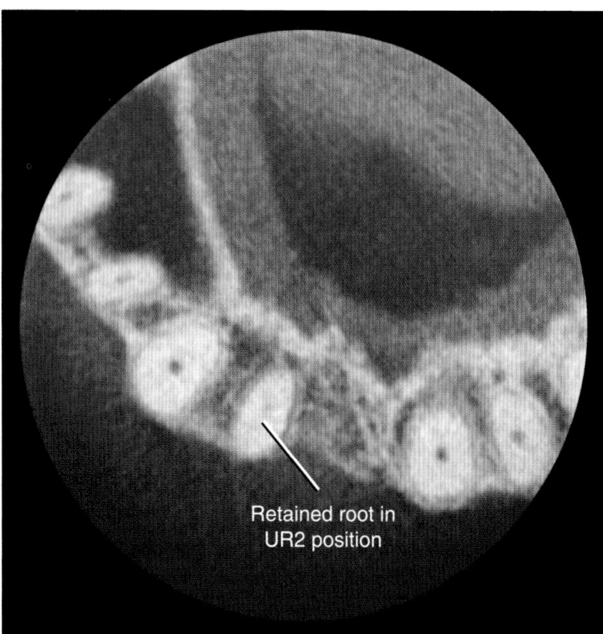

• **Fig. 69.7** Cone beam computed tomography (CBCT) image of the axial slice in the upper right incisors region to show bone width and the presence of the retained root.

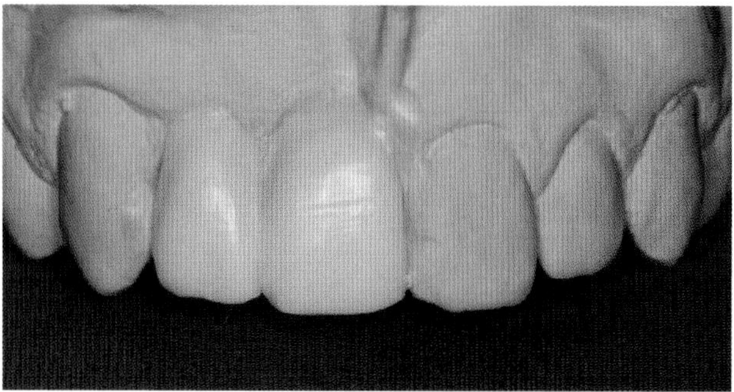

• **Fig. 69.8** Clinical photograph of a diagnostic wax-up of the missing upper right incisors.

ideal for dental practice, an example is shown in Fig. 69.7. The advantages are that the volume of bone available is known, and accurate measurements can be made. With the use of planning programs, implant length and diameters can be selected. It can also be used in the planning to construct a 3D surgical guide to aid surgical implant placement.

Diagnostic Set-Up

To help decide the size and shape of the replacement teeth, a diagnostic wax-up can be created. On a study cast, the teeth are waxed up as a guide, as shown in Fig. 69.8. The set-up should establish the height and width of the crowns and their emergence profile and provide an estimate of the level of soft tissue coverage. The set-up could be made in wax or as digitally generated images, both of which can be difficult for the patient to visualize, appreciate and comment on. It is preferable to try something in the patient's mouth. If a screw-retained implant restoration is planned, it is important that this is replicated in the wax-up because the palatal aspect will be more bulky compared with that of a natural tooth. A putty index of the wax-up is then taken and filled with a temporary crown material and positioned in the mouth. Once set, this can be trimmed to allow the patient to visualize what could be achieved in the definitive restoration. It is important here to ensure that the patient realizes the lack of soft tissue papillae and colour match. The potential gingival discrepancy at the apex and the amount of lip support may not be depicted accurately. This stage is of paramount importance in terms of managing the patient's expectations about the outcome of the final treatment. Conversations must be recorded accurately in the patient's notes.

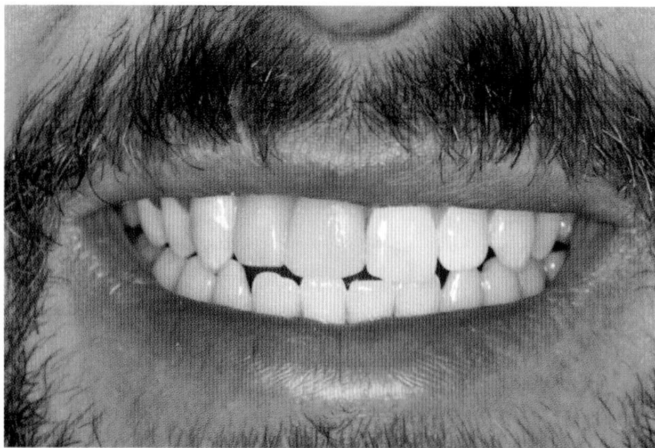

• **Fig. 69.9** Intraoral clinical anterior of the maxilla showing a diagnostic wax-up on a cast that has been transferred to the patient by using acrylic provisional material.

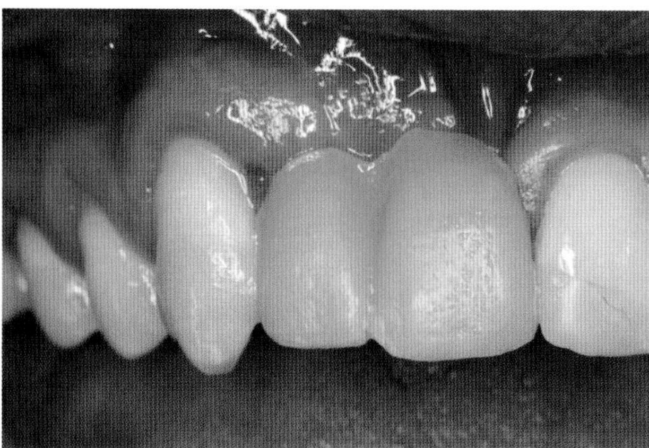

• **Fig. 69.10** Intraoral clinical anterior view of the maxilla showing intraoral wax-up demonstrating gingival the discrepancy, lack of papillae and width and height of the crowns.

Diagnosis

◆ What are Your Provisional Diagnoses?

- Missing upper right incisor
- Missing upper right incisor
- Retained root of upper right incisor

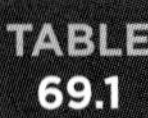

TABLE 69.1 Options Available To Replace Missing Teeth

Removable Prosthesis	Fixed Conventional	Fixed, Implant-Supported
Able to provide good aesthetics; does not involve surgery or preparation of remaining teeth. It will, however, result in further gingival coverage. Stability could be improved by making it more tooth-supported, which would involve rest seat preparations and clasping teeth, which may be visible. This will offer less gingival coverage than a mucosa-borne acrylic denture, but more than a fixed option. Oral hygiene must be optimal to prevent further plaque biofilm accumulation.	**Adhesive** A minimal preparation bridge is possible. Little/no tooth preparation involved. A two-unit span makes the design more complicated: fixed-fixed or two-cantilever designs available. Also, the upper left central incisor was involved in the initial trauma and has a large resin composite restoration, which reduces the enamel surface area for bonding. Survival rates of 8 years or more may be possible. **Conventional** Conventional bridge work would involve preparation of the unrestored upper right canine. Biologically more destructive. Survival rates of 15 years documented.	Implant restorations would require two implants, either linked or separate, depending on diagnostic wax-up and final implant placement. This option requires elective surgery, provisionalization and multiple visits. Discussion on long-term maintenance and complications if there is medical history of smoking and uncontrolled diabetes. More expensive option.

Treatment

◆ How Could You Replace the Missing Teeth?

See Table 69.1.

Whichever option is selected, the patient should be made aware of the need of ongoing lifelong maintenance and the responsibility to maintain meticulous oral hygiene and preventive home care.

Medico-Legal Considerations

Good record keeping of the clinical findings and discussions with the patient are essential. An implant option should be discussed with the patient even if you are not the clinician providing the treatment. When discussing implant options, it is important to clarify that this option is not a lifelong solution and that the restoration has a limited life expectancy, as in other treatment options. The basic treatment sequence should be discussed, as follows.

Examination

- Completion of any necessary ongoing disease control/prevention, dental treatment, extractions, periodontal treatment, restoration of teeth and preventive maintenance
- Diagnostic set-up with specialized radiographs, if needed
- Discussion/documentation of treatment options
- Construction of any provisional or transitional restorations, as required
- Construction of a surgical stent for implant placement
- Surgical placement of implants
- Adequate time to be allowed for healing and osseointegration
- Prosthodontic phase, which may include provisional restoration prior to definitive restoration
- Maintenance

This discussion should emphasize the complicated nature of treatment and also the time frame.

If a referral is to be made, it is important that you refer your patient to someone with suitable skills in implant treatment and that the patient keeps you updated of ongoing treatment. A discussion should be had about who will provide ongoing maintenance and management of complications that may occur during and after treatment. The patient must be fully engaged throughout these discussions and the procedures.

Case 70

Domiciliary Care

ELLIE HEIDARI

Summary

A 60-year-old female patient has called your practice with regard to a possible broken complete upper acrylic denture. She mentions that she dropped the denture and can now see a fracture line in the middle of it but that it is still intact. She is afraid that the denture, fitted 3 years ago, will shortly break in half. Your patient started attending the practice a few years ago but has been an irregular attender. In the last several weeks, she has been living in a care home because of complications associated with her hip replacement operation. As a result, she is now unable to travel to your practice and, thus, requires a domiciliary visit to a care home. She is otherwise fit and healthy with well-controlled blood pressure.

History

Complaint

The patient dropped her maxillary denture 3 weeks ago and has noted a line in the middle of the denture base. She is anxious that it might break in two. She also has noticed that her mouth is comparatively dry since she started her medication. She takes numerous sips of water during the day.

Medical History

She has a history of osteoporosis, and she had a recent surgery for her fractured hip. She is currently having a course of physiotherapy. The pain is controlled with fast-acting opioids (tramadol tablets) that she usually takes three to four times a day. Her American Society of Anaesthesiologists (ASA) score varies from II to III and depends on her current medical condition and how well controlled it is. Her hypertension had previously been controlled with angiotensin-converting enzyme (ACE) medication (lisinopril, an ACE inhibitor) and now has stopped. Her most recent blood pressure reading was 155/85 mm Hg.

Dental History

This patient is an irregular attender. Her Modified Dental Anxiety Scale (MDAS) score is 10.

Social History

The patient's carers at the nursing home are currently supporting her with self-care. Her daughter visits her daily and is involved in her care. The patient is currently unable to leave the care home and has limited mobility.

Problem

◆ How Can You Provide Dental Treatment for This Patient?

You and your oral healthcare team can assess this patient's dental needs by visiting her in the care home and provide domiciliary care while she is recovering from her operation. Prior to your visit, it is important to contact the care home and involve the care manager, who might wish to involve the patient's daughter. The care (support) workers will advise you about a suitable time for all parties involved (the care home staff, the patient and the patient's daughter). Try to avoid busy times (e.g. lunch and visiting times) if you wish to get full support from the care home staff.

Part 1: The Processes and Procedures of Domiciliary Care Provision

◆ What is the Definition of Domiciliary Oral Healthcare?

The British Society for Disability and Oral Health guidance for the Domiciliary Oral Healthcare Service (2009) describes domiciliary oral healthcare 'as a service that reaches out to care for those who cannot reach a service themselves. Domiciliary care is intended to include oral health care and dental treatment carried out in an environment where a patient is resident either permanently or temporarily, as opposed to that care which is delivered in dental clinics or mobile units'.

◆ Who Can Provide Domiciliary Oral Healthcare?

Domiciliary care may be provided via the general dental service (GDS), salaried primary dental care service (SPDCS) or, occasionally, the hospital dental service (HDS).

◆ Why is It Important That You Provide Domiciliary Oral Healthcare for Your Patient?

Although this patient's mobility might be limited temporarily, she has equal rights to the same high-quality oral health care as when she was able bodied and fully mobile. You need

TABLE 70.1 A Range of Guidance or Relevant Documents for Provision of Domiciliary Care in the UK

The Guidance	Relevant Website
National Health Service (NHS) England: *Guides for Commissioning Dental Specialties – Special Care Dentistry September (2015)*	https://www.england.nhs.uk/commissioning/wp-content/uploads/sites/12/2015/09/guid-comms-specl-care-dentstry.pdf
The Equality Act (2010)	https://www.legislation.gov.uk/ukpga/2010/15
NHS England: *Mental Capacity Act (2014). A Guide for Clinical Commissioning Groups and other Commissioners of Healthcare Services on Commissioning for Compliance*	https://www.england.nhs.uk/wp-content/uploads/2014/09/guide-for-clinical-commissioning.pdf
The Department of Health, The NHS Constitution: *The NHS belongs to us all (2010)*	http://www.yas.nhs.uk/AboutUs/docs/NHS_Constitution_201.pdf
Public Health England and Department of Health: *Delivery of Better Oral Health: an Evidence-Based Toolkit for Prevention,* 3rd edition.	https://www.gov.uk/government/uploads/system/uploads/attachment_data/file/605266/Delivering_better_oral_health.pdf
General Dental Council: *Standards (2015)* and *Scope of Practice (2013)* General Dental Council, London (2013): *Standards for the Dental Team*	https://www.gdc-uk.org/professionals/standards/team
General Dental Council, London (2012): *Preparing for Practice*	https://www.gdc-uk.org/professionals/students-and-trainees/learning-outcomes
British Society for Disability and Oral Health: *Guidelines for the Delivery of a Domiciliary Oral Healthcare Service (2009)*	http://www.bsdh.org/documents/BSDH_Domiciliary_Guidelines_August_2009.pdf
Scottish Government (2007b): *The National Care Standards*	http://www.gov.scot/Publications/2002/09/15395/10815
National Institute for Clinical Excellence (NICE)	https://www.nice.org.uk/guidance/conditions-and-diseases/oral-and-dental-health#pathways
NICE (2016): *Oral health for Adults in Care Homes* and *Oral Health Promotion: General Dental Practice (2015)*	https://www.nice.org.uk/guidance/ng48
Social Care Institute for Excellence: *Deprivation of Liberty Safeguards (DoLS) at a glance*	https://www.scie.org.uk/mca/dols/at-a-glance
NHS England: *Safeguarding adults*	https://www.england.nhs.uk/wp-content/uploads/2017/02/adult-pocket-guide.pdf

to provide unbiased dental care, considering the individual's needs, demands and expectations. You can always contact your local specialist services for advice/support with her individualized care plan, when necessary. You should be aware of available local specialist dental services (including the local community dental services [CDS]) and how to contact them.

What Information Does the General Dental Council 'Standards for the Dental Team' Provide With Regard To a Patient's Health and Wellbeing?

The General Dental Council (GDC) 1.6.3 standard mentions that 'you must consider patients' disabilities and make reasonable adjustments to allow them to receive care which meets their needs. If you cannot make reasonable adjustments to treat a patient safely, you should consider referring them to a colleague'. The GDC standard 1 (includes patient expectations and put patient's best interest first) states that 'all aspects of their health and well-being will be considered and they will receive dental care that is appropriate for them'.

What Other Laws, Standards and Guidance are Relevant for Provision of Domiciliary Oral Healthcare?

Table 70.1 Outlines the current guidance and references. These are few of many that you need to be aware of.

The information contained in the tabulated documents is useful. You should visit the relevant websites regularly to ensure that you have access to the latest and updated versions of guidance.

What Would Be Your Next Steps Now That You are Aware of Your Responsibilities?

You need to follow your local domiciliary protocol (Fig. 70.1). The protocol will contain vital information about your acceptance criteria, patient care pathway, data security and patient confidentiality.

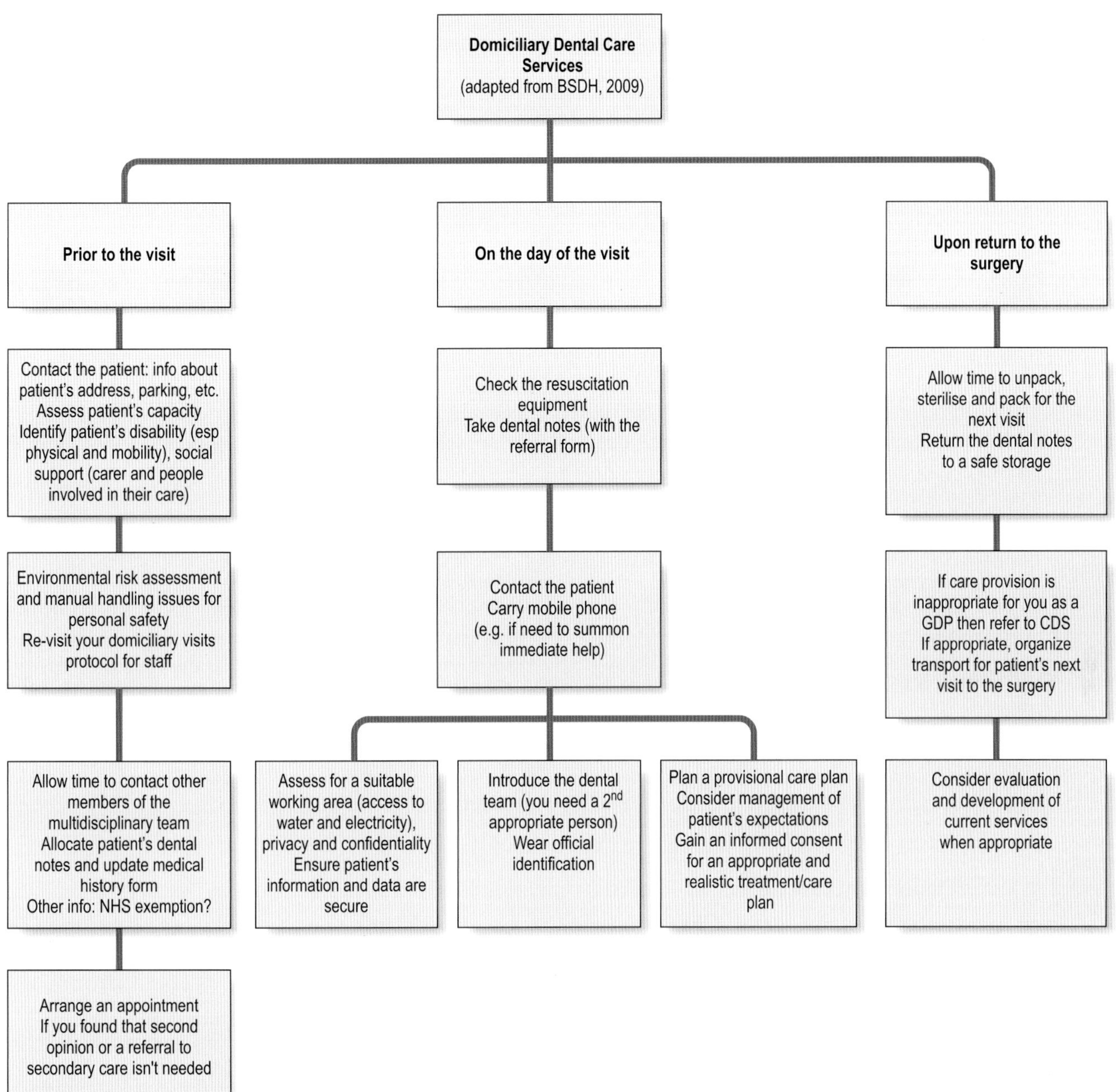

• **Fig. 70.1** An example of patient care pathway adapted from a domiciliary care protocol.

◆ How Can You Ensure Patient Confidentiality and Avoid a Medico-Legal Allegation?

The GDC standards set out in 'Standards for the Dental Team' important principles that you need to be aware of and to practise accordingly. A review of standards 3 (Obtain valid consent), 4 (Maintain and protect patients' information), 6 (Work with colleagues in a way that serves the interests of patients), 7 (Maintain, develop and work within your professional knowledge and skills) and 8 (Raise concerns if patients are at risk) is recommended prior to your visit. Note that the medical/dental defence organisations also can provide useful documents for your information.

An example of how you can protect patient data (when you provide domiciliary care) is having an encrypted and password-protected laptop that will be stored in a secure location during the domiciliary visit and afterwards. For more information about data protection, see the Information Commissioner's office (ICO) (Table 70.2) and the EU General Data Protection Regulation (GDPR, 2018) websites.

◆ What Questions Will You Ask When You Contact Your Patient?

In general, you can explore issues regarding the patient's ability to attend the surgery, and once there, the ability to be transferred to the surgery's dental chair. If possible, arrange transport for the patient to attend the surgery (see Fig. 70.1). You can enquire about transport arrangement by liaising and seeking advice from your local CDS.

However, in this case, because it is impractical for the patient to attend your dental surgery, you need to know if/when she can return to the surgery. You may want to assess the likelihood of the patient's ability (e.g. recover fully from her operation) to return to the surgery for her future dental appointments. The information gained during this encounter (from the patient's medical history, her capacity assessment, support, etc.) will enable you to decide whether you should refer the patient to a specialist dental service (e.g. CDS) or make reasonable adjustments to provide the needed care yourself. You need to prioritize the patient's care (urgent or on a waiting list) once you have accepted the responsibility to provide care for your patient.

This is also the time to gather information about the patient's request. Is she requesting a new denture? In some cases, the patient's family members are keen on getting her a new denture, and you need to discuss different treatment options with the patient and the carer(s) before your visit. In this case, the patient wishes to keep her denture and repair it, if necessary.

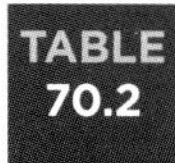

TABLE 70.2 The Information Commissioner's Office (ICO) – Website for Data Protection Self-Assessment

The Guideline	Relevant Website
The Information Commissioner's Office (ICO): *Data protection self-assessment*	https://ico.org.uk/for-organisations/resources-and-support/data-protection-self-assessment/

◆ Now That You Have Decided To Provide Care, What Equipment Do You Require for the Visit?

You need to have available portable prosthetic kits because you are anticipating that the denture might need repairs. See the list of relevant items and other kits that have been adapted from various documents and guidance and what might be required for this domiciliary visit (see Tables 70.1 and 70.2; Tables 70.3 and 70.4).

◆ What is the Care Quality Commission's Position About Purchasing an Automated External Defibrillator?

The Care Quality Commission (CQC) mentions that 'where an automated external defibrillator (AED) is not available, we would expect to see a robust and realistic risk assessment detailing how an AED could be accessed in a timely manner, as the emergency services may not always be able to respond in the critical first few minutes of an acute cardiac arrest'.

◆ Would You Need To Pay an Extra Charge for Carrying Medical Oxygen?

Not usually. The Health and Safety Executive (HSE) recommends reviewing the documents on the Management of Health and Safety at Work Regulations and the Provision and Use of Workplace Equipment Regulations. The HSE instructs that 'a car insurance company should be informed if a vehicle is being used to transport medical oxygen. There is normally no additional charge for the carriage of D size cylinders'.

TABLE 70.3 A List of Domiciliary Care Items

Administrative Items	Routine Care Kit	Emergency Kit	Infection Control Kits
Identification badge Appointment diary Appointment cards Patient's dental record Forms: Medical history Consent Referral Laboratory FP 17's Postoperative instruction leaflets Prescription pad British National Formulary (BNF) and Prescribing in the Dental Practice section of the BNF Mobile phone Pen A–Z route map/satellite navigation system Money for parking Health promotion literature List of contact phone numbers	General kit Examination kit Disposable equipment Portable: Units Suction Handpieces (rechargeable) Light source Heat source Three-in-one CoaguChek Glucometer Blood pressure machine Carry boxes Trolley Topical anaesthetic cream/spray Local anaesthetic cartridges *Note:* You can make other kits such as restorative, periodontal, prosthetic and surgical kits	Airway and breathing as well as circulation Oral airways: Equipment to provide intermittent positive pressure Self-inflating bag with reservoir or oxygen masks with reservoir Pocket mask with oxygen port Oropharyngeal airways sizes 0, 1, 2, 3, 4 *Note:* An oropharyngeal airway size is based on the distance from the maxillary incisors to the angle of the mandible. Oxygen tubing Portable source of oxygen cylinders CD size Portable independently powered suction with appropriate suction tips and tubing (e.g. Yankauer) Emergency drugs kit and single-use sterile syringes Automated external defibrillator (AED). *Note*: All clinical areas should have immediate access to AED.	Personal protective equipment (PPE) (e.g. gloves, aprons, eye protection) Protective spectacles for patient Cling film and plastic covers Disinfection wipes Paper towels, rolls, tissues Alcohol gel Waste bags: yellow bags Sharp bins: disposable equipment items Carrying boxes (one for clean instruments and one for contaminated instruments) Scissors Local guidance for transportation of instruments

◆ How Can You Ensure Safe Transportation of Medical Oxygen?

The HSE requires that 'measures have been taken to prevent any leakage of contents in normal conditions of carriage'. The Guidelines are available online at http://www.hse.gov.uk/cdg/manual/commonproblems/medicalgases.htm.

The following measures, for example, can be taken:

1. The cylinder valve is properly closed
2. The equipment is carried securely in the vehicle
3. The equipment is carried in purpose-made bags or cases
4. The equipment is removed from the vehicle as soon as possible.

TABLE 70.4 A List of Relevant Documents To Consider for Provision of Domiciliary Care

The Guidance	Relevant Website
Resuscitation Council (UK): *Resuscitation Guidelines (2015)*	https://www.resus.org.uk/resuscitation-guidelines/ and https://www.resus.org.uk/resuscitation-guidelines/adult-basic-life-support-and-automated-external-defibrillation/
The Scottish National Dental Advisory Committee (NDAC): Emergency Drugs and Equipment in Primary Dental Care *(2015)*	http://www.scottishdental.org/wp-content/uploads/2015/01/Emergency-Drugs-and-Equipment-in-Primary-Dental-Care-2015.pdf

◆ How Would You Perform Risk Assessment for Provision of Domiciliary Healthcare?

The Scottish National Dental Advisory Committee (NDAC) document entitled: *Emergency Drugs and Equipment in Primary Dental Care (2015)* considered three risk areas:

1. **The nature of the dental care.** Some dental procedures such as examinations and the construction of dentures are essentially noninvasive and will carry a much lower risk. This current case and your first visit to the care home would fall into this category.
2. **The patient's medical history and any possible/likely causes of collapse or reaction to treatment.** Your patient's medical history indicates ASA levels II and III, and the patient presents with low levels of dental anxiety.
3. **The physical environment** and any possible risks related to this (Fig. 70.2).

◆ How Does the Scottish National Dental Advisory Committee Categorize the Risks?

There are three risk categories: low, moderate and significant (Table 70.5).

◆ What Areas Do You Need To Consider in Your Risk Assessment of the Physical Environment?

You need to visit your local rules and policies (see Fig. 70.1) and do an environmental risk assessment (see Fig. 70.2). Note that you also need to ask your patient about her smoking status, mobility (transfer to a chair from her own bed) and pets.

Once in the patient's care home, you need to identify an area where you can examine her safely while respecting her privacy. The empty visiting rooms with table and chairs are

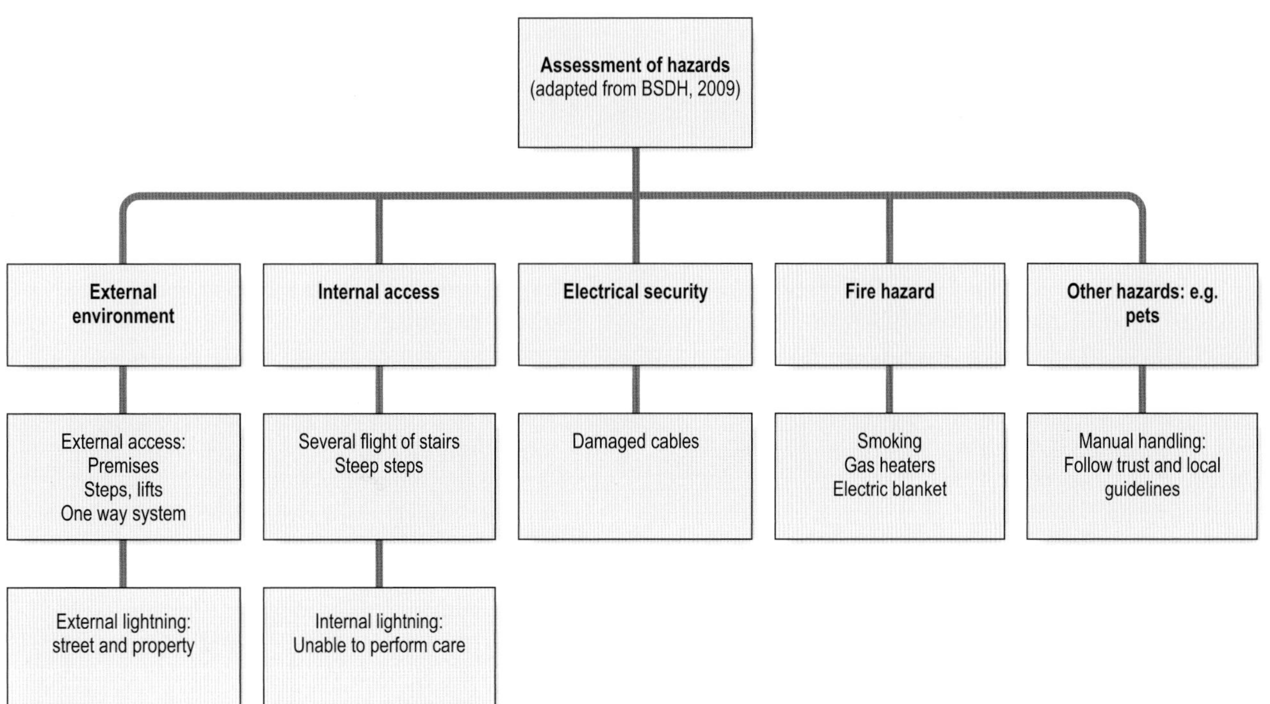

• **Fig. 70.2** An example of an environmental risk assessment.

TABLE 70.5 Risk Categories Adapted From the Scottish National Dental Advisory Committee (NDAC) 2015 Document

Risk Category	Actions
Low risk	Noninvasive dental procedure (examinations and the construction of dentures)
Moderate risk	Depends on: the nature of the dental care and if it is invasive, patient's dental anxiety; learning disabilities classification (e.g. severe); the need for clinical holding (depends on patient's ability to communicate and co-operate); support from carers; patient's medical history; comorbidities and prognosis of medical conditions/other areas that can lead to risk of patient collapse
Significant risk	The above-mentioned risks as well as physical environmental risks

usually suitable areas. The area needs to have good lightning, and access to a sink is essential. A table where you can set up for an examination is recommended. You and your dental nurse must ensure that you will not compromise infection control measures while on this visit (see Health Technical Memorandum (HTM 01-05) for more information). Fig. 70.2 provides details of different hazards areas that need to be considered prior to the visit.

◆ Can You Visit Your Patient Alone?

No. The GDC standard 6.2.5 (Standards for the Dental Team) outlines that 'if you are providing treatment in a care or domiciliary setting, you should be supported by a GDC registrant or an appropriately trained care professional'. It is important that you utilize your staff's skill mix, show flexibility and work as part of an extended team.

◆ What are the Main Skills That You and Your Staff Require for Domiciliary Care Provision?

The British Society for Disability and Oral Health Guidelines for the Delivery of a Domiciliary Oral Healthcare Service (2009) describe the required skills with the acronym 'CAMPING':

- Communication
- Assertiveness and anticipation
- Manual handling and map reading
- Planning and time management
- Improvization
- Networking and liaison
- Gerontology; medical condition, associated problems and medical emergencies

In addition to demonstrating an understanding of the guidance already mentioned, especially that relevant to special care dentistry, staff members need to have up-to-date training in manual handling, basic (or intermediate) life support, safeguarding and obtaining informed consent. The oral healthcare team need to also be aware of legal and ethical issues and be familiar with guidelines relevant to special care dentistry as part of their continuous professional development training (CPDT).

◆ What Should You Do the Day Before the Scheduled Appointment?

You can contact the patient (see Fig. 70.1 and Table 70.3) to ensure that she is well and is expecting your visit. She may want to have her daughter present at the time of your visit.

The care home staff can provide information (see Fig. 70.2) about the care home (e.g. preferred visiting times), any possible hazards and its external facilities (parking, lifts, etc.). A suitable space to set up for a dental examination can be discussed at this time to ensure that a room is kept free for your visit. It will also give you an opportunity to update the patient's medical history on your records and contact the patient's general medial practitioner, if necessary. You and your dental nurse can prepare the kits needed for this visit (see Table 70.3) at this time.

Part 2: Care Planning for This Case

You need to find a suitable working area, if not done so previously. It must be ensured that infection control requirements have been met with regard to the working area, that the patient's dignity and privacy are duly considered and that the patient can be seated comfortably. The quality of lightning will also have an impact on your treatment. See Part 1 above for details on assessing the environment and why a second appropriate person must be present at this visit.

◆ What Steps Should You Take When You Examine This Patient?

You should follow the same principles of care planning and examination as for a patient visit to your surgery. In the GDC Scope of Practice document, it is mentioned that dentists are able to 'prescribe and provide fixed and removable prostheses'.

◆ What Information Can Be Included in the History of Denture Wearing?

Your previous dental records have confirmed that the patient is edentulous. You can assess that the patient still has the capacity to inform you about her decisions at this visit (see Table 70.1). In this part of history taking, you want to establish the following factors:

- Any other complaints regarding the denture besides the hairline fracture (e.g. problems with speech, looseness, aesthetics or eating)?
- Denture's function prior to hairline fracture?
- Has this denture fractured before? If so, when? How many times?
- The patient's expectations of the care (even her daughter's expectations).

TABLE 70.6 Outlines Features and Methods To Investigate Before Deciding About a Possible Need for a Denture Replacement

Feature	What To Investigate
The existing denture	Clean the current denture, and assess it: The severity and the extent of the crack. Is the fracture line 'clean'? Assess signs of wear and examine fit. Adequate denture hygiene: Is there trapped food debris or plaque creating an environment for denture stomatitis?
Soft tissue	Facial asymmetry, atrophy or hypertrophy
Mucosal quality	Visually assess presence of ulcers, stomatitis, pathology Palpate the ridges: has there been any fibrous change?
Quality and quantity of saliva	Xerostomia (dry mouth) can have an impact on denture retention. Patient might also have altered taste perceptions. In this case, her dry mouth is caused by her medications.
Hard tissue	Examine visually and palpate the presence of tori, inter-ridge space contour. An assessment of ridge: Degree of residual ridge resorption, tenderness, etc. Fibrous/flabby ridges (suggestive of bone loss) or sharp edge ridges. Assess mucosa support for the denture and to identify undercut ridges
Muscular control of the mouth	Can have an impact on patient's ability to cope with a denture and denture's stability Decreased chewing ability

- When was this current denture made? Is this the same one that was fitted 3 years ago? How many sets of dentures does she have?
- Her current views about wearing a denture? Can she manage without her dentures, especially if it is sent for repair?
- Any cost-related issues?
- Dietary habits?
- Other contributing causes (e.g. fatigue)? Any other possible reason.

Examination

Extraoral Examination

There is no lymphadenopathy. You can examine the tissues, the temporomandibular joint and the muscles of mastication.

In this case, the patient dropped her denture in the sink while she was cleaning it. Before your planned examination, you need to consider the factors listed in Table 70.6.

Intraoral Examination

The patient is edentulous. You need to assess dryness of mucosa (see Table 70.6) and the denture's stability and retention caused by xerostomia because of the opioid's side effect. An assessment of the denture in situ to identify displacement during facial movement and appearance (if possible) is important for making a decision about future care planning for the patient.

Assess the denture intraorally:

- For tissue damage. In this case, the damaged denture base (only a hairline fracture) is unlikely to have caused damage to soft tissue and the surrounding oral tissue.
- Check the extension of the complete upper denture and examine stability and if the fit is adequate.
- Assess retention (peripheral seal, tissue fit, if possible), stability (muscle and occlusal imbalance) and support.
- Check if a lower denture is present. Also, assess retention, support and stability. Then, if possible, assess the dentures as functional units, and check occlusion and freeway space.

You need to communicate to the patient and her daughter (if the patient wishes) the rationale behind your care plan after you have completed your examination. You need to provide care to:

- Prevent the current denture from breaking
- Improve oral health
- Avoid future trauma.

Care Plan

◆ What Would Your Provisional Care Plan Be?

The GDC standards describe a holistic approach as when clinicians 'take account of patients' overall health, their psychological and social needs, their long-term oral health needs and their desired outcomes'.

You have the following care options:

- No care provided – the patient has already mentioned that she is anxious about future fracture of the denture, and so she will not accept this option.
- Repair – the patient might also find the option of repair of her existing denture more desirable because it is the least invasive option. If the patient agrees, You can consider to make copy dentures and add her name to the denture(s).
- Review.

◆ What Advice Will You Give the Patient and Her Carers Before Leaving?

At your next visit, the denture will be fitted. Advise the patient to clean her dentures over a water-filled sink in the future. Inform the patient that once you have fitted the repaired denture and assessed it (extraorally and intraorally), there is a risk of another fracture if the denture has been repaired in cold-cure acrylic. She can then decide if and when she wishes to have a new complete denture in the future. She will also be reviewed after some time to ensure that she is coping with her denture(s).

After completion of your treatment, you need to ensure that your working area is clean and that you have left your contact details with the care home. You might wish to enquire about the care home's visiting dentist. Fig. 70.1 (see Part 1) outlines steps to be taken on your return to the surgery.

◆ What Information Can Be Included in an Oral Health Care Plan for Patients in Care Homes?

It would be useful to write an oral health care plan for this patient, outlining oral hygiene procedures, denture care routines (e.g. advice on cleaning and use of a denture brush) and when the next dental visit is recommended. The patient will need periodic (annual) assessment of denture quality, health of the supporting tissues, oral lesions and bone loss, and oral health status. The role of carers in assisting and supporting this patient with her oral health (e.g. need for supervision for denture removal/cleaning) can be outlined after obtaining the patient's permission. Discussions about denture adhesives may be required. You can visit the National Institute for Clinical Excellence (NICE) website for more information about oral health assessment tools and a daily mouth care plan.

Final Thoughts

You must present a rational approach to commissioner about a need for domiciliary services. This can entail identifying health needs of your specific community (e.g. highlighting the findings of an oral health needs assessment), service gaps, potential for redesigning services and the level of resources required.

Domiciliary services can improve access to care especially for older people in residential and nursing care homes. It causes minimal interruption to the patient's day and can addresses issues such as transportation problems and missed appointments.

Consider carefully available options for arranging to see the patient in a dental surgery as you might not be able to offer a more comprehensive dental treatment on a domiciliary visit.

Ensure that you have updated risk assessments and standard operating procedures.

Please bear in mind that a denture set can get lost in residential and nursing care homes, therefore consider copy dentures and ask the lab to add your patient's name.

Consider involving the care home staff in oral health care training.

It is important to record your oral health advice and the care you have provided in the residential and nursing care homes' patient's records.

Case 71

Managing Complaints

LEN D'CRUZ

Summary

A 29-year-old patient attends your clinic with pain from his lower left quadrant.

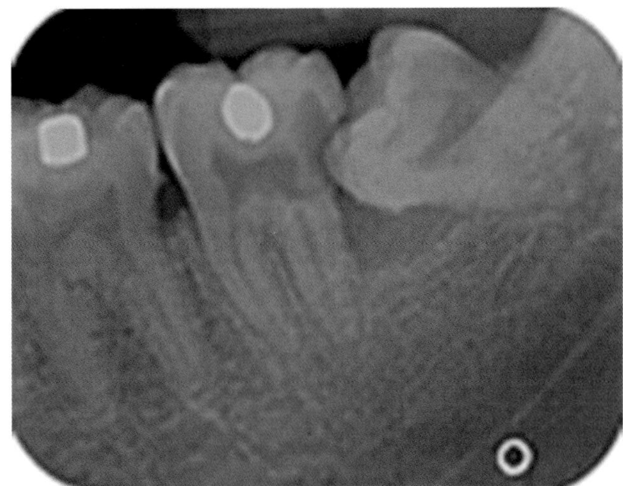

• **Fig. 71.1** A periapical radiograph of the left lower quadrant showing the mesio-angular impaction of the lower left third molar.

History

Complaint

He points to the lower left second and third molar area, saying he has had a bad taste from the tooth.

History of Complaint

The tooth has been hurting on and off for the past month or so but has got worse over the last few days. The tooth is sensitive to hot and cold, and it has started to ache spontaneously. It is occasionally tender on biting. He is also getting food caught there. Previously, he had been advised that a wisdom tooth was erupting there, but he has had no previous problems. He is going on a cruise with his fiancée in a few weeks' time and wants to get this sorted out before that.

Medical History

The patient is medically fit and healthy.

Examination

Extraoral Examination

Nothing abnormal is noted.

Intraoral Examination

The patient is fully dentate, with a small number of existing clinically sound restorations. The lower left third molar is mesio-angularly impacted against the lower left second molar. There is some food packing and plaque debris between these two teeth. There is a periodontal probing depth of 5 mm associated with this area, distal to the lower left second molar. The tooth does not respond to thermal or electric sensibility tests.

◆ What Radiographs Would You Take?

The periapical radiograph in Fig. 71.1 shows the following:

- An extensive distal radiolucency is associated with the lower second molar tooth, most likely caused by caries.
- The third molar is mesio-angularly impacted, and there is vertical bone loss up to two-thirds of the distal root of the second molar.
- The third molar is not close to the inferior dental (ID) canal, and it has a conical root.
- There are radiopaque restorations present coronally in the lower left first molar and lower left second molar, probably amalgam.
- There is distal calculus associated with the lower left first molar and some alveolar crestal bone loss.

Diagnosis

- Irreversible pulpitis in lower left second molar
- Vertical localized bone loss distally to the lower left second molar caused by impaction of third molar
- Mesio-angular impaction of the third molar
- Calculus in lower left first molar with concomitant bone loss.

Treatment Options

A number of options are available, and all will need to be discussed to obtain valid consent from the patient. It will depend on operator skills in oral surgery and endodontics as well as the patient's preferences and expectations. It will depend on access to both these specialist services if the operator does not feel confident, competent or trained to definitively manage the lower left second and third molars.

Lower Left Second Molar

◆ Is This Tooth Restorable?

Access to the distal aspect of the tooth to reach the carious tissue to remove it and allow the patient to maintain the restored tooth afterwards is hindered severely by the presence of the mesio-angularly impacted third molar.

The lower left second molar may, however, be restorable after root canal treatment if the lower left third molar is removed.

There is still significant loss of tooth structure, and a protective indirect coronal restoration will be required in the form of a full-coverage crown.

There is bone loss distally, but any pocketing may resolve after the extraction of lower left third molar.

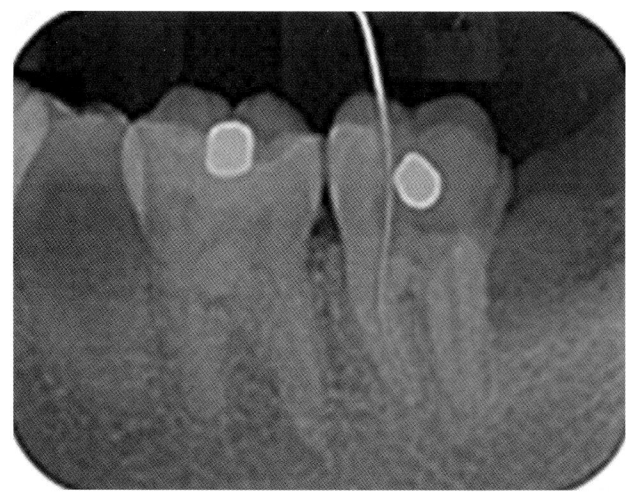

• **Fig. 71.2** A periapical radiograph of the lower left second molar, with a filling in one of the mesial canals.

◆ How Complex is the Endodontic Procedure?

This would be considered a Tier 1 endodontic procedure in the National Health Service (NHS) if there are no other complicating factors such as limited mouth opening or local difficulty in placing a rubber dam.

An alternative option would be to extract the lower left second molar and allow the third molar to erupt. It would remain in its near horizontal position but could be uprighted with orthodontic treatment and brought into reasonable approximation to the lower left first molar. This would need a potential orthodontic opinion, and tooth movement after extraction is not guaranteed.

Lower Left Third Molar

This currently nonfunctional tooth could be extracted to allow access to and treatment of the lower left second molar.

The third molar is impacted against the second molar, and its removal may require a surgical approach. However, the favourable conical-shaped roots and the potential buccal inclination of the impaction may allow careful nonsurgical elevation/rotation displacement of the tooth in trained hands. If the operator lacks the confidence, training or competence (GDC Standards for the Dental Team 7.2.1) to extract this tooth, this will need to be discussed with the patient and a suitable oral surgery referral made.

Standard 7.2 You must work within your knowledge, skills, professional competence and abilities (Standards for the Dental Team General Dental Council https://www.gdc-uk.org/professionals/standards)

Standard 7.2.1 You must only carry out a task or a type of treatment if you are appropriately trained, competent, confident and indemnified. Training can take many different forms. You must be sure that you have undertaken training which is appropriate for you and equips you with the appropriate knowledge and skills to perform a task safely.

Standard 7.2.2 You should only deliver treatment and care if you are confident that you have had the necessary training and are competent to do so. If you are not confident to provide treatment, you must refer the patient to an appropriately trained colleague.

The availability of NHS or private services will influence how soon the treatment could be carried out and whether or not this would delay the treatment of the lower left second molar. The patient is in pain, and so even if this tooth is scheduled for extraction, the pain should be addressed, and this means pulp extirpation of the second molar and a suitable provisional dressing.

Alternatively, both lower left second and third molars could be removed. Even though this might be the endpoint of care if the restorative treatment to both teeth fails, it is not necessarily an advisable first option because the patient will be left with little posterior support in the lower left quadrant. If patients are in pain, they sometimes may wish for immediate extraction to alleviate their symptoms, but consideration must be given to the final irreversible consequences of such a care plan.

Treatment Provided

In this case, the third molar was extracted uneventfully by a colleague of the operator in the same practice.

Molar endodontics was commenced on lower left second molar subsequently. A rubber dam was not used, as can be seen in the radiograph (Fig. 71.2). This is an ill-advised approach because there are obvious risks of the operator dropping the instrument and the patient swallowing or inhaling the handheld instruments. This would be considered negligent and indefensible medico-legally. There may be merit in preparing the access cavity without the rubber dam in place to help with its orientation when the tooth is rotated or tilted. Once the access cavity is cut and the canal orifices located, a rubber dam must be applied before handheld instruments such as files are used. Saliva contamination should be

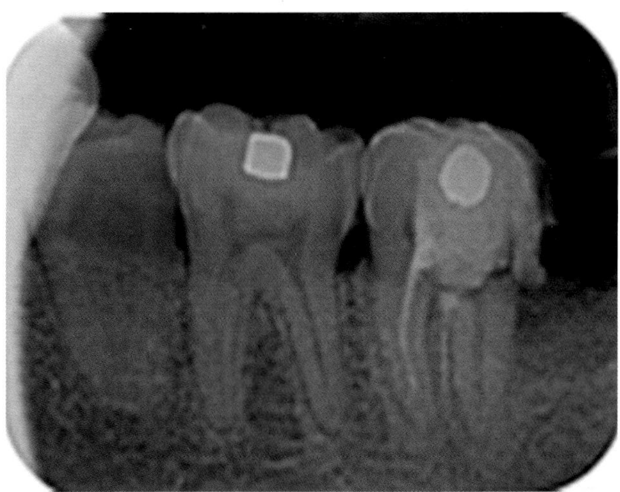

• **Fig. 71.3** A periapical radiograph after obturation of lower left second molar showing unfilled canals and perforation through the furcation area. There also appears to be a poorly condensed coronal restoration with a distal marginal discrepancy.

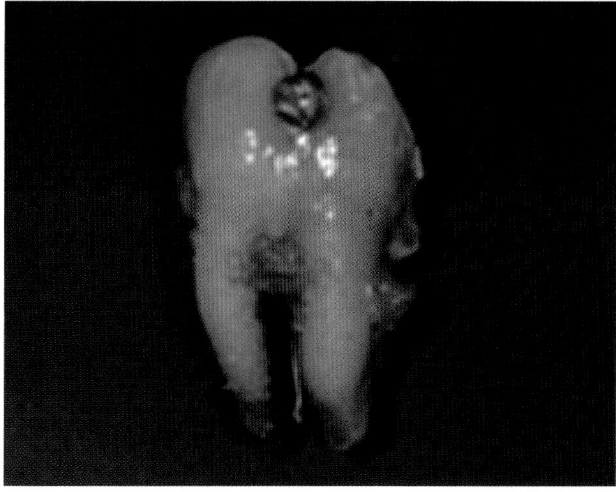

• **Fig. 71.4** Photograph from buccal aspect of the extracted lower left second molar immediately after surgery.

avoided. In this case, because the tooth was in good alignment with the rest of the dental arch, rubber dam placement was indicated from the outset.

A rubber dam was then placed and the root canal treatment completed.

Unfortunately, it was only on completion of the root canal procedure that the operator realized that the distal canal had not been filled and that a perforation was evident. This was noted on viewing the postobturation radiograph (Fig. 71.3).

The patient was informed immediately and the options of reviewing the tooth discussed, referring the patient for a specialist endodontic opinion or extraction of the tooth. With the patient's consent, the lower left second molar was extracted (Fig. 71.4).

The operator apologized and accepted responsibility for the perforation and the less-than-ideal treatment provided.

When something goes wrong, it is always important to analyse why it happened to learn from the event and reduce the chances of the error occurring again. Such events can be analysed in a number of ways, one of which is a root cause analysis (RCA – Table 71.1). This can be accomplished by adopting a clinical perspective in looking at the technical and clinical aspects of the incident as well as the dento-legal and contextual aspects, and this brings into play other human factors concerning all those involved.

Complaint

Not surprisingly, the patient was upset about losing two teeth within a very short time when he had had no other dental problems previously.

He wrote in a letter of complaint demanding to know why this had happened and why he had not been given the option of a referral for an endodontic procedure, if the operator felt it was difficult or beyond his or her capabilities.

◆ How Do You Deal with a Written Complaint?

No one ever likes receiving a complaint and particularly not in these circumstances when the care provided has led to the loss of a tooth. The first thing to do is to contact your indemnity organization for assistance. This will almost certainly be considered a case that the organization would want to settle on your behalf if the patient makes a claim for compensation against you.

Your vulnerabilities will be assessed by using a three-stage approach. To establish clinical negligence, the following three things must be established:

1. There is a duty of care between you and the patient.
2. The duty of care was breached.
3. The breach of duty directly resulted in losses (causation).

As soon as you have agreed to treat the patient, duty of care comes into existence. *Breach of duty* refers to doing something a reasonable dentist would not have done or not doing something a reasonable dentist would have done. In this case, a reasonably skilled dentist would not have perforated the tooth. Losses, that is, extraction of the tooth, have resulted from the perforation.

Manging the Complaint

The GDC expects patient complaints to be dealt with quickly and professionally and every practice to have a written complaint process.

A number of templates are available from organizations such as the British Dental Association. The process will depend on the part of the UK in which you are practising because the response times to the complaint will vary. The essential components of a complaint process are outlined in Table 71.2.

The GDC standards Section 5 say that you must:

5.1 Make sure that there is an effective complaints procedure readily available for patients to use and follow at all times
5.2 Respect a patient's right to complain
5.3 Give patients who complain a prompt and constructive response.

TABLE 71.1 An Example of a Root Cause Analysis of This Case

Root Cause Analysis Question	Reflection
What happened?	The lower left second molar was perforated during root canal treatment, a root canal missed and the tooth was extracted.
How did it happen?	The dento-legal aspects revolve around the issues of consent –failure to advise the patient of the alternatives clearly, including referral to a specialist for the root canal treatment, failing to advise the patient of the complexity and, in this case, the operator's own limited experience of complex molar endodontics.
Why did it happen?	Failure in communication
What can you do differently?	Before the procedure starts, you need to explain what is planned, how it will be done and the risks and benefits of the treatment provided. The patient should be offered the option of a referral if you think it is beyond your skill and ability either before or at any time during the procedure. When things go wrong, it is important to be open and honest and offer a clear explanation of what happened and why, and this should be followed by a discussion of what will happen next and the options. The patient needs to be reassured that his or her problem will be sorted out as quickly as possible. At an early stage, a decision about costs, if any are involved, needs to be discussed. A consideration of waiving fees or refunding any money paid should also be considered.

TABLE 71.2 The Steps in the Process of Handling a Patient Complaint

Making a complaint	A leaflet should be produced, with the name of the complaints manager identified and his or her hours of work at the practice. It must be clear that the complaint can be made in person, on the phone or via email or post. The time to acknowledge the complaint should be identified (e.g. 3 working days in England and Northern Ireland).
Investigating a complaint	Who will deal with the investigation and how long it will take to respond with a substantive response should be specified. If the complaint contains clinical issues, the practitioner who provided the treatment will be asked for his or her input, and this should be explained in the complaints leaflet. This should include what the investigation will cover (e.g. an explanation, conclusions reached and any details of remedial action taken or to be taken). The leaflet should also specify how learning from the complaint will be put into place at the practice.
If the patient is not satisfied	Addresses of whom to contact in the event the complainant remains unhappy – those of the dental complaints service and the ombudsman.

It is worth reading the detailed guidance in Section 5 of GDC standards on this aspect. The GDC advises that if a complaint is justified, then you should offer a fair solution. This may include offering to put things right at your own expense if you have made a mistake (GDC Standard 5.3.9).

If the individual is an NHS patient, he or she has the right to complain through the NHS system. In England, this is operated by NHS England. The patient has the right to complain to the practice, but if he or she does not want the practice to deal with it, then NHS England can investigate the matter. The practice will be expected to direct a letter to the patient but send it first to NHS England to ensure that all the points raised by the complainant are addressed, an apology and, where appropriate, a practical solutions are offered, an explanation of the events is given, and an action plan is prepared to prevent it from happening again.

If the patient remains unhappy, then he or she should be directed to other avenues such as the relevant ombudsman for health services complaints or the dental complaints service for complaints about private treatment.

Case 72

Loose Dentures/Resorbed Ridge Form

JONATHAN TURNER AND DAVID R. RADFORD

Summary

You are a new dentist at the practice and have been working there for just 3 months. Your nurse tells you that your next patient on the morning list has been having problems with a complete denture worn over a mandibular partial denture for the last 6 months. The previous dentist had had no luck with constructing satisfactory new dentures, and so the patient has been booked in with you for 30 minutes for new primary impressions.

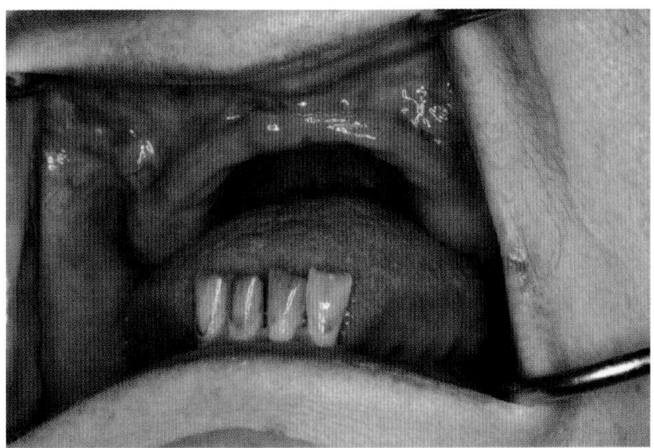

• **Fig. 72.1** An intraoral anterior view of the patient in question, showing the maxillary ridge form and remaining mandibular dentition. The anterior maxillary ridge is relatively mobile on palpation.

◆ What is Going To Be Your Strategy for the Appointment?

1. You will look through the patient's records (before your nurse invites the patient into the surgery) to see what the previous dentist has assessed and tried to achieve with the dentures made.
2. You check the medical history and note that the patient is on antidepressants, but you will update this when you see the patient. The previous dentist does not appear to have undertaken or recorded a comprehensive history, simply getting on with the technical aspects of making new dentures because the previous ones had 'failed'.

You decide, correctly, to perform a more comprehensive history taking and examination. If this is straightforward, it would be appropriate to record some primary impressions at this visit. However, if not, you will need to spend the time to properly assess the clinical situation (Tables 72.1 and 72.2). This is important because you need to try to determine if your new dentures can really improve the situation and what changes you would need to make to ensure any resolution of the cause of the problems. It is imperative not to be tempted to 'dive in' and start treatment when you have not ascertained the cause of the problem(s) and thought about how to resolve these, with discussions involving the patient throughout this process. In this way, the patient is taken along the decision-making process and can be involved in his overall care. This will increase the patient's perception of the value of the care he is receiving and his responsibilities as part of his care delivery pathway. This approach also helps reduce the risk of miscommunication between the dentist and the patient and ensure that all expectations from both sides are managed appropriately. In this way, the risk of medico-legal issues arising later is significantly diminished. All the conversations and decision-making processes must be documented contemporaneously.

◆ What are You Going To Check in Your History Taking?

1. The current problems experienced by the patient and previous denture-wearing history
2. Is the patient having problems only with the upper or lower denture, or both?
3. Is the patient experiencing looseness of the denture because of lack of stability/retention of the lower denture?
4. Is the static or functional retention of the upper complete denture poor?

You note from the previous records that the dentist tried to add a new post-dam to the maxillary denture in self-cure acrylic, but this had made the situation worse. This puzzles you.

The patient tells you that he has never got on with a lower partial denture but has previously managed with an upper complete denture satisfactorily.

◆ What Can You See in Fig. 72.1 That May Affect the Prognosis of the Dentures?

There appears to be an anterior maxillary fibrous, 'flabby' ridge, and the lower anterior teeth have overerupted somewhat over time. The fibrous ridge will affect the support of the upper denture (see Table 72.2), and as a result of the occlusal force anteriorly with the overerupted anterior teeth, this will tend to break the posterior border seal of the maxillary plate. The previous dentist tried to improve the seal by adding a new post-dam, but that made the denture even less retentive.

TABLE 72.1 Specific Prosthetic-Related Factors That Require Assessment

What Needs Assessing?	How Will You Assess?
Residual ridge – maxillary	Is there any anterior fibrous change ('flabby ridge')? What is the extent of this?
Residual ridge – mandibular	Are the ridges very resorbed, and are they knife edge?
Prognosis of remaining natural teeth	Oral hygiene and periodontal status. Presence of caries and caries risk Condition of existing restorations Sensibility and periapical status of potential denture abutment teeth
Occlusion	Are the natural teeth overerupted, or are they in an unfavourable position? How do they occlude with existing denture?
Existing dentures	Retention, support, stability Carefully assess base extensions, occlusal planes and occlusion
Saliva	Assess the quality and quantity of the saliva
Patient's expectations	Are these realistic? Retention of a complete denture over opposing natural teeth is always likely to be compromised.

TABLE 72.2 Specific Prosthetic Problems and Their Solutions

Problem	Solutions
Anterior fibrous change of maxillary ridge	You may wish to strive for a mucostatic impression of the anterior ridge if there is a support problem caused by the fibrous change. You can use alginate in a generously spaced and perforated special tray or a window tray with a light-bodied silicone or zinc-oxide eugenol (see below for more information).
Poor prognosis of remaining natural teeth	Extraction may be indicated if their presence is likely to severely reduce the chances of success of the upper denture. Retaining roots and using them as overdenture abutments may be an alternative option to help maintain alveolar bone height.
Unfavourable occlusion	If the lower teeth are overerupted, root treatment, decoronation and use as overdenture abutments may be considered.
Existing dentures	If you have identified errors with the existing dentures, take care to ensure that these errors are not repeated with your new dentures – for example, underextended bases.
Patient's expectations	You must communicate clearly to the patient (at the assessment visit) the problems associated with a complete-over-partial denture and what can and cannot be achieved.

◆ What is a Possible Reason for the Inadequacy of the New Post-Dam?

If your previous colleague had overbuilt the post-dam in acrylic, it would prevent the denture from seating properly, thus reducing overall mucosal contact. Close mucosal contact and an adequate saliva flow are vital for retention. This is why noting from the medical history that the patient is on antidepressants may affect your management because the use of many types can lead to hyposalivation as a side effect.

You can see some papillary hyperplasia on the posterior aspect of the palate and possible enlargement of the tuberosities. This is always difficult to tell unless sequential study models of the upper arch are available because it might just appear exaggerated as a result of the resorption of the anterior maxillary ridge. The above factors (tuberosity enlargement, hyperplasia and fibrous change), together with the overerupted anterior teeth and resorption of the mandibular ridge, are sometimes referred to as 'combination syndrome'. Use of this classification is not particularly helpful, however, because these factors are rarely all present simultaneously, and even if they are, it is not actually a 'syndrome'. Combined with a dry mouth, as a consequence of the use of antidepressants, the above factors will lead to difficulty with denture retention.

Other features that you should have observed are the angular cheilitis and the denture-induced hyperplasia in the labial sulcus of the 43/34 upper left and upper right canine and first premolar region. There is plaque and calculus associated with the lower incisors, and so it would be appropriate to undertake a basic periodontal examination (BPE) score and, if indicated, a probing chart for these teeth.

◆ What are the Prosthetic Difficulties of Using the Lower Incisors for Retention and Support of a Lower Partial Denture?

1. These teeth tend not to offer a useful undercut below the survey line for direct retention with clasps.

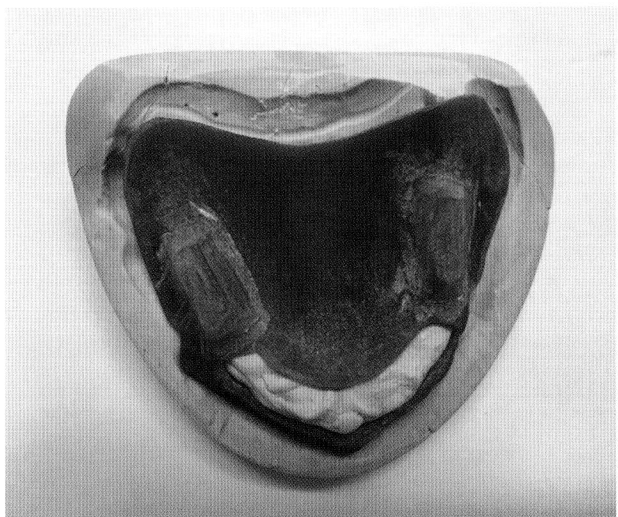

• **Fig. 72.2** The maxillary tray is close fitting on the model, with the anterior window for the fibrous anterior ridge showing.

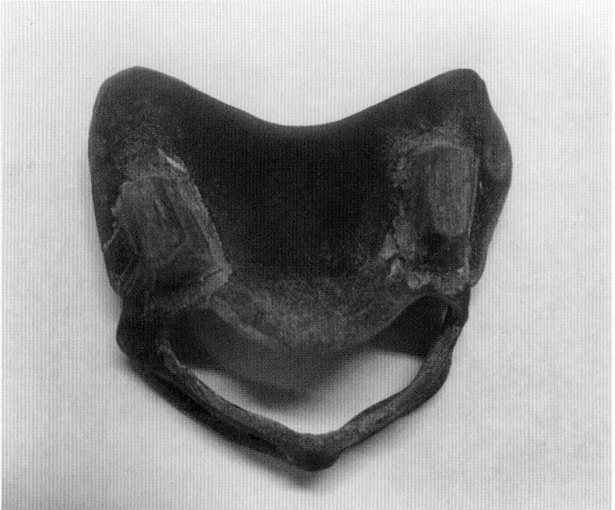

• **Fig. 72.3** A special tray showing the open window constructed from light-cured laboratory special tray material. Note the bilateral stub handles, for the operator's fingers to stabilize the tray while recording the impression.

2. If clasps are used, aesthetics may be compromised.
3. These teeth tend to have short roots and less favourable root morphology compared with the lower canine teeth.
4. These teeth do not have pronounced cingula, and so factor 3 precludes them from offering optimal tooth support.

Prosthetic Management of the Upper Fibrous Ridge

Mucostatic impressions for upper fibrous ridges have to be recorded with great care as to not cause displacement of the ridge. Special trays with an anterior open window have been advocated (Figs 72.2 and 72.3) or an impression with greater relief over the ridge anteriorly, used with alginate, might be satisfactory. The aim of the impression is to avoid displacing the fibrous, mobile section of the maxillary ridge during the recording of the impression, or this will lead to both soreness and reduced stability of the final denture.

Assessing the Current Dentures

The patient has lost the lower plate but will look for it at home. In function, the upper complete denture appears to have reasonable retention but as soon as the patient occludes, the denture displaces upwards and forwards and then loses all retention. Also, when the patient moves into lateral excursions, the denture likewise displaces. Your diagnosis is of good static retention, but poor functional retention. The borders of the denture seem reasonable, and they also appear well rounded and to be filling the lateral aspect of the sulcus. You fear that your impressions might not produce a base as good as the current one. You are also concerned that unless the patient wears a lower partial denture, you will not be able to provide an occlusion that can stabilize the upper denture. You decide to consult your colleague, and she takes a look and concurs that it would be appropriate in this case to refer the patient to the regional restorative consultant because she feels that the patient's care is outside the scope of primary dental care. You can now see the value of a proper assessment because without it, you would be struggling with this for the next 4 months.

Not Another Complete-Over-Partial Denture Case!

Your fourth patient of the morning list is another complete-over-partial denture case. The patient is complaining that the upper denture, which had been made by a clinical dental technician (CDT) 4 years ago, is getting loose. Other than that, she has been very happy with her dentures.

◆ What Do You Observe in This Image of the Patient in the Rest Position?

See Fig. 72.4.

There would appear to be a significant lack of intermaxillary clearance between the lower teeth and the upper alveolar ridge. If this really is the case, there is no room for a maxillary complete denture that gives the patient any freeway space.

◆ What are Your Options?

1. To do as in the previous case and ask for advice from a more experienced dentist or specialist
2. To go ahead, if the patient has not had previous denture difficulties caused by lack of freeway space. See the earlier case with a problem with overdentures.
3. If the teeth have a poor prognosis, consider extractions of the hopeless teeth and a lower complete overdenture on two devitalized, endodontically treated canine teeth.
4. If all the lower teeth have a hopeless prognosis, consider extractions (a clearance) and immediate complete dentures.

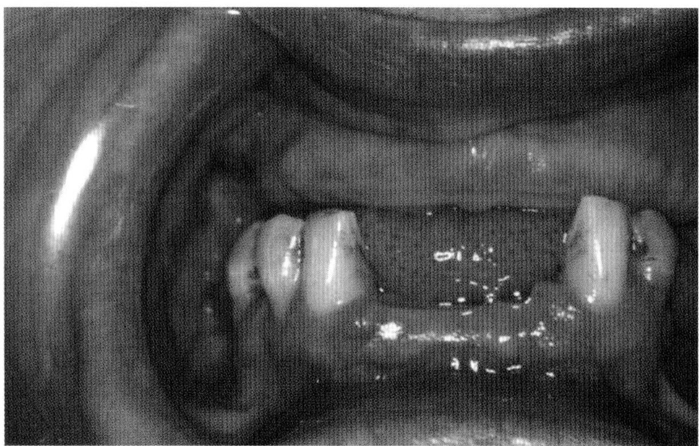

• **Fig. 72.4** Anterior intraoral view showing the patient's edentate maxillary ridge and remaining mandibular teeth.

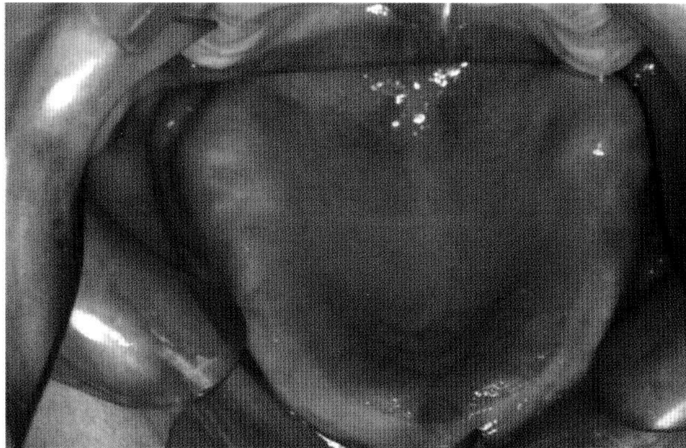

• **Fig. 72.5** A mirrored, occlusal intraoral view of the maxillary ridge and palatal contour.

5. Consider implant-supported and retained lower overdenture.

◆ What Do You Observe in This Image of the Upper Alveolar Ridge?

See Fig. 72.5.

The ridge is well formed, with no evidence of fibrous replacement, and the tuberosities are well developed, with distinct hamular notches bilaterally.

◆ What is the Significance of These Observations?

1. The ridge will offer good support and stability. The hamular notch area is an area of displaceable tissue that forms part of the post-dam, normally positioned along/within the vibrating line/area.
2. The recording of the hamular notch on the impression demarks the full posterior extent of the tuberosity.
3. The denture, if built to the depth of the hamular notch, affords a reduction in the anterior displacement of a denture.

Fig. 72.6 shows a well-constructed upper complete denture. Note the occlusal refinement of the premolar teeth to accommodate the lower natural teeth in occlusion and excursive movements.

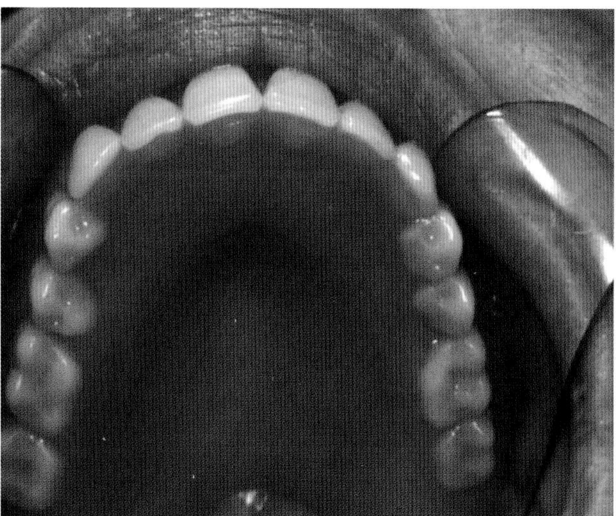

• **Fig. 72.6** An occlusal intraoral view of the patient's current maxillary complete denture in place.

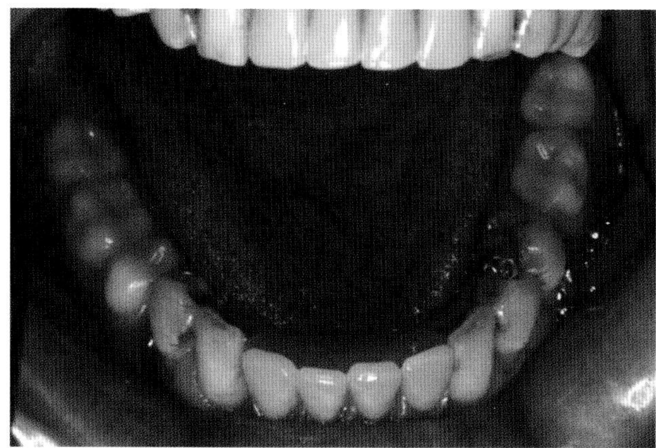

• **Fig. 72.7** A well-retained and stable mandibular denture not showing any signs of occlusal wear.

The patient's lower metal-based partial denture shows no significant wear (Fig. 72.7) and is well retained and supported.

◆ What are Your Management Options?

1. Leave these dentures for another 6 months, by which time the upper denture will probably be looser and less satisfactory but you will feel more experienced with providing dentures in general practice.
2. Refer the patient to a CDT.
3. Construct new upper and lower dentures despite the lower denture being satisfactory. A replacement lower may be considered if the current lower tooth positions are likely to adversely affect the occlusal plane or tooth positions of the new upper denture.
4. Reline the upper complete denture either chairside or by sending an impression, in the denture, to the laboratory requesting relining.
5. Construct a new upper complete denture against the lower current partial denture, either from the first principles or by using a replica block/copy denture technique.

You discuss this case with your senior colleague at your next routine case discussion session, and the colleague advises you that the laboratory does not like doing copy dentures and suggests not to reline the current denture.

◆ Considering Fig. 72.5, Why is This Good Advice?

There would already appear to be a reduced intermaxillary clearance, and relining will only increase the vertical dimension more, which means that you run the risk of severely compromising the current denture. This risk is probably even greater with a chairside relining, unless you are very experienced and skilled. Thus you decide to make a new complete upper denture against the existing lower denture. At each stage, you check that you are not deviating away from the current denture too much by comparing your impressions and wax try-in extraorally with the previous denture on the bracket table.

The Last Patient of the Morning ...

The care plan for the last patient you see was made by you in your first week in the new practice. You are concerned because you did not really assess the clinical scenario fully at that time and just got on with making the new denture – a classic error. You have stabilized the periodontitis in the lower arch with the help of the practice hygienist and have constructed the new upper complete denture (Fig. 72.8). The patient is very happy with the retention and stability of the denture and loves the appearance of the bold teeth and the midline diastema, just like he remembers how his natural teeth looked.

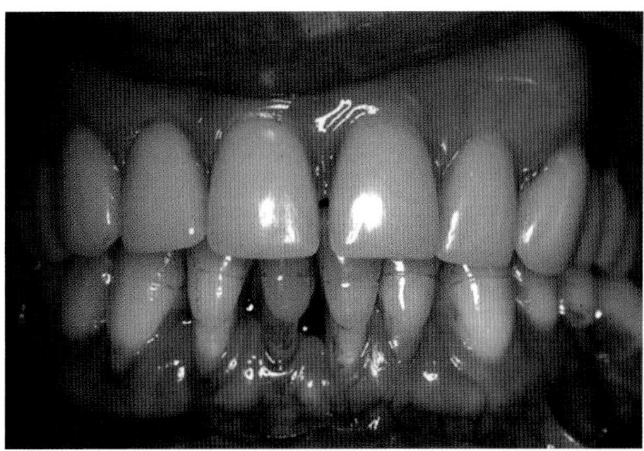

• **Fig. 72.8** An anterior intraoral view of the maxillary complete denture in occlusion with the natural mandibular dentition.

Conclusions

Not all complete-over-partial dentures placed over natural teeth are overwhelmingly challenging. However, with this series of cases, you have learnt the importance of performing a thorough assessment prior to committing yourself to a particular treatment and of recording the primary impressions. Also, you have become aware that management of patient expectations, by carefully communicating what you can realistically achieve, is crucial to successful clinical and medico-legal outcomes. Perhaps you got away with your errors in the last case of the morning because of your skill and judgment applied subsequently – or was it just good luck?

Case 73

'Invisible Custom-Made Braces'

DIRK BISTER

Summary

Here, two orthodontic treatment modalities using customized orthodontic appliances – lingual fixed appliances and aligners – are compared side by side. Both options provide treatment with minimal aesthetic impact on the patient during treatment, and both can be custom-made for the patient. For the lingual fixed appliances, a class II division 2 malocclusion with an asymmetrical buccal segment relationship is shown. The orthodontic treatment was complex and included a unilateral change of the buccal segment relationship. DW LingualSystems was used in this case. This is compared with a mild class II malocclusion treated with aligners (Align Technology), and in this case, no change in the occlusion was planned.

SUMMARY (CASE 1)

A 22-year-old patient presented with bimaxillary retroclination, an increased traumatic overbite, and crowding affecting both the upper and lower arches. The buccal segment relationship on the right was over half unit post-normal but was normal on the left. There was a subsequent lower centre line shift to the right-hand side. The upper lateral incisors were mesio-labially rotated. In the UK, the Index of Orthodontic Treatment Need (IOTN) is used to assess eligibility for treatment free of charge at the point of delivery (https://www.nhs.uk/conditions/Orthodontics/). The IOTN for this patient was 4f, which means that there was traumatic overbite, which provided the health component for qualification. Information on IOTN can be found at https://www.bos.org.uk/Public-Patients/Orthodontics-for-Children-Teens/Fact-File-FAQ/What-Is-The-IOTN.

History

Complaint

The patient complained about irregular teeth and an uncomfortable bite.

History of Complaint

Not relevant.

Examination

Extraoral Examination

On extraoral examination, the patient had a mild class II appearance. The smile line was high, and there was gingival exposure measuring 2 mm.

Intraoral Examination

Both upper lateral incisors were mesio-labially rotated, the left one more so than the right. There was crowding, particularly affecting the lower right central incisor, which was lingual to the line of the arch. The upper arch was also moderately crowded with both upper central incisors retroclined. Both upper lateral incisors were slightly small, indicating a tooth size discrepancy.

The buccal segment relationship on the right-hand side was just over half-unit class II post-normal on the first molar, but was a full-unit class II on the premolars. The buccal segment relationship on the patient's left-hand side was class I. The lower centre line was deviated to the patient's right-hand side by approximately half a lower incisor width Fig. 73.1.

◆ What Specific Questions Would You Ask the Patient?

The patients' main complaint needs to be assessed carefully. The dental health component of this malocclusion is comparatively low, although this patient is acceptable for National Health Service (NHS) orthodontic care under current commissioning guidance (see above); this, however, does not apply to treatment with customized appliances.

◆ What Further Investigations are Required?

Radiographs taken for orthodontic purposes include a dental panoramic tomogram (DPT). The radiograph showed the presence of impacted lower wisdom teeth and did not reveal any other abnormalities.

SUMMARY (CASE 2)

A 38-year-old patient presented with a mild class II incisor relationship, with a slightly increased overjet and mild irregularity mainly affecting the upper right central incisor, which was retroclined and the upper left central incisor which was labial. In the mandible, crowding was more pronounced, with the lower right canine slightly lingual to the line of the arch and residual crowding affecting the lower incisors Fig. 73.5.

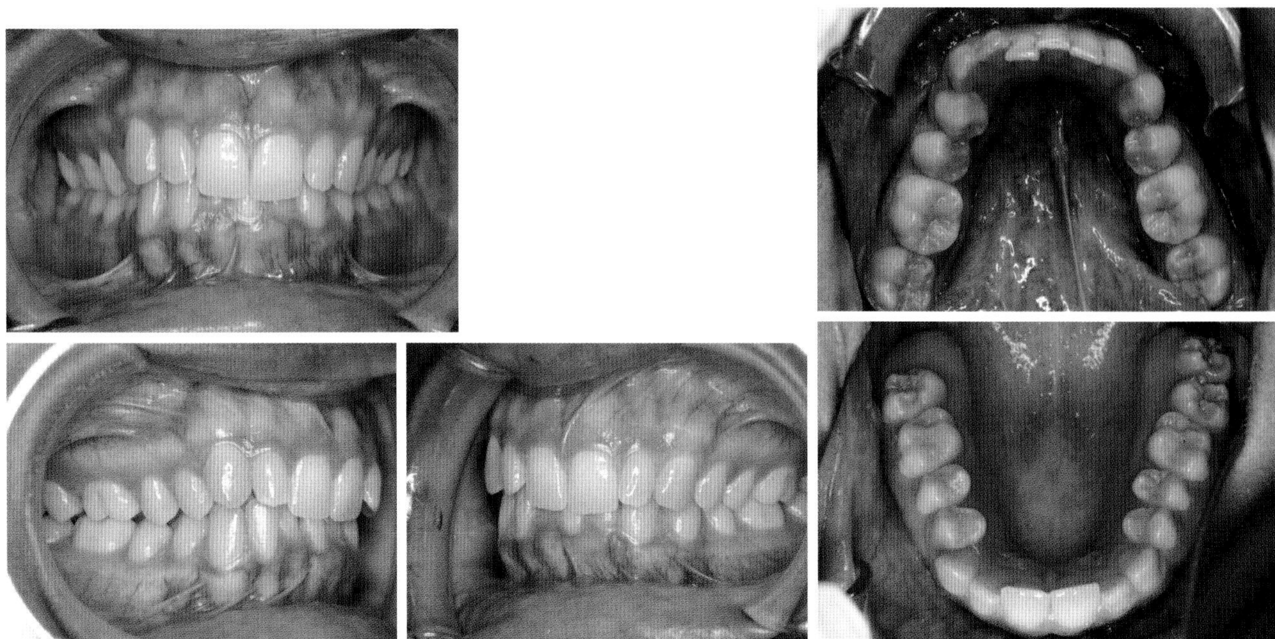

• **Fig. 73.1** Intraoral photographs of patient 1 at start of treatment. Top left: Frontal view. The increased overbite is clearly visible as is the centre line discrepancy. Lower left: Right buccal view. The buccal segment relationship is over half-unit class II on the right and the rotation of the upper left lateral incisor is visible. Lower middle: Left buccal view. The buccal segment is class I on the left-hand side; the irregularity of the upper right lateral incisor is visible. Top right and lower right images: Occlusal views. There is mild irregularity of the labial segments and overerupted and retroclined upper central incisors. The upper right canine is buccal to the line of the arch.

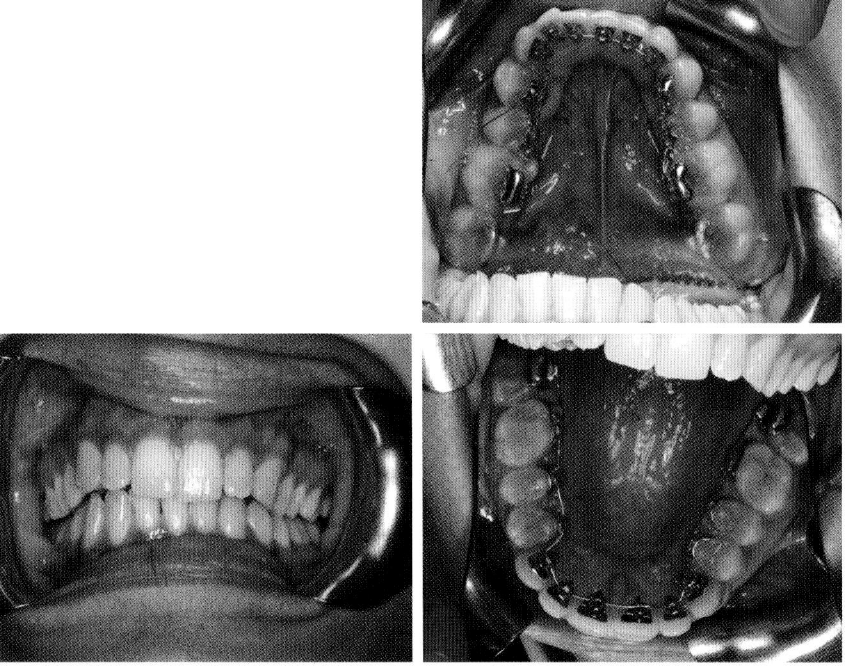

• **Fig. 73.2** Patient 1 with lingual fixed appliances fitted on day of bond-up. Left: Frontal view. The brace is not visible. There is immediate opening of the bite; this is an effect of the appliance itself and not of the treatment mechanics at this stage. Top right and lower right: Occlusal views. The fixed appliances encompass the second molars. The arch wire is, however, not extended to the second molars; this helps the patient adapt better to the brace.

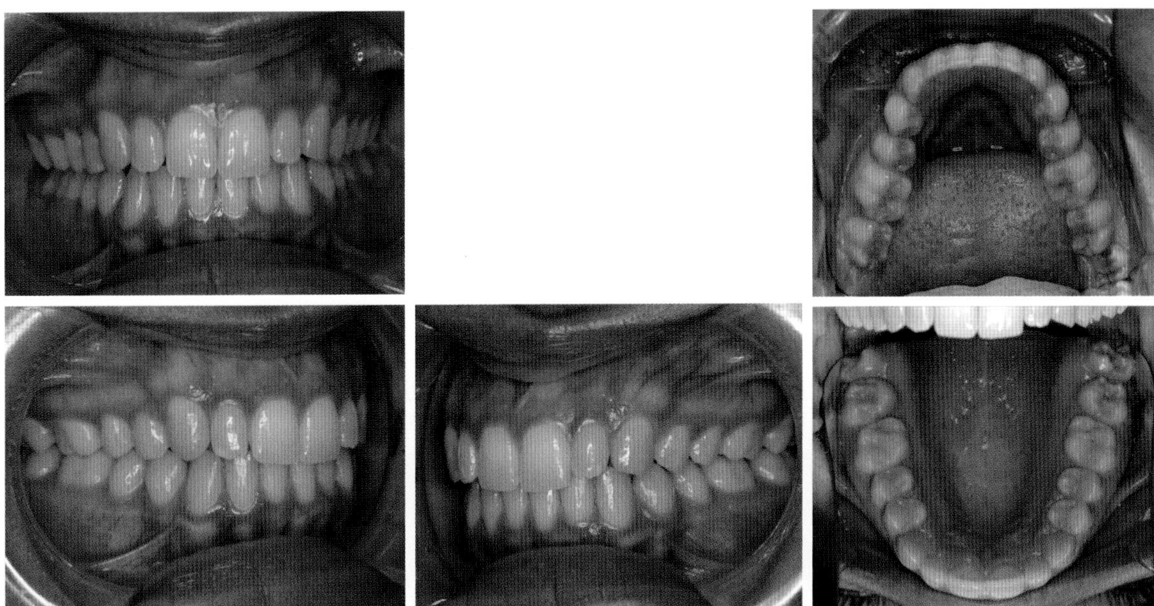

• **Fig. 73.3** Patient 1 at the end of treatment. Top left: Frontal view. The overbite is normal, and the centre lines are now coincident. Lower left: Right buccal view. The buccal segment relationship is now class I on the right-hand side. Lower middle: Left buccal view. The buccal segment is class I on the left-hand side. Top right and lower right: Occlusal views. The centre lines are corrected, the overbite and overjet are normal and the upper and lower arches are well aligned.

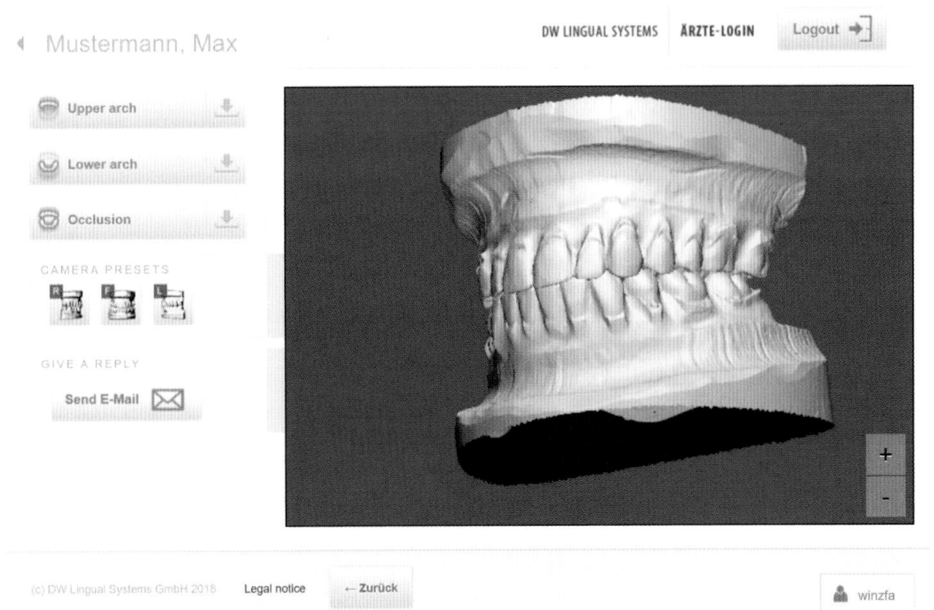

• **Fig. 73.4** Screenshot of a dental digital set-up (DW Lingualsystems). These images can be rotated and manipulated on the computer, and this improves the ability to formulate an effective treatment plan. The images can also be used for obtaining consent from patients.

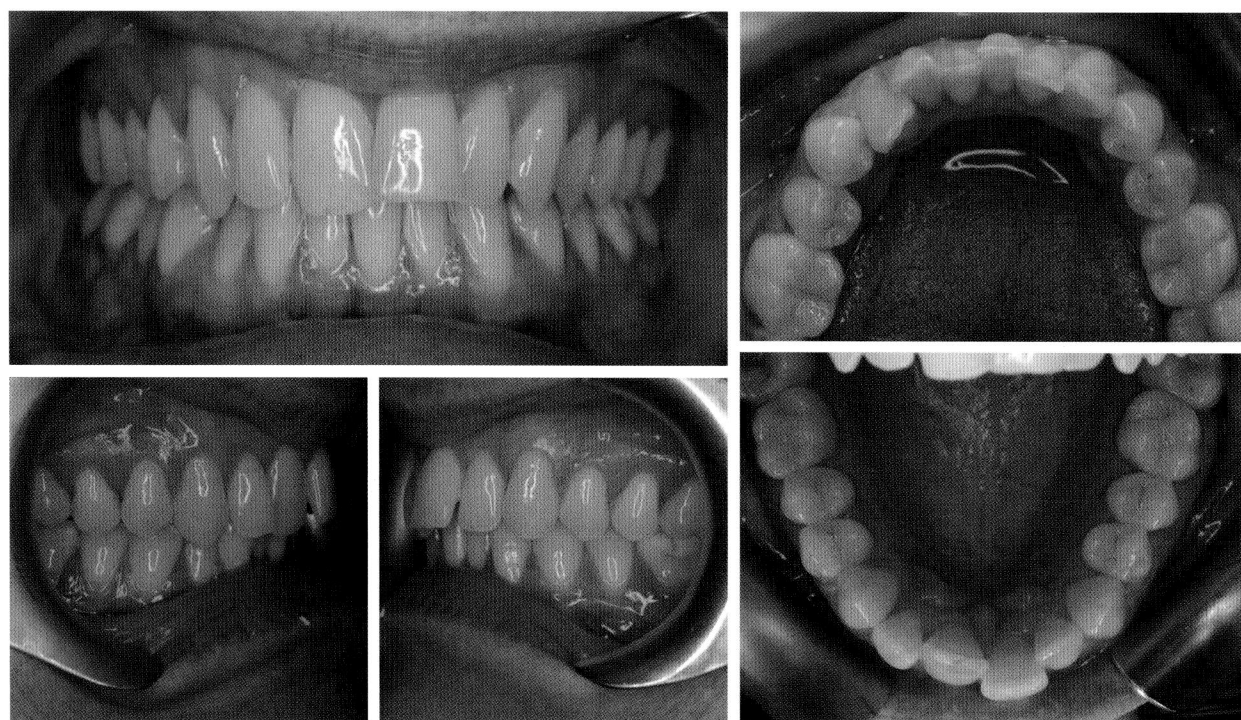

• **Fig. 73.5** Intraoral photographs of patient 2 at the start of treatment. Top left: Frontal view. The overbite is within normal limits, and there is a small discrepancy in the centre lines. Lower left: Right buccal view. The buccal segment relationship is slightly post normal. The irregularity of the upper incisors is visible. Lower middle: Left buccal view. The buccal segment is class I on the left-hand side; the irregularity of the upper incisors is visible. Top right and lower right: Occlusal views. There is mild irregularity of the upper labial segments, and the irregularity in the lower arch is more pronounced.

History

Complaint

The patient complained about irregular teeth.

History of Complaint

Not relevant.

Examination

Extraoral Examination

On extraoral examination, the patient had a class I (normal) appearance.

Intraoral Examination

The patient presented with a lower centre line shift to the right, by half a lower incisor width. The buccal segment relationship was class I on the left and mildly class II on the right. The curve of Spee in the lower arch was increased.

◆ What Further Investigations are Required?

For align technology, the submission of radiographic records, photographic records and a polyvinylsiloxane impression with corresponding occlusal records are required. The company then provides a virtual set-up (also known as Clincheck). Subsequently, the aligners are delivered and small attachments are provided for teeth to facilitate movement. These attachments can be seen in Figs 73.7 and 73.8.

Care Planning

Nonextraction management was planned for both cases. Both patients requested treatment with an orthodontic brace that has the least visible impact during treatment. The decision was made to use custom-made lingual fixed appliances for one and aligners for the other.

'Invisible' braces are widely publicized to patients and to dentists, and this is appealing to both general dentists and specialists; there are several reasons for this (Table 73.1).

The two examples of 'invisible braces' chosen are transparent aligner-type appliances and lingual appliances. The latter are fixed appliances that are attached to the inner surface of teeth.

The former (aligners) are transparent and removable and must be worn nearly full time to be effective. Some manufacturers use fixed attachments in combination with the aligners, as shown in case 2.

The appeal, for the nonspecialist practitioner in particular, is that both types of appliances appear to require little specialist knowledge to provide patient care. Both types of orthodontic braces usually require either a three-dimensional intraoral scan or polyvinyl siloxane impressions, including a record of the occlusal relationship; photographic records; and initial radiographic records. These are sent to the respective company to manufacture the orthodontic appliance.

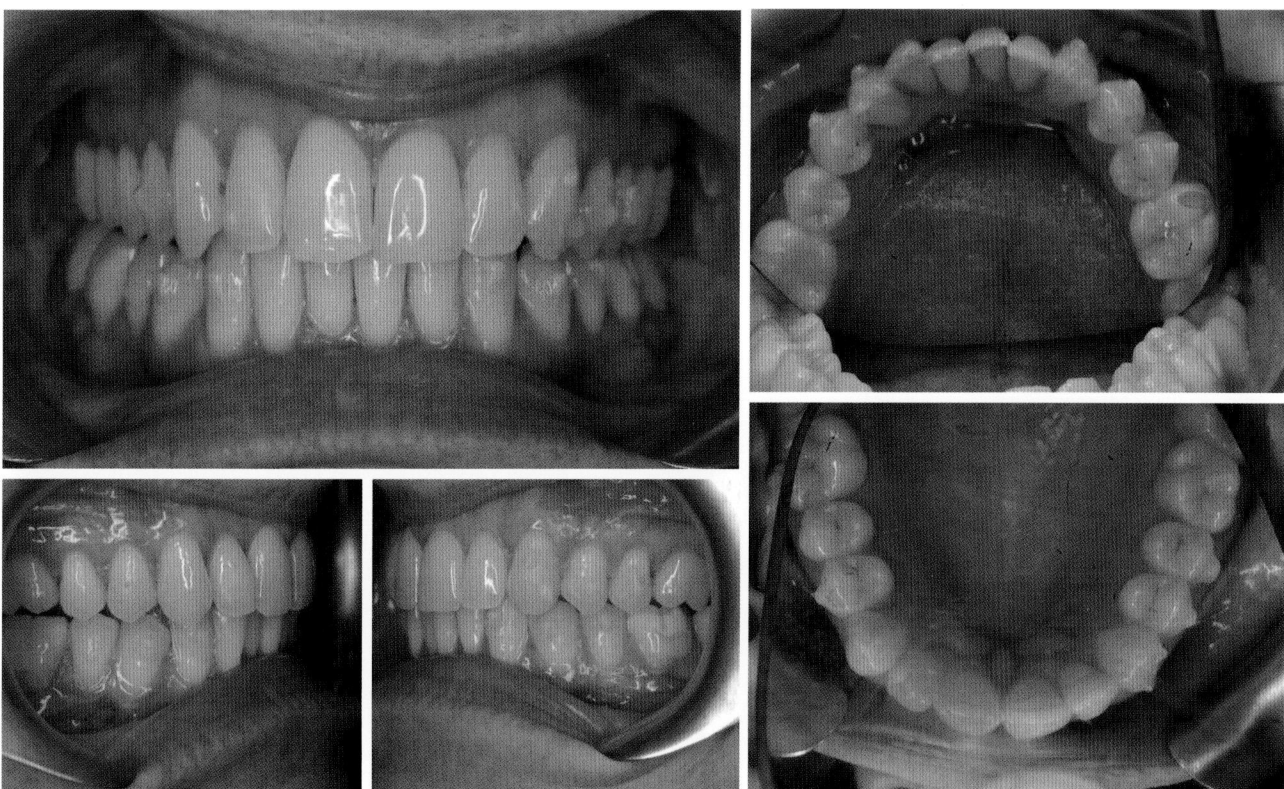

• **Fig. 73.6** Patient 2. Outcome after the last aligner of the first series. The teeth are not fully aligned yet, and the attachments are visible. Top left: Frontal view. The overbite has reduced, and the discrepancy in the centre lines is unchanged (as planned). Lower left: Right buccal view. The buccal segment relationship is still slightly post normal. Alignment of the upper incisors has significantly improved. The posterior occlusion is less interdigitated; this is to be expected at this stage. Lower middle: Left buccal view. The buccal segment is class I on the left-hand side; but the occlusion is slightly less interdigitated. Top right and lower right: Occlusal views. The upper labial segment alignment has improved a lot; the irregularity of the lower labial segment arch is still more pronounced.

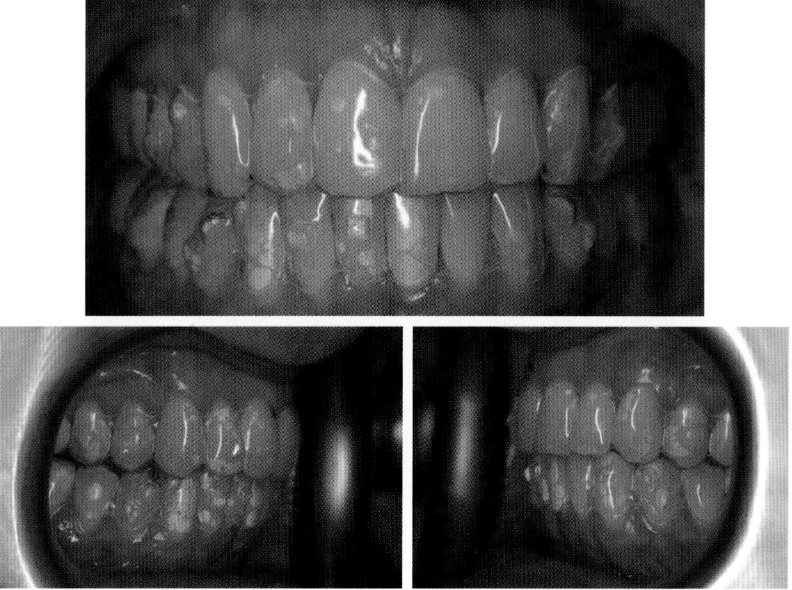

• **Fig. 73.7** Patient 2 with new refinement aligner fitted. Top: Frontal view. The attachments fit the aligners well. The condensation will soon disperse as the saliva wets the aligner. Lower left: Right buccal view. This makes it clear why aligners cause a change in the posterior occlusion. Lower right: Left buccal view.

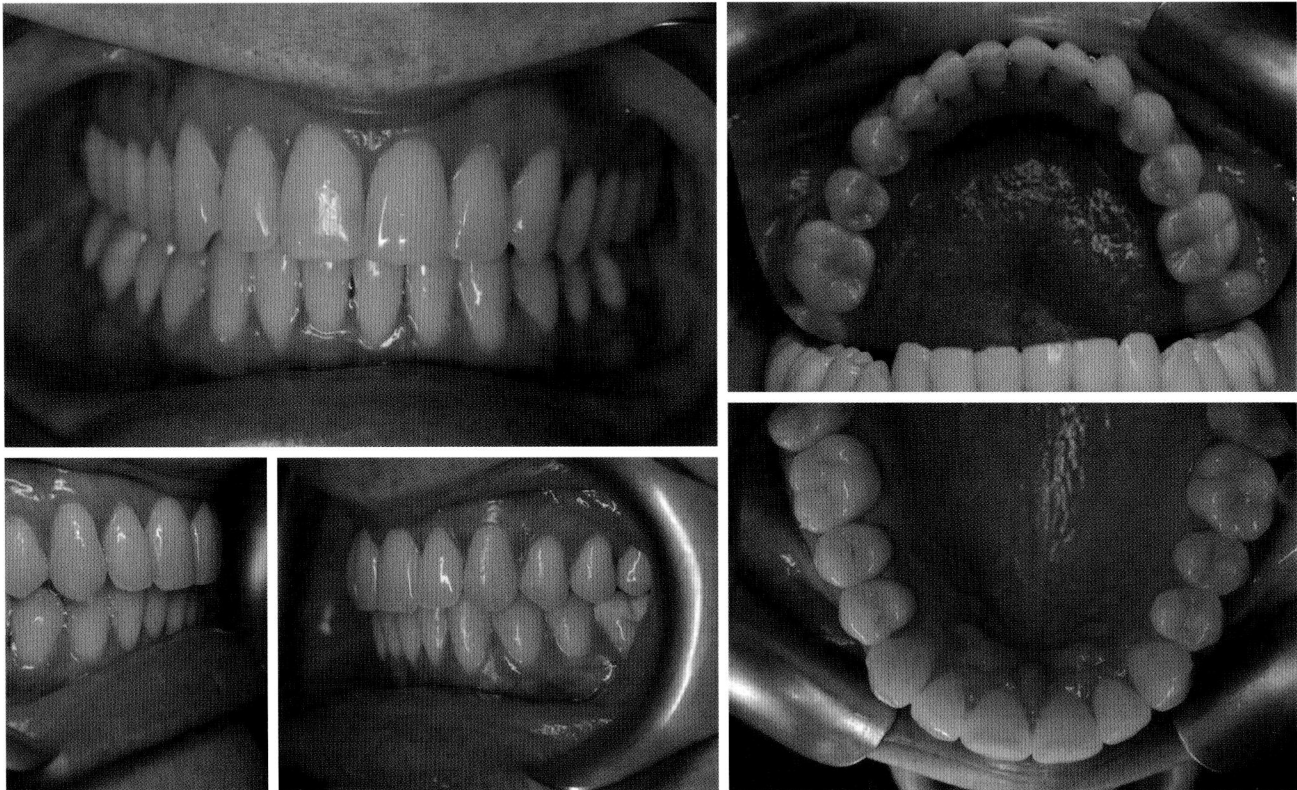

• **Fig. 73.8** Patient 2. Outcome after incisal tip adjustment and fixed lower retainer. Top left: Frontal view. The overbite is reduced and normal, and there is some improvement of the centre lines. Complete correction of the latter was not planned. Lower left: Right buccal view. The buccal segment relationship has not changed much, and the interdigitation is slightly reduced. Lower middle: Left buccal view. The buccal segment is class I on the left-hand side. Top right and lower right: Occlusal views. The labial segments are well aligned.

TABLE 73.1 Features of Lingual and Aligner 'Invisible' Orthodontic Appliances

	Lingual Appliances	Aligners
Custom-made	Can be customized or prefabricated Virtual set-up on request	Always
Silicone impressions/3D scan	In case of a customized appliance	Usually
Virtual set-up	At operators' request	Depends on manufacturer
Requires labial attachments	Rarely (e.g. for use of intermaxillary elastics)	Depends on brand used

At the company, trained personnel will produce the individualized appliance. Some manufacturers provide the dentists with 'virtual set-ups' that are designed to help visualize the desired treatment outcome. The virtual set-up can also be used as a tool for obtaining consent from patients. The patient, the dentist and the company jointly agree to the proposed care plan.

Dentists can determine/modify the care plan before the appliances are made, and this makes them responsible for the care provided. However, depending on the dentist's preferences, the manufacturer may suggest an orthodontic care plan. It is important to note that the dentist should be in a position to assess the care plan critically before committing to treating the patient. In other words, the responsibility for patient care ultimately lies with the dentist/practitioner and not with the company or other third party (e.g. advisor provided by the company). This clearly has medico-legal implications.

Another consideration is the time it takes to submit the records and to evaluate and potentially modify the proposed care plan; all these factors need to be considered in the overall cost of the orthodontic treatment.

Once the care plan has been finalized, the dentist agrees to pay the fees for the appliance. This may require a significant upfront payment. Currently, both types of 'invisible' appliances are mailed to dentists, who will then deliver them to patients to commence treatment, either by indirectly bonding the appliance to the teeth or by delivering the aligners and fitting the necessary attachments, where required.

Consent

Obtaining valid consent is one of the nine principles dental professionals must follow at all times. This should include a detailed description of what to expect during treatment (e.g. discomfort, initial speech impediment, compliance) and diet advice.

In case 1, the patient was required to wear intermaxillary elastics for a prolonged period to correct the class II buccal segment relationship and the increased overbite. It requires expertise to judge whether correction of the class II buccal segment relationship on the right and the overbite correction can be achieved through wearing of elastics or whether other treatment approaches should be considered. It is likely that an increased overjet with incomplete overbite would ensue if the upper and lower labial segments are aligned without correcting the buccal segment relationship. The alignment and the overbite reduction are not likely to be stable over the long term unless normal overjet and overbite are achieved.

In case 2, nearly full-time wear of the aligners was necessary to achieve the desired treatment outcome. Interproximal enamel reduction and attachments were required.

Potential Legal Issues and Pitfalls

Custom-made appliances (e.g. labial or lingual fixed appliances as well as removable appliances [aligners]) usually require payment to the manufacturer before treatment commences. The upfront costs for the dentist can approach £2000, depending on the appliance.

In an ideal set-up, which is usually undertaken, the dentist is required to assess and, if necessary, modify the care plan *before* the appliances are manufactured. It is important that the operator is aware of the relative strength and weaknesses of the different appliance systems; biomechanics can vary considerably. It is also important to note that patient consent should be obtained for long-term retention of the orthodontic outcome, particularly if the aesthetic concerns were the initiator for treatment.

Practitioners may be more easily persuaded to commence orthodontic treatment if custom-made appliances are used; the implication is that specialist training and knowledge may not be required to the same extent as for fixed labial appliances to achieve the desired treatment outcomes. Inadequate training may lead to discrepancies between patient expectations and treatment outcomes.

Treatment and Outcomes

For patient 1, the treatment time was 18 months. Intermaxillary elastic wear started early in treatment, and correction of the centre lines and buccal segment relationships were achieved. The overjet and overbite were normalized, and the upper and lower labial segments were well aligned. The retention regimen encompassed vacuum-formed retainers on a full-time basis for 3 months. This allows the gingival tissues to recover from orthodontic treatment and the occlusion to settle. Fixed retention can also be considered but is not usually provided or maintained by general dental practitioners because this knowledge is not part of the undergraduate curriculum for orthodontics. Treatment of patient 1 was expected to take longer than that of patient 2 because the treatment aims were more complex.

For patient 2, the overall treatment time was 12 months. Initially, 14 aligners were provided. After 7 months, impressions for orthodontic 'refinement' were taken, and seven more aligners were provided. The teeth were aligned successfully, and, as planned, occlusion had not changed significantly.

Retention needs to be planed for the long term, particularly for alignment of the labial segments. In case 1, we would not expect relapse of the buccal segment relationship, but alignment and overbite are likely to require maintenance over the long term. The need for commitment to maintenance and knowledge of the costs associated with it must be made clear to the patient, particularly when orthodontics is undertaken for aesthetic purposes. These costs can be significant. It is also worth remembering that fixed retainers are not infallible and re-treatment may become necessary at some stage, depending on the patients' requirements.

Case 74

Swollen Lips

MARTYN ORMOND, ESTHER HULLAH AND MICHAEL ESCUDIER

Summary

A 29-year-old man presents with swollen lips and generalized oral soreness. What is your diagnosis?

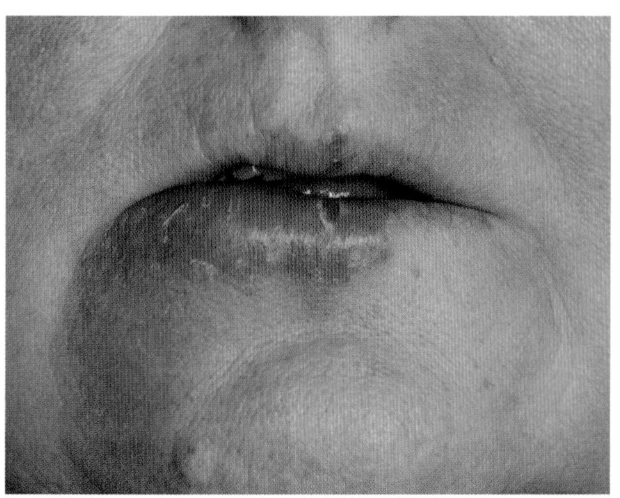

• **Fig. 74.1** The appearance of the patient's lips.

History

Complaint

The patient reports intermittent lip swelling and a sore mouth for the last 6 months.

History of Complaint

The lip swelling developed slowly, with no obvious precipitating event, around 6 months ago at a time when he was otherwise well. The swelling fluctuates in size, and he is unable to identify any specific triggers. In addition to the lip swelling, he also reports persistent oral soreness and mouth ulcers. There is no previous history of lip swelling, oral soreness or mouth ulcers.

Medical History

The patient has asthma, for which he uses a salbutamol inhaler. He also has hay fever, which he manages with daily oral antihistamine drugs during the spring months.

Examination

Extraoral Examination

The extraoral appearance of the lips are shown in Fig. 74.1.

◆ Describe What You See

The lower lip is enlarged and rounded, with the vermilion rolled outwards. The vermilion shows patchy erythema and cracking, with a fissure close to the midline. There is an area of erythema spreading outwards and downwards on the right cheek. The vermilion border has lost its definition. The upper lip appears largely normal in size, but there is a small midline fissure.

The lower lip is not tender but feels soft and rubbery. You undertake examination of the neck and conclude that there is no cervical lymphadenopathy.

Intraoral Examination

◆ The Intraoral Appearance is Shown in Fig. 74.2. Describe What You See

The buccal mucosa is swollen bilaterally. It looks soft and oedematous. On the patient's right (Fig. 74.2a), the surface has formed slightly projecting, rounded nodules separated by fissures, which can be described as having a cobblestone appearance. On the left buccal mucosa (Fig. 74.2b), there is more generalized swelling with two folds.

If you could examine the patient, you would find that there is also gingival swelling around the posterior teeth and deep fissures along the lower buccal sulci, with linear ulcers in their depths.

◆ What is the Most Likely Diagnosis, and Why?

Given the patient's age, history and clinical findings, the most likely diagnosis is orofacial granulomatosis (OFG). This condition typically develops before the third decade of life and is thought to affect both genders equally. Lip swelling affects the majority of patients, with each episode lasting days to weeks. Over time, the lips may become firm and persistently swollen. The perioral skin may become red, dry, itchy or cracked, with some patients developing angular cheilitis.

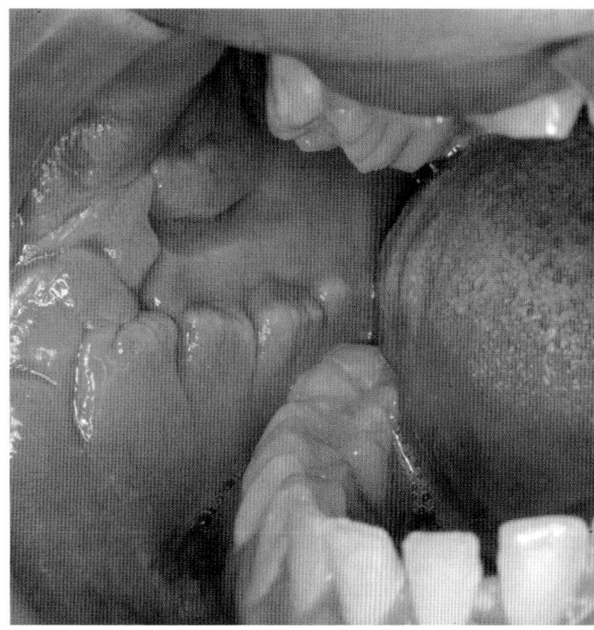
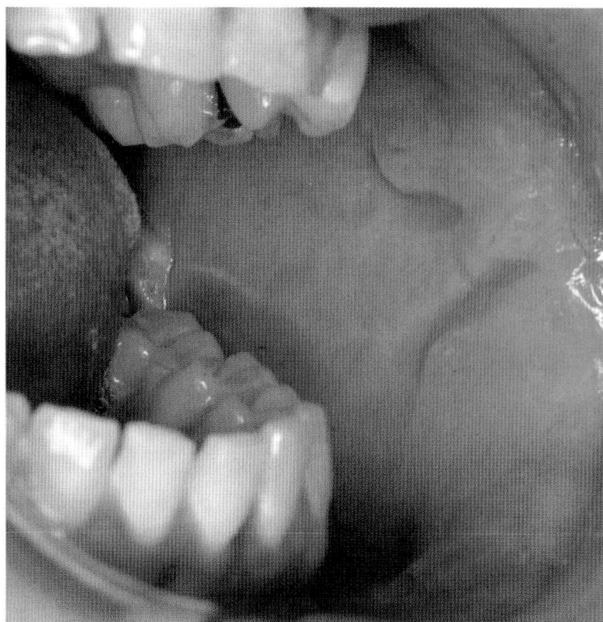

• **Fig. 74.2** The right **(a)** and left **(b)** intraoral appearance.

The intraoral findings vary among patients but include generalized swelling of the labial and buccal mucosae, often with a cobblestone pattern, or more localized tags. Linear ulcers with raised margins may be found in the buccal sulcus. Less commonly, patients may experience aphthous-like ulcers. The gingivae often show localised or generalised swelling and erytihema.

This clinical picture is so typical that few other diagnoses need to be considered unless investigations confirm an alternative diagnosis.

◆ What Other Causes of Recurrent Generalized Lip Swelling Might You Consider? Explain Why.

Other possible causes of recurrent generalized lip swelling, together with features relevant to diagnosis, are listed in Table 74.1.

◆ What Further Questions Would You Ask the Patient To Reach a Working Diagnosis?

What is the Duration of the Episodes of Swelling? The lip swelling of OFG would be expected to last days to weeks before resolving. Acute inflammatory causes such as angioedema resolve in 48 hours.

Is There Complete Resolution Between Episodes? OFG, Crohn's disease and Melkersson-Rosenthal syndrome may initially resolve between episodes, although the swelling may become permanent after months or years.

Are There Bowel Symptoms? If Crohn's disease is present, there would be abdominal pain, diarrhoea and frequency of bowel movements, possibly weight loss and perianal discomfort. However, mild disease may be asymptomatic.

Is There Shortness of Breath or a Chronic Cough? These might indicate lung involvement in sarcoidosis.

Is There an Associated Rash? Episodes of angioedema are usually associated with urticarial rashes ('hives') elsewhere on the body. Erythema nodosum, producing painful subcutaneous nodules, is seen in both Crohn's disease and sarcoidosis.

Is There a History of Allergy? About 80% of patients with OFG have a history of atopy (hay fever, asthma or eczema). Angioedema is also usually allergic in nature.

On further questioning, the patient confirms that the swelling develops over a number of hours. He also suggests that his symptoms may occasionally be triggered by certain foods. The swelling lasts for days before resolving slowly. He does not report any gastrointestinal disturbance, and there is no family history of inflammatory bowel disease. All other family members are well. His asthma is well controlled, and there is no history of hospital admissiosn. He has been assessed in an allergy clinic, where his hay fever was found to be caused by tree pollen.

Investigations

◆ What Investigations Might You Consider? Why?

Possible further investigations are listed in Table 74.2.

In this case, a swab was taken from the commissure and surrounding skin. Culture revealed Staphylococcus aureus, which was sensitive to fusidic acid. Full blood count and haematinic screen, complement and C1-esterase inhibitor levels, and serum angiotensin-converting enzyme (ACE) were all within normal limits. A decision was made to perform a biopsy.

◆ Where Should the Biopsy Be Taken From?

The pathogenesis of orofacial granulomatosis and oral Crohn's disease is granulomatous inflammation in tissues. To prove this, a deep biopsy is required because granulomas may be few and widely scattered, sometimes deep in tissues. The best tissues to sample are mucosal tags and linear ulcers, or a deep biopsy of the buccal mucosa may be performed. Unless it is the only site involved, biopsy of the lip is best avoided because any scarring on the labial mucosa will be visible, and thus unacceptable to the patient.

TABLE 74.1 Other Possible Causes of Lip Swelling

Cause	Features
Crohn's disease	Crohn's disease is a granulomatous autoinflammatory disease, which can affect any part of the gastrointestinal tract, including the mouth. It often presents between adolescence and the third decade. When Crohn's disease affects the mouth, oral signs and symptoms are indistinguishable from OFG, and a relationship exists between the two diseases. Some patients presenting with apparent OFG will have undiagnosed Crohn's disease at presentation or may develop it several years later. If bowel involvement is present or develops, Crohn's disease is the appropriate diagnosis. If not, the disease is called *orofacial granulomatosis.*
Melkersson-Rosenthal syndrome	This very rare syndrome is a combination of orofacial granulomatosis with a fissured tongue and recurrent facial palsy. Its relationship to OFG, Crohn's disease and sarcoidosis is unclear, but it is a clinically distinctive combination of features.
Hereditary angioedema	The familial disease hereditary angioedema causes recurrent swelling of lips and other parts of the body and is caused either by lack of C1-esterase in the complement cascade, or other activating defects of the bradykinin system. This disease appears an unlikely diagnosis in this case because, like allergic angioedema (see below), the swelling develops and resolves in 24 hours. Also, the intraoral features seen in this case would not be present.
Sarcoidosis	Sarcoidosis is unlikely in this case because it rarely affects the lips. It is most common in adults, with a peak incidence between ages 20 and 29 years and affects both genders. It is characterized by granulomatous inflammation, which can involve any organ, although the respiratory tract, skin and lymph nodes are typically affected first. Patients would usually report symptoms, such as shortness of breath, related to involvement of these multiple organs. Oral involvement is usually gingival, and lip swelling is very rare.
Angioedema	Angioedema is a type 1 hypersensitivity reaction characterized by transitory swelling, often of the orofacial tissues. The swelling develops quickly over minutes to hours and, importantly, typically resolves completely within 48 hours. Although the lip swelling is similar to that in OFG, the intraoral signs would not be present.
Other causes of acute lip swelling	Conditions such as trauma, oedema and cellulitis resulting from dental infection can be discounted on the basis of lack of symptoms and the repeated swelling over many months.
Other diseases in the lip	Mucous extravasation cysts, salivary tumours and other lip diseases do not produce generalized swelling and are not associated with any of the intraoral features present in this case.

TABLE 74.2 Relevant Investigations

Swab for microbiological culture from the left and right commissures	The patient has some erythema of the right commissure and may have angular cheilitis, partly as a result of swelling allowing saliva to leak to the commissure and skin. The softened skin is easily infected by *Candida* species, *Staphylococcus aureus,* or both. Culture and sensitivity will provide definitive diagnosis and inform prescription of the correct antimicrobial agent.
Biopsy	A biopsy may not be required in cases where the presentation is clearly typical. However, a biopsy will exclude other causes definitively.
Blood tests	These include a full blood count and a haematinic screen (iron, vitamin B_{12} and folate levels). Anaemia might suggest malabsorption and therefore possibly Crohn's disease. Serum angiotensin-converting enzyme (ACE) levels are raised in sarcoidosis. Complement and C1-esterase inhibitor levels are reduced in hereditary angioedema.
Referral for a medical gastrointestinal examination	Any suggestion of bowel symptoms merits referral for investigations for Crohn's disease.

◆ The Biopsy Specimen is Shown in Fig. 74.3. What Do You See?

At low power, left, the mucosa looks largely normal because the swelling is caused by oedema, and the tissue fluid present cannot be seen. The main feature is the presence of numerous clusters of inflammatory cells. There are up to 11 clusters of inflammatory cells at all levels in the mucosa, and three are shown by arrows.

On the right, a high-power view from the top right of the left-hand-side image shows the clusters to be granulomas. Granulomas comprise epithelioid macrophages, seen as a sheet of pale pink cells (M) surrounded by a cuff of

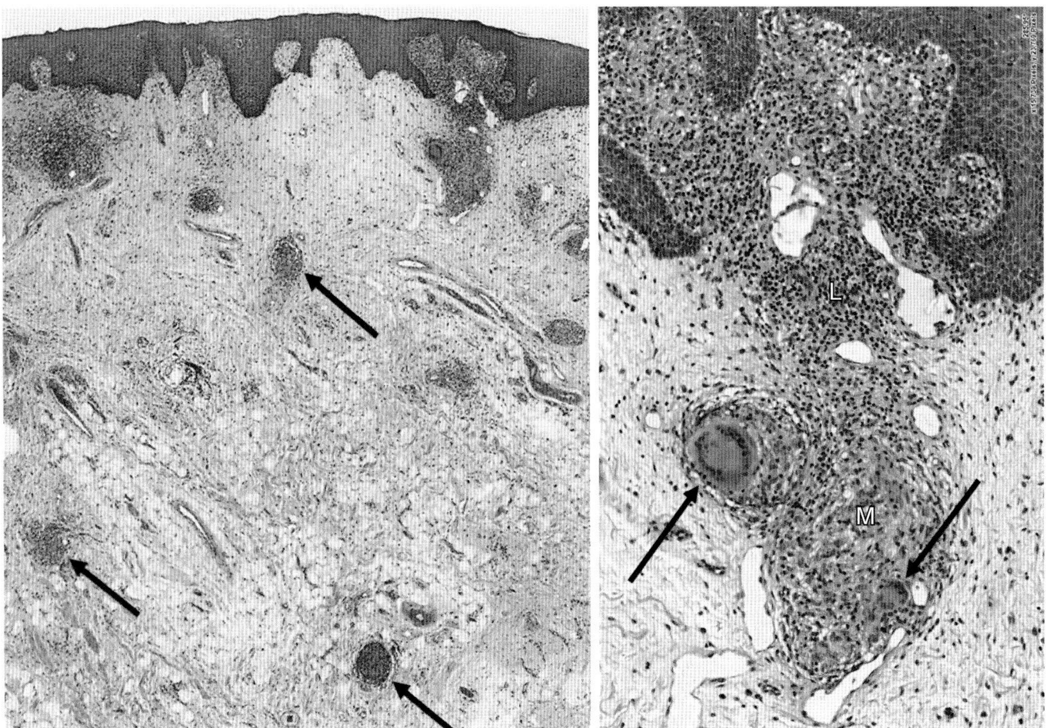

• **Fig. 74.3** Biopsy specimen of the buccal mucosa.

lymphocytes (L). Multinucleate giant cells are also present in some granulomas (arrowed).

◆ How Do You Interpret the Findings? How Does It Aid in the Diagnosis?

There is granulomatous inflammation in the mucosa, consistent with orofacial granulomatosis, Crohn's disease or sarcoidosis. These cannot be differentiated through biopsy.

◆ Does the Presence of Granulomatous Inflammation Raise the Possibility of Other Diseases?

In theory yes, but these other diseases do not cause this clinical presentation. For example, tuberculosis, deep mycoses, and foreign body reactions are all characterized by granulomatous inflammation. Additional histological features are usually present in these other diseases: caseation in tuberculosis, fungi in mycoses and foreign material in foreign body reactions. Therefore these diseases do not need to be considered in this case.

Diagnosis

◆ What is Your Diagnosis?

Because there are several similar conditions compatible with the clinical presentation and results of investigations in this case, a working, rather than a definitive, diagnosis of orofacial granulomatosis is appropriate.

The patient needs to be kept under review to see whether he develops bowel symptoms or signs that would lead to a diagnosis of Crohn's disease, or facial paralysis for a diagnosis of Melkersson-Rosenthal syndrome.

Treatment

◆ What are the Management Options?

This patient requires treatment in a specialist centre.

Fusidic acid cream should be prescribed for the angular cheilitis.

All patients need to be informed about the nature of the disease and that its progression is unpredictable. Lip swelling is disfiguring, and it is important to ask the patient about social interactions and his mood in case psychological support is needed.

No one treatment is ideal for every patient with orofacial granulomatosis, and so this patient may need to try several treatment approaches. A significant number of patients respond to dietary manipulation on the basis that the disease may be a hypersensitivity reaction to dietary components, particularly cinnamon and benzoate compounds. Avoidance of these is reported to induce a response in up to 70% of patients. The diet can be difficult to adhere to and should be managed through a dietician.

Topical corticosteroids, such as prednisolone or fluticasone mouthwashes, can be useful, particularly in patients with oral ulcers. Occasionally, treatment may include intralesional corticosteroids injection into the swollen lips or systemic corticosteroids or immunosuppressive drugs for more severe disease.

Further Advice

An example of a patient information leaflet from the British Society of Oral Medicine can be found at http://www.bsom.org.uk/ under patient information.

Case 75

Failing Implant Restoration

KALPESH A. BAVISHA

Summary

A 40-year-old woman presents with recession around an implant-retained crown and feels the implant tooth is loose. What are the treatment options and their likely chances of success?

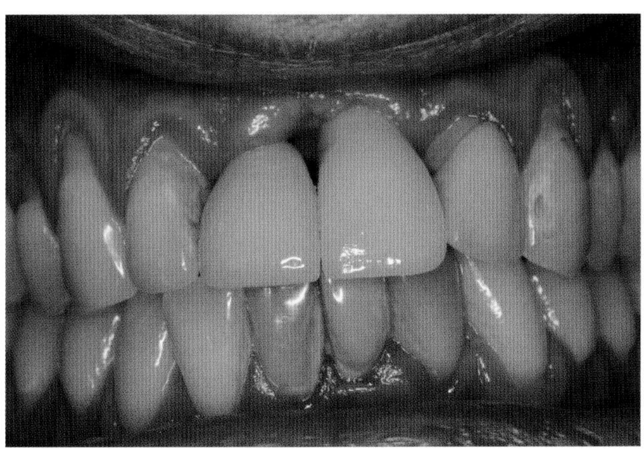

• **Fig. 75.1** Intraoral clinical photograph – anterior view in the intercuspal occlusal position.

History

Complaint

The patient feels that the gum between her upper front teeth is disappearing and that the teeth feel loose. She has no pain.

History of Complaint

The patient has noticed the gum shrinking for the past several months.

Dental History

The patient had single implant crowns to replace the maxillary central anterior teeth 7 years ago. She attends her dentist every 6 months for regular review consultations.

Medical History

The patient is otherwise fit and well.

Examination

Extraoral Examination

The temporomandibular joints appear normal, and no submental, submandibular or cervical lymph nodes are palpable.

Intraoral Examination

The patient lifts up her lip and shows you her upper front teeth.

◆ The Appearance of the Dentition with the Implant-Retained Crowns is Shown in Fig. 75.1. What Can You Deduce From the Clinical Appearance?

The upper right and upper left central incisors are implant-retained crowns; the upper left lateral incisor tooth is also crowned.

The gingival papilla between the maxillary central incisors is missing. The teeth appear generally stained and discoloured. Calculus deposits are noted on the teeth surfaces, especially the gingival margins of the mandibular anterior incisors, upper right canine and lower left canine.

There is slight erythema of the entire attached gingiva, as well as gingival recession associated with the natural dentition. The gingiva appears swollen and inflamed. This is most probably caused by a combination of poor oral hygiene and plaque accumulation. Gingival recession is present around the canines and premolars and may be a consequence of not only a plaque-associated inflammation but also an unfavourable tooth-to-bone volume ratio. This ratio can result in thin buccal bone overlying the teeth, increasing the risk of gingival recession in some patients.

The soft tissue architecture around the maxillary implant restorations is not ideal anatomically, but it does not look inflamed clinically. There is marginal gingival inflammation around the maxillary lateral incisors, with a broad rounded gingival margin and little stippling.

It is important to establish whether a full-sized interdental papilla was present when the implant crowns were fitted. This can be done by measuring the space between the tip of the papilla and the corresponding contact point of the crown. Photographs after crown placement are also an invaluable aid.

Investigations

◆ What Investigations Would You Carry Out, and Why?

Periodontal Examination. Before picking up a periodontal probe, it is advisable to place gentle finger pressure on the buccal soft tissue overlying the implants. There should be no bleeding or exudate, and this procedure should not cause any discomfort to the patient. This procedure will also offer an insight into the level and origin of any mobility of either isolated teeth or a dento-alveolar segment.

It is important to recognize the different types of peri-implant inflammation. Inflammation of the peri-implant mucosae has been termed *peri-implant mucositis* because no anatomical periodontal ligament is present adjacent to the implant surface. This is different from peri-implantitis, which is a more tissue-destructive disease that results in the loss of bone around an implant.

The examination should include accurate recording of probing depths and gingival bleeding. Probing around implants is similar to probing around teeth. The junctional epithelium is delicate and can be breached by the periodontal probe. The underlying connective tissue offers less resistance than the fibre bundles found associated with the natural dentition. In general, the probe will stop short of the bone margin by approximately 1 mm.

Standard periodontal probes can be used. Around healthy implant tissues, the probing depth should be less than 4 mm, with no or minimal bleeding.

Probing around implant restorations can be difficult to perform clinically. The bulbosity/emergence profile of the restoration may not allow accurate recording of probing depths. Removal of a screw-retained restoration is not recommended for routine probing around implants and is not feasible with cement-retained restorations.

If there is an increase in probing depth, gingival hyperplasia, purulent exudate and/or copious bleeding, it may be best to make an early referral for further investigation. This referral would be to your local specialist prosthodontist, implantologist or, ideally, the clinician who originally placed the implants. A more detailed examination will require removal of a screw-retained restoration.

For cemented implant restorations, excess cement left on the implant or abutment surfaces will allow plaque to accumulate and result in inflammation of the peri-implant tissues, just as in indirect restorations cemented onto the natural dentition. It is important to ensure that excess cement is not the cause of the inflammation. It would be unlikely in this case because the restorations have been in place for several years and because inflamed tissues are a recent finding.

Check the mobility of the implant-supported restorations. It is rare for an implant to feel loose. Even with significant bone loss, an implant restoration can still feel firm. It is important to distinguish a loose crown, which is a more common occurrence. A loose crown may be caused by a loose abutment screw, a screw fracture or debonding of a cemented crown.

On performing these investigations, you discover a 7mm probing depth associated with the upper left central incisor and a probing depth of 4 mm with the upper right central incisor, generalized marginal gingivitis with bleeding on probing and plaque accumulation around the crown margins. No mobility is noted because the crowns appear firm.

If there is any concern about an implant-supported restoration, it is advisable to obtain plain film radiographs (see later).

Occlusal Examination. It is important in single implant-supported restorations that the natural teeth are the first teeth in contact. An easy way to determine this is with the use of Shimstock foil, which has a thickness of 8 µm. In the intercuspal position, the natural teeth should hold the Shimstock foil. Between the implant restoration and the opposing contact, it should be possible to drag the Shimstock foil through without tearing it. Asking the patient to clench hard will result in the Shimstock foil being held firmly between the implant restoration and the opposing contact.

Radiographic Examination of the Upper Incisors. Periapical radiographs, taken using a paralleling technique and beam-aiming device, are required to:

- **Evaluate marginal bone levels.** With implant restorations it is important to establish baseline radiographs. Whether this should be done at the time of implant placement or during fitting of the final restoration is still being debated. The frequency and timing of taking radiographs is also controversial. Usually, a radiograph is taken after 1 year of implant function and can be repeated 2 years later. Subsequent timing can be of decreasing frequency and related more to clinical need. Where there is evidence of a change in bone levels, the frequency of taking radiographs may need to be increased. In describing bone loss, it may be useful to describe the extent of bone in relation to the radiographically visible implant threads. Depending on the system, the implant may have micro-threads, macro-threads or both. If possible, stating the number of threads exposed may allow for a better comparison of radiographs because these are a fixed reference point.
- **Abutment fit and crown margin fit.** If unsure about the fit of an abutment or screw-retained crown, a radiograph can confirm whether it is fully seated. For an abutment, there should be no space between the abutment and the wall of the implant when utilizing an internal connection, as seen in Fig. 75.2.

- **Presence of subgingival deposits calculus and/or cement.** Cement, if radiolucent, may not be seen on the radiograph.
- **Absence of continuous radiolucency around the implant.** Because there is no lamina dura around an implant, there should be no radiolucency around the implant. Radiolucency around an implant is likely to be a result of failure of osseointegration of the implant and the surrounding alveolar bone.

◆ The Periapical Radiographs are Shown in Fig. 75.2. What Do You See?

The detailed radiographic report is explained in Table 75.1.

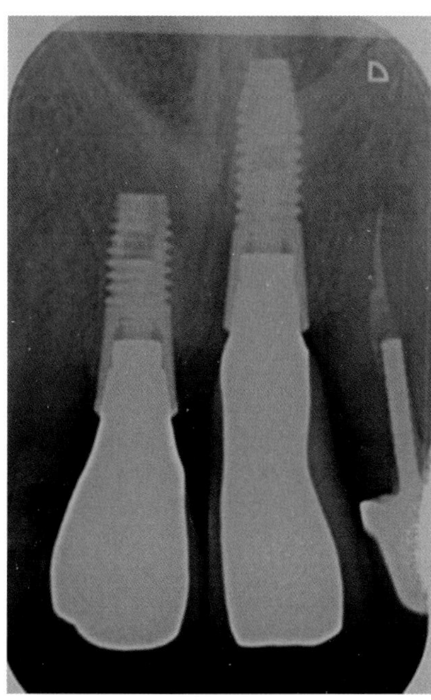

• **Fig. 75.2** Periapical radiograph of the implant restorations upper right and left central incisors using a paralleling technique.

Diagnosis

◆ What are Your Provisional Diagnoses?

See Table 75.2.

- Peri-implantitis associated with poor plaque control
- A previous history of periodontitis
- Chronic gingivitis
- Inadequate root canal filling of the upper left lateral incisor.

Treatment

◆ How Would You Manage These Conditions?

Nonsurgical Management. The management of peri-implantitis involves oral hygiene instruction as well as supra- and subgingival debridement.

◆ Is Special Equipment Required for Cleaning Around Implant Restorations?

No. Conventional instruments can be used with care to remove biofilm without causing damage. Aim to improve the patient's level of plaque control with careful oral hygiene instruction/advice.

Check for any potential occlusal causes and take measures to make it easier for the patient to clean the restoration; also, aim to improve access, embrasure contour, and emergence profile.

Titanium instruments can be used to prevent scratching of the implant surface. Some advocate the use of plastic instruments to prevent damage, but these instruments can be difficult to use, and it is more important to ensure that the biofilm and any more tenacious deposits have been removed.

Surfaces that are difficult to clean include the implant surface because of the naturally rough surface and the presence of threads. If needed, greater access and the use of specialized titanium brushes and burs, with direct access and a surgical approach, may be required.

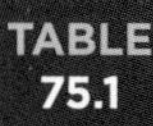

TABLE 75.1 Radiographic Findings of the Periapical Radiograph Shown in Fig. 75.2

Upper Right Central Incisor Implant	Upper Left Central Incisor Implant	Upper Left Lateral Incisor
Bone loss; only micro-threads exposed. Difficult to count micro-threads. On the mesial aspect, radiolucency is seen with 60% of the micro-threads. On the distal aspect, radiolucency seen with 50% of the micro-threads. Short implant. Crown abutment fit – no space detected. Screw-retained restoration – no screw fracture/no subgingival deposits.	Longer implant. Bone loss; threads exposed. On the mesial aspect, radiolucency is seen with all the micro-threads and up to three of the micro-threads. On the distal aspect, radiolucency is seen with all the micro-threads and with two of the macro-threads. Effects of bone loss greater then that of the upper right central incisor. Crown abutment fit – no space detected. Screw-retained restoration – no screw fracture/no subgingival deposits.	Root-filled, with material extruding through the apex. Space between the post and the apical root filling material. Post-core crown. Radiolucent area around post. Post preparation possibly too wide. Also, post preparation does not appear to follow root canal anatomy. Radiolucent area between crown margin and tooth surface.

TABLE 75.2 Radiological Diagnosis

Upper Right Central Incisor Implant	Upper Left Central Incisor Implant	Upper Left Lateral Incisor
Perimucositis or peri-implantitis. Clinically, maximum probing depth is 4 mm. Even in the absence of previous radiographs, there is an indication of bone loss. It would be unusual to place an implant with half the micro-threads not being placed in bone. Thus a diagnosis of peri-implantitis could be justified.	Peri-implantitis. A diagnosis of peri-implantitis means that the inflammatory response has caused obvious bone loss. Usually, there is associated gingival inflammation but is not always the case. In Fig. 75.1, the gingival tissues do not appear inflamed. Probing depths increased to greater than 5 mm. Peri-implantitis can be most commonly bacterially induced. With implant-retained restorations, an occlusal factor should not be ruled out.	Inadequate root filling. Absence of coronal seal. Despite this, there does not appear to be a visible periapical radiolucent area.

Surgical Management (Carried Out by a Specialist). Aim to have direct access to all of the implant exposed surfaces. A soft tissue flap is raised under local anaesthesia, with the aim of allowing removal of the biofilm. Several techniques are available to do this, including the use of ultrasonic instrumentation, specialized titanium micro-brushes, drilling of the implant surface to remove the threads, chemical debridement or even bone grafting. This surgical intervention may result in the implant threads becoming visible, compromising the final aesthetics.

The importance of an early diagnosis of peri-implantitis is important, and early specialist referral is recommended to prevent further bone loss and any subsequent implant loss. As shown in this case, the clinical signs are not always accurate indicators of the extent of the disease.

Most implant-supported restorations with perimucositis can be managed in a straightforward manner with routine oral hygiene measures. The patient should be instructed on how best to clean around the implant restoration by using routine brushing and interproximal cleaning techniques. Assess whether the patient is physically able to clean the restorations or whether cleaning procedures need to be modified to allow the patient to clean with ease. This should have been considered at the planning stage before treatment execution. Implant restorations require additional maintenance. Implants are designed to allow maximum osseointegration. Their surfaces, however, are not easy to clean once they become contaminated. Early intervention when disease is suspected, and with specialist referral when necessary, is key. A failing implant may not result in any significant clinical signs or symptoms. These changes may be only detectable with probing the tissues around the implant and taking and interpreting appropriate radiographs. A late diagnosis of a failing implant is likely to result in further surgery for the patient, a compromise in aesthetics and, at worst, removal of the implant, all of which may result in medico-legal action. Patients should be aware of the need for regular maintenance at home and at the clinic.

Medico-Legal Issues

Accurate recording of clinical findings and patient discussions is essential. In this case, documentation, including previous probing depths and periapical radiographs, are indispensable to demonstrate the progressive disease process. The patient should be encouraged to maintain a meticulous oral hygiene regimen, and appropriate referral to a suitably qualified clinician for the management of peri-implantitis is recommended.

In summary, the General Dental Council, UK recommends:

- Maintaining detailed and extensive clinical records
- Completing the initial phases of history, examination and investigations robustly
- Recording a diagnosis
- Providing an individualized written treatment plan that includes details of the need for treatment, the treatment options (the risks and benefits), the phases of treatment, the costs of treatment and the expected normal sequelae of surgery
- Considering referral at an early stage, particularly if reparative surgery is required.

Index

A
Abrasion
  defined, 340
  features, 344b
Abscess, 180
Abutment teeth, 193
Access cavities, 268f
Aciclovir, 159
Acidic food, 341
Acid regurgitation, 341
Acrylic palatal coverage, 137
Acute necrotizing ulcerative gingivitis, 158
Acute osteomyelitis, 128
Acute periodontitis, 63
Adhesive bridge, 194
Adhesive bridgework, 282
Adrenaline/epinephrine, 16–17
Advanced Life Support (ALS), 76
Advanced periodontitis
  diagnosis, 208–213, 209t
  examination, 207–208, 208f
  grading, 212t
  history, 207
  investigations, 208, 211f
  management, 213–217
  stability assessment, 212t
  staging, 212t
  treatment, 214t
Adverse reaction
  causes, 203
  differential diagnosis, 204–206
  history, 203–204
  myocardial infarction, 203
  vasovagal attack, 203
Alcoholism, 341–342
Alveolar ridge, 238–239
Alzheimer's disease (AD)
  definition, 35–38
  dementia different from, 35
  examination, 35–38
  history, 35
Ameloblastoma, types of, 13t
Amelogenesis imperfecta, 317
Anaesthesia, 143–144, 145f, 204t
Analgesia, 53–57
Anaphylaxis, 206
  drugs, 18f
  hypersensitivity, 16
  pathogenesis, 16
  risk, 17
  signs and symptoms, 15–16
Angina bullosa haemorrhagica (ABH), 229
Ankylosis, 98
Antibiotic prophylaxis, 247–248
Anticoagulation
  diagnosis, 246
  endocarditis, 249
  examination, 246
  guidelines, 248
  haemostasis, 249
  history, 245–246
  INR test, 245–246
  investigations, 246
  postextraction bleeding, 249
  postoperative, 249–250
  treatment, 247–249
Antral cyst, 300
Anxiety, 204
Anxiety management, 223–226
  anaesthesia, 223
  diagnosis, 223
  guidelines, 224
  history, 223
  investigation, 223
  methods, 224t
  prognosis, 226
  treatment, 225–226
Arthrography, 49
Autism
  causes, 232
  communication aids, 234
  examination, 231–235, 231f
  history, 231
  medical conditions, 232
  sensory processing problems, 232
Avulsed central incisor
  examination, 148
  history, 147–148
  investigations, 148, 148f
  long-term prognosis, 150
  replantation complications, 150t
  treatment, 148–149, 148f

B
Basic Life Support (BLS), 76
Basic Periodontal Examination (BPE), 208
Behçet's disease, 109
Benign neoplasms, 60
Biological width, 346
Biopsy
  dry mouth, 42–43
  facial swelling, child, 355
Biopsy *(Continued)*
  gingival swelling, 60, 61t
  mouth opening, 336f
  multilocular radiolucency, 12–13, 12f
  neck swelling, 112
  numb lips, 93
  palate swelling, 312t, 313
  sore mouth, 188–190, 190f
  tongue, white patch on, 259
Bisphosphonate drug, 131–132
Biting, pain on, 63–66
  differential diagnosis, 64
  examination, 63f, 64
  history, 63–64
  investigations, 64, 65t
  treatment, 64–66, 65t
Blisters. *See* Sore mouth with blisters
Branchial cysts, 112
Branchial/lymphoepithelial cysts, 112
Breath, shortness of
  diagnosis, 15–16, 16f
  examination, 15, 15f
  history, 15
  treatment, 16–17
Bridge designs, 283–284, 283f
  debonding, 242–243
  examination, 237–239
  history, 237
  minimal-preparation bridge, 240–242
  removable prosthesis, 240
  replacement options, 238t
  treatment, 239–243
Bridge, failed, 193–196
  examination, 193–194
  factors, 196t
  history, 193
  investigations, 194, 195t
  treatment, 194–196, 195f

C
CAD/CAM fixed prosthodontics
  clinical stages, 70, 71t, 72f
  conventional impressions, 73–74, 74t
  diagnosis, 67–68
  examination, 67, 68f
  guidelines, 74
  history, 67
  intraoral scanning systems, 73, 73t
  investigations, 67, 69t, 70f
  treatment, 68–74
Calipers method, 137

Note: Page numbers followed by "f" indicates figures, "t" indicates tables, and "b" indicates boxes.

'Camouflage' orthodontics, 288
Cancrum oris, 128
Care, sequence of, 3t
Caries, autism, 234
Caries, high rate
  diagnosis, 2
  examination, 1
  history, 1
  investigations, 1–2
  management, 2–7
  medico-legal considerations, 7
Carious dentine
  excavation techniques, 53t
  histological layers, 54t
  pulp–dentine complex responses, 54t
  removal of, 53
Carious lesions, 184
  diagnosis, 52
  examination, 51, 51f
  history, 51
  investigations, 51–52
  minimally invasive operative treatment, 53–57
  treatment, 52–53
Causative allergen, 17
Causative tooth, 65t
Cavity
  appropriate choices, 57
  'linings', 56–57
  restore materials, 57
Cementation, 242
Cephalometric analysis, 28
Child abuse, 199, 202
Children, difficult, 79–84
  behaviour management strategies, 82, 83t
  examination, 81–84, 81f
  history, 79–81
  milestone, 80b
  treatments, 82f
Child's behaviour, 232
Chlorphenamine, 17
Chronic hyperplastic candidosis, 252
Chronic osteomyelitis, 128
Class III malocclusion, 288
Collapse, sudden, 75–78
  causes, 75, 76t
  examination, 75–77
  history, 75
  prognosis, 77
  signs and symptoms, 76t
Consent, irregular teeth, 421
Conventional cantilever bridge, 69
Conventional fixed–fixed bridge, 69–70
Conventional impressions, 73–74, 74t
Cracked teeth/cusps restoration, 65t
Cranial nerve function, 90, 91t
Crossbite, anterior
  diagnosis, 287
  examination, 287, 288f
  history, 287
  legal issues and pitfalls, 289
  long-term outcome, 290
Crossbite, anterior *(Continued)*
  prognostic factors, 290
  treatment, 287–290

D

Dahl approach, 346–347
Dehydration, 40
Dementia
  Alzheimer's disease (AD), 35
  capacity assessment, 37t
  dental considerations, 37–38
  dental origin pain, 38
  management, 36
  medical conditions, 36
  relative prevalence rates, 36t
  signs and symptoms, 35–36, 38
  stages, 36, 36t
  treatment, 36–37
Dental caries, 317
Dental discolouration caries, 153t
Dental implants, 30
Dental panoramic tomogram (DPT), 29, 287
Dentigerous cyst, 12, 299
Dentine caries
  detector dyes, 55
  excavation techniques, 53t
  histological layers, 54t
  pulp–dentine complex responses, 54t
  removal of, 53
Diabetes, 207
Diet
  advice, 7t
  analysis, 4–5, 234–235
  unusual, 232
Digital intraoral scans, 73–74, 74t
Direct immunofluorescence (DIF), 230
Direct restorative materials, 57t
Discoloured teeth
  causes, 151–153, 152t–153t
  developmental defects, 153t
  diagnosis, 154
  examination, 151–153, 151f
  history, 151
  investigations, 154–155
  management options, 155t
  prognosis, 155
  treatment, 152, 155
Discomfort from pericoronitis, 234
Displacement, 28
Dividers method, 137
Domiciliary care
  care plan, 403–404
  Care Quality Commission (CQC), 400
  denture wearing, 402–403
  examination, 403
  history, 397
  medico-legal allegation, 399
  oral healthcare, 397
  problem, 397–403
Drugs
  autism, 233
Drugs *(Continued)*
  extraction, pain after, 86
  hypoglycaemia, 125f
  xerostomia, 40
Dry mouth
  causes, 40
  diagnosis, 43
  examination, 39–40, 39f
  history, 39
  investigations, 40–43, 41t
  treatment, 43
Dry socket, 86
  risk factors, 86, 86t
  treatment, 86

E

Eating disorders, 341
Electro-galvanic pain, 63
Endodontic problem
  examination, 265, 265f
  history, 265
  investigations, 266–267, 267f–268f
  treatment, 267–270, 269f
Endodontic treatment, failed
  CBCT, 368t
  diagnosis, 365
  examination, 365
  history, 365
  investigations, 365
  treatment, 367, 367f
Erosive tooth wear
  diagnosis, 342
  differential diagnosis, 340–342
  examination, 339–340, 339f
  history, 339
  investigations, 341
  treatment, 342
Erythema multiforme (EM), 158
Erythematous areas, 16
External root resorption, 97
Extraction, complicated
  antiretroviral drugs and drugs, 332t
  diagnosis, 330
  examination, 329–330, 329f
  history, 329
  treatment, 330–332
Extraction, pain after
  diagnosis, 85–87, 85f
  examination, 85, 85f
  history, 85
  investigations, 86
  treatment, 86
Extraoral dry time (EODT), 147
Extrinsic dental discoloration, 153t

F

Facial injury
  diagnosis, 199, 200t
  examination, 197–198, 197f–198f
  history, 197
  investigations, 198–199, 199f
  treatment, 199–202, 201f

Facial swelling, child
aetiology, 355–356
causes, 354t
diagnosis, 355
differential diagnosis, 355, 355t
examination, 353, 353f
history, 353
treatment, 356
False xerostomia, 40
Felypressin, 205–206
Fibrous epulis, 60
Final caries excavation, 56f
First permanent molars
care planning, 185–186
diagnosis, 184, 318
differential diagnosis, 317
examination, 183–184, 315–316
features, 184t
history, 183, 315
investigations, 184–185, 317
possible restorative options, 319t
prognosis, 319
treatment, 318–319
Fistula formation, 362
Fluorosis, 317
Fractured incisors, 219–222
Fractured mandible, 86
Fractured spiral filler fragment, 267–270
Frey's syndrome, 360
Frictional keratosis, 252
Fungiform papillae, 9

G

Gap between front teeth, 303–310
advantages and disadvantages, 307t
diagnosis, 304–305
examination, 303–304, 304f
history, 303
investigations, 304, 304f
medico-legal issues, 309
treatment, 305–309
Gastrointestinal disease, 109
Gastro-oesophageal reflux disease, 341
General Dental Council (GDC), 330
General dental practitioner (GDP), 30
Giant cell lesion, 11
Gingival fibroepithelial polyp/nodule, 60
Gingival recession
clinical assessments, 22t
diagnosis, 22–25
examination, 21–22, 21f
history, 21
investigations, 22
treatment, 23–25, 24t
Gingival swelling
diagnosis, 61
differential diagnosis, 60
examination, 59–60, 59f
history, 59
investigations, 60, 61t
treatment, 60–61

H

Halitosis, 85
Hamartomas, 60
Headache
causes, 371–374, 373t
differential diagnosis, 374
history, 369–374, 369f
main cranial nerve neuralgias, 372t
temporomandibular disorders, 371
Hemisected/root-resected teeth, 215
Hepatitis B
antibodies, 177t
antigens, 177t
prophylaxis, 176
Hepatitis C, 176
prophylaxis, 176
Herpes simplex virus (HSV), 160
Hidden occlusal caries, 184
Hidden sugar, 5
High caries susceptibility, 68
Human Immunodeficiency Virus (HIV), risk factors for, 175, 175t
Hydrocortisone, 17
Hypersensitivity, 16, 205
Hypodontia, 28
Hypoglycaemia, 123–126
causes, 124t
examination, 123
history, 123
symptoms and signs, 124t
treatment, 123–124

I

Idiopathic molar–incisor hypomineralization, 317
Immediate Life Support (ILS), 76
Implant planning
cone beam computed tomography, 393–394
diagnosis, 394
edentulous space, 392
examination, 391–393, 391f
history, 391
investigations, 393–394
medico-legal considerations, 395
prosthesis, 392–393
treatment, 395
Implant-supported restorations, 282–283
Implant tooth
diagnosis, 429
examination, 427–428
history, 427
investigations, 428–429
medico-legal issues, 430
treatment, 429–430
Incisors, central, 117–122
examination, 117–118, 118f
history, 117
investigations, 118–119, 118f
treatment, 119–120
Incisors, fractured, 219–222
diagnoses, 220–222, 221f
examination, 219–220, 219f
history, 219
investigations, 220, 221f
replacement, 222t
Incisors, missing, 27–34
care planning, 29–31
consent, 31–32
diagnosis, 29
diagnostic tools, 29–31, 30f
examination, 27f, 28–29
history, 27–28
investigations, 29
legal issues and pitfalls, 32
long-term outcome, 33
treatment, 29–31
Incisors, missing upper lateral, 277–286
care plan, 279–285
examination, 277, 280f
history, 277
investigations, 277–279, 279b
orthodontic treatment, 279–282
root resorption, 278–279
treatment, 279–285, 280b–281b
Index of Orthodontic Treatment Need (IOTN), 29
Inflammatory/postinflammatory pigmentation, 188
Inflammatory root resorption, 97
Internal root resorption, 97
Intraoral scanning systems, 73, 73t
Intravascular injection, 204
Intravenous fluid, 17
Intrinsic dental discolouration, 153t
Invisible braces
examination, 415
history, 415
legal issues and pitfalls, 421
treatment, 421
Irregular teeth
care planning, 418–421
consent, 421
examination, 418
history, 418

J

Joint hypermobility, 50

L

Langerhans' cell
definition, 295
histiocytosis, 295, 296t
Latex hypersensitivity, 206
Lichen planus (LP), 188, 228, 252
Lichenoid reaction, 188, 252
Lidocaine, 205
Lip swelling
causes, 425t
diagnosis, 426
examination, 423–424

Lip swelling *(Continued)*
history, 423
investigations, 424–426, 425t
treatment, 426
Lips, numb
causes, 90, 90t
diagnosis, 94
differential diagnosis, 92–94
examination, 89f, 90–92
history, 89–90, 89f
investigations, 92
sensory nerve supply, 89–90, 89f
Local flap design, 105t
Localized periodontitis
diagnosis, 295
differential diagnosis, 292–293
examination, 291–292
history, 291
investigations, 292–293
treatment, 295–296
Loose anterior tooth
diagnosis, 97–98
examination, 95–96
history, 95
investigations, 96–97, 97t
treatment, 98–99
Loose dentures
current dentures, 411
management options, 412–413
specific prosthetic-related factors, 410t
strategy, 409–411
upper fibrous ridge, 411
Loss, tooth. *See* Tooth loss, eating
Lower left second molar
complaint, 407–408
diagnosis, 405
examination, 405
history, 405
treatment, 406–407
treatment options, 405–406
Lupus erythematosus (Le), 188
Luxation injuries, 120t
Lymphoepithelial cysts, 112

M
Magnetic resonance imaging (MRI), 49
Malignant neoplasms, 12, 60
Malocclusion, 30
Mandibular impacted third molars (MITMs), 139–146
coronectomy complications, 146t
examination, 139–140, 139t
extractions, 143
history, 139
investigations, 140–145
removal complications, 144t
Winter's lines techniques, 143
Mandibular right first molar, 5
Maxillary right second molar, 51
Mean cell volume (MCV), 109
Medication-related osteonecrosis (MRONJ), 86
Metastatic malignancy, 112
Mild fluorosis, 317
Mild periodontal disease susceptibility, 68
Mobile lower incisors, 234
Mobility, 262
Moderate erosive tooth wear susceptibility, 68
Molar endodontic treatment
causes, 263t
diagnosis, 262
examination, 261–262
history, 261, 261t
investigations, 262
root canal treatment, 264t
treatment, 262–264
Mouth opening
diagnosis, 334–335
examination, 333–334, 333f
history, 333
investigations, 335
treatment, 335–337, 336t
Mouth ulcers, 107–110. *See also* Dry mouth; Painful mouth; Sore mouth
diagnosis, 109–110
examination, 107f, 108–109
features, 108t
history, 107–108
treatment, 110, 110t
Mucous membrane pemphigoid (MMP), 227–228
Multilocular radiolucency
diagnosis, 13, 13t
differential diagnosis, 11–12
examination, 9–10, 9f
history, 9
investigations, 10–11, 10f–11f
treatment, 13–14

N
National Health Services (NHS), 32
Neck swelling, 357–364
causes, 112, 113t
diagnosis, 112, 358
differential diagnosis, 112
examination, 111–112, 357–358, 357f
history, 111, 357
investigations, 112–116, 114t, 358–360, 358t
prognosis, 116
techniques, 113t–114t
treatment, 116, 360–362
Necrosis, 129
Necrotizing periodontitis, 128
Neoplastic lesion, 96
Nerve palsy, 362
New spring cantilever bridge, 194
Non–insulin-dependent diabetes mellitus (NIDDM), 124
Nonverbal communication, 232
Nucleotide reverse transcriptase inhibitors (NRTIs), 331

O
Occipito-mental view, 103
Occlusal caries, 1
Occlusal examination, 428
Occlusion, 220, 242
implant planning, 393
Odontogenic keratocyst, 12
Odontogenic tumours, 60, 299
Oral blisters, 229
Oral cancer
diagnosis, 321
examination, 321, 321f
history, 321
investigations, 322–323
radiotherapy, 324–325, 325t
staging, 322t
surgery, 324–325, 325t
treatment, 322, 325–327
treatment planning, 323–325
Tumour–Node–Metastasis (TNM), 322t
Oral hygiene, 213
advice, 213
regimen, 207
Oroantral communication, 105–106
Oroantral fistula (OAF)
aetiology, 102
definition, 102
diagnosis, 103
differential diagnosis, 101–102
examination, 101, 101f
factors, 102
history, 101
investigations, 102–103, 102t
oroantral communication, 105–106
signs and symptoms, 102
treatment, 103–105
Orthodontic consent, 32
Osteitis, 128
Osteoarthrosis, 46
Osteomyelitis, 128
Osteonecrosis, 128, 132
Osteoradionecrosis, 86
Overdentures, 135–138
diagnosis, 137–138
examination, 135–137, 136f, 136t
history, 135

P
Painful mouth
diagnosis, 158
examination, 157–158
final outcome, 160
history, 157
investigations, 158, 159t
prognosis, 159–160
treatment, 158–159
Palate swelling, 311–314
diagnosis, 314
differential diagnosis, 311–312
examination, 311, 311f
history, 311

Palate swelling *(Continued)*
investigations, 312–314
prognosis, 314
treatment, 313f–314f, 314
Palpation, 262
Papillomas, 60
Parotid ultrasound, dry mouth, 42
Pemphigus (PV), 228
Percussion sounds of teeth, 118
Percutaneous injury
diseases, 173–178
history, 173–178
positive patients, 176t
postexposure prophylaxis, 173
Pericoronitis
diagnosis, 179–181
examination, 179
history, 179
lower third molars, 181t
patient condition, 180–181
treatment, 181–182
Periodontal probing, 262
Peripheral giant cell granuloma, 60
Periradicular radiolucency, 266
Potential abutment teeth, 238–239
Premolar-to-premolar occlusion, 213
Prilocaine, 205–206
Primary herpetic gingivostomatitis, 157–158
Prosthodontic consent, 32
Pulpal pain, 63
Pulpitis, 183
Pulpotomy, 221
Pyogenic granuloma, 60

R
Radicular cyst, 299–300
Radiographs
advanced periodontitis, 211f, 214t
anticoagulation, 246
avulsed central incisor, 148
bridge design, 239
bridge, failed, 195
caries, 2t, 2
carious lesion, 51–52, 52f
endodontic problem, 266
endodontic treatment, failed, 366t
facial injury, 198–199
facial swelling, child, 354t
first permanent molars, 184
gingival recession, 22
implant planning, 393
implant tooth, 428–429
incisor, central, 118
incisors, fractured, 220
incisors, missing, 29
incisors, missing upper lateral, 278
localized periodontitis, 292–293
loose anterior tooth, 96–97
mandibular impacted third molars (MITMs), 140–145, 140t
molar endodontic treatment, 262
mouth opening, 337

Radiographs *(Continued)*
multilocular radiolucency, 10–11, 10t
neck swelling, 112
numb lips, 89
oroantral fistula (OAF), 105
swollen face, 271–272
toothache, 298, 350
tooth loss, eating, 128
tooth wear, 344b
trismus, 49
X-rays, 163t, 164f
Rare vesiculobullous conditions, 229
Rarer odontogenic tumours, 12
Recession, 22–23, 25, 25f
Recurrent aphthous stomatitis (RAS), 109, 110t
Replacement options
conventional cantilever bridge, 98–99
minimal preparation adhesive bridge, 98
Replacement root resorption, 98
Resin-bonded bridges, 30
Resin composite build-up, 221
Resorption, 96
causes, 98
features, 98
Restorations
assessment training, 382
classifying restorative failure, 382–383
clinical quality, 382
diagnosis, 386
examination, 381, 382f
failing restorations assessment, 381–386
hickel restorative assessment system, 383–386
history, 381
medico-legal issues, 388
mesial box, 56
minimum-intervention treatment options, 386–388
refurbish, 386, 387f
repair, 387–388
replace, 388
reseal, 387
rubber dam, 53
Retained root fragments, 86
Root canal treatment, 185
Root fracture, 96
Root morphology, 266
Rubber dam, 53
Rumination, 341–342

S
Salbutamol, 16
Salivary gland
diagnosis, 41
dry mouth, 42–43
minimally invasive techniques, 358t
swelling, 43
Self-mutilation, 234
Sensation test, 90–91
Sensibility testing, 118, 148, 262
Sialolithiasis, 360–362

Single tooth implant, 70, 99, 194
Sinus, 262
Sinus papilla, 60
Sjögren's syndrome, 40, 41t
Smoker's keratosis, 252
Smoking, 207
Smoking cessation, 109
Sodium lauryl sulphate (SLS), 191
Sore mouth
autoantibody screen, 189
diagnosis, 190–191
examination, 187–188, 187f
history, 187
investigations, 188–190
microbiological tests, 189
oral symptoms, 191
treatment options, 191t
Sore mouth with blisters
diagnosis, 230
differential diagnosis, 227–229
examination, 227, 227f
history, 227
investigations, 229t
treatment, 230
Special trays, lower/upper
dental care plan, 170t
first patient, 167
diagnosis, 167–168
handle faults, 169f
history, 167
solutions, 168–169
second patient, 169
examination, 170
history, 169–170
solution, 170–172
Squamous cell carcinoma, 252
Stepwise excavation, 56
Sublingual keratosis, 252
Supernumerary teeth, 298
Surgical crown lengthening
alternatives, 346
definition, 345–346
disadvantages, 346
Swollen face
causes, 272b
diagnosis, 272–273
examination, 271, 271f
history, 271
investigations, 271–272
treatment, 273–276

T
Temporary restorative materials, 4t
Temporomandibular joint (TMJ)
CAD/CAM, 67
causes, 46–47
ginglymo-arthroidal joint, 47
internal derangement, 46
joints click, 47, 48f
joints lock in internal derangement, 47
myofascial pain, 46–47
synovitis, 47

Tissue injuries, 120t
Tongue, white patch on
diagnosis, 255, 259
differential diagnosis, 251–253, 257–258
examination, 251, 251f, 257, 257f
history, 251, 257
investigations, 253–255, 258–259
leucoplakia, 252
prognosis, 255
treatment, 255, 259–260
Toothache
diagnosis, 350–352
differential diagnosis, 299–300
examination, 297, 297f, 349–350
history, 297, 349
investigations, 298–299, 301–302, 301f, 350
surgical procedures, 301t
treatment, 300–301
Tooth decay
diagnosis, 376–378, 377f
examination, 375–376, 375f
history, 375
investigations, 378
osteoradionecrosis, risk factors for, 378t
treatment, 378–379
Tooth loss, eating
diagnosis, 127–129
examination, 127
history, 127
investigations, 129–130
treatment, 130–132, 130f
Tooth wear
aetiological factors, 344b
care planning, 345–346, 346f
diagnosis, 344–345
examination, 343–344, 343f
history, 343
investigations, 344, 344f
medico-legal issues, 347–348
stages, 347t
treatment, 346–347
Trigeminal neuralgia, 63
Trismus
causes, 46
differential diagnosis, 45–47
examination, 45, 45f
history, 45
investigations, 47–49
treatment, 49–50
Tuberculosis, 112
Tumour–Node–Metastasis (TNM), 322t

U
Ultrasonography, 49
Unsuspected lesion, 96
Upper central incisor displacement, 117–122
differential diagnoses, 118–119
examination, 117–118, 118f
history, 117
investigations, 118–119, 118f
treatment, 119–120
Upper removable appliance, 288–289
Urticarial rash, 15

V
Varicella-zoster virus (VSV) infection, 159
Verbal communication, 232
Vitality
caries, 1
toothache, 298

W
Warfarin, 245, 248, 250
Wear. *See* Toothwear
WHARFE (mnemonic), 142
White patches. *See* Tongue, white patch on
Wide-needle biopsy, 313t
Willis Bite Gauge, 137
Winter's lines techniques, 143
World Health Organization (WHO), 208

X
Xerostomia
causes, 40
false xerostomia, 40–43
true xerostomia, 40–43
X-rays
digital radiography, 165
dose limitation methods, 162t
guiding principles, 161–165
history, 161–165, 161t
quality assurance programme, 163
regulations, 165

Z
Zygoma, 219
Zygomatic arch, 334t